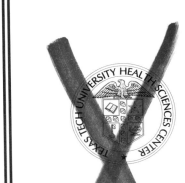

D1307228

ADVANCES IN NEUROLOGY
Volume 90

Advances in Neurology

INTERNATIONAL ADVISORY BOARD

ADVANCES IN NEUROLOGY
Volume 90

Neurological Complications of Pregnancy
Second Edition

Editors

Brian Hainline, M.D.

Department of Neurology
New York University School of Medicine;
Departments of Neurology and Integrative Pain Medicine
ProHEALTH Care Associates
Lake Success, New York, U.S.A.

Orrin Devinsky, M.D.

Departments of Neurology, Neurosurgery, and Psychiatry
New York University School of Medicine
New York, New York, U.S.A.

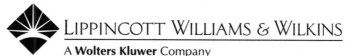

LIPPINCOTT WILLIAMS & WILKINS
A **Wolters Kluwer** Company
Philadelphia · Baltimore · New York · London
Buenos Aires · Hong Kong · Sydney · Tokyo

Acquisitions Editor: Anne M. Sydor
Developmental Editor: Mildred G. Ramos
Production Editor: Melanie Bennitt
Manufacturing Manager: Colin Warnock
Cover Designer: Patricia Gast
Compositor: Lippincott Williams & Wilkins Desktop Division
Printer: Maple Press

© 2002 by **LIPPINCOTT WILLIAMS & WILKINS**
530 Walnut Street
Philadelphia, PA 19106 USA
LWW.com

Printed in the USA

Library of Congress Cataloging-in-Publication Data
ISBN: 0-7817-3621-8
ISSN: 0091-3952

Care has been taken to confirm the accuracy of the information presented and to describe generally accepted practices. However, the authors, editors, and publisher are not responsible for errors or omissions or for any consequences from application of the information in this book and make no warranty, expressed or implied, with respect to the currency, completeness, or accuracy of the contents of the publication. Application of this information in a particular situation remains the professional responsibility of the practitioner.

The authors, editors, and publisher have exerted every effort to ensure that drug selection and dosage set forth in this text are in accordance with current recommendations and practice at the time of publication. However, in view of ongoing research, changes in government regulations, and the constant flow of information relating to drug therapy and drug reactions, the reader is urged to check the package insert for each drug for any change in indications and dosage and for added warnings and precautions. This is particularly important when the recommended agent is a new or infrequently employed drug.

Some drugs and medical devices presented in this publication have Food and Drug Administration (FDA) clearance for limited use in restricted research settings. It is the responsibility of the health care provider to ascertain the FDA status of each drug or device planned for use in their clinical practice.

10 9 8 7 6 5 4 3 2 1

Advances in Neurology Series

Vol. 51:   Alzheimer's Disease: *R. J. Wurtman, S. Corkin, J. H. Growdon, and E. Ritter-Walker, editors*. 308 pp., 1990.
Vol. 50:   Dystonia 2: *S. Fahn, C. D. Marsden, and D. B. Calne, editors*. 688 pp., 1988.
Vol. 49:   Facial Dyskinesias: *J. Jankovic and E. Tolosa, editors*. 560 pp., 1988.
Vol. 48:   Molecular Genetics of Neurological and Neuromuscular Disease: *S. DiDonato, S. DiMauro, A. Mamoli, and L. P. Rowland, editors*. 288 pp., 1987.
Vol. 47:   Functional Recovery in Neurological Disease: *S. G. Waxman, editor*. 640 pp., 1987.
Vol. 46:   Intensive Neurodiagnostic Monitoring: *R. J. Gumnit, editor*. 336 pp., 1987.
Vol. 45:   Parkinson's Disease: *M. D. Yahr and K. J. Bergmann, editors*. 640 pp., 1987.
Vol. 44:   Basic Mechanisms of the Epilepsies: Molecular and Cellular Approaches: *A. V. Delgado-Escueta, A. A. Ward, Jr., D. M. Woodbury, and R. J. Porter, editors*. 1,120 pp., 1986.
Vol. 43:   Myoclonus: *S. Fahn, C. D. Marsden, and M. H. VanWoert, editors*. 752 pp., 1986.
Vol. 42:   Progress in Aphasiology: *F. C. Rose, editor*. 384 pp., 1984.
Vol. 41:   The Olivopontocerebellar Atrophies: *R. C. Duvoisin and A. Plaitakis, editors*. 304 pp., 1984.
Vol. 40:   Parkinson-Specific Motor and Mental Disorders, Role of Pallidum: Pathophysiological, Biochemical, and Therapeutic Aspects: *R. G. Hassler and J. F. Christ, editors*. 601 pp., 1984.
Vol. 39:   Motor Control Mechanisms in Health and Disease: *J. E. Desmedt, editor*. 1,224 pp., 1983.
Vol. 38:   The Dementias: *R. Mayeux and W. G. Rosen, editors*. 288 pp., 1983.
Vol. 37:   Experimental Therapeutics of Movement Disorders: *S. Fahn, D. B. Calne, and I. Shoulson, editors*. 339 pp., 1983.
Vol. 36:   Human Motor Neuron Diseases: *L. P. Rowland, editor*. 592 pp., 1982.
Vol. 35:   Gilles de la Tourette Syndrome: *A. J. Friedhoff and T. N. Chase, editors*. 476 pp., 1982.
Vol. 34:   Status Epilepticus: Mechanism of Brain Damage and Treatment: *A. V. Delgado-Escueta, C. G. Wasterlain, D. M. Treiman, and R. J. Porter, editors*. 579 pp., 1983.
Vol. 33:   Headache: Physiopathological and Clinical Concepts: *M. Critchley, A. Friedman, S. Gorini, and F. Sicuteri, editors*. 438 pp., 1982.
Vol. 32:   Clinical Applications of Evoked Potentials in Neurology: *J. Courjon, F. Manguiere, and M. Revol, editors*. 592 pp., 1982.
Vol. 31:   Demyelinating Diseases: Basic and Clinical Electrophysiology: *S. Waxman and J. Murdoch Ritchie, editors*. 544 pp., 1981.
Vol. 30:   Diagnosis and Treatment of Brain Ischemia: *A. L. Carney and E. M. Anderson, editors*. 424 pp., 1981.
Vol. 29:   Neurofibromatosis: *V. M. Riccardi and J. J. Mulvilhill, editors*. 288 pp., 1981.
Vol. 28:   Brain Edema: *J. Cervós-Navarro and R. Ferszt, editors*. 539 pp., 1980.
Vol. 27:   Antiepileptic Drugs: Mechanisms of Action: *G. H. Glaser, J. K. Penry, and D. M. Woodbury, editors*. 728 pp., 1980.
Vol. 26:   Cerebral Hypoxia and Its Consequences: *S. Fahn, J. N. Davis, and L. P. Rowland, editors*. 454 pp., 1979.
Vol. 25:   Cerebrovascular Disorders and Stroke: *M. Goldstein, L. Bolis, C. Fieschi, S. Gorini, and C. H. Millikan, editors*. 412 pp., 1979.
Vol. 24:   The Extrapyramidal System and Its Disorders: *L. J. Poirier, T. L. Sourkes, and P. Bédard, editors*. 552 pp., 1979.
Vol. 23:   Huntington's Chorea: *T. N. Chase, N. S. Wexler, and A. Barbeau, editors*. 864 pp., 1979.
Vol. 22:   Complications of Nervous System Trauma: *R. A. Thompson and J. R. Green, editors*. 454 pp., 1979.
Vol. 21:   The Inherited Ataxia: Biochemical, Viral, and Pathological Studies: *R. A. Kark, R. Rosenberg, and L. Schut, editors*. 450 pp., 1978.
Vol. 20:   Pathology of Cerebrospinal Microcirculation: *J. Cervós-Navarro, E. Betz, G. Ebhardt, R. Ferszt, and R. Wüllenweber, editors*. 636 pp., 1978.
Vol. 19:   Neurological Epidemiology: Principles and Clinical Applications: *B. S. Schoenberg, editor*. 672 pp., 1978.
Vol. 18:   Hemi-Inattention and Hemisphere Specialization: *E. A. Weinstein and R. P. Friedland, editors*. 176 pp., 1977.
Vol. 17:   Treatment of Neuromuscular Diseases: *R. C. Griggs and R. T. Moxley, editors*. 370 pp., 1977.
Vol. 16:   Stroke: *R. A. Thompson and J. R. Green, editors*. 250 pp., 1977.
Vol. 15:   Neoplasia in the Central Nervous System: *R. A. Thompson and J. R. Green, editors*. 394 pp., 1976.
Vol. 14:   Dystonia: *R. Eldridge and S. Fahn, editors*. 510 pp., 1976.
Vol. 13:   Current Reviews: *W. J. Friedlander, editor*. 400 pp., 1975.
Vol. 12:   Physiology and Pathology of Dendrites: *G. W. Kreutzberg, editor*. 524 pp., 1975.
Vol. 11:   Complex Partial Seizures and Their Treatment: *J. K. Penry and D. D. Daly, editors*. 486 pp., 1975.
Vol. 10:   Private Models of Neurological Disorders: *B. S. Meldrum and C. D. Marsden, editors*. 270 pp., 1975.
Vol. 9:   Dopaminergic Mechanisms: *D. B. Calne, T. N. Chase, and A. Barbeau, editors*. 452 pp., 1975.

To our children—
Our teachers,
Our love

Contents

Contributing Authors

Machelle H. Allen, MD
Department of Obstetrics and Gynecology
New York University School of Medicine
Bellevue Hospital
550 First Avenue
New York, New York 10016
U.S.A.

Vicky Bassi, MD
University of Florida College of Medicine
1600 S.W. Archer Road
Gainesville, Florida 32610
U.S.A.

H. Richard Beresford, MD, JD
Department of Neurology
University of Rochester School of Medicine
601 Elmwood Avenue, Box 673
Rochester, New York 14642
U.S.A.

Aleksandar Berić, MD
Department of Neurology
New York University School of Medicine
Hospital for Joint Diseases
550 First Avenue
New York, New York 10016
U.S.A.

Danielle Chiaravalloti, MSN, RN, CS
The Women's Center at Premier HealthCare
YAI/National Institute for People with Disabilities
589 Broadway, 2nd floor
New York, New York 10012
U.S.A.

Stuart D. Cook, MD
Department of Neurosciences
UMDNJ/New Jersey Medical School
185 South Orange Avenue
Newark, New Jersey 07102
U.S.A.

Lisa M. DeAngelis, MD
Department of Neurology
Memorial Sloan-Kettering Cancer Center
1275 York Avenue
New York, New York 10021
U.S.A.

Orrin Devinsky, MD
Departments of Neurology, Neurosurgery, and
*   Psychiatry*
New York University School of Medicine
403 East 34th Street, 4th Floor
New York, New York 10016
U.S.A.

J. Donald Easton, MD
Department of Neurology
Brown University/Rhode Island Hospital
110 Lockwood Street, #324
Providence, Rhode Island 02903
U.S.A.

Edward Feldmann, MD
Department of Neurosciences
Brown University School of Medicine;
Department of Neurology
Rhode Island Hospital
593 Eddy Street
Providence, Rhode Island 02903
U.S.A.

James M. Gilchrist, MD
Department of Neurosciences
Brown University School of Medicine;
Department of Neurology
Rhode Island Hospital
593 Eddy Street
Providence, Rhode Island 02903
U.S.A.

Martin Goldstein, MD
Department of Neurology
New York Hospital—Cornell Medical Center;
Department of Neurology and Neuroscience
Cornell Medical College
525 East 68th Street
New York, New York 10021
U.S.A.

Brian Hainline, MD
Department of Neurology
New York University School of Medicine;
Departments of Neurology and Integrative Pain
*   Medicine*
ProHEALTH Care Associates
2800 Marcus Avenue
Lake Success, New York 11042
U.S.A.

Richard T. Johnson, MD
Department of Neurology
Johns Hopkins Hospital
600 North Wolfe Street, Meyer 6
Baltimore, Maryland 21287
U.S.A.

Barry D. Jordan, MD, MPH
Department of Neurology
Weill Medical College of Cornell University;
Brain Injury Program
Burke Rehabilitation Hospital
785 Mamaroneck Avenue
White Plains, New York 10605
U.S.A.

Peter W. Kaplan, FRCP
Department of Neurology
Johns Hopkins University School of Medicine and
Johns Hopkins Bayview Medical Center
4940 Eastern Avenue, B Building, Room 123
Baltimore, Maryland 21224
U.S.A.

Stephan A. Mayer, MD
Division of Critical Care Neurology
Neurological Institute
New York Presbyterian Hospital, Columbia-
  Presbyterian Medical Center
710 West 168th Street, Unit 39
New York, New York 10032
U.S.A.

Adam S. Mednick, MD, PhD
Neurological Associates of New Haven, P.C.
330 Orchard Street, Suite 216
New Haven, Connecticut 06511
U.S.A.

Mary T. Miceli, RN
Department of Neurology
New York University School of Medicine
560 First Avenue, Rivergate 4th Floor
New York, New York 10016
U.S.A.

Alireza Minagar, MD
Department of Neurology
University of Maryland School of Medicine
655 West Baltimore Street
Baltimore, Maryland 21201
U.S.A.

Joan T. Moroney, MD, MRCPI
Department of Neurosciences
Royal College of Surgeons, Ireland;
Department of Neurology
Beaumont Hospital
Beaumont Road
Dublin, 9 Ireland

Meheroz H. Rabadi, MD, MRCPI
Department of Neurology
Weill Medical College of Cornell University;
Department of Neurorehabilitation
Burke Rehabilitation Hospital
785 Mamaroneck Avenue
White Plains, New York 10605
U.S.A.

Alejandro Rabinstein, MD
Department of Neurology
University of Maryland School of Medicine
655 West Baltimore Street
Baltimore, Maryland 21201
U.S.A.

Steven M. Rosman, PhD
Division of Complementary Medicine
ProHEALTH Care Associates
2 ProHEALTH Plaza
Lake Success, New York 11042
U.S.A.

Lisa R. Sammaritano, MD
Department of Internal Medicine
Weill Medical College of Cornell University;
Division of Rheumatology
Hospital for Special Surgery
535 East 70th Street
New York, New York 10021
U.S.A.

Steven C. Schachter, MD
Department of Neurology
Harvard Medical School and
Beth Israel Deaconess Medical Center
330 Brookline Avenue, K-478
Boston, Massachusetts 02215
U.S.A.

Richard B. Schwartz, MD, PhD
Department of Radiology
Harvard Medical School;
Division of Neuroradiology
Brigham and Women's Hospital
75 Francis Street
Boston, Massachusetts 02115
U.S.A.

Debra Shabas, MD
Department of Neurology
New York University Medical Center;
The Women's Center at Premier HealthCare
460 West 34th Street
New York, New York 10001
U.S.A.

Lisa M. Shulman, MD
Department of Neurology
University of Maryland School of Medicine
22 South Greene Street
Baltimore, Maryland 21201
U.S.A.

William J. Weiner, MD
Department of Neurology
University of Maryland School of Medicine
22 South Greene Street
Baltimore, Maryland 21201
U.S.A.

Janet L. Wilterdink, MD
Department of Clinical Neurosciences
Brown University Medical School;
Department of Neurology
Rhode Island Hospital
110 Lockwood Street, #324
Providence, Rhode Island 02903
U.S.A.

Mark S. Yerby, MD, MPH
Oregon Comprehensive Epilepsy Program
2455 N.W. Marshall, Suite 14
Portland, Oregon 97210
U.S.A.

Bruce K. Young, MD
Department of Obstetrics and Gynecology
New York University Medical Center
530 First Avenue, 5G
New York, New York 10016
U.S.A.

Preface

Physicians and allied health care providers participate in the potentially greatest joy of humanity—assisting a child safely through the voyage of fetal development and birth. Uncertainty, fear, and pain may supplant joy when a pregnant woman develops a neurological condition. In addition, some women with chronic neurological conditions may forego becoming pregnant for fear that their own health or that of their child will be compromised. Health care providers can counsel and guide patients with knowledge and compassion. Our second edition seeks to meet these challenges.

Neurological emergencies during pregnancy require prompt recognition and treatment. Pregnant patients suffering with a cerebrovascular accident, eclampsia, brain tumor, head trauma, or other life-threatening conditions must be managed with meticulous care, and our updated chapters in these areas will guide physicians in critical decision-making. Women with epilepsy have many options for safely becoming pregnant and delivering a healthy child. The chapters on endocrinology and epilepsy bring solid medical evidence to the forefront so that these patients can be appropriately counseled and treated without superstition or prejudice. Autoimmune conditions such as multiple sclerosis also are too frequently coupled with an unjustified stigma regarding the safety of pregnancy, and the meta-analyses presented regarding these disorders should reassure physicians and patients regarding the relative safety of pregnancy. Infections, especially HIV, can seriously harm the mother and developing child; guidelines regarding aggressive treatment and outcome considerations are highlighted.

Women with neuromuscular conditions and paraplegia can overcome their disabilities in many ways, including pregnancy, and we hope that our relevant chapters will guide physicians and others who must work imaginatively with these patients. The often punitive approach to women who abuse drugs and alcohol is countered with a sympathetic understanding of the human behind the disorder, challenging all health care providers to reexamine the evidence that a punitive approach brings to the mother and child. As the borders between psychiatry and neurology merge in pathophysiology and therapy, we have expanded the range of psychiatric disorders and psychopharmacologic agents covered in this edition.

Quality of life is a critical measure of medical outcome for all patients. With this in mind, we invite all health care providers to become actively involved in addressing the common ailments of low back pain and headache during pregnancy. Since patients are increasingly utilizing complementary and alternative medicine, we have added a comprehensive chapter that analyzes scientific and evidence-based studies so that health care providers can overcome their reluctance to discuss such options in a meaningful way with their patients. Imaging studies are often necessary during pregnancy, and we offer concrete guidelines for ordering such studies. Our litigious society demands a careful presentation and consideration of legal issues confronting health care providers who manage pregnant women, and we have ended our book with this important chapter.

We hope this book helps some women, answers a few questions, and stimulates many more questions.

Brian Hainline, MD
Orrin Devinsky, MD

Acknowledgments

We are indebted to many people who give us the freedom and possibility to bring a book to completion. Jerry Posner, Fred Plum, Norman Geschwind, and Joe Evans stimulated curiosity, reason, and doubt of dogma. Margie Hernandez, Danielle Beltran, April Cannon, and Marlene Amaro provided outstanding secretarial and administrative support. Anne Sydor patiently and expertly facilitated completion of this work. Roseanne Mercandetti, you bring order to our life so that we can branch out beyond our daily patient care, and we thank you for the limitless passion and compassion you carry to work and beyond. Pascale, Clotilde, Arthur, and Juliette— Deborah, Janna, and Julie,—we are here because of you.

Brian Hainline, MD
Orrin Devinsky, MD

ADVANCES IN NEUROLOGY
Volume 90

Neurological Complications of Pregnancy, Second Edition, edited by Brian Hainline and Orrin Devinsky. Lippincott Williams & Wilkins, Philadelphia © 2002.

1

Neuroradiographic Imaging: Techniques and Safety Considerations

Richard B. Schwartz

Division of Neuroradiology, Brigham and Women's Hospital, Boston, Massachusetts, U.S.A.

In November 1895, Wilhelm Roentgen, a professor of physics at the University of Wurtzburg in Germany, was experimenting with cathode ray tubes when he deduced the properties of a previously unknown form of electromagnetic radiation that penetrated soft tissue but was attenuated by bone. The ability to noninvasively image the internal structure of the body was immediately recognized to be of immense medical importance, and within months of Roentgen's announcement, diagnostic imaging using x-rays was in widespread use. *However,* researchers working with x-rays noted deleterious effects of this radiation. Thomas Edison noted "severe smarting of the eyes" after several exposures to x-ray discharges 3 months after Roentgen's announcement (1). Definitive evidence of dermatitis induced by x-ray exposure was reported in late 1896, and by 1901 animal studies demonstrated that x-ray injuries extended to deep tissues as well. Although the mechanism behind the destructive effects of x-rays was unknown at the time, the capacity of x-rays to induce cancer and cell death soon became evident. Edison's assistant, Clarence M. Dally, first lost his hand and then his life to repeated x-ray exposures. Marie Curie's premature death as a result of radiation-induced leukemia is a sobering reminder of the dangers of radiation exposure.

The first standards for radiation protection were adopted in 1921, and by 1931 international recommendations were established for exposure to the general population, radiology workers, and patients (2,3). These guidelines have been updated in the succeeding decades as our means of production and measurement of x-rays became more refined and our understanding of the detrimental effects of radiation increased. However, after almost a century of research, no consistent biologic effects of radiation in the doses employed for diagnostic imaging have been found. All radiation safety guidelines are predicated on a theoretical linear dose-effect relationship, with the only observable effects present at the high-dose range from animal studies and such human experiments as occurred at Hiroshima, Nagasaki, and Chernobyl.

The internationally accepted unit of radiation exposure is the Gray (Gy), which is a measure describing the amount of energy deposited in tissues by radiation exposure (1 joule of energy per kilogram of body tissue; 1 Gy equals 100 rad; 1cGy equals 1 rad). The average cumulative radiation doses from medical, occupational, and natural sources (cosmic rays and radioactive decay from the earth's crust) are estimated to be approximately 0.2 cGy (0.2 rad) per year. By international agreement, the allowable radiation doses are 0.5 cGy (0.5 rad) per year for the general population and 5 cGy (5 rad) per year for the radiology worker (4). By comparison, the lowest amount of acute radiation exposure that was required to produce observable clinical effects (temporary decrease in white cell and platelet counts) in Chernobyl patients was on the order of 0.5 Gy (50 rad). Although there is no limit to the dose that a patient may receive for diagnostic purposes, it is universally accepted that the radiation dose to any patient should be kept *as low as reasonably achievable* (the ALARA principle).

The pregnant patient is a special case because she is carrying an unwilling member of the general population who must be protected from excess radiation exposure. The effect of radiation on the developing conceptus is vitally important and is central to our concerns for the pregnant patient (5–11). Implantation of the zygote is affected by radiation, and the most common radiation effect at time of implantation is death of the conceptus, with a threshold of at least 5 cGy (5 rad). The embryonic stage (implantation to 8 weeks) is also a very radiosensitive time because this is the stage of organogenesis. Radiation exposure during this time is more likely to result in developmental anomalies or overall retardation of growth, with threshold doses of at least 5 cGy (5 rad). Neoplasia also can occur. Theoretically, it takes only a single point mutation to render a cell cancerous, so there is no threshold for this effect. The fetal period (second and third trimesters) is the least radiosensitive. The majority of the organ systems have by this time developed, and the primary effects of high-dose radiation are growth retardation and neoplasia. Because neuronal migration still is occurring throughout this time, functional (central nervous system-related) abnormalities such as mental retardation also may become manifest, without theoretical threshold limits.

To appreciate fully the effects of radiation on the embryo or fetus, it must be remembered that radiation-induced effects are not specific and are identical to those produced by toxins, infection, or other noxious agents (11). For example, the rate of spontaneous abortion is considered to be as high as 30% during the implantation stage, and the baseline frequency of congenital deformities is 4% to 6%. Against this background of relatively high baseline risks, it has been impossible to demonstrate any evidence of an increased incidence of mutation, neoplasm, or developmental abnormality as a result of in utero x-ray exposure in the range of usual diagnostic procedures (<0.1 cGy, or 0.1 rad) at any time of gestation. Even in the extremely unlikely event of an exposure of greater than 10 cGy (10 rad) during the first trimester, the incidence of radiation-induced abnormalities is expected to be less than 1% over baseline. Experimentally, the dose necessary to produce significant increases in deformities that would warrant termination of pregnancy is on the order of 15 cGy (15 rad), more than 10 times the maximum dose of standard diagnostic examinations. Because some radiation-induced effects, such as neoplasm or cell death, may occur from a single x-ray photon striking a single DNA molecule, it is incumbent upon us to limit the in utero radiation dose as much as possible.

TECHNIQUES

Plain Films

For 60 years, plain films and angiography were the mainstay of radiology. Plain film technique requires an anode-cathode pair that projects high-energy electrons at a tungsten target; collisions with outer shell electrons produce x-ray photons, which are projected at the patient. The differential absorption of x-rays by internal objects as a result of density differences (differential attenuation of x-ray beam) is responsible for the image, which is captured on film or on a fluoroscopic screen. At present, the indications for plain films of the skull are few; nondisplaced facial and skull fractures (excluding those of the skull base) sometimes can be seen best on plain films, but all intracranial pathology, including sinus disease, is best evaluated with computed tomography (CT). Although plain films are the most widely used means of screening for fractures of the spine, some facilities now use thin-slice CT with 3D reconstructions for this purpose (see below).

The dose to the uterus from a skull film or cervical spine film is less than 0.001 cGy (1 mrad), from a thoracic spine series up to 0.1 cGy (0.1 rad) and from a lumbar spine series up to 1.5 cGy (1.5 rad), depending on the number of views obtained (12). The exposure to the conceptus from plain films or CTs that do not directly address the abdomen or pelvis is from scatter of x-ray photons within the patient, and a lead shield on the patient blocks only a minuscule amount of airborne scatter radiation. However, the lead shield always should be used because it provides the patient with a sense that the utmost is being done to *protect* her unborn child.

Angiography

Angiography is essentially fluoroscopy performed after intraarterial injection of iodinated contrast. Permanent images are obtained with real-time filming devices (cutfilm) or by computer-aided subtraction (digital film) technique. The former provides superior anatomic detail (necessary for adequate evaluation of vascular malformations or vasculitis), but the latter requires less exposure and contrast load and is acceptable for large-vessel examinations.

The radiation dose for a typical cervical or intracranial angiogram is less than 0.001 cGy (1 mrad). However, scatter radiation from fluoroscopy is generally greater than that for plain films, and fluoroscopy delivers 1 cGy (1rad) per minute to the skin (12). Thus, the uterus may be imparted relatively large doses from procedures requiring long fluoroscopy times. In addition, iodinated contrast does cross the placenta, although no untoward effects on the fetus have been noted in animal or human studies.

Computed Tomography

CT has virtually replaced plain films for the evaluation of the intracranial and extracranial structures. In this technique, multiple anode-cathode pairs are oriented around a ring opposite scintillation detectors. Pencil-thin beams of x-ray photons penetrate the patient, and the detectors record the attenuation values of the various beams. This information is subjected to a computer-assisted reconstruction algorithm to produce a cross-sectional image with different densities of tissue assigned different shades of gray on the final film. CT is highly sensitive to blood within the brain and is the technique of choice for identifying acute intraparenchymal, subarachnoid, subdural, or epidural hemorrhage. Acute blood may be indistinguishable from brain tissue on magnetic resonance imaging (MRI). Also, CT is preferred for the uncooperative or unstable patient. Because each axial image is obtained separately, patient motion artifact is minimized, particularly on the later generation scanners, which can perform individual scans in 2 seconds or less. Patients also are accessible for monitoring and urgent care in CT. Bony structures are extremely well visualized; thus, all skull fractures should be evaluated with CT to determine possible displacement as well as to determine the presence and extent of underlying hematoma formation or brain pathology. Vertebral fractures should be examined by CT or MRI so that the possibility of associated disc herniation or epidural/intradural blood can be assessed.

The dose to the uterus from CT away from the uterus is lower than that from plain films, largely as a result of the tight collimation of the x-ray beam, which markedly curtails internal scatter. The exposure to the uterus from a standard head or cervical spine CT is less than 0.001 cGy (1 mrad), and that from a thoracic CT is about 0.02 cGy (20 mrad). However, the dose from a lumbar spine CT is approximately 0.7 cGy (700 mrad) and caution should be used in ordering this study *in pregnant patients* (12).

Myelography

Until the advent of MRI, myelography was the only means of assessing the intrathecal contents, including the spinal cord and nerve roots. It remains a valuable resource in the diagnosis of the effects of spinal trauma and spondylosis in patients with significant bony disease, and it is the only study for the evaluation of the spinal canal in patients in whom MRI is contraindicated. Myelography is performed by injecting contrast into the intrathecal space at the C1-C2 interspace or any of the interspaces between L2 and L5 under fluoroscopic guidance and obtaining plain films of the area in question. The present standard is also to perform CT through the region of interest to evaluate fully the thecal sac and neural foramina.

The dose to the uterus from a myelogram is therefore a combination of the dose of fluoroscopy, plain films, and CT scans. This amounts to 0.002–0.01 cGy (2–10 mrad) for a cervical myelogram, but on the order of 0.2 cGy (200 mrad) for a lumbar myelogram (12).

Magnetic Resonance Imaging

The advent of clinical MRI in the mid-1980s has changed the practice of neuroradiology. The ability to differentiate tissues on the basis of signal characteristics in multiple planes has made MRI invaluable in the evaluation of vascular disease, infection, demyelination, and neoplasms and has provided a means to evaluate the intrathecal and epidural spaces in the spine without myelography. The technique of magnetic resonance angiography (MRA) has helped to decrease dependence on angiography for the evaluation of cervical and intracranial vasculature. The MR technique involves placing a patient within a large-bore magnet that possesses a 0.3–4.0 T magnetic field (more recently available magnets have field strengths of more than 4 T, but these are used for research purposes primarily). The patient's protons align to that main field and process coherently (in phase). In a typical spin-echo sequence, a transient magnetic pulse is applied to the patient in the transverse (90 degree) plane, and the protons align to the new field. After this magnetic pulse is turned off, the protons realign to the main field, and a signal is generated, reflecting predominantly anatomic detail (the T1 effect). During this process, the protons, which at first spin in

phase with each other, begin to lose their coherence, and a 180-degree magnetic pulse then is applied to rephase the protons. A different signal is thereby generated, conveying information primarily reflecting the water environment surrounding the protons (the T2 effect). The various signals are coded for position using complex magnetic gradients, and an image is produced using reconstruction techniques similar to those used for CT. Gradient refocusing techniques are used to image moving protons for MRA. Using a saturation pulse that eradicates signal from blood flowing into the imaging volume from a given direction, arterial or venous flow can be selectively imaged. Arterial MRA may be used to evaluate stenoses of the cervical and large intracranial vessels and to identify aneurysms and arteriovenous malformation (AVM) larger than 3 mm in size. MR venography can be used to evaluate for venous thrombosis of large intracranial veins. Diffusion-weighted imaging is a newly developed imaging technique in which the microscopic movement of water can be assessed; special gradients are used that reduce the signal arising from mobile water protons, so that protons that are more restricted in their motion (as in acute infarction) can be specifically imaged. Diffusion-weighted imaging shows increased signal in the brain within several hours of infarction, indicating restricted diffusibility of protons in the extracellular and/or intracellular spaces.

Because MR involves the administration of electromagnetic pulses, patients with pacemakers or other electrical implants cannot be exposed to the magnet (13). Aneurysm clips composed of ferromagnetic material also are absolutely contraindicated because the magnetic field may cause them to move, with potentially disastrous consequences. However, in most medical centers, titanium or tantalum clips, which are MRI compatible, have been used routinely for the past several years. Nevertheless, unless the composition of an aneurysm clip is known with complete assurance, MR should be avoided. Large metallic orthopaedic devices are relatively contraindicated. Although they will not move in the magnetic field, they generally produce field distortions that may degrade the image. Heating of the material is another theoretic concern, although there has never been a report of a patient that was seriously injured as a result of excessive heating in an implanted metallic device. It should be remembered that all jewelry (including body rings) should be removed, if possible, prior to MR. Although skin staples theoretically are safe to image in MR magnets, a gap between the limbs of the staple may result in a burn to the skin; thus, the presence of skin staples is a relative contraindication if the patient is unconscious and unable to report skin heating (14).

MR magnets in the range of diagnostic field strengths can raise the core body temperature, but studies have shown that these changes are minor (less than 0.6°C, according to Shellock), and well within the limits of safety (14). It may be surmised that feelings of warmth occasionally reported by patients within the bore of the magnet relate more to the restricted airflow within the bore of the magnet than to the effects of the magnetic field *per se*.

Gadolinium crosses the placental barrier and is excreted through the fetal kidneys. Although no ill effects on fetal growth or renal function after birth have been demonstrated to date, gadolinium injection (as well as CT contrast) should be avoided during pregnancy unless considered to be absolutely necessary for patient care.

The majority of the studies performed to evaluate the effects of magnetic fields in various animal species have failed to show any significant genetic, developmental, or homeostatic effects. Several investigators, however, have shown effects in animals exposed to magnetic fields at a sensitive time of gestation (days 7–14 of a 3-week gestation), corresponding to the time when the neural tube and reproductive system are expected to develop. Tyndall and colleagues (15) have shown that in mice prone to ocular deformities, in utero exposure (36 minutes on day 7 of pregnancy) to 1.5 T fields doubled the frequency of these

abnormalities at birth; this group also showed that such exposure resulted in decreased crown–rump length and smaller craniofacial perimeter measures (16). Heinrichs and associates (17) reported a small but significant reduction in fetal crown–rump length, but no other toxic effects after mid-gestational exposure of genetically normal mice to a magnet with a field strength of 0.35 T. Magin and colleagues (18) found no statistically significant effect on fetal growth when pregnant mice were subjected to long-term (9 hours) exposure to high field strength (4 T) magnets; however, they did find a significant increase in the rates of intrauterine demise, stillbirths, postpartum weight levels, and the time required to acquire motor skills in these animals. Murakami and associates (19), however, showed that even a 7-day exposure of pregnant mice between days 7 and 14 of gestation to a field strength of 6.3 T did not result in a significant difference in litter size, fetal weight, intrauterine mortality rate, or external or skeletal abnormalities compared to control groups. High and colleagues (20) performed a study in which rats were exposed to two 5-week periods of exposure to a 9.4 T field—one immediately prior to breeding (during gametogenesis) and the other during the second and third trimesters of pregnancy. They found no effect on various biologic endpoints of the offspring, including gestation period, litter size, intrauterine or postnatal mortality, behavioral or physical development, or biochemical or anatomic parameters. Thus, although reports are conflicting, it appears that long duration of exposures to magnetic fields at or above the field strength used for diagnostic MR *may* have effects on developmental end-points if mammals are exposed during critical times in fetal development. It should be remembered, however, that many studies have been performed specifically to evaluate the safety of MR in pregnant human patients and health care workers, and none has revealed any demonstrable detrimental effects of exposure to diagnostic MR.

In 1996, the U.S. Food and Drug Administration (FDA) designated all field strengths below 4 T as posing a "non-significant risk," and the FDA does not require informed consent of the patient or approval by an Institutional Review Board (13). No consensus has been reached concerning imaging of pregnant patients, but based on the above data, it would be prudent to avoid exposure of the embryo or fetus to high magnetic fields in the first or second trimesters of pregnancy unless absolutely indicated. Overall, however, it is clear that because MRI does not generate ionizing radiation, it is perforce safer for the conceptus than any x-ray study, regardless of the amount of ionizing radiation imparted to the uterus.

At the Brigham and Women's Hospital, more than 60 pregnant patients have been examined with MR of the brain or spine over the past decade. Most of these patients were studied with MR after the second trimester; several patients in the emergency or critical care setting were studied in the second trimester. The neuroradiologic findings included intracranial hemorrhage due to AVM, aneurysm, and cavernous angioma; hypertensive encephalopathy due to the preeclampsia-eclampsia syndrome; tumors that enlarged during pregnancy (which included meningiomas and pituitary adenomas); arterial thrombosis with infarction; and superior sagittal sinus thrombosis with venous infarction (21). Several patients had incidental findings unrelated to pregnancy, including glioblastoma multiforme, metastatic melanoma, pineal astrocytoma, sacral mass, and disc herniation. All patients initially underwent head CT followed by MRI, except for those patients with presumed pituitary mass, sacral tumor, venous thrombosis, and disc herniation, who underwent only MRI. No patient received iodinated contrast during CT or gadolinium during MRI. All patients with intracranial hemorrhages underwent angiography and surgery to remove the vascular malformations. Healthy babies were born in all of the above cases, and thus far all children for whom follow-up is available are developing normally. In this same time period, one woman was in her first trimester of pregnancy when she was involved in a serious automobile accident and sustained serious internal injuries that required assessment with angiography. She underwent several interventional and operative procedures. She had received, in total, an estimated 10 cGy (10 rad) to her abdomen and pelvis during her evaluation, and she chose to terminate her pregnancy.

RECOMMENDATIONS

Head CT, used judiciously, is relatively safe during pregnancy and is the study of choice for head trauma as well as for the evaluation of acute nontraumatic subarachnoid, subdural, or intraparenchymal hemorrhage. Cervical spine plain films and CT also carry little risk. Thoracic and lumbar plain films or CT, however, should be avoided in any patient who is or may be pregnant, unless absolutely necessary. Lumbar myelography is contraindicated. For examination of the lower spine and for all other nontraumatic or nonhemorrhagic craniospinal pathology, MRI is the study of choice. MRI should also be the first test used to evaluate any suspected vascular pathology, but when necessary, angiography is considered reasonably safe in the pregnant patient, as long as fluoroscopy time and contrast load are kept to a minimum.

In conclusion, the following guidelines may be helpful. When faced with a patient who is or may be pregnant and has a neurologic problem:

1. Determine the necessity of a radiologic examination and the potential risks involved.
2. If possible, perform the examination only during the first 10 days post menses, or if the patient is pregnant, delay the examination until the third trimester or preferably postpartum.
3. Determine the most efficacious use of radiation for the problem.
4. Use MRI if possible.
5. Avoid direct exposure to the abdomen and pelvis. Offer a lead shield to the patients for all examinations.
6. Avoid contrast agents.

7. Do not avoid radiologic testing purely for the sake of the pregnancy. Remember that you are responsible for providing the best possible care for the patient. The risk to the pregnant patient of not having an indicated radiologic examination is also an indirect risk to the fetus.

8. If significant exposure is incurred by a pregnant patient, have a radiation biologist (usually *stationed* in the radiology department) review the radiology examination history carefully so that an accurate dose estimate can be ascertained.

9. The decision to terminate a pregnancy because of excessive radiation exposure is an extremely complex issue and is dependent on many factors, including the amount and timing of the exposure to the embryo or fetus, the hazard to the expectant mother of continuing the pregnancy, the ethnic and religious background of the family, and the state laws pertaining to legal abortion. Because any increased risk of malformation is considered to be negligible unless radiation doses exceed 10 cGy (10 rad), the amount of exposure that an embryo or fetus would likely receive from diagnostic procedures is well below the level for which a therapeutic abortion should be considered. Be aware of all the potential issues. For instance, patients have tried to use the concerns over radiation exposure as a reason to terminate an unwanted pregnancy.

10. Consent forms are neither required nor recommended. The patient should be informed verbally that any radiologic examinations ordered during pregnancy are considered necessary for her medical care. She also should be informed that the risks to the fetus associated with ionizing radiation from CT/plain films are very low and that there are no known risks to humans from MRI. This should be discussed with an air of reassurance, and the patient then should be given the option of declining the study. In our experience, having the patient sign a consent form increases the perceived risks of the procedure and adds needlessly to her concerns during and after the examination.

ACKNOWLEDGMENT

I would like to thank Martin A. Samuels, M.D., for his help in the preparation of this manuscript.

REFERENCES

1. Eisenberg RL. *Radiology: an illustrated history.* St. Louis: Mosby-Year Book, 1992.
2. Shapiro J. *Radiation protection: a guide for scientists and physicians.* 3rd ed. Cambridge: Harvard University Press, 1990.
3. Taylor LS. *Radiation protection standards.* Cleveland: CRC Press, 1971.
4. Hall EJ. *Radiobiology for the radiologist.* 3rd ed. Philadelphia: JB Lippincott, 1988.
5. Brent, RL. The effect of embryonic and fetal exposure to x-ray, microwaves, and ultrasound: counseling the pregnant patient about these risks. *Semin Oncol* 1989; 16:347–368.
6. Glaze S, Schneiders N, Bushong SC. A computer-assisted procedure for estimating patient exposure and fetal dose in radiographic examinations. *Radiology* 1982; 145:187–190.
7. Mattison DR, Angtuaco T. Magnetic resonance imaging in prenatal diagnosis. *Clin Obstet Gynecol* 1988; 31:353–389.
8. Mossman KL. Imaging the pregnant patient. *Postgrad Radiol* 1988;8:215-23.
9. National Council on Radiation Protection and Measurements. *Review of NCRP radiation dose limit for embryo and fetus in occupationally-exposed women.* NCRP Report No. 53. Bethesda, MD, 1977.
10. National Council on Radiation Protection and Measurements. *Medical radiation exposure of pregnant and potentially pregnant women.* NCRP Report No. 53. Bethesda, MD, 1977.
11. Wagner LK, Hayman LA. Pregnancy and women radiologists. *Radiology* 1982;145:559–562.
12. Judy PE, Zimmerman RE. Dose to critical organs. In: McNeil BJ, Abrams HL, eds. *Brigham and Women's Hospital handbook of diagnostic imaging.* Boston: Little, Brown, 1986.
13. Schenck JF. Safety of strong, static magnetic fields. *J Magn Reson Imaging* 2000;12:2–19.
14. Shellock FG. Radiofrequency energy-induced heating during MR procedures: a review. *J Magn Reson Imaging* 2000;12:30–36.
15. Tyndall DA, Sulik KK. Effects of magnetic resonance imaging on eye development in the C57BL/6J mouse. *Teratology* 1991;43:263–275.
16. Tyndall DA. Effects on craniofacial size and crown-rump length in C57BL/6 mice in 1.5 T fields. *Oral Surg Oral Med Oral Pathol* 1993;76:655–660.
17. Heinrichs WL, Fong P, Flannery M, et al. Midgestational exposure of pregnant BALB/c mice to magnetic resonance imaging conditions. *Magn Reson Imaging* 1988;6:305–311.

18. Magin RL, Lee JK, Klintsova A, Carnes KI, et al. Biological effects of long-duration, high-field (4 T) MRI on growth and development in the mouse. *J Magn Reson Imaging* 2000;12:140–149.

19. Murakami J, Torii Y, Masuda K. Fetal development of mice following intrauterine exposure to a static magnetic field of 6.3 T. *Magn Reson Imaging* 1992;10:433–437.

20. High WB, Sikora J, Ugurbil K, et al. Subchronic in vivo effects of a high static magnetic field (9.4 T) in rats. *J Magn Reson Imaging* 2000;12:122–139.

21. Mantello MT, Schwartz RB, Jones KM, et al. Pictorial essay: imaging of neurologic complications associated with pregnancy. *AJR Am J Roentgenol* 1993;160: 843–848.

Neurological Complications of Pregnancy, Second Edition, edited by Brian Hainline and Orrin Devinsky. Lippincott Williams & Wilkins, Philadelphia © 2002.

2

Low Back Pain

Brian Hainline

Neurology and Integrative Pain Medicine, ProHEALTH Care Associates, Lake Success, New York, U.S.A.

Low back pain is widely recognized as a common accompaniment of pregnancy. Although most obstetric textbooks recognize back pain as a pregnancy-related problem, the related issues of etiology and management often are addressed superficially. In addition, women may be told simply to accept back pain as an expected burden of pregnancy. However, there are various causes of low back pain in pregnancy, and management should be based on the pathogenesis of the patient's pain.

BIOMECHANICS OF PREGNANCY

Lumbar Spine

The weight of the body normally is transmitted down the entire vertebral column to the sacrum. In standing, increasing direct compressive load is transmitted from the cervical to the lumbar spine. The vertebral column adapts to this weight-bearing stress through an increasing mass of the caudal vertebral bodies. The vertebral column can be considered as compromising superimposed functional units, with each unit compromising two segments. The anterior portion of the vertebral column is a supporting, weight-bearing, shock-absorbing, and flexible structure. The principal components of this anterior segment are the vertebral body and the intervertebral disc. The posterior segment of the vertebral column is a nonweight-bearing structure that contains and protects the nervous system and also serves to direct the movement of the functional unit as a whole (1). The principal components of the posterior segment are the pedicles, the facets, and the facet articular cartilage.

The normal vertebral column has developed three curves: the cervical lordosis, thoracic kyphosis, and lumbar lordosis. These curves develop as an adaptation to assuming an upright posture during infancy. All three curves must meet in a midline center of gravity to balance the weight distribution of the curves and to counter the eccentric loading of each curve (1). Although the caudal lumbar vertebral bodies are larger than the other vertebral bodies, the load on the lower lumbar discs is higher because the center of gravity is anterior to the intervertebral disc at this level, with a corresponding flexion on the vertebral column counterbalanced by ligaments and back-muscle forces (2). Increased load, combined with the lordotic angle, causes an increasing shearing force on the caudal lumbar intervertebral discs, making these discs more vulnerable to degenerative changes and disc herniations.

Pregnancy is a physiologic condition that necessitates postural adjustments to maintain a balanced, erect posture. During normal pregnancy with a single fetus, the body weight increases by approximately 12 kg. From a biomechanical viewpoint, the increasing weight and increasingly protuberant abdomen are the major characteristics of a pregnant woman. After 12 weeks, the uterus is too large to remain within the true pelvis. Thereafter, the uterus touches the anterior abdominal wall, displaces the intestines laterally and superiorly, and ascends further into the abdominal cavity (3). Consequently, the center of gravity is displaced upward, forward, and laterally, and the pregnant woman must make postural adjustments. In addition, the expanding uterus stretches the muscles of the abdominal wall and lowers muscle tone, thereby diminishing the contribution of these muscles to maintaining an upright posture (4).

Traditionally, the posture of a pregnant woman is viewed as that of a progressive increase in lumbar lordosis as a compensation for the progressive anterior displacement of the center of gravity (1,4–10). However, other authors have determined that with the increasing body weight of pregnancy, the line of the center of gravity moves backward and approximates caudally to the ankle joint. This is accomplished by an entire backward movement of the vertebral column with either no change or a flattening of the lumbar lordosis (3,11). The literature is virtually silent regarding strict biomechanical measurements of the lumbar spine and the influence of biomechanical changes on the development of back pain during pregnancy.

Hummel (3) states that the majority of pregnant women have displacement of the whole vertebral column backward by way of translatory and rotatory movement. This occurs predominantly after the thirtieth week, with no significant change in the lumbar lordosis. Hummel distinguishes between nulliparous and primiparous women. In both, the spine straightens before the thirtieth week of pregnancy. In nulliparous women, the lumbar lordosis becomes more exaggerated during the last 10 weeks of pregnancy, whereas the entire spine remains generally straightened throughout the entire pregnancy in primiparous women. Hummel concludes that the widely accepted view of an increased lumbar lordosis during pregnancy may be a perceptual misinterpretation because of the change of spatial orientation of the spine.

Ligamentous Laxity

The pelvis must adapt to the enlarging uterus and to the eventual descent of the child through the birth canal during labor. This adaptation is largely accomplished biomechanically through ligament relaxation. Estrogen causes a proliferation of connective tissue, and the hormone relaxin mediates softening and vascularization of this proliferative connective tissue (7,12). Relaxin is a peptide hormone of the insulin-like growth family, and it is thought to be responsible in part for progressive ligamentous laxity during pregnancy. Relaxin blood concentrations increase ten-fold during pregnancy, but there is not a consensus regarding the trimester during which maximum levels occur (7,12). In a prospective study of relaxin levels among pregnant women, Kristiansson and colleagues (12) demonstrated peak levels during the twelfth week, followed by a decline in serum levels to about 50% of the peak value in the seventeenth week through delivery.

Joint laxity increases can be measured in multiple joints (13) and are more prominent in multigravida than primigravida patients. The most notable biomechanical effects occur at the symphysis pubis and sacroiliac joints. The width of the symphysis pubis increases from 0.5 mm to 12 mm, and vertical displacement of the symphysis may result (7,8,11,13, 14). The most notable increase occurs during the last trimester, and the symphysis width gradually returns to normal between 3 and 5 months after delivery (13). The diastasis of the symphysis resulting from the width changes may be associated with secondary changes in the periosteum. Also, progressive symphysis widening causes rotatory stress on the sacroiliac joints (8).

Normally, the sacroiliac joint is an extremely stable joint marked by reinforcement from powerful ligaments anteriorly and posteriorly. Furthermore, the articular surfaces are so curved and sigmoid in their direction that movement within the joint is limited (1). Ligamentous laxity can be associated with minor subluxation of the sacroiliac joints. The rotatory stress across the pelvis rim resulting from the widening of the symphysis pubis can cause further movement within the sacroiliac joint.

Relaxin also may cause an increase in laxity of the lumbar intervertebral joints, although this has not been demonstrated directly (15). Such laxity theoretically could allow an even further exaggeration of the lumbar lordosis, thereby increasing further the shearing stress placed on the lower intervertebral discs. Relaxin may directly affect the collagen of the facet joint capsules, as well as the collagen of the annulus, thereby reducing the stability of the lumbar spine (16). This may predispose parous women to spondylolisthesis, which is almost twice as high in parous than in nulliparous women (17).

INCIDENCE OF BACK PAIN DURING PREGNANCY

Low back pain is ubiquitous during pregnancy. When discussing low back pain, a distinction must be made among several variables: type of pain; time of onset during pregnancy; time of onset during the day; precipitating and palliative features; correlation with body mechanics; correlation with prior pregnancy; correlation with any complications during pregnancy, including excessive weight gain; correlation with physical examination; and correlation with prior history of back pain. Unfortunately, these variables are not uniformly addressed in the few prospective studies of low back pain during pregnancy. Several studies, however, provide important insight into this problem.

Although some authors indicate that back pain may occur in up to 90% of pregnant women (18,19), the literature most consistently sites an incidence rate of approximately 50% (20–23). Peak onset of back pain occurs between the 5th and 7th months (21,24,25). Between 10% and 30% of back-pain sufferers describe their pain as severe or incapacitating (19,22,23). These facts should serve to remind obstetricians and other primary health care providers not to simply dismiss back pain as a

normal accompaniment of pregnancy; a woman's functioning and well-being may be seriously compromised because of such pain. In addition to the sometimes underrecognized severity of low back pain, several studies also shed important light on the diversity of presentation of low back pain during pregnancy. Nwuga (19) demonstrated a correlation between low back pain and pregnancy with advancing age and parity; 60% of patients had peak low back pain during the evening and 30% had peak pain at night. Mantle (23) similarly noted a correlation of low back pain with advancing age and parity. Both Mantle and Nwuga stress that the patients who underwent antenatal training had less back pain than those who had not (19,23). Mantle noticed no correlation between back pain and obesity, total weight, weight gain during pregnancy, patient height, or baby's birthweight (23).

Fast (21) found that 67% of patients with low back pain had night backache while lying in bed and 36% of those questioned had such severe pain that they were awakened from sleep. There was no correlation between back pain and age, race, weight before pregnancy, weight gain during pregnancy, patient's height, number of prior pregnancies or deliveries, or back pain before pregnancy.

Berg (22) prospectively studied 862 pregnant patients by way of questionnaire during weeks 20 to 35. A total of 9% had such severe pain that they could not continue their professional or household work, and when these patients were examined from a musculoskeletal point of view, the majority suffered from posterior pelvic pain or dysfunction of the sacroiliac joints.

The above studies demonstrate that back pain is common during pregnancy, is often severe, and frequently occurs during the evening or nighttime. In general, age and parity are associated with more frequent and severe pain. Most incident studies are done by way of questionnaire. The relationship between back pain, physical examination findings, and biomechanical factors must be studied further to provide better insight to this common problem.

ETIOLOGY OF BACK PAIN DURING PREGNANCY

Posterior Pelvic Pain

The pelvis undergoes considerable biomechanical changes during pregnancy because of the development of ligamentous laxity in the symphysis pubis and sacroiliac joints. The role of the sacroiliac joint in low back pain syndromes, in general, is unclear (1). The controversy results in part from the fact that both lumbar disc disease and sacroiliac dysfunction can cause low back pain with referred pain down one or both legs, and both syndromes can be treated successfully with similar conservative measures (1,7). Furthermore, some women have radiographic demonstration of great mobility and diastasis of the symphysis pubis or sacroiliac joint and have no symptoms, whereas others have minimal radiographic changes with considerable symptoms (7,26).

In Berg's (22) prospective study of pregnant women, 9% of the patients that had incapacitating pain underwent an orthoneurologic exam by an orthopedic surgeon and answered a follow-up questionnaire 6 to 12 months after delivery. The physical examination in Berg's study was done while patients were standing, walking, and lying down. The presence and degree of scoliosis and tilting of the pelvis, postural asymmetry of the pelvis, and asymmetry of the spine were recorded. In addition, functional and provocative tests of the sacroiliac and lumbar spine were performed. Whereas forward flexion and straight-leg raising may be indicative of lumbar disc referred pain, Berg (22) and Ostgaard (27) have demonstrated that posterior pelvic pain or sacroiliac dysfunction can be demonstrated with the following provocative maneuvers. Ventral gapping test is positive if pain is provoked at the sacroiliac joint when the pelvis is manually pressed apart. The dorsal gapping test is positive if pain is produced when the pelvis is pressed together. The sacroiliac joint fixation test is positive if one posterior superior spine is lower than the other and the position reverses on forward flexion. Patrick's test is positive if pain is produced after one heel is placed on the opposite knee

and the leg is rotated outward while the patient is recumbent. Derbolowski's test is positive if the positions of the medial malleoli change in relation to one another with the patient sitting and lying supine. Two-thirds of the 79 patients in Berg's study who underwent such an examination had clinical evidence of sacroiliac dysfunction (22). Patients with sacroiliac dysfunction had low back pain for a significantly longer time than those women who had low back pain without sacroiliac dysfunction. Most women with sacroiliac dysfunction had symptoms several months postpartum.

It may be simplistic to state that such provocative tests only stress the sacroiliac joint, and this is why Ostgaard (27) has proposed the terminology "posterior pelvic pain." Both Berg and Ostgaard have demonstrated that the majority of musculoskeletal low back pain in pregnancy is a result of posterior pelvic pain. Such patients typically have back pain for a significantly longer time than those women who had back pain without posterior pelvic pain. Most women with posterior pelvic pain have symptoms that remain symptomatic several months postpartum. The relationship of posterior pelvic pain to pubic symphysis pain is unclear, and further research is needed to clarify this matter (27,28).

Although posterior pelvic pain is approximately four times as prevalent as other causes of musculoskeletal low back pain during pregnancy (18), there remains a paucity of data with regard to predisposing biomechanical factors to musculoskeletal pain. There are no prospective studies that address detailed physical examinations and biomechanical analyses in asymptomatic or mildly symptomatic individuals. Thus, the influence of posture and biomechanics *per se,* as well as other contributing factors, remains unknown. Despite these shortcomings, there is convincing evidence that posterior pelvic pain is a common cause of low back pain in pregnant women.

Lumbar Disc Disease

If most pregnant women developed a significant increase in lumbar lordosis, one would expect a significant increase in lumbar disc disease among gravida women. An exaggerated lumbar lordosis is associated with an increase in sacral angulation and shearing stress across the lower back. Some authors (7,15,29) have suggested that women are more prone to lumbar disc disease, but the available data are not convincing.

Walde (7) states that the symptoms of sacroiliac pain and lumbar disc disease can be indistinguishable, including radiating "sciatica-like pain." He points out that some clinical and autopsy surveys have demonstrated more frequent degenerative changes in the lumbar discs in women than in men. However, no correlation is made with prior pregnancies or with symptoms of low back pain or sciatica during pregnancy.

O'Connell (15) observed that the postural stress during pregnancy and the mechanical stress during labor predispose women of childbearing years to lumbar disc disease. He postulates that mechanical and postural stress coupled with possible effects of relaxin on the ligaments of the lumbar and vertebral discs cause lumbar degenerative disc disease and subsequent lumbar disc herniation. To test his hypothesis, he studied 1,100 consecutive, surgically proven cases of lumbar disc protrusions. Of the patients, 347 were women and two-thirds were in their childbearing years. Lumbar disc symptoms developed in 39% of patients who had been pregnant; in 25% of these cases, women developed such symptoms during two or more pregnancies. This study is limited because no control data are available, the patient population is selective, and no correlation is made between biomechanical or physical measurements during pregnancy.

Kelsey and colleagues (29) also suggested that the mechanical stress of pregnancy coupled with intervertebral ligamentous laxity predispose to lumbar disc disease in women. The authors present epidemiologic data demonstrating an association between pregnancy and herniated lumbar discs, and they suggest that this association increases in multiparous women. However, the data are derived from symptoms and signs elicited by nonmedically trained personnel, and no correlation is made between the physical exam or biomechanical measures.

LaBan and associates (26) identified five pregnant patients with symptoms and signs of a herniated lumbar disc in a series of 48,760 consecutive deliveries. All patients had confirmed clinical and electromyographic signs, and all patients had surgically proven herniated lumbar discs. Although this study often is cited to show that lumbar disc disease is unusual during pregnancy, LaBan studied only women who had advanced clinical signs. No mention is made of symptoms and signs in other patients, and it is not clear how closely patients were followed during pregnancy or after delivery for clinical manifestations of lumbar disc disease. In the five symptomatic patients, no correlation is made with postural or biomechanical considerations.

In summary, the incidence of lumbar disc disease during pregnancy is not known. No prospective, well-designed study has addressed this problem. Specifically, no prospective study has analyzed pertinent clinical factors, postural changes, physical examinations, and relevant laboratory data in an attempt to assess the true incidence of lumbar disc disease in pregnancy.

Lumbar Pain

Lumbar pain describes a more nonspecific entity, and it is differentiated from posterior pelvic pain and lumbar disc disease. Uncomplicated lumbar pain occurs over the area of the lumbar spine, with or without radiating pain into the leg. Clinical presentation is not dissimilar from lumbar pain experienced by women who are not pregnant, and it is generally aggravated by activities such as prolonged standing, sitting, or repetitive lifting (18). Posterior pelvic pain provocative maneuvers and mechanical stretch pain are not positive physical examination findings. The examination may demonstrate erector spinae muscle tenderness.

Lumbar pain shows a stronger link with back pain prior to pregnancy than does posterior pelvic pain (22,27,28). Although the abdominal musculature often is emphasized as an important etiologic factor in lumbar pain, Fast (32) demonstrated no correlation between abdominal muscle insufficiency and lumbar pain. Although the ability to perform a sit-up is significantly decreased in pregnant women compared to nonpregnant women, there is no statistical correlation between the sit-up performance and lumbar pain.

Lumbar pain may be correlated with dysfunction of the back muscles, especially the erector spinae. Sihvonen and associates (33) note that pre-pregnancy lumbar pain predicts renewed pain during pregnancy, and they tested the hypothesis that back-muscle dysfunction is a causative factor. They studied 32 pregnant women and compared them to 21 healthy pregnant controls. Visual analogue scale and disability questionnaires were completed, and back-muscle activities were recorded by surface electromyography and movement sensors. The authors demonstrated a significant correlation between disturbance in the relaxation of back muscles during forward flexion with current and later pain scores during pregnancy. The results of this simple functional screening test suggest that simple diagnostic tools may be valuable in identifying mothers with a high risk of pregnancy-related lumbar pain.

Venous Congestion

Epidemiologic studies of back pain in pregnancy demonstrate that back pain frequently occurs during the evening or at nighttime. We can speculate that evening back pain should be expected from musculoskeletal dysfunction. Muscle fatigue occurs most commonly in the evening, thereby not allowing the pregnant patient to uphold a proper posture and straining further the lumbar paraspinal muscles. Progressive muscle fatigue, muscle spasm, or both may worsen lumbar pain, lumbar disc disease pain, and posterior pelvic pain.

Although nighttime low back pain also may be unrelated to musculoskeletal pain, Fast (34) speculates that some factor other than musculoskeletal pain or posterior pelvic pain accounts for the large number of patients who suffer from night back pain. The following scenario is proposed: water retention during pregnancy can lead to secondary increase in blood volume and extracellular fluid retention. The blood flow to and from pelvic organs increases considerably. Concomitant with these changes, the enlarging uterus can compress the inferior vena cava and aorta when the pregnant woman is lying in the supine position. Vena cava compression can be as rostral as the uterine fundus and will cause blood flow to be routed to the ascending lumbar veins, the vertebral venous plexus, the paraspinal veins, and the azygous system. At nighttime, when such changes are more likely to occur, the venous volume already is increased because of redistribution from the extracellular space. All of these factors can cause venous engorgement, with a significant increase in venous pressure to structures subserved by the circulation, such as the vertebral bodies. This increased venous pressure can cause edema and stasis in key neurovascular structures, with subsequent stagnant hypoxemia and metabolic disturbances of neural elements, resulting in pain.

Some clinical observations support Fast's hypothesis of night back pain. During menstruation, women commonly develop low back pain. Transuterine pelvic venography demonstrates pelvic venous congestion during menstruation. Reginald (35) demonstrated that dihydroergotamine, a venoconstrictor, lessens venous congestion while improving the menstruating patient's symptoms of low back pain. Similarly, patients with symptomatic lumbar stenosis and congestive heart failure can have an exacerbation of nighttime lumbar stenosis symptoms during periods of worsening heart failure, and symptoms abate progressively once heart failure is improved (36).

In summary, nighttime low back pain may be caused by venous congestion and may be unrelated to any underlying musculoskeletal dysfunction. Treatment directed at the musculoskeletal system will be ineffective, whereas patient education and positional changes at night are likely to improve symptoms. In patients with refractory nighttime low back pain and no obvious skeletal pathology, pathologic venous congestion, including proximal venous thrombosis, should be considered.

Labor Pain

Labor is characterized by forceful uterine contractions, with associated contractions of the abdominal and low back muscles, occasionally with lumbar paraspinal muscle spasm. Intraabdominal pressure increases, and this causes an increase in lumbar intradiscal pressure and pressure across the symphysis pubis and sacroiliac joints. Thus, preexisting musculoskeletal pain may become exacerbated during labor, although this has not been well substantiated in the medical literature. Labor back pain may be unrelated to more classic musculoskeletal dysfunction, and in a substantial number of women, the back pain of labor is the most severe aspect of labor pain (37).

Melzack has studied the low back pain of labor (37,38,39). Approximately three-fourths of patients have low back pain during labor. Of the patients with low back pain, 44% state that continuous low back pain is more severe than contraction low back pain, and 33% of patients state that continuous low back pain is the worst pain of labor. There is a significant correlation between continuous labor low back pain and back pain during menstruation, which suggests that both share a common underlying mechanism.

The cause of continuous low back pain during labor is not certain. Possible explanations include (21,34,37–39):

1. Traction and pressure on the adnexa and parietal peritoneum
2. Pressure and stretch of the bladder, urethra, rectum, and other pain-sensitive structures in the pelvis
3. Pressure on one or more roots of the lumbosacral plexus
4. Reflex skeletal muscle spasm and vasospasm of those structures supplied by the same spinal cord segments supplying the uterus
5. Excessive prostaglandin production, thereby producing more intense contractions and secondary referred back pain
6. Inferior vena cava compression and subsequent venous stasis changes

POSTPARTUM BACK PAIN

Postpartum low back pain is less well studied than back pain during pregnancy. The incidence of postpartum low back pain is uncertain, although it may be relatively common. Some of the biomechanical factors predisposing women to low back pain during pregnancy are in effect for several months after delivery. Ligamentous laxity may persist for 3 to 5 months (8,12), thereby causing persistent vulnerability to posterior pelvic pain. Postural changes do not immediately correct postpartum (3), and diminished abdominal and paraspinal muscle tone, coupled with bending and lifting a newborn, may predispose to lumbar pain.

Brynhildsen (40) prospectively studied pregnant women who developed low back pain during pregnancy. Women with severe low back pain during pregnancy have an extremely high risk for experiencing a new episode of severe low back pain during another pregnancy and when not pregnant. Although this study hints that severe low back pain may be a prognostic indicator of prolonged postpartum back pain, the etiology of severe low back pain during pregnancy was not defined. Ostgaard and Andersson (41) found that persistent postpartum back pain correlated with back pain before pregnancy, the presence of back pain during pregnancy, physically heavy work and multiple pregnancies. Physically heavy work has the strongest association with persistent, postpartum back pain at 12 months.

SCOLIOSIS

Up to 10% of women of childbearing age may have some degree of scoliosis (42). Because the incidence of progressive idiopathic scoliosis is approximately eight times higher in female patients than in male patients, the possibility that there is an adverse relationship between pregnancy and scoliosis has been considered (42). Women with scoliosis may refrain from becoming pregnant, either because of their own fear or because of the fear of their primary health care provider.

Earlier literature is divided regarding progression, or lack thereof, of idiopathic scoliosis as a result of pregnancy (43–48). Furthermore, discussion of pregnancy and scoliosis often was limited to obstetric complications of patients suffering with severe kyphoscoliosis.

In a comprehensive study on the effects of pregnancy on patients with idiopathic scoliosis, Betz and colleagues (49) investigated the possibility that pregnancy increases the risk of progression of scoliotic curve. Charts, radiographs, and other pertinent data on 355 women who had reached skeletal maturity were reviewed and analyzed; 175 patients who had at least one pregnancy were compared with 180 patients who had never been pregnant. The groups were comparable with regard to treatment and degree of scoliosis and were analyzed with regard to the degree of curve, including 30 degrees or less, 31 to 49 degrees, and 50 degrees or more. In all subcategories, pregnancy was noted to have no adverse effect on scoliosis, and patients were not found to have an increased risk of progression of scoliosis curvature. Seventy-seven percent of patients reported having backache during pregnancy, and 12% considered the pain to have been severe, consistent with patients without scoliosis. Spinal anesthesia could not be administered successfully in two deliveries because of problems related to scoliosis (49).

With regard to patients who have undergone corrective surgery, Betz (49) found that no patient who had been treated surgically showed progression in the fused portion of the spine, and only 2 of the 18 patients who had undergone a fusion had significant progression in the unfused portion of the spine. Orvomaa and colleagues (50) studied 142 pregnancies in 146 patients who underwent Harrington rod placement for treatment of idiopathic scoliosis. They found no significant increase in either the fused scoliotic curvature or the remaining unfused curvatures as a result of pregnancy.

In a retrospective chart review, Visscher and colleagues (51) examined for possible adverse reproductive outcomes in scoliosis patients. Patients were compared to appropriate age-match controls, and no difference was noted in the rate of stillbirths, spontaneous abortions, or pregnancy complications. Premature births occur more commonly in scoliosis patients than in controls. The authors speculate that women with scoliosis may be predisposed to premature births as a result of a malpositioning of the uterus from the spinal deformity or from the more generalized effective prior x-ray exposure. Women who had undergone spinal surgery had an even higher risk of premature births than women who had other forms of scoliosis treatment.

In summary, there is no justifiable reason to discourage women with scoliosis from becoming pregnant, including women who have undergone corrective surgery. Such patients do not place themselves at risk from a musculoskeletal point of view, nor from the point of view of other complications during pregnancy. Other than low birthweight, reproductive outcomes are similar to patients without scoliosis.

MANAGEMENT

General Principles

Low back pain in pregnancy is most likely to result from posterior pelvic pain, and other considerations include lumbar pain, lumbar disc disease, and venous congestion. Understanding the pathogenesis of low back pain in the individual patient is the cornerstone of proper management.

Although low back pain during pregnancy is commonplace, preventative measures may be neglected because they are not perceived as important. However, there is ample evidence in the medical literature that preventative measures are highly effective in helping to manage most cases of low back pain in pregnancy (18,19,52–54). Women contemplating pregnancy should have a clear understanding of the possible causes of low back pain in pregnancy, and they should be encouraged to perform some type of daily low back exercise. For women with a prior history of low back pain, her obstetrician or primary health care provider should have a thorough understanding of the cause of the low back pain, and appropriate treatment and rehabilitation should be initiated. If there is any doubt, the patient should be referred to a specialist so that further corrective measures can be undertaken. Untreated, preexisting low back pain, regardless of cause, is likely to worsen during pregnancy. There are no contraindications to performing appropriate spinal surgery and later becoming pregnant (50,51).

Simple preventative measures can be generalized for all potential low back problems during pregnancy. All women who are contemplating having children and all pregnant patients should be questioned about a history of low back problems. If a significant history exists, verify that the patient has been appropriately managed for her condition and understands the risk of developing recurrent symptoms during pregnancy.

Some general preventative guidelines hold true for all pregnant women. Proper posture, exercise, and awareness of good low back mechanics will benefit all patients. Pregnant women should understand not only that they may gain about 12 kg, but also that the distribution of weight gain will affect their normal center of gravity and therefore may place more stress on the lower back. Pregnant women also should understand that an additional component of low back stress occurs because of normal hormonal changes. Once the patient understands the concept of low back pain, she is better able to follow through with preventative measures.

Proper posture is the foundation of preventing undue musculoskeletal stress during pregnancy. We have witnessed a laissez-faire attitude about the importance of posture and the necessity of proper maintenance of the supporting muscles of the back. Women's fashion often dictates biomechanically unsound wardrobes and can create a situation in which someone unwittingly may become a poor subject for the normal process of pregnancy.

For pregnant women, maintaining proper posture throughout the day must be stressed, as opposed to occasionally ensuring their posture is correct while walking. A neutral lumbar lordosis should be the goal of the pregnant patient. This means that she should try to avoid developing either an excessive swayback (i.e., excessive lumbar lordosis) or roundback (i.e., a reversal of the lumbar lordosis). The patient should try to ensure that her posture is proper by periodically looking into a full-length mirror and making any corrective measures needed.

Some activities are more likely to accentuate lumbar lordosis and should be avoided. Wearing high-heeled shoes is inadvisable during pregnancy because they cause the sacrum to tilt downward, thereby increasing the lumbosacral angle and lumbar lordosis. When patients stand for a prolonged period, they have a tendency to throw their shoulders back and tilt the pelvis down, again accentuating the lumbar lordosis. A simple measure such as placing one foot on a footstool will relax the iliopsoas and subsequently tilt the pelvis forward, thereby reducing the strain on the lumbar spine and paraspinal muscles. Similarly, when patients are sitting for a prolonged period, elevating one foot onto a low stool will relieve traction on the pelvis by relaxing the iliopsoas and flattening the lumbar curve, thereby relieving lumbar muscular strain. In some patients who develop posterior pelvic pain, pelvic instability necessitates modification of corrective measures such as raising one foot on a stool. In such patients, this may lead to asymmetric loading of the pelvis, and low back pain symptoms may be exacerbated.

Ideally, the pregnant woman should sit in a firm, straight-back chair in which the hips and knees may be flexed with no strain and with both feet touching the floor. The back of the chair should support the low back 4 to 6 inches from the seat and permit a flat lumbar curve. Chairs without a firm back support or that arch forward at the lumbar curve can excessively strain the hamstring and paraspinal muscles. In low chairs, such as in an automobile, the hamstrings are similarly taut and may place excessive traction on the pelvis, causing rotation and strain on the lumbar spine (1). Low back-support cushions are designed to correct sitting postures that excessively strain the lumbar spine, and patients often obtain relief when using such devices (18,52).

Proper lifting is an essential aspect of low back care. The knees always must be flexed before lifting, and the object to be lifted should be held close to the body. The woman should stand upright by using the leg muscles, and the glutei and abdominal muscles should be holding the pelvis neutral. If the lumbar lordosis is regained prematurely with the upper body ahead of the center of gravity, the erector spinae muscles will perform inefficiently and there will be excessive strain on the lumbar spine. Proper lifting techniques are more likely to be neglected when patients act in haste or when they are excessively fatigued. Posture is important when lying supine as well. The mattress should be firm, or a bed board should be under the mattress to prevent sagging. Patients may benefit from placing a pillow under their knees or between their legs when lying on their side.

Stress management and methods of relaxation may be quite helpful in relieving low back pain (52). Frequently, emotional and physical stress results in excessive contraction of the lumbar paraspinal muscles, leading to muscular strain. Such strain can in turn cause sustained muscle spasms, which can potentiate all causes of musculoskeletal low back pain. Even if lumbar spasm is not causing or aggravating lumbar disc disease or posterior pelvic pain, such spasm can in and of itself be painful and will lead to excessive muscular fatigue. This in turn will increase the propensity toward faulty body posture and mechanics, which then may potentiate any underlying

musculoskeletal dysfunction. This leads to a potential chronic cycle of low back pain.

Walde (7) has identified several relief factors for low back pain in pregnancy. All have a similar underlying current: posture is addressed, positions are changed, and lumbar strain is minimized. The following measures, listed in order of decreasing effectiveness, are cited as ways to reduce low back pain in pregnant patients (7,18,52):

1. Placing a cushion or lumbar support behind the back when sitting
2. Changing from standing or sitting to lying down
3. Changing from standing to sitting
4. Taking analgesics
5. Taking hot water baths
6. Placing a hot water bottle in the low back
7. Changing from a lying or sitting position to standing
8. Walking

Although these recommendations are rather general, the important point is that pregnant women who suffer from low back pain should be willing to try simple maneuvers to relieve pain. Not only may such maneuvers be successful, but they also may prevent a chronic cycle of low back pain.

The exercise regimen to prevent or minimize low back symptoms in pregnant is simple and nonstrenuous. The pelvic tilt is the mainstay of exercise for pregnant women (7,18,19,52). The patient lies supine with hips and knees flexed and both feet flat on the floor. She then presses the lower back against the floor by contracting both the abdominal and gluteal muscles. This completes the first part of the pelvic tilt and may be all that some patients tolerate. For the second part, the pregnant woman raises the buttocks from the floor while not permitting the lower back to leave the floor (which could result in hyperextension of the lumbar spine rather than the desired reversal of lumbar lordosis). The patient then may begin slow, rhythmic elevation of the pelvis with the lower back remaining flat against the floor. The pelvic tilts serve several purposes: the lumbar lordosis is flattened; the gluteal and abdominal muscles are strengthened; and the patient begins to understand the kinesthetic concept of pelvic tilting, which can be applied to the sitting and upright positions.

Other simple exercises are useful. In all, the patient begins from the initial position of the pelvic tilt with the back flat against the floor. The patient should breathe slowly and in a relaxed manner throughout the exercises. These exercises include: (i) modified sit-ups, in which the patient raises the head and shoulder slowly from the ground to a 30-degree angle, holds the position for several seconds, and then slowly returns to the floor; (ii) hamstring stretch, in which the patient slowly extends and raises one leg to approximately 90 degrees, then alternates with the other leg; and (iii) hip flexion, in which the patient slowly brings one knee to the chest, then alternates with the other, then brings both knees together. These exercises may become more dif-

ficult during the latter months of pregnancy, and undue pressure should not be exerted against the abdominal wall.

If there are no contraindications, fast walking and swimming are excellent aerobic exercises that also serve to strengthen the supporting lumbar paraspinal muscles. Indeed, water gymnastics may be performed during the second half of pregnancy without an increased risk of urinary or vaginal infections. When compared to a control group, pregnant patients participating in water gymnastics had a lower incidence of low back pain and fewer numbers of sick-leave days (55).

Some patients may complain of moderate or severe low back pain, and these patients deserve special attention (Fig. 2.1). If the clinical suspicion is that low back pain occurs primarily at nighttime, the treatment simply may be to instruct the patient to lie on her left side so that compression of the inferior vena cava is avoided. If there is a clinical suspicion of

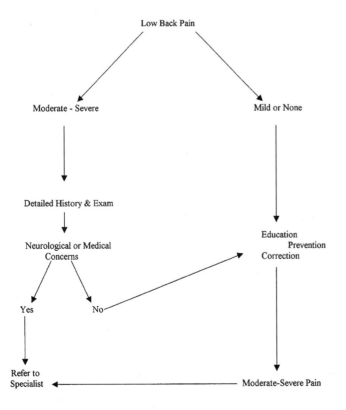

FIG. 2.1. Algorithm for low back pain management during pregnancy.

musculoskeletal low back pain, the clinician must attempt to distinguish among the more likely causes of such pain: posterior pelvic pain, lumbar pain, or lumbar disc disease.

The physical exam will complement the history, and a detailed history and exam should be performed for patients who do not respond to simple corrective measures and for all patients who complain of severe back pain. The examination should include a careful note of posture as well as mechanical stress maneuvers of the sacroiliac joint and lumbar spine. A directed neurologic exam should be performed to rule out nerve root or peripheral nerve entrapment. If there is a suspicion of any type of worrisome neurologic or medical condition, the patient should be referred to an appropriate specialist.

Refractory Pain

Posterior Pelvic Pain

Patients with persistent posterior pelvic pain may require short-term bed rest. Jarring physical activity may need to be avoided, and asymmetric pelvic loading, such as stair-climbing, may need to be significantly curtailed (18). A trochanteric or sacral belt helps to stabilize pelvic instability (22). This belt straps around the pelvis and minimizes movement in the sacroiliac and symphysis pubis. A trial injection of corticosteroids and short-acting local anesthetic into the sacroiliac joint may provide symptomatic relief, and this then should be followed by an exercise program.

Mobilization by an experienced practitioner may be highly efficacious in treating posterior pelvic pain during pregnancy (56–59). There are no well-designed, prospective trials of chiropractic during pregnancy, and it is a mistaken notion that mobilization is only performed by chiropractors. Indeed, there are many additional specialists who are well trained in simple mobilization techniques, including osteopathic physicians, physiatrists, and physical therapists. The cornerstone of posterior pelvic mobilization involves rotational manipulation of the sacroiliac joint and incidentally the lumbar spine, using the femur as a lever. With the patient

supine on a firm examination table, the leg on the painful side is placed with the hip flexed to 90 degrees and the knee flexed to 45 degrees with the heel resting on the opposite knee. The practitioner is positioned on the side contralateral to the raised leg with one hand on the shoulder ipsilateral to the raised leg, and the other hand placed on the lateral aspect of the raised knee. Pressure then is gradually applied to adduct the hip as far as possible, finishing with a thrust (58). When symptomatic relief is obtained, the patient then should be encouraged to follow through with the exercise regimen outlined above.

Lumbar Disc Disease

Patients with symptomatic lumbar disc disease who have failed the above preventative and exercise program may require short-term bed rest to diminish intradiscal pressure and alleviate symptoms. Bed rest should not be prolonged. A lumbar corset may help to further minimize intradiscal pressure. The corset gives support to the lumbar spine ligaments and paraspinal muscles and prevents hyperextension of the lumbar lordosis. Acupuncture and massage therapy may provide symptomatic relief (see Chapter 22).

With refractory pain, the patient should be evaluated further, and she may require diagnostic imaging by way of an magnetic resonance imaging (MRI) study (see Chapter 1). Lumbar epidural corticosteroids may be administered safely for moderate to large symptomatic disc herniations, although fluoroscopy should be avoided. Surgery for lumbar disc disease during pregnancy should be reserved for patients who have acutely lost control of bowel or bladder function or who have developed acute paralysis of muscles supplied by the corresponding entrapped nerve root. Partial muscle weakness is not an absolute indication for lumbar decompressive surgery.

Case Report

A thirty-year old primigravida presented with severe low back pain and numbness radiating down the posterolateral aspect of the left leg. She had no prior history of low back pain, and she did not recall any sudden incident that led to the development of pain during her 6th month of pregnancy. She failed 3 days of bed rest, analgesics by way of acetaminophen, and outpatient physical therapy.

Pertinent physical examination revealed a normal cervical and lumbar lordosis, normal thoracic kyphosis, and no scoliosis. There was no trigger-point tenderness in the paraspinal musculature or sacroiliac joints. Trunk flexion at 30 degrees reproduced the patient's pain, and other aspects of trunk range of motion were normal. Sacroiliac provocative tests were negative. Straight-leg raising was positive on the left at 30 degrees and crossed straight-leg raising was positive on the right at 50 degrees. The segmental neurologic exam revealed a decrease to pinprick in a left L5 distribution, and the left extensor hallucis longus motor power was 3/5. Other segmental neurologic function was normal. The patient underwent a diagnostic MRI of the lumbar spine, and this revealed a moderately large posterolateral disc herniation at L4–L5, with moderate compression of the thecal sac and left L5 nerve root. Because the pain was refractory, the patient underwent a series of three lumbar epidural corticosteroid injections, and she obtained moderate pain relief. She then began a program of acupuncture and simple exercises, and her pain remained well controlled for the remainder of her pregnancy. With concern that the disc herniation was quite large and potentially unstable, vaginal delivery was not recommended. She delivered uneventfully by way of cesarean section.

Labor Pain

For patients who prefer not to be managed by way of narcotic analgesics or epidural anesthesia, other options are available for refractory labor pain. Repositioning may be an important component of alleviating continuous low back pain of labor. Biofeedback has been employed successfully to help reduce refractory low back pain during labor (see Chapter 22). Intracutaneous sterile water injections have been utilized as an effective strategy for relieving low back pain during labor (60,61), and such injections are superior to back massage, mobilization, or transcutaneous electrical nerve stimulation (61).

CONCLUSION

Management of low back pain during pregnancy should be guided, as much as possible, by the pathogenesis of the pain. In mild to moderate low back pain, education and simple exercises often provide symptomatic relief. More severe pain may require more specialized treatment. All pregnant patients with low back pain deserve some management plan, and the guiding principle should begin with an acknowledgment that low back pain is not a trivial matter for the pregnant woman.

REFERENCES

1. Cailliet R. *Low back pain syndrome.* Philadelphia: FA Davis Co., 1995.
2. White AA, Panjabi MM. *Clinical biomechanics of the spine.* Philadelphia: JB Lippincott Co., 1978.
3. Hummel P. *Changes in posture during pregnancy.* Philadelphia: WB Saunders, 1987.
4. Fitzhugh ML, Newton M. Posture in pregnancy. *Am J Obstet Gynecol* 1963;85:1091–1095.
5. Bushnell LF. The postural pains of pregnancy. I: Parietal neuralgia of pregnancy. *West J Surg* 1949;57:123–127.
6. Young J. Relaxation of the pelvic joints in pregnancy: pelvic arthropathy of pregnancy. *J Obstet Gynaecol Br Em* 1940;47:493–524.
7. Walde J. Obstetrical and gynaecological back and pelvic pains, especially those contracted during pregnancy. *Acta Obstet Gynecol Scand* 1962;41:11–53.
8. Spankus JD. The cause and treatment of low back pain during pregnancy. *Wis Med J* 1965;64:303–304.
9. Rhodes P. Posture in obstetrics. *Physiotherapy* 1967;53: 158–163.
10. Schafer RC. Clinical biomechanics: musculoskeletal actions and reactions. Baltimore: Williams and Wilkins, 1983.
11. Fries EC, Hellebrandt, FA. The influence of pregnancy on the location of the center of gravity, postural stability, and body alignment. *Am J Obstet Gynecol* 1943;46:374–380.
12. Kristiansson P, Svardsudd K, von Schoultz B. Serum relaxin, symphyseal pain, and back pain during pregnancy. *Am J Obstet Gynecol* 1996;175:1342–1347.
13. Calguneri M, Bird HA, Wright V. Changes in joint laxity occurring during pregnancy. *Ann Rheum Dis* 1982; 41:126–128.
14. Abramson D, Roberts SM, Wilson PD. Relaxation of

pelvic joints in pregnancy. *Surg Gynecol Obstet* 1934; 58:595–613.

15. O'Connell, JEA. Lumbar disc protrusions in pregnancy. *J Neurol Neurosurg Psychiat* 1960;23:138–141.

16. Gunzburg R, Hutton WC, Crane G, et al. Role of the capsulo-ligamentous structures in rotation and combined flexion-rotation of the lumbar spine. *J Spinal Disord* 1992;5:1–7.

17. Sanderson PL, Fraser RD. The influence of pregnancy on the development of degenerative spondylolisthesis. *J Bone Joint Surg* 1996;78:951–954.

18. Perkins J, Hammer RL, Loubert PV. Identification and management of pregnancy-related low back pain. *J Nurse Midwifery* 1998;43:331–340.

19. Nwuga VCB. Pregnancy and back pain among upper class Nigerian women. *Aust J Physiother* 1982;28:8–11.

20. Orvieto R, Achiron A, Ben-Rafael Z, et al. Low-back pain of pregnancy. *Acta Obstet Gynecol Scand* 1994;73: 209–214.

21. Fast A, Shapiro D, Ducommun EJ, et al. Low-back pain in pregnancy. *Spine* 1987;12:368–371.

22. Berg G, Hammar M, Moller-Nielsen J, et al. Low back pain during pregnancy. *Obstet Gynecol* 1988;71:71–75.

23. Mantle MJ, Greenwood RM, Currey HL. Backache in pregnancy. *Rheumatol Rehabil* 1977;16:95–101.

24. Kristiansson P, Svardsudd K, von Schoultz B. Back pain during pregnancy: a prospective study. *Spine* 1996;21: 702–709.

25. Mens JM, Vleeming A, Stoeckart R, et al. Understanding peripartum pelvic pain. Implications of a patient survey. *Spine* 1996;21:1363–1370.

26. LaBan MM, Perrin JCS, Latimer, FR. Pregnancy and the herniated lumbar disc. *Arch Phys Med Rehabil* 1983;64:319–321.

27. Ostgaard HC, Zetherstrom G, Roos-Hansson E. Reduction of back and posterior pelvic pain in pregnancy. *Spine* 1994;19:894–900.

28. Ostgaard HC. Assessment and treatment of low back pain in working pregnant women. *Semin Perinatol* 1996;21:61–69.

29. Kelsey JL, Greenberg RA, Hardy RJ, et al. Pregnancy and the syndrome of herniated lumbar intervertebral disc: an epidemiologic study. *Yale J Biol Med* 1975; 48:361–368.

30. Garmel SH, Guzelian GA, D'Alton JG, et al. Lumbar disk disease in pregnancy. *Obstet Gynecol* 1997;89: 821–822.

31. LaBan MM, Viola S, Williams DA, et al. Magnetic resonance imaging of the lumbar herniated disc in pregnancy. *Am J Phys Med Rehabil* 1995;74:59–61.

32. Fast A, Weiss L, Ducommun EJ, et al. Low-back pain in pregnancy. Abdominal muscles, sit-up performance, and back pain. *Spine* 1990;15:28–30.

33. Sihvonen T, Huttunen M, Makkonen M, et al. Functional changes in back muscle activity correlate with pain intensity and prediction of low back pain during pregnancy. *Arch Phys Med Rehabil* 1998;79: 1210–1212.

34. Fast A, Weiss L, Parikh S, et al. Night backache in pregnancy. Hypothetical pathophysiological mechanisms. *Am J Phys Med Rehabil* 1989;68:227–229.

35. Reginald RW, Beard RW, Kooner JS, et al. Intravenous dihydroergotamine to relieve pelvic congestion with pain in young women. *Lancet* 1987;2(8555):351–353.

36. LaBan MM, Wesolowski J. Night pain associated with diminished cardiopulmonary compliance. A concomitant of lumbar spine stenosis and degenerative spondylolisthesis. *Am J Phys Med Rehabil* 1988;67: 155–160.

37. Melzack R, Schaffelberg D. Low-back pain during labor. *Am J Obstet Gynecol* 1987;156:901–905.

38. Melzack R, Kinch R, Dobkin P, et al. Severity of labour pain: influence of physical as well as psychologic variables. *Can Med Assoc J* 1984;130:579–581.

39. Melzack, R, Belanger E. Labour pain: correlations with menstrual pain and acute low-back pain before and during pregnancy. *Pain* 1989;36:225–229.

40. Brynhildsen J, Hansson ASA, Persson A, et al. Follow-up of patients with low back pain during pregnancy. *Obstet Gynecol* 1998;91:182–186.

41. Ostgaard HC, Andersson GBJ. Postpartum low-back pain. *Spine* 1992;17:53–55.

42. Rogala EJ, Drummond DS, Gurr J. Scoliosis: incidence and natural history. A prospective epidemiological study. *J Bone Joint Surg* 1978;60:173–176.

43. Keim, HA. *The adolescent spine.* New York: Springer-Verlag New York, 1982;104–109.

44. Berman AT, Cohen DL, Schwentker EP. The effects of pregnancy on idiopathic scoliosis. A preliminary report on eight cases and a review of the literature. *Spine* 1982; 7:76–77.

45. Nachemson A, Cochran TP, Irstam L, et al. Pregnancy after scoliosis treatment. *Orthop Trans* 1982;6:5.

46. Blount WP, Mellencamp DD. The effects of pregnancy on idiopathic scoliosis. *J Bone Joint Surg Am* 1980;62: 1083–1087.

47. Carr WA, Moe JH, Winter RB, et al. Treatment of idiopathic scoliosis in the Milwaukee brace. *J Bone Joint Surg Am* 1980;62:599–612.

48. Bunnell WP. A study of the natural history of idiopathic scoliosis. *Orthop Trans* 1983;7:6.

49. Betz RR, Bunnell WP, Lambrecht-Mulier E. Scoliosis and pregnancy. *J Bone Joint Surg Am* 1987;69:90–96.

50. Orvomaa E, Hiilesmaa V, Poussa M, et al. Pregnancy and delivery in patients operated by the Harrington method for idiopathic scoliosis. *Eur Spine J* 1997;6: 304–307.

51. Visscher W, Lonstein JE, Hoffman DA, et al. Reproductive outcomes in scoliosis patients. *Spine* 1988;13: 1096–1098.

52. Mantle MJ, Holmes J, Currey HL. Backache in pregnancy II: prophylactic influence of back care classes. *Rheumatol Rehabil* 1981;20:227–232.

53. Ostgaard HC. Assessment and treatment of low back pain in working pregnant women. *Semin Perinatol* 1996;20:61–69.

54. Alexander JT, McCormick PC. Pregnancy and discogenic disease of the spine. *Neurosurg Clin N Am* 1993; 4:153–159.

55. Kihlstrand M, Stenman B, Nilsson S, et al. Water-gymnastics reduced the intensity of back/low back pain in pregnant women. *Acta Obstet Gynecol Scand* 1999;78: 180–185.

56. Rungee JL. Low back pain during pregnancy. *Orthopedics* 1993;16:1339–1344.

57. McIntyre IN, Broadhurst NA. Effective treatment of low back pain in pregnancy. *Aust Fam Physician* 1996; 25:S65–S67.

58. Daly JM, Frame PS, Rapoza PA. Sacroiliac subluxation: a common, treatable cause of low-back pain in pregnancy. *Fam Pract Res J* 1991;11:149–159.

59. Davidson JH. Manipulation for low back pain. *Br Med J* 1978;2:1644.

60. Martensson L, Wallin G. Labour pain treated with cutaneous injections of sterile water: a randomised controlled trial. *Br J Obstet Gynaecol* 1999;106:663–667.

61. Labrecque M, Nouwen A, Bergeron M, et al. A randomized controlled trial of nonpharmacologic approaches for relief of low back pain during labor. *J Fam Pract* 1999;48:259–263.

Neurological Complications of Pregnancy, Second Edition, edited by Brian Hainline and Orrin Devinsky. Lippincott Williams & Wilkins, Philadelphia © 2002.

3

Migraine and Other Headache Conditions

Brian Hainline

Neurology and Integrative Pain Medicine, ProHEALTH Care Associates, Lake Success, New York, U.S.A.

Headache is an almost universal phenomenon. The lifetime prevalence of headache in women is 99% (1). More than 90% of headache patients suffer with either migraine or tension-type headache (2–4). Migraine is a common condition, affecting at least 11% of the adult population. Whereas males and females are affected equally prepuberty, there is an approximate 3 to 1 ratio of migraine in favor of females after puberty (1,5–10). Approximately 18% of women suffer with migraine (11), and the vast majority of women with migraine or tension-type headache are of childbearing age. This has profound implications for women who are contemplating pregnancy or who become pregnant.

Because the majority of migraine or tension-type headache sufferers have intermittent headache, and because the headaches may be severe, a woman may unwittingly take a medication to control headache while pregnant. During pregnancy, the serious negative impact of migraine on quality of life may be dismissed by a treating physician or primary health care provider because the cause of the headache is "benign." Within that line of reasoning, the practitioner may simply ask the patient to accept the fate of migraine. Because one always must balance the risk versus benefit of treating any medical condition, especially during pregnancy, it is reassuring there are many strategies and approaches to headache management that are safe to the mother and developing fetus. The purpose of

this chapter is to explore diagnosis and management strategies of migraine in particular, while presenting an overview of other headache conditions that may occur during pregnancy.

MIGRAINE

Definition

Migraine is a chronic medical condition in which the patient has a neurobiological predisposition to developing severe headache, often with associated nausea, vomiting, photophobia, phonophobia, and aura. Headache pain is usually unilateral, pulsating, and moderately severe. The headache may last anywhere from hours to days at a time, and it typically progresses in a crescendo pattern. Migraine without aura is characterized by recurrent headache pain without any visual or neurologic symptoms. Migraine with aura is characterized by the development of visual or neurologic symptom that progresses over a period of 5 to 20 minutes and lasts less than 60 minutes, followed by the migraine headache. Most commonly, the aura is a visual disturbance, often a scintillating scotoma that can progress from the corner of a visual field to encompass most of the vision and that occasionally is followed by visual field loss. Other auras can include hemibody numbness, tingling, weakness, or speech and language changes (12).

Migraine headache can be debilitating, necessitating prolonged bed rest. In some patients, nausea and vomiting are even more distressing than the headache itself. The majority of migraine patients have a genetic predisposition to such headaches. In many patients, specific triggers can be identified (Table 3.1). These triggers include foods that can activate the serotonergic system, perfumes, light, hormonal fluctuations, and stress (13). Because there has been such emphasis on migraine as a neurobiological order, the importance of unresolved stress sometimes is minimized in migraine treatment. Furthermore, some patients seek to minimize the role of stress, seeking instead a more classic allopathic explanation for their condition.

Because migraine is a chronic condition, new-onset migraine must be diagnosed with certainty. This is especially so during pregnancy. Many conditions can mimic migraine

TABLE 3.1. *Potential migraine triggers*

Diet
  Aged cheeses
  Alcohol
  Artificial sweeteners
  Caffeine excess/withdrawal
  Chocolate
  Citrus fruits
  Monosodium glutamate (MSG)
  Nitrates and nitrites
  Nuts
  Skipped meals
Environment
  High altitude
  Schedule changes
  Sleeping-pattern changes
  Travel across time zones
  Weather/seasonal changes
Hormones
  Hormone replacement therapy
  Menses
  Oral contraceptives
  Ovulation
Sensory stimuli
  Bright or flickering lights
  Loud noises
  Perfumes
Stress
  Crisis
  Job or personal stress
  Letdown periods
  Loss (death, separation, divorce)
  Unresolved conflicts

(14–24) or can produce neurologic symptoms with headache as one pathophysiologic manifestation. For example, vascular malformations may produce focal neurologic symptomatology that mimic aura and may be followed by severe headache. The headache of increased intracranial pressure, with or without cerebral venous thrombosis, initially may mimic migraine. Therefore, in new-onset migraine, it is critical to obtain a thorough history and perform a physical examination, and a specialist should be consulted if there is any diagnostic uncertainty.

Hormonal Considerations

That the ratio of migraine changes so considerably at puberty onset provides strong evidence that female hormones play a role in this disorder. Epstein and colleagues (25) surveyed 142 patients with migraine who recalled both their age of menarche and age of onset of migraine; 24 of 131 patients recalled that their headache began in the same year as menarche. Most patients noted no direct connection between migraine, age of puberty, and subsequent menarche. Patients who presented with migraine onset at the time of menarche subsequently were more likely to have menstrual-related migraine and to have relief of migraine during pregnancy.

From a more casual perspective, the majority of women with migraine link their attacks to menstruation, but a closer examination reveals that true menstrual migraine is less common than what is commonly believed. True menstrual migraine is defined as migraine attack confined to 24 hours before or 48 hours after the start of menses. Using such criteria, approximately 14% of women develop true menstrual migraine, and the vast majority have migraine without aura (25,26).

Estrogen is the hormone that most significantly influences menstrual migraine. Somerville (27–29) studied women who suffered with menstrual migraine, and he exogenously manipulated both estrogen and progesterone levels. He noted that falling estrogen levels were a significant trigger in the development of migraine. With estradiol replacement, the migraine attack was postponed. Once exogenous estradiol levels fell, migraine recurred. Somerville postulates that estrogen somehow primes the cerebral vasculature to be more susceptible to neurochemicals such as serotonin. If high estrogen levels are induced by exogenous hormone, migraine attacks can be prevented with considerable success. If progesterone is added for withdrawal bleeding, migraine attacks do not occur. Thus, in a subgroup of patients, prolonged high levels of estrogen considerably diminish or abolish migraine attacks.

Prolonged high-dose estrogen administration is not a practical alternative to migraine treatment and would likely only be effective in patients with true menstrual migraine. With regard to the more common clinical use of the birth control pill, there is not a clear-cut or predictable pattern of headache that emerges following such use (30–33). Headache is one of the most common complaints of women who first begin taking the birth control pill, but these headaches are not necessarily migrainous in nature. For migraineurs who begin taking the birth control pill, up to 49% notice an increase in their attacks. During the drug-free interval of the cycle, established migraineurs show a trend toward an increased incidence of migraine attacks. This is not seen for patients who develop new-onset migraine following oral contraceptive use. Some established migraine patients note improvement with beginning oral contraceptive use. Thus, although hormonal influences are an important aspect of migraine, for many patients, other factors are more critical in determining migraine frequency and severity.

Pregnancy Considerations

Investigations on headache during pregnancy are limited, and studies that are most frequently cited were published prior to the International Headache Society formal classification system of headache in 1988. For patients who suffer with menstrual migraine, there is clear evidence that these patients im-

prove considerably during pregnancy. Because pregnancy is associated with up to a 100-fold increase in estradiol levels (29) and because these levels are likely to be stable, these clinical data are in keeping with Somerville's experimental data.

Even for established migraineurs who do not have true menstrual migraine, 70% to 80% improve considerably or remit completely during pregnancy (34–37). The headache pattern may change as well. Maggioni and colleagues (38) found that 12 patients out of 149 studied converted from migraine with aura to migraine without aura during pregnancy. A smaller percentage of patients converted from migraine without aura to tension-type headaches. Only 1 patient out of 149 developed new-onset headache during pregnancy.

The literature is very consistent regarding the improvement of the majority of migraineurs during pregnancy. It also can be stated that new-onset migraine during pregnancy is unusual, and in the author's opinion, such a diagnosis must be made very cautiously. Callaghan (39) noted that migraine often begins during pregnancy, with an incidence corresponding to the general population, but subsequent studies have refuted Callaghan's data, both on diagnostic and epidemiologic grounds.

Chancellor (40) also has stated that new-onset migraine is not uncommon during pregnancy, and such cases always involve migraine with aura. He studied nine women who developed migraine with aura during pregnancy. However, a more careful analysis of his data demonstrates that four patients developed thrombocytopenia, two suffered with pre-eclampsia, and one had a threatened abortion. Coagulation and immunologic studies were not performed. Chancellor stresses the benign nature of migraine with aura during pregnancy, but three patients were lost to follow-up, and the underlying mechanism accounting for the patient's neurologic and hematologic abnormalities were not fully explored.

With more uniform diagnostic standards available, large studies have not demonstrated new-onset migraine during pregnancy (41–43). Because pregnant women are more vulnerable to developing a hypercoagulable state than nonpregnant women, transient neurologic symptoms in association with headache must be fully investigated for possible brain ischemia. Thus, for true migraine sufferers, they are more likely than not to have a reprieve during pregnancy.

Regarding complications of migraineurs during pregnancy, migraine does not represent a risk factor for neurologic or other medical complications during pregnancy or labor. Furthermore, studies have demonstrated unequivocally that there is no increased risk of fetus viability or fetal malformations in migraineurs (4,44). As physicians and health care practitioners, we can confidently reassure our migraine patients that their medical condition is not a hindrance to a safe pregnancy.

Management

New-Onset Migraine

The most important historical feature in a pregnant patient with a headache is a prior history of headache. Patients who present with new-onset headache, with or without neurologic symptoms, should receive an appropriate evaluation before being diagnosed with migraine, which should include inclusion and exclusion criteria. In assessing for new-onset migraine, the clinician must weigh clinical judgment versus interventions that may be psychologically distressing to the mother or potentially harmful to the developing fetus. If a pregnant woman presents with a crescendo, unilateral, or bilateral severe pounding headache and has other symptoms typical of migraine, a detailed history and neurologic exam must be performed. If the patient has no neurologic symptoms or signs and the headache subsequently resolves, she can be followed clinically without performing extensive diagnostic tests. If the headache becomes progressive or recurrent, however, then a brain imaging study should be performed.

Magnetic resonance imaging (MRI) is the test of choice. (See Chapter 1.) Sequential sagittal images should be performed to assess the patency of the superior sagittal sinus.

Pregnant women who have new-onset headache with visual or neurologic symptoms must also be evaluated with a careful history and examination. New-onset migraine with aura during pregnancy may represent an underlying hypercoagulable state. Again, clinical judgment must guide the clinician, but unless the history is unequivocal, strong consideration should be given to assessing for a hypercoagulable state. This includes checking a complete blood count and platelet count, prothrombin and partial thromboplastin time, anticardiolipin antibody, fibrinogen, clotting factors, protein C, protein S, and antithrombin III assays (see Chapter 5). Serious consideration also must be given to performing a brain MRI to rule out an occult vascular anomaly.

Other headaches may mimic migraine and are discussed later in this chapter. Mild headaches that are bifrontal or bitemporal may simply be tension-type headache. Any type of progressive headache may represent a more serious underlying medical condition and must be investigated thoroughly. Once a diagnosis of migraine without or with aura is secured, management options are the same as for established migraineurs.

Established Migraine: Nonpharmacologic Strategies

Nonpharmacologic treatment is preferred if patients do not have debilitating headaches. Any medication potentially harms the developing fetus. As a start, a detailed search should be made for environmental triggers (Table 3.1). Most established migraineurs have already performed such a search, but it is surprising in day-to-day clinical practice how many patients are unaware of true environmental triggers.

Stress management and relaxation techniques should be employed when possible. There is some benefit to biofeedback and other relaxation strategies in migraine management (45). Because many pregnant women may be learning relaxation strategies, especially with regard to labor and delivery, this becomes an ideal time to utilize a single strategy for more than one treatment. Biofeedback has demonstrated efficacy in reducing labor pain (see Chapter 22) and in reducing the frequency and severity of headache (45). Biofeedback is a process in which the patient is hooked up to a computerized device while receiving constant data regarding physiologic measures such as skin temperature or muscle tone. The patient learns to progressively change her physiology by focusing on muscle tone or skin temperature, and thereby she learns a type of relaxation response that can be practiced on a daily basis.

Acupuncture is another nonpharmacologic strategy that should be considered for patients who suffer with migraine during pregnancy. Although prospective studies for migraine during pregnancy are lacking, the author's experience is that acupuncture does benefit some patients who suffer with migraine, especially if there is a concomitant tension-type headache component. Massage therapy, meditative exercises such as yoga and t'ai chi, and manual physical therapy with a focus on myofascial release and craniosacral technique

are also strategies to consider, although they do not have proven efficacy in clinical studies. Unfortunately, the literature is rather silent regarding nonpharmacologic treatment of migraine during pregnancy.

Established Migraine: Pharmacologic Strategies

If medications are used, potential fetal toxicity must be considered. Table 3.2 is a reference guide for drug categories used during pregnancy. When utilizing medications, Category A and B drugs should be used if at all possible, and when necessary, category C drugs may be employed. Category D drugs are associated with known fetal risk and should be avoided. Category X drugs are contraindicated. When headaches are periodic, medication should be taken only for specific migraine attacks. Prophylactic or preventive medication should be employed only when migraines occur with such regularity that quality of life is significantly impaired.

The goal of symptomatic pharmacologic treatment is to reduce the severity and duration of an individual migraine attack. For headaches that do not respond to nonpharmacologic treatment, symptomatic medication

TABLE 3.2. *Fetal drug risk categories*

Category A:	Controlled studies in women fail to demonstrate a risk to the fetus in the first trimester (and there is no evidence of a risk in later trimesters), and the possibility of fetal harm appears remote.
Category B:	Either animal-reproduction studies have not demonstrated a fetal risk but there are no controlled studies in pregnant women or animal-reproduction studies have shown an adverse effect (other than a decrease in fertility) that was not confirmed in controlled studies in women in the first trimester (and there is no evidence of a risk in later trimesters).
Category C:	Either studies in animals have revealed adverse effects on the fetus (teratogenic or embryocidal or other) and there are no controlled studies in women or studies in women and animals are not available. Drugs should be given only if the potential benefit justifies the potential risk to the fetus.
Category D:	There is positive evidence of human fetal risk, but the benefits from use in pregnant women may be acceptable despite the risk (e.g., if the drug is needed in a life-threatening situation or for a serious disease for which safer drugs cannot be used or are ineffective).
Category X:	Studies in animals or human beings have demonstrated fetal abnormalities or there is evidence of fetal risk based on human experience or both, and the risk of the use of the drug in pregnant women clearly outweighs any possible benefit. The drug is contraindicated in women who are or may become pregnant.
Subscript M:	Manufacturer rating in professional literature.

From Briggs GC, Freeman RK, Yaffe JJ. *Drugs in pregnancy and lactation: a reference guide to fetal and neonatal risk.* 5th ed. Baltimore: Williams & Wilkins, 1998, with permission.

should begin with simple analgesics. This includes acetaminophen, with or without a mild narcotic. Nonsteroidal anti-inflammatory drugs also can be used safely during the first and second trimester, but as term approaches, these medications are contraindicated. The practitioner must be cognizant of the fact that nausea and vomiting can be as disabling as the headache itself, and with this in mind, antiemetics in combination with a simple analgesic may be highly effective.

Table 3.3 lists commonly used drugs for headache treatment and includes the risk factors as well as clinically documented effectiveness, when available. First-line symptomatic treatment should include acetaminophen alone. There is no convincing evidence of teratogenic effects of moderate-dose acetaminophen. Acetaminophen may be used in conjunction with caffeine, especially doses less than 300 mg per day. Such doses of caffeine also do not pose a measurable risk to the fetus, although high doses may be associated with spontaneous abortion or low birthweight.

Aspirin and other nonsteroidal anti-inflammatory drugs generally can be safely employed

TABLE 3.3. *Migraine medication: efficacy and fetal risk*

Symptomatic treatment	Efficacy (ref. 11)	Fetal risk (ref. 61)
Mild analgesics		
Acetaminophen	1+	B
Aspirin	2+	C[a]
Caffeine	2+	B
NSAIDS		
Celecoxib	—	C$_m$
Diclofenac	2+	B[a]
Flurbiprofen	2+	B$_m$[a]
Ibuprofen	2+	B[a]
Indomethacin	2+	B[a]
Ketorolac IM	2+	C$_m$[a]
Naprosyn/Naproxen	2+	B$_m$[a]
Rofecoxib	—	C$_m$
Narcotics		
Butorphanol	3+	B[b]
Codeine	2+	C[b]
Meperidine	—	B[b]
Methadone	—	B[b]
Morphine	—	B[b]
Antiemetics		
Chlorpromazine	2+	C
Metoclopramide	1+	B$_m$
Prochlorperazine	1+/2+	D
Barbiturates		
Butalbitol	3+	C[b]
Corticosteroids		
Dexamethasone	—	C
Hydrocortisone/Prednisone	—	B
Triptans		
Naratriptan	2+	C$_m$
Rizatriptan	3+	C$_m$
Sumatriptan	3+	C$_m$
Zolmitriptan	3+	C$_m$
Ergot alkaloids		
Dihydroergotamine SQ/IV	3+	X$_m$
Ergotamine	2+	D
Dihydroergotamine nasal spray	2+	X$_m$
Other		
Lidocaine nasal spray	—	C

continued on next page

Prophylactic treatment	Efficacy	Fetal risk
β-blockers		
Atenolol	2+	D_m
Metoprolol	3+	$C_m{}^c$
Nadolol	3+	$C_m{}^c$
Propanolol	3+	$C_m{}^c$
Timolol	1+	$C_m{}^c$
Antidepressants		
Tricyclic		
Amitriptyline	3+	D
Doxepin	1+	C
Imipramine	1+	D
Nortriptyline	3+	D
Protriptyline	2+	C
SSRI		
Fluoxetine	1+	B_m
Fluvoxamine	1+	C_m
Paroxetine	1+	B_m
Sertraline	1+	B_m
Monoamine oxidase inhibitors		
Phenelzine	3+	C
Other antidepressants		
Buproprion	1+	B_m
Mirtazepine	1+	C_m
Trazodone	1+	C_m
Venlafaxine	1+	C_m
Calcium channel blockers		
Nimodipine	2+	C_m
Verapamil	2+	C_m
Antiepileptics		
Divalproex sodium/sodium valproate	3+	D
Gabapentin	2+	C_m
Topiramate	2+	C_m
Serotonin antagonists		
Cyproheptadine	1+	B_m
Methysergide	3+	D_m
Other		
Feverfew	1+	D
Magnesium	1+	B
Vitamin B_2	2+	C^d

Efficacy:
—, not established
1+, somewhat effective
2+, effective
3+, very effective
Fetal risk: see Table 3.2
[a]Category D in 3rd trimester
[b]Category D if prolonged use or high doses at term
[c]Category D in 2nd and 3rd trimester
[d]Category D in migraine prophylaxis doses

during the first two trimesters. In the third trimester, nonsteroidal anti-inflammatory drugs may inhibit labor, decrease amniotic fluid volume, and increase the risk of bleeding. Aspirin and nonsteroidal anti-inflammatory drugs also may have a detrimental effect on the hemostasis of the newborn close to term (46). These medications, when prescribed, can be used alone or in conjunction with low-dose caffeine during the first two trimesters (47). The general strategy is that such medication should be given at the very beginning of a migraine attack because they are then more likely to have a stabilizing effect on a prostaglandin-induced inflammatory cascade, which is an important component of migraine pain.

Antiemetics should be employed at the beginning of migraine attacks for patients who suffer with moderate to severe nausea and vomiting in association with migraine (48). Metoclopramide, alone or in conjunction with simple analgesics, is generally safe during pregnancy (46). Patients may require antiemetics in the form of a suppository. The role of ginger has been well established for nausea and vomiting in pregnancy, but its role in migraine is not well documented (see Chapter 22).

For patients who do not respond to simple analgesics, more potent narcotic analgesics may be employed (47). Prolonged narcotic use is associated with maternal and neonatal addiction, but judicious, intermittent narcotic use is generally safe. Indiscriminate use of codeine, especially during the first and second trimester, has been associated with cleft lip, cleft palate, inguinal hernia, hip dislocation, and cardiopulmonary defects. Other narcotics are probably not teratogenic.

Barbiturates are sometimes employed for acute migraine management, and as with narcotics, their use must be limited to intermittent pulse therapy (46,47). Fetal dependence and neonatal withdrawal can occur equally with barbiturates and narcotics. Butalbital was commonly employed prior to the development of more specific antimigraine drugs and often is used in conjunction with caffeine and either acetaminophen or aspirin. Short-acting benzodiazepine such as lorazepam may be employed, especially when migraine is associated with considerable anxiety.

Ergotamines are contraindicated during pregnancy. At the time of conception, ergotamine and dihydroergotamine can lead to implant failure. In a developing fetus, cleft palates and bilateral limb defects are noted in animal studies exposed to ergotamine. Ergotamines also have a potent uterogenic effect, which may lead to premature labor. Ergotamine is also a strongly vasoconstrictive drug, which may cause fetal hypoxia (46,47,49).

With the advent of the new generation of migraine-specific drugs known as triptans, it is not surprising that several migraineurs have been exposed to these medications during their first trimester of pregnancy. Triptan medications are more highly specific serotonin agonists, and their development revolutionized the treatment of migraine. Many hailed these medications as miracle drugs because patients who previously suffered severely with migraine attacks had complete or near-complete resolution of migraine symptomatology within 1 to 2 hours of taking the triptan medication.

Approximately 15% of a single dose of sumatriptan crosses into the fetal compartment over a period of 4 hours, and only the parent drug crosses the placenta (50). The mechanism of transfer is passive, and the rate of transfer is equal in both directions. In several large database analyses, sumatriptan exposure during pregnancy has been compared to controls. Olesen and colleagues (51) identified 34 patients who were exposed to sumatriptan during pregnancy, and they were compared to 15,955 healthy women and 89 migraine controls. The odds ratio for having a newborn with low birthweight was increased for all migraine patients who delivered at term, compared with the outcome of healthy pregnant patients without migraine. Sumatriptan exposure during pregnancy was associated with an increased risk of preterm delivery and low birthweight, but it was unclear if this reflected chance or the impact of disease severity itself.

O'Quinn and colleagues (52) assessed the results of 76 first-trimester exposures to sumatriptan and found no differences in pregnancy outcome when compared to patients who had not used medication. Kallen and Lygner (53) identified 658 women who had used sumatriptan during pregnancy. There was a slight increase in preterm and low-birthweight infants, but the results were not statistically significant. There was no increase in the rate of congenital malformations. Other studies confirm the apparent lack of increased risk in major birth defects for sumatriptan-exposed pregnancies, including during organogenesis (54–56). Thus, although sumatriptan is not recommended as a treatment option for migraine during pregnancy, patients who have taken sumatriptan should be reassured that they have likely not exposed their infant to any significant risk.

For patients who have more refractory migraine, the clinician must consider prophylactic medication in an attempt to reduce the frequency and severity of regularly recurrent headache. The most commonly used prophylactic medications are beta-blockers and antidepressant medications. If a patient has a co-existing illness that requires treatment, a drug that can treat both disorders should be used. For example, beta-blockers treat hypertension and migraine, and antidepressants can treat comorbid depression.

Propranolol is the most widely used beta-blocker for prophylactic migraine treatment. Fetal and neonatal adverse effects have been reported with propranolol use, but it is unclear if this represents the effects of a comorbid disease. Daily doses of less than 160 mg are probably not associated with serious complications (46,47), but higher doses will more likely be associated with intrauterine growth retardation, bradycardia, and respiratory depression (57–60).

Antidepressants often are effective as prophylactic agents, especially when there is associated depression or anxiety. There is considerable experience with the use of tricyclic antidepressants, especially amitriptyline and nortriptyline, but limb-reduction anomalies have been reported, although not confirmed (46,47). The collaborative perinatal project found no increase in congenital malformations in pregnant women treated with amitriptyline during the first trimester (61). Selective serotonin reuptake inhibitors such as fluoxetine also may be effective as prophylactic agents, although they are probably less efficacious than tricyclic antidepressants (11). There is no evidence of teratogenicity, spontaneous abortion, or other fetal complications in patients taking fluoxetine during the first trimester (61).

Anticonvulsants are sometimes utilized as prophylactic agents, but they should be avoided during pregnancy. Women with epilepsy who take anticonvulsants during pregnancy have double the general population risk of malformations. Valproic acid (divalproate sodium) is the only Food and Drug Administration-approved anticonvulsant medication for prophylactic migraine treatment, and the absolute risk of producing a child with a neural tube defect when exposure occurs between day 17 and day 30 is 1% to 2%. Lamotrigine more recently has been studied as a migraine prophylactic agent, and a drug registry study noted no increase in fetal complications for pregnant women exposed to lamotrigine; however, the small numbers do not justify using this medication for migraine prophylaxis (54,62).

Calcium channel blockers also may be efficacious for migraine, but their use should be limited to patients who suffer concomitant hypertension. There are no adequate well-controlled studies of verapamil or other calcium channel blockers in pregnant women (47).

OTHER HEADACHE CONDITIONS

Tension-Type Headache

Definition

Tension-type headaches are recurrent headache episodes lasting minutes to days. The pain is typically pressing or tightening in quality, of mild to moderate severity, and bilateral in location and patients generally do not feel unwell. Nausea is absent but photophobia or phonophobia may be present (12). Tension-type headaches result in part from involuntary tightening of muscles, but there is likely a biological continuum between tension-type headache and migraine (63). There is a paucity of data on the incidence of tension-type headache during pregnancy. Maggioni and associates (38) studied 430 women by way of questionnaire, and they documented that 126 women were primary headache sufferers (29.3%). Of these, 33 had tension-type headache. In the tension-type headache group, approximately 80% showed complete remission or greater than 50% decrease in the number of attacks. The improvement was more evident after the end of the first trimester.

Tension-type headaches may develop in conjunction with low back pain or neck pain as a continuum of myofascial pain. Anxiety and psychologic stress during pregnancy also may contribute to tension-type headache. Such patients do not develop neurologic symptoms, and pain generally is relieved with bed rest, relaxation therapy, or simple analgesics. New-onset, refractory, tension-type headache during pregnancy is a diagnosis of exclusion.

Management

The focus of treatment in pregnant patients with tension-type headaches should be behavioral and postural modification. Gentle exercise should be prescribed as warranted, and mild analgesics such as acetaminophen can be used periodically. As with migraine, the focus of treatment should be nonpharmacologic strategy, and modalities similar to those outlined above should be employed. Pharmacologic strategies should focus on simple analgesics and rarely narcotic analgesics.

Brain Hemorrhage

Subarachnoid hemorrhage is characterized by the sudden onset of a severe, incapacitating headache. Unlike migraine and tension-type headache, the headache is not crescendo and it is not unilateral. Subarachnoid hemorrhage is a medical emergency. Patients may present with headache alone, but also may rapidly develop neurologic signs, stupor, or coma and may even die. Subarachnoid hemorrhage accounts for 50% of intracranial bleeding during pregnancy, and there is a 50% mortality rate in subarachnoid hemorrhage (64). The majority result from a ruptured cerebral aneurysm or arterial venous malformation, although eclampsia, drug use, disseminated intravascular coagulation, and other coagulopathies need to be considered (65,66) (see Chapter 6). In the so-called sentinel bleeds, in

which the aneurysm does not completely rupture, subarachnoid hemorrhage will present as headache alone. Even in sentinel bleeds, the headache is characteristically abrupt and severe. Any pregnant patient who presents with new onset of precipitous, severe headache should be evaluated for subarachnoid hemorrhage.

Intracerebral hemorrhage also usually presents with sudden, severe headache, and rapidly progressive neurologic signs often accompany the headache. Most cases of intracerebral hemorrhage during pregnancy result from hypertension, especially in the setting of eclampsia (see Chapter 6). Other causes include arterial venous malformation, cerebral venous thrombosis, and alcohol and cocaine abuse (65–67). Patients with highly vascular brain tumors also may develop intracerebral hemorrhage during pregnancy because estrogen may have a pathologic vasoactive effect on the abnormal blood vessels (see Chapter 12). Intracerebral hemorrhage is a medical emergency that may progress rapidly to stupor, coma, and death (18,20,65,68–71).

In any patient who develops new onset of severe headache during pregnancy, diagnostic workup must begin immediately. Brain computed tomography (CT) scan is the imaging study of choice because brain MRI is less sensitive for acute blood. (See Chapter 1.) If the brain CT scan is unrevealing, lumbar puncture must be performed to assess for subarachnoid blood. Patients with subarachnoid or intracerebral hemorrhage require management by a neurologic and neurosurgical team in an intensive care unit setting.

Cerebral Venous Thrombosis

Pregnancy increases the risk of stroke in young women by 13-fold, and the most common cerebrovascular accident during pregnancy is cerebral venous thrombosis (14,24) (see Chapter 5). Most women with cerebral venous thrombosis present with neurologic symptoms and signs, but thrombosis of the superior sagittal sinus may manifest as a progressively severe headache without focal symptomatology (72–74). With superior sagittal sinus thrombosis, intracranial hypertension may develop, and patients will manifest a progressively severe global headache resistant to analgesics. If thrombosis progresses, neurologic symptoms and signs will develop.

Cerebral venous thrombosis is usually a result of an underlying hypercoagulable state and develops in 1 out of 2,500 to 1 out of 10,000 deliveries (14,21,22). Clotting factors and fibrinogen increase during pregnancy, and antithrombin III, plasminogen activity, and protein-S levels decrease (see Chapter 5). Platelets may become hypercoagulable. Approximately 5% of patients who develop cerebral venous thrombosis in pregnancy present as having pseudotumor cerebri (74). It is important to distinguish between cerebral venous thrombosis and pseudotumor cerebri because the management differs considerably. Patients who develop new-onset headache that is global in nature and that becomes progressively severe must undergo a brain MRI study. Although a sagittal image may delineate thrombosis of the superior sagittal sinus, specialized venous and arterial images also should be obtained when there is any doubt in the diagnosis. Heparin may be used as a treatment when necessary. Heparin does not cross the placenta, has a short half-life, and can be used safely during pregnancy by subcutaneous or intravenous administration (see Chapter 9).

Pseudotumor Cerebri

Pseudotumor cerebri is a syndrome characterized by global headache secondary to increased intracranial hypertension (75). Its cause is unknown, but it may be related to either increased cerebrospinal fluid production or decreased cerebrospinal fluid resorption through the arachnoid villi (76). Patients develop progressively severe headache that often worsens when the patient is recumbent. Blurred vision, visual loss, and horizontal diplopia result if intracranial hypertension progresses (77).

Pseudotumor cerebri occurs more commonly in obese women of childbearing age (78,79). Up to 12% of patients with pseudotumor cerebri may become pregnant (15, 80–82), and pseudotumor cerebri may develop during any trimester (19,35,83,84). The available literature does not document any increased risk from pseudotumor cerebri to the pregnant patient or the developing fetus. Visual outcome is the same for pregnant and nonpregnant patients. Subsequent pregnancy does not increase the risk of recurrent pseudotumor cerebri relative to nonpregnant patients with this syndrome (15,85).

Patients who present with new-onset progressively severe headache must undergo a brain MRI study, and cerebral venous thrombosis must be excluded. If imaging studies are unremarkable, a diagnostic lumbar puncture should be performed. Patients with pseudotumor cerebri have a pathologically elevated opening pressure.

Pseudotumor cerebri must be differentiated from cerebral venous thrombosis. If headache pain is not intolerable, papilledema is mild, and formal visual field and visual acuity testing are normal, patients can be followed conservatively and treated with mild analgesics. Patients must be instructed to report any new visual symptoms, and formal ophthalmologic and visual field testing must be performed on a regular basis (86). For patients who develop progressive symptoms, a short course of corticosteroids may lead to clinical improvement; prednisone is the medication of choice. With intolerable headache or vision loss, patients must be treated with either serial lumbar punctures or a lumboperitoneal shunt.

Brain Tumor

Patients who present with new-onset headache often fear that they have a brain tumor. However, brain tumors usually present with neurologic symptoms or signs. Less than half of patients develop headache, and they are often not severe (17). Although classic medical teaching equates early-morning headache with brain tumor, clinical evidence indicates that such headaches usually are not observed in patients with brain tumors. Pregnancy does not increase the risk of developing a brain tumor, although pregnancy may adversely affect highly vascular tumors, acoustic neuromas, or meningiomas. (See Chapter 12.) Treatment should be dictated by the patient's overall clinical condition, and patients should be managed by a neuro-oncologist.

Sinusitis

Sinus headaches are overdiagnosed. Chronic sinusitis is not a cause of headache. Patients who report frequent sinus headaches often have misdiagnosed themselves, and a closer examination indicates that these patients suffer with recurrent tension-type headache, migraine, or both (12). Acute sinusitis is usually easy to recognize, especially for acute frontal or maxillary sinusitis. Patients have localized pain, and they may be febrile and appear ill. Acute sphenoid sinusitis is more difficult to diagnose, and pain may develop referred to the occipital area, the vertex, the frontal region, or behind the eyes (87). Some cases of acute sinusitis may be obvious, and imaging studies are not required. Antibiotic treatment is appropriate, and patients should respond briskly to treatment (88,89).

Postpartum Headache

The incidence of postpartum headache is not known, and the medical literature is rather silent on this condition. In two separate studies, Stein and colleagues (90) documented that headache occurs most frequently on days 2 to 6 postpartum. Approximately 40% of women develop postpartum headache, and risk factors include a previous personal or family history of migraine and premenstrual migraine. These headaches are usually milder and more frequently bilateral than are typical migraine headaches. There is no correlation with depression or mood changes during the puerperium (91). Given the hormonal fluctuations that develop rapidly postpartum, one pathophysiologic factor may be a precipitous decline in estrogen levels (8). This is in keeping with clinical data cited previously.

A possible underdiagnosed cause of postpartum headache may be from an inadvertent puncture of the dural sac during spinal anesthesia. Obstetric patients may be more likely to suffer accidental dural puncture than nonobstetric patients (92). The incidence of this complication varies with the experience of the anesthesiologist and ranges from 0.5% to 2.5% in teaching hospitals (93). When unintentional dural puncture occurs, 30% to 70% of patients develop postdural headache (94), often referred to as post-lumbar puncture headache in the neurology literature.

Evans and associates (94) report that for obstetric spinal anesthesia, the average frequency of post-lumbar puncture headache is 18%. Besides the experience of the anesthesiologist, risk factors include the following (94–100):

1. Needle size: with dural puncture, the incidence of post-lumbar headache is 40% with a 20- to 22-gauge needle, and 5% to 12% with a 24- to 27-gauge needle.
2. Direction of bevel: if the spinal needle is inserted parallel to the dural fibers, which are longitudinally oriented structures of collagen and elastin, 24% of patients will develop a post-lumbar puncture headache compared to 70% of patients whose dural puncture is perpendicular to these fibers.
3. Placement of the stylet before withdrawing the needle: post-lumbar puncture headache is reported in 16% of patients without reinsertion of the stylet compared to 5% of patients in whom the stylet was replaced before withdrawing the spinal needle.
4. Needle design: atraumatic needles commonly are used by anesthesiologists (101), and post-lumbar puncture headaches develop much less frequently when such a noncutting needle is used.

The amount of spinal fluid removed and the duration of recumbency following dural puncture has no effect on the development of a post-lumbar puncture headache.

Post-lumbar puncture headaches are usually self-limited, and patients obtain relief when they are recumbent. However, this is not always practical for the mother with a newborn, who may wish to be upright when caring for her infant. These headaches usually are distinguished from other types of headaches in that immediate relief is obtained with lying down. For refractory patients, a blood patch may be performed. This involves removal of a small amount of the patient's own blood and inserting it into the epidural space at the level of the dural puncture. This technique can be utilized safely and successfully, and 85% to 90% of patients obtain symptomatic relief within 1 to 24 hours; 90% of patients who fail an initial blood patch will respond to a second patch (94). Pain medications are not an appropriate treatment for post-lumbar puncture headaches because the cause of the headache is persistent cerebrospinal fluid leakage with less buoyancy protection of the brain and other neural structures.

SUMMARY

Migraine and other headache conditions are relatively common during pregnancy. Physicians and other primary health care providers should not assume that because a patient presents with headache alone, such symptoms can be taken lightly. Most patients do not develop new-onset headache during pregnancy, and all patients who do develop such a condition must be evaluated thoroughly. Similarly, patients who develop any change in their headache condition must undergo a careful evaluation. Fig. 3.1 is an algorithm to aid in evaluating pregnant patients with headache. Postpartum headaches also must be evaluated and treated appropriately.

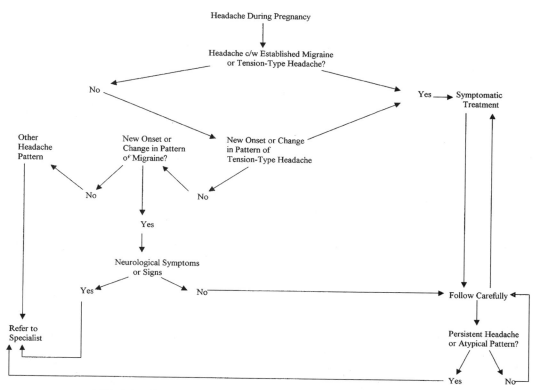

FIG. 3.1. Algorithm for headache management during pregnancy.

In most cases of headache during pregnancy and postpartum, the patient is suffering with a benign medical condition. Even so, quality of life is an important consideration in preserving the patient's physical and emotional well-being (102,103). A stepwise approach to symptomatic treatment should be provided for all patients. A high index of suspicion for nonbenign causes of headache will assist in decreasing morbidity and mortality to the mother and fetus.

REFERENCES

1. Rasmussen BK, Jensen R, Schroll M, et al. Epidemiology of headache in a general population—a prevalence study. *J Clin Epidemiol* 1991;44:1147-1157.
2. Lance JW, Curran DA, Anthony M. Investigations into the mechanism and treatment of chronic headache. *Med J Aust* 1965;2:909–914.
3. Leviton A. Epidemiology of headache. In: Schoenberg BS, ed. *Advances in neurology,* Vol 39. New York: Raven Press, 1978:341–353.
4. Wainscott G, Sullivan FM, Volans GN, et al. The outcome of pregnancy in women suffering from migraine. *Postgrad Med J* 1978;54:98–102.
5. Deubner DC. An epidemiologic study of migraine and headache in 10–20 year-olds. *Headache* 1977;17:173–180.
6. Linet MS, Stewart WF, Celentano DD, et al. An epidemiologic study of headache among adolescents and young adults. *JAMA* 1989;261:2211–2216.
7. Sparks JP. The incidence of migraine in school children. A survey by the medical officers of school association. *Practitioner* 1978;221:407–411.
8. Stang PE, Yanagihara T, Swanson JW, et al. Incidence of migraine headache: a population-based study in Olmsted County, Minnesota. *Neurology* 1992;42:1657–1662.
9. Stewart WF, Lipton RB, Celentano DD, et al. Prevalence of migraine headache in the United States. Relation to age, income, race, and other socioeconomic factors. *JAMA* 1992;267:64–69.
10. Waters WE, O'Connor PJ. Epidemiology of headache and migraine in women. *J Neurol Neurosurg Psychiatry* 1971;34:148–153.
11. Silberstein SD. Practice parameter: evidence-based guidelines for migraine headache (an evidence-based review): report of the Quality Standards Subcommittee of the American Academy of Neurology. *Neurology* 2000;55:754–762.
12. Classification and diagnostic criteria for headache disorders, cranial neuralgias and facial pain. Headache Classification Committee of the International Headache Society. *Cephalalgia* 1988;8:1–96.
13. Goadsby PJ, Edvinsson L. The trigeminovascular system and migraine: studies characterizing cerebrovascular and neuropeptide changes seen in humans and cats. *Ann Neurol* 1993;33:48–56.
14. Cross JN, Castro PO, Jennett WB. Cerebral strokes associated with pregnancy and the puerperium. *Br Med J* 1968;3:214–218.
15. Digre KB, Varner MW, Corbett JJ. Pseudotumor cerebri and pregnancy. *Neurology* 1984;34:721–729.
16. Edmeads J. Headaches and head pains associated with disease of the cervical spine. *Med Clin North Am* 1978;62:533–544.
17. Forsyth PA, Posner JB. Headaches in patients with brain tumors: a study of 111 patients. *Neurology* 1993;43:1678–1683.
18. Minielly R, Yuzpe AA, Drake CG. Subarachnoid hemorrhage secondary to ruptured cerebral aneurysm in pregnancy. *Obstet Gynecol* 1979;53:64–70.
19. Nickerson CW, Kirk RF. Recurrent pseudotumor cerebri in pregnancy. *Obstet Gynecol* 1965;26:811–813.
20. Sadasivan B, Malik G, Lee C, et al. Vascular malformations and pregnancy. *Surg Neurol* 1990;33:305–313.
21. Simolke GA, Cox SM, Cunningham FG. Cerebrovascular accidents complicating pregnancy and the puerperium. *Obstet Gynecol* 1991;78:37–42.
22. Srinivasan K. Cerebral venous and arterial thrombosis in pregnancy and puerperium: a study of 135 patients. *Angiology* 1983;34:731–746.
23. Tietjen GE. Migraine and antiphospholipid antibodies. *Cephalalgia* 1992;12:69–74.
24. Wiebers DO. Ischemic cerebrovascular complications of pregnancy. *Arch Neurol* 1985;42:1106–1113.
25. Epstein MT, Hockaday JM, Hockaday TD. Migraine and reproductive hormones throughout the menstrual cycle. *Lancet* 1975;1:543–548.
26. Singh M. Progesterone in migraine. *Lancet* 1947;1:745.
27. Somerville BW. The role of estradiol withdrawal in the etiology of menstrual migraine. *Neurology* 1972;22:355–365.
28. Somerville BW. Estrogen-withdrawal migraine. I. Duration of exposure required and attempted prophylaxis by premenstrual estrogen administration. *Neurology* 1975;25:239–244.
29. Somerville BW. Estrogen-withdrawal migraine. II. Attempted prophylaxis by continuous estradiol administration. *Neurology* 1975;25:245–250.
30. Mears E, Grant ECG. "Anovlar" as an oral contraceptive. *Br Med J* 1962;75:5297.
31. Whitty CW, Hockaday JM, Whitty MM. The effect of oral contraceptives on migraine. *Lancet* 1966;1:856–859.
32. Phillips BM. Contraceptive drugs and migraine. *Br Med J* 1968;299.
33. Nilsson A, Jacobsen L, Ingemanson CA. Side effects of an oral contraceptive with particular attention to menstrual symptoms and sexual adaptation. *Acta Obstet Gynecol Scand* 1967;45:537–56.
34. Bousser MG, Ratinahirana H, Darbois Y. Migraine and pregnancy: a prospective study in 703 women after delivery. *Neurology* 1990;40:437.
35. Greet M. Benign intracranial hypertension: V. Menstrual dysfunction. *Neurology* 1964;14:668–673.
36. Lance JW, Anthony M. Some clinical aspects of migraine. A prospective survey of 500 patients. *Arch Neurol* 1966;15:356–361.
37. Somerville BW. A study of migraine in pregnancy. *Neurology* 1972;22:824–828.
38. Maggioni F, Alessi C, Maggino T, et al. Headache in pregnancy. *Cephalgia* 1997;17:765–769.

39. Callaghan N. The migraine syndrome in pregnancy. *Neurology* 1968;18:197–201.

40. Chancellor AM, Wroe SJ, Cull RE. Migraine occurring for the first time in pregnancy. *Headache* 1990;30:224–227.

41. Bousser MG, Ratinahirana H, Darbois X. Migraine in pregnancy: a prospective study in 703 women after delivery. *Neurology* 1990;40:437.

42. Aube M. Migraine in pregnancy. *Neurology* 1999;53: S26–S28.

43. Paulson GW. Headaches in women, including women who are pregnant. *Am J Obstet Gynecol* 1995;173: 1734–1741.

44. Uknis A, Silberstein SD. Review article: migraine and pregnancy. *Headache* 1991;31:372–374.

45. Rapoport AM. Emerging nonspecific migraine therapies: targets and unmet needs. *Headache* 1999;39: S27–S34.

46. Pfaffenrath V, Rehm M. Migraine in pregnancy. *Drug Saf* 1998;19:383—388.

47. Silberstein SD. Migraine and pregnancy. *Neurol Clin* 1997;15:209–231.

48. Kallen B. Hyperemesis during pregnancy and delivery outcome: a registry study. *Eur J Obstet Gynecol Reprod Biol* 1987;26:291–302.

49. Hosking SP. Ergotamine use in pregnancy. *Aust NZ J Obstet Gynaecol* 1996;36:2:159–160.

50. Schenker S, Yang Y, Perez A, et al. Sumatriptan (imitrex) treatment by the human placenta (43941). *Proc Soc Exp Biol Med* 1995;210:213–220.

51. Olesen C, Steffensen FH, Sorenson HT, et al. Pregnancy outcome following prescription for sumatriptan. *Headache* 2000;40:20–24.

52. O'Quinn S, Ephross SA, Williams V, et al. Pregnancy and perinatal outcomes in migraineurs using sumatriptan: a prospective study. *Arch Gynecol Obstet* 1999;263: 7–12.

53. Kallen B, Lygner PE. Delivery outcome in women who used drugs for migraine during pregnancy with special references to sumatriptan. *Headache* 2001;41: 351–356.

54. Reiff-Eldridge R, Heffner CR, Ephross SA, et al. Monitoring pregnancy outcomes after prenatal drug exposure through prospective pregnancy registries: a pharmaceutical company commitment. *Am J Obstet Gynecol* 2000;182:159–163.

55. Pastore LM, Hertz-Picciotto I, Beaumont JJ. Risk of stillbirth from medications, illnesses and medical procedures. *Paediatr Perinat Epidemiol* 1999;13: 421–430.

56. Shuhaiber S, Pastuszak A, Schick B, et al. Pregnancy outcome following first trimester exposure to sumatriptan. *Neurology* 1998;51:581–583.

57. Featherstone HJ. Fetal demise in a migraine patient on propranolol. *Headache* 1983;23:213–214.

58. Hughes HE, Goldstein DA. Birth defects following maternal exposure to ergotamine, beta blockers, and caffeine. *J Med Genet* 1998;25:396–399.

59. Pruyn SC, Phelan JP, Buchanan GC. Long-term propranolol therapy in pregnancy: maternal and fetal outcome. *Am J Obstet Gynecol* 1979;135:485–489.

60. Repke JT. Pharmacologic management of hypertension in pregnancy. In: Niebyl JR, ed. *Drug use in pregnancy,* 2nd ed. Philadelphia: Lea & Febiger 1988: 55–65.

61. Briggs GC, Freeman RK, Yaffe JJ. *Drugs in pregnancy and lactation: a reference guide to fetal and neonatal risk,* 5th ed. Baltimore: Williams & Wilkins, 1998.

62. Gilmore J, Pennell PB, Stern BJ. Medication use during pregnancy for neurologic conditions. *Neurol Clin* 1998;16:189–206.

63. Sheftell FD. Chronic daily headache. *Neurology* 1992; 42:32–36.

64. Barno A, Freeman DW. Maternal deaths due to spontaneous subarachnoid hemorrhage. *Am J Obstet Gynecol* 1976;125:384–392.

65. Henderson CE, Torbey M. Rupture of intracranial aneurysm associated with cocaine use during pregnancy. *Am J Perinatol* 1988;5:142–143.

66. Hillbom K, Kaste M. Alcohol intoxication: a risk factor for primary subarachnoid hemorrhage. *Neurology* 1982;32:706–711.

67. Mercado A, Johnson G, Calver D, et al. Cocaine, pregnancy, and postpartum intracerebral hemorrhage. *Obstet Gynecol* 1989;73:467–468.

68. Carmel P, Swift D. Spontaneous intracranial hemorrhage occurring during pregnancy. In: Kaufman H, ed, *Intracerebral hematomas.* New York: Raven Press, 1992:117–125.

69. Dias MS, Sekhar LN. Intracranial hemorrhage from aneurysms and arteriovenous malformations during pregnancy and the puerperium. *Neurosurgery* 1990; 27:855–866.

70. Robinson JL, Hall CJ, Sedzimir CB. Subarachnoid hemorrhage in pregnancy. *J Neurosurg* 1972:36:27–33.

71. Robinson JL, Hall CJ, Sedzimir CB. Arteriovenous malformations, aneurysms, and pregnancy. *J Neurosurg* 1974;41:63–70.

72. Bousser MG, Chiras J, Bories J, et al. Cerebral venous thrombosis-a review of 38 cases. *Stroke* 1985;16: 199–213.

73. Bousser MG. Cerebral venous thrombosis: diagnosis and management. *J Neurol* 2000;247:252–258.

74. Panagariya A, Maru A. Cerebral venous thrombosis in pregnancy and puerperium-a prospective study. *J Assoc Physicians India* 1998;46:748.

75. Ahlskog JE, O'Neill BP. Pseudotumor cerebri. *Ann Int Med* 1982;97:249–256.

76. Rottenberg DA, Foley KM, Posner JB. Hypothesis: the pathogenesis of pseudotumor cerebri. *Med Hypotheses* 1980;6:913–918.

77. Rush JA. Pseudotumor cerebri: clinical profile and visual outcome in 63 patients. *Mayo Clin Proc* 1980;55: 541–546.

78. Weisberg LA. Benign intracranial hypertension. *Medicine* 1975;54:197–207.

79. Wilson DH, Garden WJ. Benign intracranial hypertension with particular reference to its occurrence in fat young women. *Can Med Assoc J* 1966;95:102–105.

80. Bulens C, DeVries WA, Van Crevel H. Benign intracranial hypertension. *J Neurol Sci* 1979;40: 147–157.

81. Rush JA. Pseudotumor cerebri. *Mayo Clin Proc* 1980; 55:541–546.

82. Weisberg LA. The syndrome of increased intracranial pressure without localizing signs: a reappraisal. *Neurology* 1975;25:85–88.

83. Foley J. Benign forms of intracranial hypertension: "Toxic" and "otitic" hydrocephalus. *Brain* 1955;78: 1–41.

84. Donaldson JO. *Neurology of pregnancy,* 2nd ed. Philadelphia: WB Saunders Co., 1978:185–216

85. Arseni C, Simoca I, Jipescu I, et al. Pseudotumor cerebri: risk factors, clinical course, prognostic criteria. *Rom J Neurol Psychiatry* 1992;30:115–132.

86. Wall M, George D. Visual loss in pseudotumor cerebri: incidence and defects related to visual field strategy. *Arch Neurol* 1987;44:170–175.

87. Lew D, Southwick FS, Montgomery WW, et al. Sphenoid sinusitis: a review of 30 cases. *N Engl J Med* 1983;19:1149–1154.

88. Silberstein SD. Headaches and women: treatment of the pregnant and lactating migraineur. *Headache* 1993;33:533–540.

89. Dzhabbarov KK, Muminov AI. Characteristics of the course and treatment of inflammatory nasal and paranasal sinus diseases in pregnancy. *Vestn Otorinolaringol* 1993;5-6:42–45.

90. Stein G, Morton J. Marsh A, et al. Headache after childbirth. *Acta Neurol Scand* 1984;69:74–79.

91. Stein GS. Headaches in the first post partum week and their relationship to migraine. *Headache* 1981;21:201–205.

92. Spencer HC. Postural puncture headache: what matters in technique. *Regional Anesthesia and Pain Medicine* 1988;23:374–379.

93. Smedstad KG. Dealing with post-dural puncture headache—is it different in obstetrics? *Can J Anaesth* 1998;45:6–9.

94. Evans RW, Armon C, Frohman EM, et al. Assessment: prevention of post-lumbar puncture headaches. *Neurology* 2000;55:909–914.

95. Angle P, Thompson D, Halpern S, et al. Second stage pushing correlates with headache after unintentional dural puncture in parturients. *Can J Anesth* 1999;46:861–866.

96. Richardson MG, Wissler RN. The effects of needle bevel orientation during epidural catheter insertion in laboring parturients. *Anesth Analg* 1999;88:352–356.

97. Hopkinson JM, Samaan AK, Russell IF, et al. A comparative multicentre trial of spinal needles for caesarean section. *Anaesthesia* 1997;52:998–1014.

98. Sinclair M, Simmons S, Cyna A. Incidents in obstetrics anaesthesia and analgesia: An analysis of 5000 aims reports. *Anaesth Intensive Care* 1999;27:275–281.

99. Mansi ML. Prevention of postpartum postspinal headache. *J Am Osteopath Assoc* 1982;81:496–499.

100. Hwang JJ, Ho ST, Wang JJ, et al. Post dural puncture headache in cesarean section: comparison of 25-gauge whitacre with 25- and 26-gauge quincke needles. *Acta Anaesthesiol Sin* 1997;35:33–37.

101. Birnbach DJ, Kuroda MM, Sternman D, et al. Use of atraumatic spinal needles among neurologists in the United States. *Headache* 2001;41:385–390.

102. Terwindt GM, Ferrari MD, Tijhuis M. The impact of migraine on quality of life in the general population. *Neurology* 2000;55:624–629.

103. Holmes WF, MacGregor A, Dodick D. Migraine-related disability: impact and implications for sufferers' lives and clinical issues. *Neurology* 2001;56:S13–S19.

Neurological Complications of Pregnancy, Second Edition, edited by Brian Hainline and Orrin Devinsky. Lippincott Williams & Wilkins, Philadelphia © 2002.

4

Neurologic Aspects of Eclampsia

Peter W. Kaplan

Department of Neurology, Johns Hopkins Bayview Medical Center, and Johns Hopkins University School of Medicine, Baltimore, Maryland, U.S.A.

Several early references to problems in pregnancy and childbirth can be found in ancient Egyptian, Chinese, Greek, and Indian literature (1). Egyptian sources mention amulets worn to ward off convulsions during childbirth, but more specifically, the Kahun Papyrus (200 BC) and Hippocrates in the 4th century BC refer to seizures or convulsions during pregnancy (2,3). It was only in the 18th century, however, that a distinction was made between eclamptic seizures and epilepsy (4), and even medical reports from the turn of the century use the term eclampsia for seizures occurring outside pregnancy.

The conditions of preeclampsia and eclampsia as we know them today refer to a continuum of disorders that exclusively affect women after the twentieth week of pregnancy. The principal (although not invariable) characteristic is one of pregnancy-induced hypertension, but other characteristics include proteinuria and generalized edema, producing the classic triad of preeclampsia. Eclampsia is defined by the appearance of seizures. To be eclampsia, this particular triad of clinical features cannot be attributable to other causes such as epilepsy, kidney disease, or preexisting hypertension.

The incidence of preeclampsia varies according to social, economic, geographic, and other demographic factors. Although throughout the world preeclampsia–eclampsia is a significant cause of perinatal morbidity and death, the incidence of eclampsia has de-creased in the West with improved antenatal care. In Western or developed countries, the incidence is approximately 1 in 2,300 deliveries, contrasting with 1 in 100 to 1 in 1,700 pregnancies in developing countries (5,6). About 50,000 maternal deaths yearly can be attributed to eclampsia, and it remains a leading cause of maternal mortality in the United Kingdom, Scandinavia, and the United States (7). In the United States, 6% of pregnant women may develop preeclampsia, with the incidence increasing to 15–20% of black primigravidas and to approximately 30% in twin pregnancies (8). Maternal age older than age 35 years, extrauterine pregnancies, and multiple pregnancies, as well as low social economic class, are risk factors. The risk of eclampsia increases with subsequent pregnancies if present in prior pregnancies; one series noted a 47% incidence in the second pregnancy (9).

DEFINITION

The essential characteristic of preeclampsia is pregnancy-induced hypertension, although it need not invariably be present throughout pregnancy. Hypertension is defined as a relative increase of more than 15 mm/Hg in diastolic blood pressure or greater than 30 mm/Hg in systolic blood pressure over the values obtained before pregnancy or in early pregnancy. When antenatal information is not available, a repeated absolute measurement of at least 140/90 mm/Hg during pregnancy is regarded as "hypertensive" (10). Typically, there may be proteinuria (defined as ≥300 mg of protein per day; ≤1+ proteinuria on two separate occasions, 6 hours apart by dipstick testing) and/or marked edema involving the face and hands (11).

As with many syndromes, all features of the triad may not be present in this pathophysiologic continuum, and absence of one or more classic features should not deter diagnosis. The appearance of the defining feature of eclampsia—the convulsion—is frequently unrelated to the degree of preeclampsia. At one extreme, seizures may supervene when few signs of preeclampsia are present and often when edema, hypertension, or proteinuria are absent. In up to 20% of patients, one of the three features of the triad may be absent at the time of seizures (12). In some post-partum patients, seizures may occur with no heralding features of preeclampsia.

PATHOPHYSIOLOGY

The pathophysiologic process(es) underlying preeclampsia involve(s) multisystem abnormalities. No single unifying mechanism can be implicated, but multiorgan vasospasm with endothelial dysfunction is a significant contributor. The neuropeptide neurokinin B, produced by the placenta, induces pressor activity and may well be a cause of hypertension and preeclampsia (13).

The causes of vasospasm are not entirely understood, but increased vascular responsiveness to circulating catecholamines and angiotensin likely contribute to renal insufficiency, proteinuria, hypoalbuminemia, edema, and hypertension. In addition, coagulopathies with hemoconcentration and hepatic dysfunction may supervene. The shrinking intravascular volume contributes to a decrease in cardiac output and renal function that may in turn affect uteroplacental perfusion, delaying/retarding fetal growth. Morbidity is further increased by the constellation of clinical abnormalities that includes *h*emolysis, *e*levated *l*iver enzymes, *l*ow *p*latelets (HELLP)

syndrome (14). Vascular and endothelial damage have been ascribed to cytotoxic mediators secreted by the trophoblast. A deficient fetal–placental circulation is associated with increased vascular pressor sensitivity that leads to vasospasm, multisystem organ ischemia, and an abnormal coagulation cascade, in turn triggering disseminated intravascular coagulation. Kidney abnormalities include glomerular endotheliocytosis with increased production of endothelin, fibronectin, and von Willebrand factor (15).

One of the principal sites of abnormality involves the developing placenta and placental bed. Because preeclampsia may occur with hydatidiform mole (in the absence of a fetus), the "placental," as opposed to "fetal," nature of the disease becomes apparent (16).

With normal pregnancies, the cytotrophoblast migrates through the inner-third of the myometrium via the decidua. This trophoblastic invasion replaces the endothelial lining, internal elastic laminae, and muscular layers, deafferenting the spiral arteries of the placenta. In so doing, the cytotrophoblasts come to resemble the endothelial cells of the spiral arteries by transforming their adhesion receptor phenotype (17). The transformation of the nonpregnant spiral artery system converts the developing vascular supply to the fetus to a "low-pressure" system, which is advantageous to the fetus and placenta. With preeclampsia, there is a failure of trophoblastic invasion of the spiral arteries and hence failure of transformation to a low-pressure system, resulting in placental and fetal ischemia. This causes more widespread maternal multiorgan damage because of the release of mediators which induce more widespread vascular endothelial damage and hypoxia. The abnormal myometrial vessels are substantially smaller than those in normal pregnancy, and fewer are invaded by trophoblast (18).

Growing evidence suggests that a mitochondrial defect can impair cytotrophoblastic invasion and differentiation (19), based on observations in women with preeclampsia with particular mitochondrial dysfunction (20). Mitochondrial mutations may affect either nuclear or mitochondrial genomes, which during mitochondrial segregation and division may result in varying amounts of wild-type and mutant mitochondria in the daughter cells (19). As a rule, mitochondrial disease has a predilection for syncytial tissues with specialized function and high metabolic demands (21). These mitochondrial defects disturb normal placentation during pregnancy. In *mito*chondrial *e*ncephalomyopathy with *l*actic *a*cidosis and *s*troke-like episodes (MELAS), large amounts of mutant mitochondrial DNA are found in the placenta (22). Searching for a genetic model has been problematic because none of the genetic models explains the pattern of inheritance. There are higher incidences of the disease in the immediate blood relatives, particularly those in a direct line from mother to daughter (23,24). The existing lack of concordance might be explained by the different proportions of mutated and wild-type DNA segregating to siblings or twins, resulting in different cytoplasmic phenotypes (25). The cytoplasmic genome is transmitted by the maternal oocyte, whose cytoplasm excludes the male sperm mitochondria, suggesting a female pattern of inheritance (26). Genetic differences are linked to alterations in morphology and function (e.g., mitochondrial swelling and loss of cristae indicate a systemic metabolic dysfunction associated with decreased cytochrome oxidase) (27).

Recent observations indicate that a decrease in oxygen tension by as little as 2% may adversely affect cytotrophoblast invasion and differentiation (28). It has been hypothesized that with dysfunctional oxygen-using organelles (mitochondria), impaired cytotrophoblastic behavior can occur at normal oxygen tensions (18). Mitochondria are also the site of endothelial nitric oxide synthetase, where it affects respiration-dependent processes such as ion transport and energy formation (29). This chromosomal locus is implicated in pregnancy-induced hypertension (30).

A more unifying explanation of multisystem dysfunction derives from the observations by Roberts and associates of a widespread maternal endothelial dysfunction (31). Abnormal endothelial control of vascular tone contributes to hypertension and impaired endothelial permeability and can result in fluid retention and edema, whereas abnormal endothelial elaboration of coagulation factors results in clotting dysfunction, which, along with hypoperfusion of the liver, further triggers HELLP.

Recent work by Redman and colleagues has led to the hypothesis that the intravascular inflammatory response underlies the preeclamptic process (32). The authors suggest that there is an excessive inflammatory stimulus proportional, in part, to placental size, and hence inflammatory burden, in keeping with the observation that preeclampsia occurs more frequently in multiple gestations and with increasing placental size near term. The uteroplacental arterial insufficiency, as noted above, increases the release of inflammatory factors, which might activate leukocytes or stimulate proinflammatory cytokine production. These all increase the intensity of the proinflammatory stimulus. In this way, the placenta generates signals that may excite a more generalized inflammatory response in the mother. This universal maternal intravascular inflammatory response in pregnancy may decompensate in certain instances, such as from excessive placental stimulus or excessive maternal response.

The inflammatory response is part of the normal pregnancy, and thus differences between normal pregnancy and preeclampsia may be less marked than those between normal pregnancy and the nonpregnant state. The pathophysiologic process, therefore, reflects an exaggeration of changes that normally occur in pregnancy, and the investigators suggest that the problem lies not with preeclampsia but with the physiology of pregnancy itself. This heightened impairment of the inflammatory process as normal pregnancy progresses might be adversely affected by a number of factors that include genetic, toxic, septic, or other components. These insults may interfere with the normal downward regulation of components of the immune activation system that serve to keep inflammatory reactions in check. Such a dynamic is another example of the maternal–fetal "genetic conflict" (33).

NEUROPATHOPHYSIOLOGY

The specific neurologic consequences of preeclampsia–eclampsia also are under debate. Head computed tomography (CT), angiography, and transcranial Doppler ultrasound (TCD) reveal cerebral vasospasm (34–38), which, along with hypertensive encephalopathy, may cause seizures in eclampsia. The cerebral insults thus arise from contributions both from cerebral vasoconstriction (and consequent underperfusion) as well as the effects of hypertensive insult leading to cerebral hyperperfusion and encephalopathy. The cerebral perfusion autoregulatory curve in young women lies to the left of the autoregulatory curve of chronic hypertensives, perhaps explaining why these changes may occur with lesser increases in blood pressure. The middle cerebral artery contributing blood flow in the parietal regions may fail to constrict when blood pressure rises, reflecting a focal failure in autoregulation. This, along with the relative paucity of sympathetic control of the basilar arterial system, subjects the parieto-occipital regions to the greatest effect of the failure of autoregulation and hypertensive insult. Not surprisingly, frequent neurologic features consist of abnormalities of vision.

Magnesium sulfate may act by increasing vasodilatation by countering calcium-dependent arterial vasoconstriction (39). Transcranial and retinal Doppler arterial ultrasonography have revealed a decrease in middle cerebral and orbital artery pulsatility (40). The failure of phenytoin to dilate cerebral vasculature as well as its known antiepileptic effect further support the concept that the eclamptic seizure is triggered by cerebrovascular-mediated damage, rather than a specific effect on an epileptic process (41).

Despite the multiplicity of organ involvement, neurologic manifestations often are sudden but transient. An increasingly severe headache may last for days with superimposed visual hallucinations, the perception of flashing lights (from whence the name "eclampsia" is derived), and blindness that is usually reversible. This may progress to confusion and the appearance of seizures and coma. With regard to the visual axis in particular, the process may involve the retinal arterioles, causing dilatation and transvascular exudates, hemorrhages, or even retinal detachment. Raised intracerebral pressure may cause papilledema. The posterior cortical watershed zones may be affected by microhemorrhages and infarctions, as well as by subcortical edema (41). Almost any part of the cerebral hemisphere may be involved, however, resulting in pareses and aphasia.

Seizures may start focally, but generalized tonic-clonic seizures usually are seen. The interictal electroencephalogram (EEG) is abnormal in about 80% of patients (42), usually showing diffuse slowing in about half of patients or focal slowing in a quarter of patients. Epileptiform spikes are seen in about 14% (42). Although the EEG usually normalizes shortly after delivery, some abnormalities may persist for several weeks or even months (43). Seizures usually supervene before childbirth, but up to 40% of all eclamptic seizures occur before women get medical treatment (6, 44,45). Late postpartum seizures (those occurring after 48 hours) are seen in 16% (46).

Systemic and intracerebral hypertension as well as vasoconstriction play an important role. Recent studies using TCD have confirmed reports of magnetic resonance imaging (MRI), angiography, and conventional angiography imaging studies showing reversible vasospasm (47). These changes are not seen in preeclampsia or in normotensive pregnant women, indicating that the process is associated with eclampsia.

Eclampsia constitutes a significant risk factor for ischemic stroke during pregnancy and in the first 6 weeks postpartum (48) and may well account for almost half the cases of pregnancy-related strokes (49). As noted above, although some women have neurologic sequelae with eclampsia, most return to normal within days or weeks, arguing against actual cerebral ischemic necrosis.

No feature of preeclampsia is consistently present (44). Although particular signs are used to recognize and diagnose preeclampsia, the absence of even one of the cardinal triad (proteinuria, hypertension, edema) does not exclude the syndrome. Hypertension (an elemental feature of preeclampsia) may itself be absent (44,50). Waiting for all the "potentially sinister clusters of signs" to make a diagnosis would make the treating physician "too rigid in demanding that one or other (signs) must be present before there is a need for concern" (44). Other signs of preeclampsia may be present even if they do not feature in one of the "definitions" of the syndrome (44). In fact, eclampsia (defined by the appearance of a seizure) may occur before the clinical features of preeclampsia become evident. This has been the case particularly in postpartum eclampsia where hypertension, proteinuria, and edema have not been evident until the patient returns to the hospital following a seizure and when these clinical features are noted for the first time.

Although hypertension is a significant contributing feature to the neurologic features of eclampsia, particularly those that result from hypertensive encephalopathy, it is not absolutely essential to diagnosis. The reliance on the finding of hypertension for diagnosis might result in patients being mismanaged if they manifest *other* signs of preeclampsia but have no significant increase in blood pressure.

Even in the absence of hypertension, HELLP as a disorder of coagulation may, of itself, cause significant neurologic sequelae, including intracranial hemorrhage (44).

Imaging

Most women with eclampsia without focal neurologic features have normal head CT scans. MRI of the head may show evidence of cerebral edema, particularly in the anterior and posterior watershed zones and in patients with focal findings. Cerebral edema and hemorrhages of various sizes can be found in the gray-white junctions; subependymal, subarachnoid, and deep white matter regions; and in the brainstem. Virtually any part of the cerebrum can be affected. In a study involving comparison of MRIs by blinded observers, in women with eclampsia compared to those with severe preeclampsia there were focal T2-weighted signal changes in the frontal and parietal white matter, deep white matter, and brainstem in the patients with preeclampsia (51). However, in eclampsia, there were also characteristic multifocal curvilinear abnormalities at the gray-white junction of the posterior watershed zones (Fig. 4.1). Similar distribution of

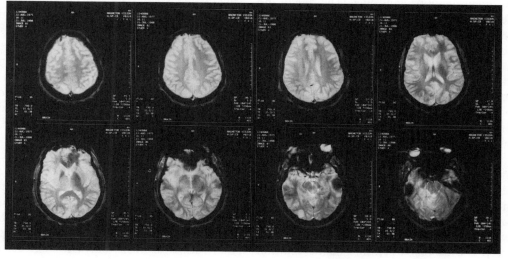

FIG. 4.1. Axial T2-weighted MRI study shows peripheral edema, particularly in the right parieto-occipital watershed zones.

abnormality has been delineated using single-photon emission computerized tomography (52). In aggregate, these different imaging modalities demonstrate the various neuropathological processes, including ischemic infarction, hemorrhage, focal cerebral edema, border-zone ischemia, and changes consistent with vasoconstrictive cerebral ischemia.

Most patients with eclampsia do not get head CT or MRI scans. Women with lateralized or focal neurologic findings may merit investigation. Treatment usually is based on clinical diagnosis without the use of imaging studies because of the urgency of delivering the baby.

Management

Eclampsia (being a progressive multisystem disorder) presents a substantial problem to clinicians because of the absence of specific diagnostic tests. Management is predicated on treatment of the clinical features and preventing complications because no directed therapy at the underlying causes exist, although new lines of research suggest potential promise (13).

The management of the woman with eclampsia falls to the obstetrician. Neurologists are consulted in the management of focal cerebral problems or coma or when seizures cannot be controlled. The role of the neurologist is to determine the nature or severity of neurologic deficits and direct the appropriate clinical investigation that will help in the management of the acute cerebral events. This may include investigation of cerebral venous thrombosis, cerebral infarction, and intracranial hemorrhage. Most of these problems are best managed in the intensive care setting.

Treatment of hypertension—in this case, malignant hypertension—again falls to the obstetrician or intensivist. Urgent therapy aimed at lowering blood pressure is mandatory, particularly when the diastolic blood pressure exceeds 100 mm Hg, maintaining the mean arterial blood pressure below 125 mm Hg but not less than 105 mm Hg. Preferred agents are nicardipine, administered parenter-

ally at 5–15 mg per hour, or labetalol given at 2–3 mg per minute. Nifedepine given orally (10 mg) may help. ACE inhibitors are not used because of their toxic effect on the fetal kidneys.

The approach to the control of seizures has been the subject of extensive controversy (53–56). Within the obstetric community in the United States, magnesium sulfate has been the mainstay of management. Initially popularized by Lazard in 1925 (57) and by Pritchard and colleagues in 1984 (58), an intravenous loading dose of 4 grams in a 20 mL solution, followed by deep intramuscular doses of 5 grams as a 50% solution given every 4 hours, is continued for a day after the last seizures (58). More contemporary protocols use an intravenous route only, with an infusion of 1 gram per hour until a day after the last seizure (59). Signs of magnesium toxicity include the loss of limb reflexes at levels of 8–12 mg per dL, followed by dysarthria, somnolence, and widespread muscular paralysis that may include the respiratory muscles. Cardiac arrest can occur above 30 mg per dL. An antidote for toxicity involves the administration of 10% calcium gluconate solution given intravenously.

In eclampsia, with regard to the prevention of current seizures, neurologists have advocated using known antiepileptic drugs, such as the benzodiazepines, or intravenous formulations of phenytoin (53–55) or fosphenytoin. Diazepam or chloradiazepoxide has been successfully used with low morbidity. An intravenous bolus of 10 mg diazepam followed by infusion of 40 mg in 500 mL of 5% dextrose is usually effective, but it may cause respiratory depression of the mother and infant. The Eclampsia Trial Collaborative Group (1995) (60) compared the efficacy of diazepam or phenytoin to magnesium sulfate in 1,687 women with eclampsia in treatment centers located predominantly in the developing world. One arm compared magnesium sulfate against diazepam; the other compared magnesium sulfate to phenytoin. Different centers administered magnesium sulfate either intravenously or intramuscularly versus an IV bolus of 10 mg of diazepam, followed by 40 mg over 24 hours. Phenytoin was given as 1 gram intravenously as a loading dose, followed by 100 mg every 6 hours for the next 24 hours. There was a 52% lower incidence of recurrent convulsions in those taking magnesium sulfate compared to diazepam; there was a 67% lower incidence when compared to phenytoin. These studies support the superiority of magnesium sulfate. Shortly later, the Parkland Memorial Trial studied 2,138 patients with preeclampsia (61) and showed that 10 of 1,089 women with preeclampsia treated with phenytoin had seizures, whereas none of 1,049 patients randomized to magnesium sulfate had seizures. Methodologic concerns with this study include the fact the seizure decrease was from 1% to 0%. Additionally, only 19% of the women had pregnancy-induced hypertension with other signs of preeclampsia, such as proteinuria. None of the 10 women who had seizures while taking phenytoin had phenytoin levels greater than 13.1 µg per mL, which represents a level in the lower "therapeutic" range (10–20 µg per mL).

More recent information suggests that the mechanism of magnesium sulfate's action is blocking vasospasm in cerebral vasculature, thus increasing cerebral blood flow and thereby preventing the ischemic insult that would engender seizures. Magnesium sulfate also increases the production of prostacyclin, (62) an endothelial vasodilator. Magnesium sulfate also may protect against endothelial cell injury from free radicals (63).

The management of raised intracranial pressure and cerebral edema follows the lines standardly used in neurointensive care management. In patients without focal findings or coma, specific neurointensive intervention rarely is needed, but urgent reduction in intracranial pressure occasionally is necessary. Such cases may benefit from intubation, hyperventilation, correction of hyponatremia, and the use of dexamethasone or mannitol.

It is unlikely that magnesium sulfate is acting as an anticonvulsant in the true sense. Although the N-methyl D-aspartate (NMDA) subtype of the glutamate receptor can be blocked by magnesium ions, thus preventing neuronal damage and seizures, animal models using penicillin-induced cortical epilepsy when compared with controls found the decrease in neuronal burst firing to be the result of natural "decay phenomenon" (64, 65).

Other animal models for seizures, including maximal electroshock, pentylenetetrazol, or lidocaine-induced seizures, showed no anticonvulsant defect of magnesium sulfate (66–68). However, given the relatively insignificant degree of blood–brain barrier disruption in these animal models, they may not be appropriate for the clinical circumstance of hypertensive encephalopathy with its more widespread breakdown of the blood–brain barrier.

CONCLUSION

Preeclampsia and eclampsia continue to be significant causes of maternal death. Neurologists have a role to play in the management of patients with eclampsia, particularly in those with recurrent seizures, raised intracranial pressure, and coma. Magnesium sulfate is the usual treatment used by obstetricians in the United States for eclamptic seizures, but in the event of failure there is also proven efficacy with diazepam and phenytoin. Recent studies shed light on the pathogenesis of hypertension in preeclampsia–eclampsia, but further studies are needed to uncover the multiplicity of pathophysiologic effects, and the role of magnesium sulfate in women without significant hypertension in preeclampsia.

ACKNOWLEDGMENT

Dr. Peter W. Kaplan has been a consultant or advisor or has done medication trials for the following pharmaceutical companies:
Novartis, Ortho-McNeil, Elan, Parke-Davis, Warner Lambert, Abbott, Glaxo-Wellcome, and U.C.B.

REFERENCES

1. Bernhart F. Geschichte, Wesen und behandlung der eklampsie. *Wien Klin Wochschr* 1939;52:1009–1013, 1036–1043.

2. Petrie JJB, MacLean PR, Robson JS. Glomerular permeability to serum proteins and high molecular weight dextrans in glomerulonephritis. *Clin Sci* 1968;34:83–95.
3. Hippocrates. *The medical works of Hippocrates.* Oxford: Blackwell Scientific Publications, 1950. Chadwick J, translator.
4. de Sauvages FBS. *Pathologia methodica, seu de cognoscendis morbis,* 3rd ed. Leyden: Fratum de Tournes, 1759:286.
5. Cunningham FG, MacDonald PC, Gant NF, et al. Hypertensive disorders in pregnancy. In: Cunningham FG, MacDonald PC, Gant NF, et al., eds. *Williams Obstetrics,* 19th ed., Norwalk, CT: Appleton & Lange, 1993:763–817.
6. Douglas K, Redman CW. Eclampsia in the United Kingdom. *Brit Med J* 1994;309:1395–1400.
7. Roberts JM, Redman CWG. Preeclampsia: more than pregnancy-induced hypertension. *Lancet* 1993;341:1447–1451.
8. Sibai BM. Preeclampsia-eclampsia. In: Sciarra JJ, ed. *Gynecology and Obstetrics 1989.* Vol. 2. Philadelphia: JB Lippincott, 1989:1–12.
9. Sibai B, el-Nazer A, Gonzalez-Ruiz A. Severe preeclampsia-eclampsia in young primigravid women: subsequent pregnancy outcome and remote prognosis. *Am J Obstet Gynecol* 1986;155:1011–1016.
10. Lenfant C, Gifford RW, Zuspan FP. Report on national high blood pressure education program working group on high blood pressure in pregnancy. *Am J Obstet Gynecol* 1990;163:1691–1712.
11. American College of Obstetricians and Gynecologists. Hypertension in pregnancy. ACOG Technical Bulletin 219. Washington, DC: 1996.
12. Porapakkam S. An epidemiologic study of eclampsia. *Obstet Gynecol* 1983;54:26–30.
13. Page NM, Woods RJ, Gardiner SM, et al. Excessive placental secretion of neurokinin B during the third trimester causes pre-eclampsia. *Nature* 2000;405:797–800.
14. Sibai BM, Ramadan MK, Chari RS, et al. Pregnancies complicated by HELLP syndrome (hemolysis, elevated liver enzymes, and low platelets): subsequent pregnancy outcome and long-term prognosis. *Am J Obstet Gynecol* 1995;172:125–129.
15. Easton JD, Mas JL, Lamy C, et al. Severe preeclampsia/eclampsia: hypertensive encephalopathy of pregnancy? *Cerebrovasc Dis* 1998;8:53–58.
16. Piering WF, Garancis JG, Becker CG, et al. Preeclampsia related to a functioning extrauterine placenta: report of a case and 25-year follow-up. *Am J Kidney Dis* 1993;21:310–313.
17. Zhou Y, Fisher SJ, Janatpour M, et al. Human cytotrophoblasts adopt a vascular phenotype as they differentiate. A strategy for successful endovascular invasion? *J Clin Invest* 1997;99:2139–2151.
18. Brosens I, Robertson WB, Dixon HG. The role of the spiral arteries in the pathogenesis of preeclampsia. *Obstet Gynecol Annu* 1972;1:177–191.
19. Widschwendter M, Schrocksnadel H, Mortl MG. Opinion: Pre-eclampsia: a disorder of placental mitochondria? *Mol Med Today* 1998;4:286–291.
20. Torbergsen T, Oian P, Mathiesen E, et al. Preeclampsia—a mitochondrial disease? *Acta Obstet Gynecol Scand* 1989;68:145–148.
21. Clarke A. Mitochondrial genome: defects, disease, and evolution. *J Med Genet* 1990;27:451–456.
22. Suomalainen A, Majander A, Pihko H, et al. Quantification of tRNA3243(Leu) point mutation of mitochondrial DNA in MELAS patients and its effects on mitochondrial transcription. *Hum Mol Genet* 1993;2:525–534.
23. Cooper DW, Brennecke SP, Wilton AN. Genetics of preeclampsia. *Hypertens Pregn* 1993;12:1–23.
24. Cooper DW, Hill JA, Chesley LC, et al. Genetic control of susceptibility to eclampsia and miscarriage. *Br J Obstet Gynaecol* 1988;95:644–653.
25. Folgero T, Storbakk N, Torbergsen T, et al. Mutations in mitochondrial transfer ribonucleic acid genes in preeclampsia. *Am J Obstet Gynecol* 1996;174:1626–1630.
26. Kaneda H, Hayashi J, Takahama S, et al. Elimination of paternal mitochondrial DNA in intraspecific crosses during early mouse embryogenesis. *Proc Natl Acad Sci USA* 1995;92:4542–4546.
27. Furui T, Kurauchi O, Tanaka M, et al. Decrease in cytochrome c oxidase and cytochrome oxidase subunit 1 messenger RNA levels in preeclamptic pregnancies. *Obstet Gynecol* 1994;84:283–288.
28. Genbacev O, Joslin R, Damsky CH, et al. Hypoxia alters early gestation human cytotrophoblast differentiation/invasion *in vitro* and models the placental defects that occur in preeclampsia. *J Clin Invest* 1996;97:540–550.
29. Ghafourifar P, Richter C. Nitric oxide synthase activity in mitochondria. *FEBS Lett* 1997;418:291–296.
30. Amgrimsson R, Hayward C, Nadaud S, et al. Evidence for a familial pregnancy-induced hypertension locus in the eNOS-gene region. *Am J Hum Genet* 1997;61:354–362.
31. Roberts JM, Taylor RN, Musci TJ, et al. Preeclampsia: as endothelial cell disorder. *Am J Obstet Gynecol* 1989;161:1200–1204.
32. Redman CWG, Sacks GP, Sargent IL. Preeclampsia: an excessive maternal inflammatory response to pregnancy. *Am J Obstet Gynecol* 1999;180:499–506.
33. Haig D. Genetic conflicts in human pregnancy. *Q Rev Biol* 1993;68:495–532.
34. Raroque HG, Orrison WW, Rosenberg GA. Neurologic involvement in toxemia of pregnancy: reversible MRI lesions. *Neurology* 1980;40:167–169.
35. Crawford S, Varner MW, Digre KB, et al. Cranial magnetic resonance imaging in eclampsia. *Obstet Gynecol* 1985;70:474–477.
36. Trommer BL, Homer D, Mikhael MA. Cerebral vasospasm and eclampsia. *Stroke* 1988;19:326–329.
37. Sibai BM. Eclampsia. In: Goldstein PJ, Stern BJ, eds. *Neurological Disorders of Pregnancy,* 2nd ed. Mount Kisco, NY: Futura Publishing Co., 1992:1–24.
38. Qureshi AI, Frankel MR, Ottenlips JR, et al. Cerebral hemodynamics in preeclampsia and eclampsia. *Arch Neuro* 1996;53:1226–1231.
39. Zaret GM. Possible treatment of preeclampsia with calcium channel blocking agents. *Med Hypotheses* 1983;12:303–319.
40. Belfont MA, Moise KJ. Effect of magnesium sulfate on maternal brain blood flow in preeclampsia: a randomised placebo controlled study. *Am J Obstet Gynecol* 1992;167:661–666.
41. Sheehan HL, Lynch JB. *Pathology of toxaemia of pregnancy.* Baltimore: Williams & Wilkins, 1973.
42. Thomas SV, Somanathan N, Radhakumari R. Interictal EEG changes in eclampsia. *Electroencephalogr Clin Neurophysiol* 1995;94:271–275.

43. Sibai BM, McCubbin JH, Anderson GD, et al. Eclampsia I: observations from 67 recent cases. *Obstet Gynecol* 1981;58:609–613.
44. Redman CWG, Roberts JM. Management of pre-eclampsia. *Lancet* 1993;341:1451–1454.
45. Sibai BM. Eclampsia VI: maternal-perinatal outcome in 254 consecutive cases. *Am J Obstet Gynecol* 1990;163:1049–1055.
46. Lubarsky SL, Barton JR, Friedman SA, et al. Late postpartum eclampsia revisited. *Obstet Gynecol* 1994;83:502–505.
47. Naidu S, Payne AJ, Moodley J, et al. Randomised study assessing the effect of phenytoin and magnesium sulphate on maternal cerebral circulation in eclampsia using transcranial Doppler ultrasound. *Br J Obstet Gynaecol* 1996;103:111–116.
48. Lanska DJ, Kryscio RJ. Stroke and intracranial venous thrombosis during pregnancy and puerperium. *Neurology* 1998;51:1622–1628.
49. Sharshar T, Lamy C, Mas JL. Stroke in Pregnancy Study Group. Incidence and causes of strokes associated with pregnancy and puerperium. *Stroke* 1995;26:930–936.
50. Schwartz ML, Brenner W. Toxemia in a patient with none of the standard signs and symptoms of preeclampsia. *Obstet Gynecol* 1985;66:19S–21S.
51. Digre KB, Varner MW, Osborn AG, et al. Cranial magnetic resonance imaging in severe preeclampsia vs eclampsia. *Arch Neurol* 1993;50:399–406.
52. Schwartz RB, Jones KM, Kalina P, et al. Hypertensive encephalopathy: findings on CT, MR imaging, and SPECT imaging in 14 cases. *Am J Radiol* 1991;159:379–383.
53. Kaplan PW, Lesser RP, Fisher RS, et al. No, magnesium sulfate should not be used in treating eclamptic seizures. *Arch Neurol* 1988;45:1361.
54. Kaplan PW, Lesser RP, Fisher RS, et al. A continuing controversy: magnesium sulfate in the treatment of eclamptic seizures. *Arch Neurol* 1990;47:1031.
55. Donaldson JO. The case against magnesium sulfate for eclamptic convulsions. *Intern J Obstet Anes* 1992;1:159–166.
56. Chien PFW, Khan KS, Arnott N. Magnesium sulphate in the treatment of eclampsia and pre-eclampsia: an overview of the evidence from randomised trials. *Br J Obstet Gynaecol* 1996;103:1085–1091.
57. Lazard EM. A preliminary report on the intravenous use of magnesium sulfate in puerperal eclampsia. *Am J Obstet Gynecol* 1925;9:178–188.
58. Pritchard JA, Cunningham FG, Pritchard SA. The Parkland Hospital protocol for treatment of eclampsia: evaluation of 245 cases. *Am J Obstet Gynecol* 1984;148:951–963.
59. Zuspan FP. Problems encountered in the treatment of pregnancy-induced hypertension. A point of view. *Am J Obstet Gynecol* 1978;131:591–597.
60. Eclampsia Trial Collaborative Group. Which anticonvulsant for women with eclampsia? *Lancet* 1995;45:1455–1463.
61. Lucas L, Leveno K, Cunningham G. A comparison of magnesium sulfate with phenytoin for the prevention of eclampsia. *N Engl J Med* 1995;333:201–205.
62. Sipes SL, Weiner CP, Gellhaus TM, et al. Effects of magnesium sulfate infusion upon plasma prostaglandins in pre-eclampsia and preterm labor. *Hypertens Pregn* 1994;13:293–302.
63. Dickens BF, Weglicki Y, Li S, et al. Magnesium deficiency in vitro enhances free radical induced intracellular oxidation and cytotoxicity in endothelial cells. *FEBS Lett* 1992;311:187–191.
64. Borges LF, Gücer G. Effect of magnesium on epileptic foci. *Epilepsia* 1978;19:81–91.
65. Koontz WL, Reid KH. Effect of parenteral magnesium sulfate on penicillin-induced seizure foci in anesthetized cats. *Am J Obstet Gynecol* 1985;153:96–99.
66. Krauss GL, Kaplan PW, Fisher RS. Parenteral magnesium sulfate fails to control electroshock and pentylenetetrazol seizures in mice. *Epilepsy Res* 1989;4:201–206.
67. Link MJ. Anderson RE, Meyer FB. Effects of magnesium sulfate on pentylenetetrazol-induced status epilepticus. *Epilepsia* 1991;32:543–549.
68. Choi WW, Warner DS, Monahan DJ, et al. Effects of acute hypermagnesemia on the threshold for lidocaine-induced seizures in the rat. *Am J Obstet Gynecol* 1991;164:693–697.

Neurological Complications of Pregnancy, Second Edition, edited by Brian Hainline and Orrin Devinsky. Lippincott Williams & Wilkins, Philadelphia © 2002.

5

Cerebral Ischemia in Pregnancy

Janet L. Wilterdink and J. Donald Easton

Department of Neurology, Brown University and Rhode Island Hospital, Providence, Rhode Island, U.S.A.

EPIDEMIOLOGY

Whether pregnancy is a risk factor for ischemic stroke remains controversial. There are considerable challenges in interpreting the available epidemiologic data that associate pregnancy and stroke because of heterogeneity in study design (1). For example, not all studies differentiate between ischemic and hemorrhagic stroke. Some investigators include venous infarction with ischemic stroke, whereas some exclude it or classify it separately. The postpartum period also is variably included and, when included, is variably defined. This is critically important because recent investigators note that much if not all of pregnancy-associated stroke risk is associated with the post partum period (2–4). Case ascertainment exclusively from tertiary medical centers have obvious referral bias, whereas that which relies on International Classification of Diseases, Ninth Revision (ICD-9), codes have inherent problems in reliability. Particularly confusing in this matter is that strokes associated with eclampsia may or may not receive ICD-9 coding specific to their stroke as well as for eclampsia (2). Estimates of incidence, therefore, range considerably from 4.3 to 25.6 cases per 100,000 deliveries. Estimates of risk attributable to pregnancy similarly vary from an odds ratio of 1.3 to a 13-fold increased risk (3,5–14).

PATHOPHYSIOLOGY

Epidemiologic data aside, there are reasons to believe that pregnancy is a risk factor for ischemic stroke. Several changes in coagulation parameters are seen in pregnancy that likely represent a slightly hypercoaguable state. Fibrinogen levels as well as levels of clotting factors, V,VII,VIII,IX,X,XII, rise during pregnancy (13,15–17). Decreased antithrombin III activity, tissue plasminogen activity, and protein S levels, as well as increased platelet aggregability, are also seen in pregnancy (16,18–20). More recently it has been shown that resistance to activated protein C develops in a substantial number of women during pregnancy (21). Why these changes occur is not precisely known. Local consumption of clotting factors in the uteroplacental circulation and inhibitors of plasminogen activation produced by the placenta are believed to be at least partly responsible (16). Additionally, hormonal influences are likely to play a role because many of these changes are also seen in patients using oral contraceptives (22). In pregnancy, these changes generally are seen in the second and third trimesters and the first 2 to 4 postpartum weeks, mirroring the times of increased incidence of stroke.

Specific hypertensive disorders of pregnancy might be expected to play a role because hypertension is the single most important risk factor for ischemic stroke in general. In fact, in the National Hospital Discharge Survey, hypertension was shown to carry a risk ratio of 15.3 for peripartum stroke (this study did not distinguish between hemorrhage and ischemia) (13,23). Other series support a role for hypertension in pregnancy-related stroke with 30% to 47% of such patients having hypertension risk two to three times higher than the general obstetric population (3,12), whereas others have failed to demonstrate an association (2).

Cerebral venous thrombosis is the classic stroke type associated with pregnancy; however, arterial occlusion is more common, accounting for 60% to 80% of all cerebral infarctions occurring in pregnancy and the puerperium (2,5,8). The risk of pregnancy-related stroke increases as term approaches and may be even higher in the early postpartum period, particularly for cerebral venous thrombosis (2,8,10).

ARTERIAL ISCHEMIC STROKE

In most cases of arterial occlusion, pregnancy predisposes to cerebral infarction in already susceptible individuals and is rarely the only identifiable risk factor for stroke. The spectrum of identifiable causes of stroke in pregnancy appears to be similar to that in nonobstetric patients of the same age (24,25) (Table 5.1).

Diagnosis

Because many conditions that are associated with stroke also are associated with a high risk of stroke recurrence and require medical intervention specific to etiology, the diagnosis of cerebral infarction and the identification of its etiology should be pursued aggressively (Table 5.2). Pregnancy should not significantly impair or retard this process (1). To exclude hemorrhage or other structural etiology, an imaging study of the brain should be performed immediately. A computed tomography (CT) scan of the brain can be done with abdominal shielding to limit fetal exposure to radiation, which is most important in the second to fourth week of gestation. Although magnetic resonance imaging (MRI) does not use ionizing radiation, it takes longer, may be less available acutely, and is difficult to do in very ill patients. No short-term risks for the fetus have been as yet identified from the MRI procedure or from gadolinium administration (25).

A standard battery of tests should include a platelet count, complete blood count, prothrombin time, partial thromboplastin time (PTT), erythrocyte sedimentation rate, toxicology screen, serum glucose, chemistries, and an electrocardiogram. Further testing should be guided by clinical suspicion obtained from history and screening evaluation and may be quite extensive (Table 5.2).

If the cause of infarction is not quickly evident from history, screening laboratories, and noninvasive tests, most authors recommend cerebral angiography with minimal delay because the diagnostic yield is highest when done early. Angiography may be diagnostic or highly suggestive of such entities as dissection, vascular anomalies, embolism, large-vessel atherosclerosis, vasculitis, and venous occlusion and therefore may be of substantial value in guiding or limiting subsequent testing (8,24,26,95). Abdominal shielding during angiography will limit fetal exposure to radiation except during fluoroscopy-guided catheter insertion, which can be limited by skilled radiologists. Fetal monitoring is recommended. Maternal hydration avoids fetal dehydration secondary to iodine administration. If iodine is administered at 6 months, the fetus should be screened for fetal hypothyroidism at birth (25).

Management

Because the etiologies are diverse, there is no standard therapy for ischemic stroke associated with pregnancy. There are a few conditions for which *anticoagulation* is universally recommended and many others in which it is used. It generally is recommended for secondary stroke prevention after cerebral embolism from any source except infectious endocarditis and amniotic, air, or fat embolism. Anticoagulation also is used for primary stroke prevention in patients with artificial valves and valvular atrial fibrillation (24,26, 69,70). Anticoagulation also is sometimes used in patients with recurrent cerebral is-

TABLE 5.1. *Causes of arterial ischemic stroke associated with pregnancy*

Vasculopathies	Comment	References
Atherosclerosis	Even in this young group of stroke patients, the incidence of atherosclerosis is modest and increases with age. Look for classic atherosclerosis risk factors (hypertension, diabetes, tobacco use, hypercholesterolemia, and family history). Homocystinuria, a congenital condition, is associated with premature atherosclerosis. Prior neck irradiation for thyroid or throat cancers can produce stenosis in the cervical carotid arteries and increase the risk of stroke.	5, 8, 26, 27
Extracranial carotid and vertebral artery dissection	Some of these are associated with unusual trauma or that occurring during labor and delivery; others occur without apparent cause. Authors postulate that hormone-induced changes in arterial wall structure and increases in intravascular blood volume may increase susceptibility to this condition in pregnancy.	2, 3, 7, 28–30
Moyamoya disease	Characterized by a progressive stenosis of the rostral internal carotid arteries with extensive collateral development, this is associated with cerebral hemorrhage as well as infarction of the brain and retina in pregnancy.	31–33
Fibromuscular dysplasia	A nonatheromatous arteropathy occurring predominantly in women but uncommonly described in pregnancy, it may be associated with occlusive disease, arterial dissection, aneurysm, or carotid-cavernousfistula.	8, 24, 34
Vasculitides	These are uncommon conditions and are rarely described in pregnancy. Rather than classic stroke syndromes, these often produce headache or encephalopathy with multifocal neurologic deficits, reflecting their diffuse nature. These may occur quite rarely as an isolated angiitis of the nervous system, as a complication of chronic central nervous system infections (such as fungal and tubercular meningitides or herpetic infection), or as a manifestation of systemic disease (such as systemic lupus erythematosus). Stroke has occurred in pregnant patients with lupus. However, in one series 60% of prospectively followed patients with lupus experienced exacerbations during pregnancy, but only 15% of these involved the central nervous system and none produced permanent deficits.	2, 8, 24, 26, 35–37
Takayasu's arteritis	This is a chronic inflammatory arteropathy of the aorta and brachiocephalic arteries that occurs predominantly in women of childbearing age. Half of patients experience an increase of symptoms during pregnancy. Carotid occlusion, however, is a late manifestation of the disease, occurring in only 5% of patients and very infrequently during pregnancy. Sedimentation rate may increase with disease activity, and steroids may decrease the inflammatory response and arterial stenosis. Hypertension may complicate labor and delivery.	8, 24, 38, 39
Reversible arteropathy of pregnancy	This syndrome produces obtundation, multifocal neurologic deficits, and seizures. It is most common in the postpartum period (as late as 2 weeks). It may fall into the spectrum of eclampsia, although hypertension, proteinuria, and edema appear to be variable features. Hormonal and immune-mediated changes have been implicated in its pathogenesis. Clinical deficits, as well as the appearance of ischemic lesions and arteropathy on neuroimaging studies resolve more often than not, although permanent deficits and fatality occur. This led physicians to treat one reported patient aggressively with hyperosmolar, hypervolemic therapy and nimodipine. However, it is not clear that vasospasm is the underlying pathology in this disorder. Although bromocriptine and sympathomimetic agents have been implicated, this complication also occurs without offending medications.	40–50

Hematologic conditions	Comment	References
Sickle hemoglobinopathies	More than half of pregnancies in patients with sickle cell anemia are associated with a crisis, most occurring in the third trimester. Both arterial and venous occlusions as well as intracerebral hemorrhage occur. It is also associated with toxemia (in 15–30% of cases). Arterial occlusion usually occurs because of ischemic injury to the vessel wall with subsequent intimal and medial proliferation. Improvements in state-of-the-art medical and obstetric care that includes plasma exchange transfusion have decreased the very high maternal and fetal mortality.	51–53

continued on next page

TABLE 5.1. *(continued)*

	Comment	References
Hematologic conditions		
Antiphospholipid antibodies	These include the lupus anticoagulant and anticardiolipin antibody and may be present in isolation or associated with systemic lupus erythematosus (in which it causes up to 40% of strokes). They also may be in certain drugs or occur as part of Sneddon's syndrome. Antiphospholipid antibodies can lead to in situ thrombosis of cerebral arteries or veins, cardiogenic emboli, paradoxical emboli from venous thrombosis, and spontaneous abortion. Pregnancy may be a particularly high-risk time for these patients: 54% of 39 patients with antiphospholipid antibodies had at least one thrombotic episode in association with pregnancy or oral contraceptive use.	54–59
Thrombotic thrombocytopenic purpura	This occurs three times as often in pregnant and puerperial women as in other women of the same age group. Activated platelets form diffuse microthrombi that occlude terminal arterioles and produce multiple small infarcts manifesting as a fluctuating encephalopathy and focal neurologic signs. It usually presents in the second half of pregnancy and may be confused with eclampsia.	2, 8, 60
Homocystinuria	A rare recessive inborn error of metabolism, it is associated with increased risk of venous and arterial thrombosis. Vitamin supplementation may reduce risk of thrombotic complications. Pregnancy may be a high-risk period because of fetal demands for pyridoxine or folate during gestation.	61, 62
Inherited thrombophilias	These include factor V Leiden mutation, prothrombin gene mutations (both of which produce resistance to activated protein C), and deficiencies of plasma proteins C and S and antithrombin III. These recently have been recognized to be an important cause of stroke in pregnancy; 83% of 12 patients with a first cerebral ischemic event during pregnancy were found to have such conditions, compared with 17% of controls.	3, 63–68
Disseminated intravascular coagulation	This may complicate stillbirths, placental abruption, and other acute conditions of pregnancy. By causing diffuse occlusion of small and large arteries, it produces an encephalopathy with multifocal neurologic deficits.	2, 3
Cardiogenic embolism		**References**
Prosthetic valves and rheumatic valvular disease	Pregnant patients with artificial valves have a systemic embolic complication rate of 4.2% per pregnant patient year with resulting risk of morbidity to mother and fetus as well as fatality. Patients with biological prostheses and rheumatic heart disease are at lower but not negligible risk; in one series, three strokes occurred in 15 untreated patients with biological prosthetic heart valves. Anticoagulation reduces, but does not eliminate, risk.	8, 23, 69–73
Mitral valve prolapse	Present in 5% of healthy young women, its association with stroke is somewhat controversial. In one series of 42 pregnancies in 25 patients no strokes occurred. Other cases of stroke have been reported, but cause-and-effect relationships are not proven.	74–76
Subacute bacterial endocarditis	This is a serious complication of pregnancy, occurring in one series in one of 16,500 pregnancies and producing stroke in about 20%. *Streptococcus viridans* is the most common organism. A somewhat higher percentage of enterococcal infection (8%) is seen in pregnancy, usually after cesarean section or uterine curettage.	8, 77–79
Nonbacterial thrombotic endocarditis	This is associated with hypercoagulable conditions, lupus, and malignancy and can occur without apparent risk factors or with a family history of the disorder.	54, 72, 80, 81
Atrial fibrillation	This carries a 10–23% risk of embolism in pregnancy and a 2–10% risk of cerebral embolism.	8, 72, 73
Peripartum cardiomyopathy	This is a rare complication of pregnancy presenting in the last 2 months of pregnancy or 6 months postpartum, usually with congestive heart failure and occasionally with cerebral embolism. Other well-recognized causes of heart disease are absent. Older, multiparous black women seem to be at highest risk. All four chambers are enlarged and mural thrombi are common. Although the condition usually resolves, chronic heart failure develops in some.	25, 72, 82, 83

continued on next page

TABLE 5.1. (continued)

Other embolism	Comment	References
Paradoxical embolism	A patent foramen ovale is the most common intracardiac septal defect, present or potentially patent in 30% of individuals. Deep venous thrombosis in the legs is not uncommon during pregnancy and may be a source of paradoxical cerebral embolism. Other sources include pelvic and ovarian vein thrombosis. Valsalva during labor may predispose to paradoxical embolism by increasing right-sided pressures and opening interventricular or interatrial foramen.	8, 72, 84, 85
Fat embolism	Presenting with dyspnea and encephalopathy rather than a major arterial occlusive syndrome, this may occur after long bone injury, secondary to trauma or sickle cell crisis, or after injury to adipose tissue. Other described sources include degenerating placental and decidual tissue and a ruptured dermoid cyst.	86–88
Amniotic fluid embolism	This occurs just after abortion or childbirth. Older age, multiparity, or prolonged or tumultuous labor with cervical or vaginal tearing predispose to this event. The usual presentation is sudden dyspnea, cyanosis, shock, and convulsions, the latter occurring from generalized hypoxia or paradoxical embolism. Antemortem diagnosis can be made by the presence of fetal epithelial cells just above the buffy coat of settled blood withdrawn from the right atrium during central venous line placement.	3, 25, 89–91
Air embolism	During abortion, cesarean section, and complicated vaginal delivery, air may gain access to the uterine veins after entering the cervix and dissecting to the subplacental sinuses. The presentation is similar to amniotic fluid embolism with sudden apprehension, tachycardia, dyspnea, shock, coma, and death. Convulsions often occur. The cause must be recognized immediately, and the patient must be turned on the left side to trap air in the right heart from which it must be promptly aspirated.	92

Miscellaneous	Comment	References
Hypotension	Watershed cerebral infarction may result if hypotension complicates delivery either secondary to anesthesia or to massive hemmorrhage.	93
Migraine	Women of childbearing age make up 70% of migraine sufferers. During pregnancy, migraine may abate, exacerbate, or begin (rarely). Although oral contraceptive use is relatively contraindicated for migraineurs, migraine-related stroke does not appear to be increased during pregnancy.	94
Drug abuse	Although drug abuse has no particular association with pregnancy, it is an increasing and often neglected cause of cerebral infarction in young patients. Cocaine in particular, but also heroin, amphetamines, and other recreational drugs, have been associated with stroke. The mechanism of arterial occlusion is variable and includes an arteritis, embolization of foreign material, and endocarditis.	2, 24
Cryptogenic	Similar to a series of strokes in young individuals, approximately 20–35% of arterial occlusions in pregnant patients defy diagnosis.	2, 3, 26

TABLE 5.2. *Diagnostic evaluation for ischemic stroke in pregnancy*

Screening tests	Second tier testing	
CBC differential, platelet count	All patients	Cerebral angiography
ESR	?Cardiogenic or paradoxical embolism	Echocardiography, transesophageal, bubble contrast, Holter monitor, blood cultures, lower extremity ultrasound
Chemistries		
Prothrombin, partial thromboplastin times		
Blood, urine toxicology	?Hematologic condition	Assays for protein C, protein S, antithrombin III, lupus anticoagulant, resistance to activated protein C, factor V Leiden, anticardiolipin antibodies, DIC screen, homocysteine, hemoglobin electrophoresis
ECG		
Noncontrast CT scan or MRI		
	?Arterial occlusive disease	Carotid duplex, transcranial doppler, MRA, lipid profile
	?Inflammatory or infectious disease	ANA, RF, contrast-enhanced MRI, lumbar puncture and CSF analysis

CBC, complete blood cell count; ESR, erythrocyte sedimentation rate; ECG, electrocardiogram; CT, computed tomography; MRI, magnetic resonance imaging; DIC, disseminated intravascular coagulation; MRA, magnetic resonance angiography; ANA, anti-nuclear antibody; RF, rheumatoid factor; CSF, cerebrospinal fluid.

chemic events of unknown cause, with acute atherothrombotic stroke in evolution, and in documented thrombophilias (26). For patients with antiphospholipid antibodies or with prior pregnancy losses or history of thrombosis, treatment with adjusted dose heparin plus aspirin is recommended to prevent fetal loss; there are no specific data on efficacy for stroke prevention, although small series suggest that it may be effective for this as well (57,96).

Anticoagulation can be done safely in pregnancy with reasonable caution. *Warfarin* crosses the placenta and is teratogenic in the first trimester, causing, in one series, spontaneous abortions in 28.1% and embryopathy in 7.9% of 128 patients receiving anticoagulation for artificial cardiac valves (69). Fetal neurologic abnormalities associated with warfarin are rare but include agenesis of the corpus callosum and Dandy-Walker malformations and may occur with maternal use in the later trimesters. The risks of embryopathy appear highest between 6 and 12 weeks gestation; central nervous system abnormalities can occur after exposure during any trimester (96). Warfarin, with its relatively long half-life, also is unsafe near delivery because of fetal and maternal bleeding complications.

Heparin does not cross the placenta and appears to be safe for the fetus (96). It has a very short half-life and, while cumbersome, can be safely used in pregnancy by subcutaneous administration, prolonging the PTT to 1.5 to 2 times control. The major complication of heparin is hemorrhage, estimated to occur in less than 10% of pregnancies in which it is used at a rate similar to that of the general population (96,97). Heparin is rarely associated with stillbirth or prematurity, it may cause thrombocytopenia and carries a risk of maternal osteoporosis when used for more than 6 months (26,70,96). At the time of delivery the anticoagulant effect may be prolonged up to 28 hours after the last injection, leading some to recommend its discontinuation 24 hours prior to elective induction and/or careful monitoring of the PTT near delivery with use of protamine sulfate to reduce risk of bleeding (96).

Experience with *low molecular weight heparins and heparinoids* for stroke prevention in pregnancy is still limited. They appear not to cross the placenta and appear to have a lower risk of osteoporosis. Recent evidence suggests that they are safe for the fetus and, because of lower maternal complications (osteoporosis, thrombocytopenia), more convenient dosing, and less monitoring requirements, they may be favored over heparin (96).

Hence, there are three potential strategies for anticoagulation during pregnancy. Some use warfarin during weeks 13 through 32 and heparin before and afterward, whereas others recommend use of subcutaneous heparin (given twice daily adjusted for PTT twice control) or the use of low molecular weight heparin adjusted according to weight or anti-Xa level of 1.0 U per mL throughout pregnancy (26,70,96). No comparison of these approaches exist; despite the conclusions promulgated by authors, reports of ischemic events during pregnancies treated with heparin or low molecular weight heparin in individuals treated prior to pregnancy with warfarin are not persuasive that warfarin is in fact superior (56,71).

Although tissue plasminogen activator has been found effective for treatment of acute ischemic stroke presenting within 3 hours in the nonobstetric population, there are limited reports on the use of *thrombolysis* in pregnancy. The risk of maternal and fetal hemorrhage have precluded study of these agents and experience is limited to case reports within the literature—none of which are specific to the use of tissue plasminogen activator for stroke (98).

Aspirin, especially in high doses, is associated with increased fetal mortality and complications such as intrauterine growth retardation, congenital salicylate intoxication, and hemorrhagic complications. A meta-analysis and a large randomized trial have documented no increase in adverse complications from taking 60 mg to 150 mg of aspirin during the second or third trimester (96). Higher doses and use close to term are not recommended because of bleeding complications (26,99). Aspirin use in the first trimester is not known to be safe (96).

The requirements for *antibiotic prophylaxis* for uncomplicated vaginal delivery in patients with valvular disease is not established, but it is generally recommended for patients with prosthetic valves. In complicated vaginal deliveries and cesarean sections, patients with a broader range of valvular disease are treated, including patients with rheumatic heart disease and symptomatic mitral valve prolapse. Some physicians also recommend monthly injections with benzathine penicillin for women with prosthetic valves or rheumatic heart disease (26,73,78).

Corticosteroids, used in the treatment of some vasculitides, do not appear to increase fetal abnormalities. Similarly, dose-related maternal complications, diabetes, osteoporosis, and adrenal suppression do not occur any more frequently than in nonpregnant women (26,99).

Management of *increased intracranial pressure* due to acute cerebral infarction is problematic. Steroids generally are considered ineffective in this setting. Mannitol in large doses may cause dangerous dehydration in the fetus, with serious neurologic and other sequelae, but it has been given in isolated cases without reported harm. Hyperventilation does not appear to pose any significant risk (26).

There are no guidelines for the *management of labor and delivery* in the setting of ischemic stroke other than careful hemodynamic monitoring and control to avoid extremes of arterial pressure as well as hypocarbia and hypoxemia, particularly in the setting of acute stroke. Whereas some feel that this is best accomplished in cesarean section, others believe the risks to be equal in vaginal deliveries with epidural anesthesia and low forceps delivery (26,31). Advantages of epidural over general anesthesia include the ability to monitor the clinical situation immediately and a reduced risk of maternal aspiration. The use of nuclear medicine or other techniques to assess cerebrovascular reserve and thereby select the optimum approach to delivery has been suggested but has not been subjected to evaluation in a large case series or controlled trials (100).

Prognosis

The morbidity and mortality related to arterial infarction mirror the size of the infarction and neurologic condition. The underlying condition is often relevant. The reported 26% mortality rate in 31 patients in 1956–1965 (5), appears to be significantly lower today. In three small, recent series, no maternal deaths were reported, but up to 33% of patients were left with permanent neurologic deficits. Premature labor or delivery is not uncommon, and fetal mortality is reported in 10% to 20% (3,12,101).

There is a paucity of data for risk of stroke recurrence with subsequent pregnancies because physicians and patients have believed it to be a risk and avoided it. In one study of 441 young women with arterial stroke or cerebral venous thrombosis, 37 were pregnancy related. After 5 years of follow-up and 187 pregnancies, 13 women had recurrent stroke, two of which were pregnancy associated. The authors concluded that future pregnancy is not clearly contraindicated (4). Another series of three patients with stroke attributed to antiphospholipid antibodies had event-free pregnancies using aspirin and anticoagulation (57). It remains a standard practice to counsel young women with stroke to use methods of contraception other than oral contraceptives, without supporting data.

CEREBRAL VENOUS THROMBOSIS

Although cerebral venous thrombosis (CVT) does not constitute the majority of strokes in pregnancy, it is highly associated with pregnancy, in particular the puerperium. Whereas one series showed CVT to occur in as many as one in 2,500 deliveries (102), other series estimate the incidence to be less than 1 per 10,000 (5,10,13). In one series, 52 cases of puerperal CVT occurred during postpartum weeks 1 through 5; the majority (75%) occurred in weeks 2 and 3 (26,103). CVT also occurs during the third, and, less commonly, first and second trimesters (104).

Thrombosis of the sagittal sinus with secondary extension into the cortical veins, or primary thrombosis of one of the cortical veins, are the most common sites of involvement in pregnancy. Cavernous sinus thrombosis and lateral sinus thrombosis are not particularly associated with pregnancy. Thrombus in the sagittal sinus obstructs the protruding arachnoid villi, blocks uptake of spinal fluid, and produces intracranial hypertension. Cortical vein occlusion produces ischemia and edema of cerebral tissue and, when extensive, bland or hemorrhagic infarction (26,105).

The clinical syndrome of CVT is distinctive from arterial occlusive syndromes and generally presents as a progressive headache resistant to analgesia and accompanied by nausea and vomiting, blurred or double vision, and altered mentation representing increased intracranial pressure. Focal and generalized seizures and lateralizing neurologic signs, usually affecting the proximal arms and legs selectively, occur with cortical venous infarction (26,103,105).

Cesarean section has been shown to be a risk factor with a relative risk as high as 14, perhaps reflecting a surgical activation of blood clotting. Hypertension, age, and parity have been inconsistently associated. CVT is associated with systemic infection. Vomiting and dehydration, blood loss, and anemia also increase risk (13,23,103). Increasingly, thrombophilias are associated with pregnancy-related cerebral venous thrombosis (103). These include protein-S deficiency, protein-C deficiency, antithrombin III deficiency, and resistance to activated protein C (25,64,106). Hyperviscosity syndromes, sickle cell anemia, leukemia, polycythemia vera, paroxysmal nocturnal hemoglobinuria, and malignancy also are associated with CVT (25,26,105).

Diagnosis

In patients with CVT, the CT scan may show parasagittal edema, bland or hemorrhagic infarction, or, more specifically, an "empty delta sign" in which contrast enhancement of the dura around the thrombus signals thrombosis of the superior sagittal sinus. MRI is more sensitive than CT. Acute thrombus results in the absence of normal flow void on T1 sequences and produces hypointensity on long repetition time sequences. In the subacute period, the hyperintense methemoglobin appears hyperintense on T1. Time of flight and phase contrast magnetic resonance venography increase the specificity of the diagnosis (107). With contrast enhancement, the empty delta sign may be seen on MRI as well. Venous phase angiography is more sensitive than either CT or MRI. Intravenous digital subtraction imaging angiography is usually adequate and may be safer than conventional angiography when this diagnosis is specifically suspected (26,95,108).

Treatment

Although its use in CVT remains controversial, many studies have shown that anticoagulation is beneficial in patients with CVT and can be used safely with benefit even if hemorrhagic transformation is seen on CT scan. The goal of anticoagulation in this setting is to prevent extension of the thrombus; therefore, it should be used early (105,109). The use of intracranial venous thrombolysis is reserved for patients deteriorating despite conventional therapy and in specialized centers; successful use of this treatment has been reported in pregnant women (110).

Prognosis

The mortality rate of CVT may be as high as 20% to 30%. A recent series of 67 pregnancy-related CVT cases in which the mortality was only 9% suggested to the investigators that CVT associated with pregnancy is more benign than otherwise (103). The presence of coma, a rapid progression of symptoms, or recurrent seizures identifies a poor prognosis. The long-term prognosis is relatively good for survivors, with 10% to 20% having persisting deficits. The extent of cerebral involvement is obviously important, but the long-term deficit for venous infarcts is often less severe than that for arterial infarcts of similar size (26, 105,111). In one series of 77 patients (not all pregnancy related), only 14% had ongoing problems with optic atrophy, epilepsy, and/or neurologic deficits (112). In another series of

67 patients with pregnancy-related CVT, good neurologic outcome was seen in 80% (103).

Recurrence in subsequent pregnancies has been reported, but the incidence is likely to be very low (26). In a series of nine patients with a history of CVT, (two of whom originally had presented with pregnancy-related CVT), there were 16 pregnancies in follow-up with no recurrence of CVT during pregnancy or postpartum. Only four of these were given prophylactic treatment: two with aspirin and two with heparin during the pregnancy. Twelve pregnancies were uncomplicated, two ended in miscarriage, and two ended in voluntary abortion (112).

REFERENCES

1. Grosset DG, Ebrahim S, Bone I, et al. Stroke in pregnancy and the puerperium: what magnitude of risk? *J Neurol Neurosurg Psychiatry* 1995;58:129–131.
2. Kittner SJ, Stern BJ, Feeser BR, et al. Pregnancy and the risk of stroke. *New Engl J Med* 1996;335:768–774.
3. Sharshar T, Lamy C, Mas JL. Stroke in pregnancy study group. Incidence and causes of stroke associated with pregnancy and puerperium. A study in public hospitals of Ile de France. *Stroke* 1995;26:930–936.
4. Lamy C, Hamon JB, Coste J, et al. French study group on stroke in pregnancy. Ischemic stroke in young women. Risk of recurrence during subsequent pregnancies. *Neurology* 2000;55:269–274.
5. Cross J, Castro P, Jennett W. Cerebral strokes associated with pregnancy and the puerperium. *BMJ* 1968;3: 214–218.
6. Johnson S, Skre H. Transient cerebral ischemic attacks in the young and middle aged. *Stroke* 1986;17: 662–666.
7. Wiebers D, Whisnant J. The incidence of stroke among pregnant women in Rochester, Minn, 1955 through 1979. *JAMA* 1985;254:3055–3057.
8. Wiebers D. Ischemic cerebrovascular complications of pregnancy. *Arch Neurol* 1985;42:1106–1113.
9. Srinivasan K. Cerebral venous and arterial thrombosis in pregnancy and puerperium: a study of 135 patients. *Angiology* 1983;34:731–746.
10. Simolke G, Cox S, Cunningham F. Cerebrovascular accidents complicating pregnancy and the puerperium. *Obstet Gynecol* 1991;78:37–42.
11. Lidegaard O. Oral contraceptives, pregnancy and the risk of cerebral thromboembolism: the influence of diabetes, hypertension, migraine and previous thrombotic disease. *Br J Obstet Gynaecol* 1995;102: 153–159.
12. Witlin AG, Mattar F, Sibai BM. Postpartum stroke: a twenty-year experience. *Am J Obstet Gynecol* 2000; 183:83–88.
13. Lanska DL, Kryscio RJ. Peripartum stroke and intracranial venous thrombosis in the National Hospital Discharge Survey. *Obstet Gynecol* 1997;89:413–418.
14. Petitti DB, Sidney S, Quesenberry CP, et al. Incidence

of stroke and myocardial infarction in women of reproductive age. *Stroke* 1997;28:280–283.

15. Fletcher A, Alkjaersig N, Burstein R. The influence of pregnancy upon blood coagulation and plasma fibrinolytic enzyme function. *Am J Obstet Gynecol* 1979; 134:743–751.

16. Crowley J. Coagulopathy and bleeding in the parturient patient. *R I Med J* 1989;72:135–143.

17. Finley B. Acute coagulopathy in pregnancy. *Med Clin North Am* 1989;73:723–741.

18. Malm J, Laurell M, Dahlback B. Changes in the plasma levels of vitamin K-dependent proteins C and S and of C4b-binding protein during pregnancy and oral contraception. *Br J Haematol* 1988;68:437–441.

19. Pekonen F, Rasi V, Ammala M. Platelet function and coagulation in normal and preeclamptic pregnancy. *Thromb Res* 1986;43:553–560.

20. Kjellberg U, Andersson NE, Rosen S, et al. APC resistance and other haemostatic variables during pregnancy and puerperium. *Thromb Haemost* 1999;81:527–531.

21. Cumming AM, Tait RC, Fildes S, et al. Development of resistance to activated protein C during pregnancy. *Br J Haematol* 1995;90:725–727.

22. Schipper H. Sex hormones in stroke, chorea and anticonvulsant therapy. *Sem Neurol* 1988;8:181–186.

23. Lanska DJ, Kryscio RJ. Risk factors for peripartum and postpartum stroke and intracranial venous thrombosis. *Stroke* 2000;31:1274–1282.

24. Stern B. Cerebrovascular disease and pregnancy. In: Goldstein P, Stern B, eds. *Neurological disorders of pregnancy.* Mount Kisco: Futura Pub, 1992:51–84.

25. Mas JL, Lamy C. Stroke in pregnancy and the puerperium. *J Neurol* 1998;245:305–313.

26. Donaldson J. *Cerebrovascular disease. Neurology of pregnancy.* London: WB Saunders Co, 1989:137–184.

27. Amias AG. Cerebral vascular disease in pregnancy. 2. Occlusion. *J Obstet Gynaecol Br Commonw* 1970;77: 312–315.

28. Perier O, Cauchie O, Demanet J. Hematome interamurole par dissection parital. *Acta Neurol Phychiat Belg* 1964;64:1064–1074.

29. Mass SB, Cardonick E, Haas S, et al. Bilateral vertebral artery dissection causing a cerebrovascular accident in pregnancy. A case report. *J Reprod Med* 1999; 44:887–890.

30. Van de Kelft E, Kunnen J, Truyen L, et al. Postpartum dissecting aneurysm of the basilar artery. *Stroke* 1992; 23:114–116.

31. Sharma SK, Wallace DH, Gajraj NM, et al. Epidural anesthesia for a patient with moyamoya disease presenting for cesarean section. *Anesth Analg* 1994;79: 183–185.

32. Yamada T, Kasamatsu H, Nagano Y, et al. Moyamoya disease presenting as cerebral infarction after cesarean. *Obstet Gynecol* 1999;94:822–823.

33. Ushimura S, Mochizuki K, Ohashi M, et al. Sudden blindness in the fourth month of pregnancy led to diagnosis of moyamoya disease. *Ophthalmologica* 1993; 207:169–173.

34. Ezra Y, Kidron D, Beyth Y. Fibromuscular dysplasia of the carotid arteries complicating pregnancy. *Obstet Gynecol* 1989;73:840–843.

35. Farine E, Andreyko J, Lysikiewicz A, et al. Isolated angiitis of brain in pregnancy and puerperium. *Obstet Gynecol* 1984;63:586–588.

36. Mintz G, Niz J, Gutierrez G, et al. Prospective study of pregnancy in systemic lupus erythematosus. *J Rheumatol* 1986;13:732–739.

37. Suzuki Y, Kitagawa Y, Matsuoka Y, et al. Severe cerebral and systemic necrotizing vasculitis developing during pregnancy in a case of systemic lupus erythematosus. *J Rheum* 1990;17:1409–411.

38. Wong V, Wang R, Tse T. Pregnancy and Takayasu's arteritis. *Am J Med* 1983;75:597–601.

39. Ishikawa K, Matsuura S. Occlusive thromboaortopathy (Takayasu's disease) and pregnancy. Clinical course and management of 33 pregnancies and deliveries. *Am J Cardiol* 1982;50:1293–1300.

40. Brick J. Vanishing cerebrovascular disease of pregnancy. *Neurology* 1988;38:804–806.

41. Call G, Fleming M, Sealfon S, et al. Reversible cerebral segmental vasoconstriction. *Stroke* 1988;19: 1159–1170.

42. Geraghty J, Hoch D, Robert M, et al. Fatal puerperal cerebral vasospasm and stroke in a young woman. *Neurology* 1991;41:1145–1147.

43. Roh JK, Park KS. Postpartum cerebral angiopathy with intracerebral hemorrhage in a patient receiving lisuride. *Neurology* 1998;50:1152–1154.

44. Akins PT, Levy KJ, Cross AH, et al. Postpartum cerebral vasospasm treated with hypervolemic therapy. *Am J Obstet Gynecol* 1996;175:1386–1388.

45. Granier I, Garcia E, Geissler A, et al. Postpartum cerebral angiopathy associated with the administration of sumatriptan and dihydroergotamine—a case report. *Intensive Care Med* 1999;25:532–534.

46. Janssens E, Hommel M, Mounier-Vehier F, et al. Postpartum cerebral angiopathy possibly due to bromocriptine therapy. *Stroke* 1995;26:128–130.

47. Lee KH, Sohn YS, Kim SH, et al. Basilar artery vasospasm in postpartum cerebral angiopathy. *Neurology* 2000;54:2003–2005.

48. Comabella M, Alvarez-Sabin J, Rovira A, et al. Bromcriptine and postpartum cerebral angiopathy: a causal relationship? *Neurology* 1996;46:1754–1756.

49. Raps EC, Galetta SL, Broderick M, et al. Delayed peripartum vasculopathy: cerebral eclampsia revisited. *Ann Neurol* 1993;33:222–225.

50. Barinagarrementeria F, Cantu C, Balderrama J. Postpartum cerebral angiopathy with cerebral infarction due to ergonovine use. *Stroke* 1992;23:1364–1366.

51. Powars D, Sandhu M, Niland-Weiss J, et al. Pregnancy in sickle cell disease. *Obstet Gynecol* 1986;67: 217–228.

52. Grotta J, Manner C, Pettigrew L, et al. Red blood cell disorders and stroke. *Stroke* 1986;17:811–817.

53. Perry K. The diagnosis and management of hemoglobinopathies during pregnancy. *Sem Perinatol* 1990;14: 90–102.

54. Levine S, Welch K. Antiphospholipid antibodies. *Ann Neurol* 1989;26:386–389.

55. Branch D. Antiphospholipid antibodies and pregnancy: maternal implications. *Semin Perinatol* 1990; 14:139–146.

56. Hunt BJ, Khamashta M, Lakasing L, et al. Thromboprophylaxis in antiphospholipid syndrome pregnancies with previous cerebral arterial thrombotic events: is warfarin preferable? *Thromb Haemost* 1998;79: 1060–1061.

57. Langevitz P, Livneh A, Dulitzki M, et al. Outcome of

pregnancy in three patients with primary antiphospholipid syndrome after stroke. *Semin Arthritis Rheum* 1998;28:26–30.

58. Dietl J, Stroppel G, Poremba M, et al. Sneddon's syndrome and pregnancy; a case report. *Eur J Obstet Gynecol Reprod Biol* 1991;39:219–221.

59. Wilson JJ, Zahn CA, Ross SD, et al. Association of embolic stroke in pregnancy with the lupus anticoagulant. A case report. *J Reprod Med* 1986;31:725–728.

60. Upshaw J, Reidy T, Groshart K. Thrombotic thrombocytopenic purpura in pregnancy: response to plasma manipulations. *South Med J* 1985;78:677–680.

61. Calvert SM, Rand RJ. A successful pregnancy in a patient with homocystinuria and a previous near-fatal postpartum cavernous sinus thrombosis. *Br J Obstet Gynaecol* 1995;102:751–752.

62. Newman G, Mitchell JR. Homocystinuria presenting as multiple arterial occlusions. *Q J Med* 1984;53: 251–258.

63. Kupferminc MJ, Yair D, Bornstein NM, et al. Transient focal neurological deficits during pregnancy in carriers of inherited thrombophilia. *Stroke* 2000;31: 892–895.

64. Martinelli I, Landi G, Merati G, et al. Factor V gene mutation is a risk factor for cerebral venous thrombosis. *Thromb Haemost* 1996;75:393–394.

65. Lao T, Lewinsky R, Ohlsson A, et al. Factor XII deficiency and pregnancy. *Obstet Gynecol* 1991;78: 491–493.

66. Hart R, Kanter M. Hematologic disorders and ischemic stroke; a selective review. *Stroke* 1990;19:1111–1121.

67. Conrad J, Horellou M, Van Dreden P, et al. Thrombosis and pregnancy in congential deficiencies in AT III, protein C or protein S: study of 78 women. *Thromb Haemost* 1990;63:319–320.

68. Hellgren M, Svensson PJ, Dahlback B. Resistance to activated protein C as a basis for venous thromboembolism associated with pregnancy and oral contraceptives. *Am J Obstet Gynecol* 1995;173:210–213.

69. Salazar E, Zajarias A, Gutierrez N, et al. The problem of cardiac valve prostheses, anticoagulants, and pregnancy. *Circulation* 1984;70:169–177.

70. Sareli E, England M, Berk M, et al. Maternal and fetal sequelae of anticoagulation during pregnancy in patients with mechanical heart valve prostheses. *Am J Cardiol* 1989;63:1462–1465.

71. Watson WJ, Freeman J, O'Brien C, et al. Embolic stroke in a pregnant patient with a mechanical heart valve on optimal heparin therapy. *Am J Perinatol* 1996;13:371–372.

72. Awada A, al Rajeh S, Duarte R, et al. Stroke and pregnancy. *Int J Gynaecol Obstet* 1995;48:157–161.

73. Brady K, Duff P. Rheumatic heart disease in pregnancy. *Clin Obstet Gynecol* 1989;32:21–39.

74. Rayburn W, Fontana M. Mitral valve prolapse and pregnancy. *Am J Obstet Gynecol* 1981;141:9–11.

75. Anzalone S, Landi G. Lacunar infarction in a puerpera with mitral valve prolapse. *Ital J Neurol Sci* 1988;9: 515–517.

76. Bergh PA, Hollander D, Gregori CA, et al. Mitral valve prolapse and thromboembolic disease in pregnancy: a case report. *Int J Gynaecol Obstet* 1988;27:133–137.

77. Cox S, Hankins G, Leveno K, et al. Bacterial endocarditis. A serious pregnancy complication. *J Repro Med* 1988;33:671–674.

78. Kaplan EL. Prevention of bacterial endocarditis. *Circulation* 1977;56:139–143.

79. Lien J, Stander R. Subacute bacterial endocarditis following obstetric and gynecologic procedures: report of eight cases. *Obstet Gynecol* 1959;13:568–573.

80. George J, Lamb JT, Harriman DG. Cerebral embolism due to non-bacterial thrombotic endocarditis following pregnancy. *J Neurol Neurosurg Psychiatry* 1984;47: 79–80.

81. Leung KL, Milewicz DM, Phillips MD, et al. Nonbacterial thrombotic endocarditis in three members of a family. *N Engl J Med* 1997;336:1677–1678.

82. Homans D. Peripartum cardiomyopathy. *N Engl J Med* 1985;312:1432–437.

83. Hodgman M, Pessin M, Homans D. Cerebral embolism as the initial manifestation of peripartum cardiomyopathy. *Neurology* 1982;32:668–671.

84. Jones H, Caplan L, Come P, et al. Cerebral emboli of paradoxical origin. *Ann Neurol* 1983;13:314–319.

85. Effeney DJ, Krupski WC. Paradoxical embolus in pregnancy. An unusual thromboembolic event. *West J Med* 1984;140:287–288.

86. Chmel H, Bertles J. Hemoglobin S/C disease in a pregnant woman with crises and fat embolization syndrome. *Am J Med* 1975;58:563–566.

87. Jonas E. Maternal death due to fat-embolism. *J Obstet Gynaecol Br Commonw* 1961;68:479–483.

88. Prichard R. Generalized fat embolism: a complication of rupture of a dermoid cyst during labor: a case report. *Med Times* 1965;93:1359–1362.

89. Chatelain SM, Quirk JG Jr. Amniotic and thromboembolism. *Clin Obstet and Gynecol* 1990;33:473–481.

90. Mulder J. Amniotic fluid embolism: an overview and case report. *Am J Obstet Gynecol* 1985;152:430–435.

91. Price TM, Baker V, Cefalo RC. Amniotic fluid embolism. Three case reports with a review of the literature. *Obstet Gynecol Surv* 1985;40:462–475.

92. Nelson P. Pulmonary gas embolism in pregnancy and the puerperium. *Obstet Gynecol Surv* 1960;15: 449–481.

93. Connor R, Adams J. Importance of cardiomyopathy and cerebral ischaemia in the diagnosis of fatal coma in pregnancy. *J Clin Path* 1966;19:244–249.

94. Khurana R. Headache. In: Goldstein P, Stern B, eds. *Neurological disorders of pregnancy.* Mount Kisco: Futura Pub, 1992:107–124.

95. Wong C, Giuliani M, Haley E. Cerebrovascular disease and stroke in women. *Cardiology* 1990;77:80–90.

96. Ginsberg JS, Greer I, Hirsh J. Use of antithrombotic agents during pregnancy. *Chest* 2001;119:122S–131S.

97. Lavin J, Shaup T. Cardiac drugs during pregnancy. In: Rayburn W, Zuspan F, eds. *Drug therapy in pregnancy.* St Louis: Mosby Year Book, 1990:190–208.

98. Turrentine M, Braems G, Ramirez MM. Use of thrombolytics for the treatment of thromboembolic disease during pregnancy. *Obstet Gyn Surv* 1995;50: 534–541.

99. Briggs G, Bodendorfer T, Freeman R, et al. *Drugs in pregnancy and lactation: a reference guide to fetal and neonatal risk.* Baltimore: Williams and Wilkins, 1983.

100. Kume N, Hayashida K, Shimotsu Y, et al. Hyperventilation Technetium-99m-HMPAO brain SPECT in moyamoya disease to assess risk of natural childbirth. *J Nuc Med* 1997;38:1894–1897.

101. Witlin AG, Friedman SA, Egerman RS, et al. Cerebrovascular disorders complicating pregnancy—beyond eclampsia. *Am J Obstet Gynecol* 1997;176:1139–1148.

102. Carroll J, Leak D, Lee H. Cerebral thrombophlebitis in pregnancy and the puerperium. *Q J Med* 1966;35: 347–368.

103. Cantu C, Barinagarrementeria F. Cerebral venous thrombosis associated with pregnancy and puerperium. Review of 67 cases. *Stroke* 1993;24:1880–1884.

104. Lavin P, Bone I, Lamb J, et al. Intracranial venous thrombosis in the first trimester of pregnancy. *J Neurol Neurosurg Psychiatry* 1978;41:726–729.

105. Enevoldson TP, Russell RW. Cerebral venous thrombosis: new causes for an old syndrome? *Q J Med* 1990; 77:1255–1275.

106. Gokcil Z, Odabasi Z, Vural O, et al. Cerebral venous thrombosis in pregnancy: the role of protein S deficiency. *Acta Neurol Belg* 1998;98:36–38.

107. Kotsenas AL, Roth TC, Hershey BL, et al. Imaging neurologic complications of pregnancy and the puerperium. *Acad Radiol* 1999;6:243–252.

108. Estanol B, Rodriguez A, Conte G, et al. Intracranial venous thrombosis in young women. *Stroke* 1979;10: 680–684.

109. Einhaupl E, Villringer A, Meister W, et al. Heparin treatment in sinus venous thrombosis. *Lancet* 1991; 338:597–600.

110. Niwa J, Ohyama H, Matumura S, et al. Treatment of acute superior sagittal sinus thrombosis by t-PA infusion via venography—direct thrombolytic therapy in the acute phase. *Surg Neurol* 1998;49:425–429.

111. Donaldson J. Neurologic emergencies in pregnancy. *Obstet Gynecol Clin North Am* 1991;18:199–212.

112. Preter M, Tzourio C, Ameri A, et al. Long-term prognosis in cerebral venous thrombosis. Follow-up of 77 patients. *Stroke* 1996;27:243–246.

Neurological Complications of Pregnancy, Second Edition, edited by Brian Hainline and Orrin Devinsky. Lippincott Williams & Wilkins, Philadelphia © 2002.

6

Intracranial Hemorrhage

Janet L. Wilterdink and Edward Feldmann

Department of Neurology, Brown University and Rhode Island Hospital, Providence, Rhode Island, U.S.A.

EPIDEMIOLOGY

Intracranial hemorrhage (ICH) is an infrequent but serious complication of pregnancy. Various series estimate its incidence to be between 0.5 and 5 per 10,000 pregnancies (1–4). A very high associated mortality of 25% to 60% makes it responsible for a disproportionately high percentage of maternal mortality—nearly one in every ten maternal deaths (1, 5–7). In one series, it is the eighth most common cause of maternal mortality overall and the third most common cause of nonobstetric maternal mortality (5). The mortality associated with ICH in pregnancy appears unchanged in recent reports, as compared with older reports (4,8–10).

The role of pregnancy as a risk factor for ICH is controversial. Some estimate that the risk of ICH is increased five-fold in pregnant women compared to nonpregnant women of childbearing age (11), but this concept has been challenged recently (12). In Rochester, Minnesota, over the years 1955–1979, no cases of ICH were seen among 26,099 pregnancies, whereas 33 intracranial hemorrhages, unassociated with pregnancy, occurred in women of childbearing age—a rate less than two per 100,000. Of these women, 26 had a mean of 2.2 previous uncomplicated deliveries (13). The controversy is promoted by the infrequency with which ICH occurs in this age group, making population data difficult to interpret. Including the postpartum period in assessing pregnancy associated risk, Kittner and

associates found that the relative risk of ICH incurred in the 6-week postpartum period of 28.3 was higher than that (2.5) incurred during pregnancy itself (14); other investigators also stress the importance of increased ICH risk in the postpartum period (8,10).

Indirect evidence also suggests that pregnancy does increase the risk of ICH. Hemorrhage is associated with conditions specifically associated with pregnancy, such as eclampsia, metastatic choriocarcinoma, and disseminated intravascular coagulation. Aneurysmal rupture and hypertensive hemorrhage cluster in the later trimesters, suggesting that pregnancy influences their pathogenesis. Additionally, there is a relative preponderance of hypertensive intracerebral hemorrhage and subarachnoid hemorrhage from arteriovenous malformation (AVM) in pregnant patients compared with the general population (15–17).

CARDIOVASCULAR AND OTHER PHYSIOLOGIC CHANGES IN PREGNANCY

The physiology of pregnancy itself plays a potential role in increasing the risk of ICH. Hypertension is the most important risk factor for intracerebral hemorrhage in the general population and is also a risk factor for aneurysmal subarachnoid hemorrhage (18). Pregnancy is associated with a spectrum of hypertensive disease, ranging from pregnancy-induced hypertension to eclampsia. Hypertension accounts for one-third of pregnancy-related fatal intracranial hemorrhages (5) and is associated with 10% to 20% of aneurysmal subarachnoid hemorrhage in pregnancy (2,19,20). Hypertension also increases the risk of hemorrhage from AVMs (21).

Numerous other hemodynamic changes in pregnancy may promote ICH. Cardiac output increases by nearly 60% in the first half of pregnancy and remains elevated until term (22,23) (Fig. 6.1). Blood volume and venous pressure increase steadily throughout pregnancy, reaching a maximum at term, when whole blood volume is increased by 40%, red cell volume by 28%, and plasma volume by 50% (24) (Fig. 6.2). During labor, uterine contractions increase cardiac output by another 20% (24). In the second stage of labor, Valsalva produces a sharp increase in arterial blood pressure with a concomitant but briefer rise in intracranial pressure. At the end of Valsalva, the arterial wall is thus subjected to a sudden increase in transluminal pressure (25–28). The pain of labor further elevates blood pressure. Immediately postpartum, the vascular volume of the uterus decreases as well as its compressive effect on the vena cava, with a consequent increase in venous return. Depending in part on the amount of blood loss occurring in delivery, cardiovascular and hemodynamic parameters may not normalize for 2 to 6 weeks postpartum (24,29). These events combine to contribute to the risk of intracerebral hemorrhage in late pregnancy and up to 6 weeks postpartum (14).

The hormonal effects of pregnancy also may be important in the pathogenesis of ICH. Circulating estrogens are elevated in pregnancy and may dilate abnormal blood vessels, explaining the enlargement of meningiomas and skin tumors during pregnancy, as well as the increase in number and size of spider nevi, which fade away shortly after delivery. Neurologists suspect a similar hormonal effect on abnormal cerebral vascular structures, including AVMs and carotid cavernous fistulae, increasing their risk of bleeding (30–33). Furthermore, the smooth muscle of the cerebral arterial wall is similar to that of the myometrium and also may undergo some involutional change postpartum, perhaps predisposing the vessel to rupture (25,33,34).

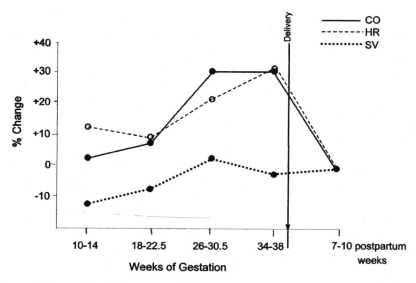

Fig. 6.1. Percent changes in cardiac output (CO), heart rate (HR), and stroke volume (SV) during gestation with the postpartum period used as a control. (Reprinted with permission from Mashini I, Albazzaz S, Fadel H, et al. Serial noninvasive evaluation of cardiovascular hemodynamics during pregnancy. *Am J Obstet Gynecol* 1987;156:1208–1213.)

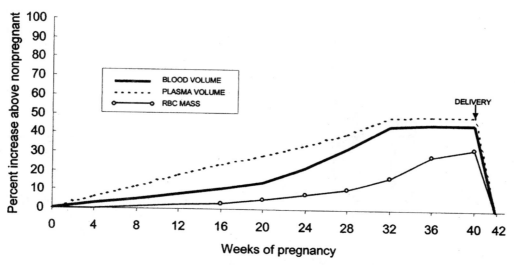

Fig. 6.2. Percent changes in blood volume, plasma volume, and red blood cell mass during pregnancy. (Reprinted with permission from Scott DE. Anemia in pregnancy. In: Wynn RM, ed. *Obstetrics and gynecology annual.* Vol. 1. New York: Appleton-Century-Crofts 1972:219.)

SUBARACHNOID HEMORRHAGE

Subarachnoid hemorrhage accounts for one-half of all intracranial bleeding in pregnancy and carries a very high risk of mortality (5).

Etiology

The majority of subarachnoid hemorrhages in pregnancy (70% to 90%) are caused by cerebral aneurysms and AVMs, in roughly equal proportion (20,35). The remainder result from a miscellany of causes including eclampsia or preeclampsia, cocaine abuse, disseminated intravascular coagulopathy, anticoagulation therapy and other bleeding diatheses, ectopic endometriosis, Moyamoya disease, vasculitis, subacute bacterial endocarditis, and choriocarcinoma (Table 6.1). In only a small percentage of patients can no cause be identified after aggressive evaluation (5,25,36–42).

Cerebral aneurysms in pregnancy are similar to those in the general population in regard to location (usually located at the major branch points in the anterior circle of Willis), and they are multiple in 5% to 20% of patients (1,26,43). There is a similar association with

hypertension, family history, and certain rare conditions: fibromuscular dysplasia, polycystic kidney disease, coarctation of the aorta, and Ehler-Danlos and Marfan syndromes (25). The relative risk of aneurysmal rupture increases with age in both pregnant and nonpregnant women of childbearing age (26).

The incidence of aneurysmal bleeding increases steadily throughout gestation and into the early postpartum period, paralleling elevations in cardiac output and blood volume. It occurs in the first trimester in 6% percent of patients, 30% in the second, 55% in the third,

TABLE 6.1. *Causes of intracranial hemorrhage in pregnancy*

Cerebral aneurysm
Arteriovenous malformation
Hypertension and eclampsia
Hemorrhagic transformation of venous or arterial
  infarction
Choriocarcinoma, other tumors
Septic embolism from bacterial endocarditis
Moyamoya disease
Cocaine, other drug abuse
Other vascular malformations: cavernous
  malformation, arteriovenous fistulae
Vasculitis or vasculopathy
Bleeding diatheses

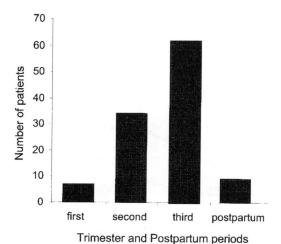

Fig. 6.3. Time of pregnancy-related aneurysmal rupture. (Data from Hunt H, Schifrin B, Suzuki K. Ruptured berry aneurysms and pregnancy. *Obstet Gynecol* 1974;43:827–36.)

and 9% in the first 6 weeks postpartum (27) (Fig. 6.3). Despite the apparent hemodynamic stress, initial aneurysmal rupture during labor and delivery is relatively rare (38,44).

In contrast to cerebral aneurysms, *arteriovenous malformations* more commonly cause subarachnoid hemorrhage in younger (18 to 25 years) rather than older (25 to 35 years) pregnant patients. Pregnant patients with AVMs are more likely than those with cerebral aneurysm to be primiparous, or, if multiparous, more likely to have a history of previously complicated pregnancies (56%). These epidemiologic differences between aneurysms and AVMs likely reflect that AVMs are congenital and aneurysms are acquired (26).

AVMs tend to bleed with equal frequency throughout pregnancy and the puerperium (Fig. 6.4) and are less often associated with hypertension (45). Because AVMs are felt to

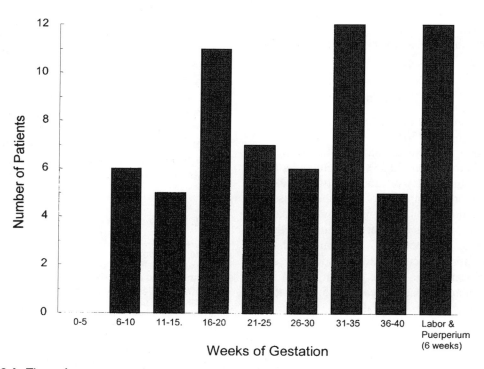

Fig. 6.4. Time of pregnancy-related arteriovenous malformation hemorrhage. (From Sadasivan B, Malki GM, Lee C, et al. Vascular malformations and pregnancy. *Surg Neurol* 1990;33:305–313, with permission from Elsevier Science.)

bleed from the venous side, increased blood volume and venous pressure is probably more important than arterial pressure in the pathogenesis of their bleeding. Labor and delivery is a high-risk period for AVM hemorrhage, when 11% of these occur (2). Cerebral AVMs are not associated with a positive family history or systemic vascular malformations.

Pregnancy appears to affect the natural history of AVMs. In pregnancy, hemorrhage is much more likely than seizure to be the presenting symptom of an AVM, whereas the opposite is true for those presenting in nonpregnant patients (44). Hemorrhage from an AVM in pregnancy is likely to be larger, with a worse prognosis and a higher rehemorrhage rate (1,33,44).

Clinical Presentation

The clinical presentation of subarachnoid hemorrhage is as dramatic in pregnancy as in the general population. Patients present with paroxysmal onset of severe headache, variably associated with meningismus or loss of consciousness. Nausea, vomiting, seizures, and focal neurologic signs may develop (25). A history of sentinel headache is present in nearly half of patients presenting with a major aneurysmal subarachnoid bleed (46).

The unwary neurologist seeing these patients must recognize that the clinical syndromes of subarachnoid hemorrhage and eclampsia overlap. Transient hypertension is common in acute subarachnoid hemorrhage, reflecting increased intracranial pressure or acute catecholamine release, and falsely suggests the diagnosis of eclampsia. Further clouding the diagnosis, proteinuria may be present in up to 30% of patients with acute subarachnoid hemorrhage, and meningismus may not be detectable in the obtunded or comatose patient (1). Additionally, subarachnoid hemorrhage may occur in the setting of eclampsia (38). A high index of suspicion for subarachnoid hemorrhage will avoid misdiagnosis or delay to diagnosis.

Complications of subarachnoid hemorrhage include vasospasm with associated ischemic stroke and rehemorrhage. Clinical vasospasm occurs in 30% to 40% of aneurysmal hemorrhages, but rarely in those due to AVMs. Subarachnoid blood, irritating arterial vessel walls, is thought to cause vasospasm, which usually becomes symptomatic with obtundation and focal neurologic deficits between a few days and 2 weeks after the initial hemorrhage. Some propose that the relative hypervolemic state of pregnancy prevents vasospasm, but this has not actually been demonstrated (47).

Rehemorrhage is associated with high mortality and morbidity, increasing the mortality of the original hemorrhage from 30% to nearly 70% (1). Rehemorrhage occurs in up to half of aneurysmal hemorrhages in both pregnant and nonpregnant patients. AVMs have a 25% risk of rehemorrhage within the same pregnancy (44,45), a rate substantially higher than the 3% to 6% annual rehemorrhage rate reported in nonpregnant individuals (48,49).

Diagnosis

Subarachnoid hemorrhage is a life-threatening condition. The risks of diagnostic tests are quite small, even in pregnancy. Standard evaluation therefore should proceed without delay. A computed tomography (CT) scan of the brain is mandatory for any patient suspected of subarachnoid hemorrhage and will confirm the diagnosis in nearly 90% of patients (47, 50). If negative or inconclusive, CT scan must be followed by lumbar puncture to detect blood or xanthochromia in the spinal fluid.

Patients in whom the diagnosis of subarachnoid hemorrhage has been confirmed should undergo angiography to identify the etiology of the hemorrhage. Four-vessel angiography is necessary because aneurysms may be multiple and AVMs may have a dual arterial blood supply. Radiologic shielding of the fetus, fetal monitoring during the procedure, and maternal hydration to reduce fetal dehydration resulting from contrast administration are recommended in addition to the normal procedure (50). If angiography is negative, a magnetic resonance imaging (MRI) scan, by all accounts safe in pregnancy, may detect AVMs that are either angiographically occult or located in the spinal cord (25,38,51). A small number of subarachnoid hemorrhages occur without identifiable vascular lesion (52). These so-called perimesencephalic subarachnoid hemorrhages have a distinctive neuroimaging appearance with restricted hemorrhage in the cisterns around the midbrain. Patients with more extensive areas of subarachnoid hemorrhage should have repeat cerebral angiography to exclude the presence of a cerebral aneurysm missed on the original study.

Treatment

Medical and surgical interventions are directed at preventing or minimizing the complications of subarachnoid hemorrhage. Medical management needs little modification in pregnancy. Careful hemodynamic monitoring and blood pressure control of the mother should occur in conjunction with careful fetal monitoring. Seizure control in subarachnoid hemorrhage takes precedence over possible teratogenic effects of anticonvulsants (45). Sedation should be performed, but it should be done cautiously to avoid fetal hypotension. Stool softeners, antitussive agents, and a darkened room also are generally recommended (25).

Treatment of elevated intracranial pressure is problematic. Steroids, although relatively safe in pregnancy, are not particularly effective in this setting. Hyperventilation, a potential cause of acid–base shifts and decreased oxygen transfer to the fetus, is believed to be safe in practice, but its beneficial effect on intracranial pressure is not sustained. Dehydrating agents, especially with osmotic agents such as mannitol, should be used cautiously because it may cause dangerous dehydration of the fetus with subsequent neurologic sequelae if severe (25,53). Increased intracranial pressure in subarachnoid hemorrhage is an extreme situation for mother and child, and these difficult treatment decisions are made on an individual basis.

Treatment of vasospasm associated with aneurysmal subarachnoid hemorrhage is not clearly defined in pregnancy. Nimodipine, used routinely for vasospasm in nonpregnant patients, is teratogenic in some animal experiments, but not clearly in humans. Clinicians should be aware that nimodipine is detectable in breast milk in concentrations relatively equivalent to plasma (54). Generally, neurologists consider that its potential maternal benefit outweighs potential fetal risks (52,55).

In aneurysmal subarachnoid hemorrhage, neurosurgical considerations generally take precedence over obstetric considerations. If the patient is not in active labor (sometimes precipitated by subarachnoid hemorrhage) or suffering from eclampsia, and if there is no fetal distress, then evaluation and subsequent surgery should proceed expediently just as if the patient were not pregnant. The decision to operate usually depends on the patient's clinical grade and the accessibility of the aneurysm. If a pregnant patient with a ruptured cerebral aneurysm is judged to be operable, clipping of the aneurysm during pregnancy is recommended. This approach significantly decreases the risk of rebleeding and maternal and fetal morbidity and mortality (1,45,47, 56). Endovascular treatment may be recommended if surgery seems to be relatively contraindicated by virtue of the patient's condition or accessibility of the aneurysm (50). Once the aneurysm has been clipped, there is no reason to modify future obstetric management of labor and delivery (25).

If a patient with subarachnoid hemorrhage goes into labor or if fetal distress or eclampsia dictate urgent delivery, emergent cesarean section is recommended, with intracranial surgery immediately following or as soon as possible thereafter (52,55,57). Cases of simultaneous neurosurgical and obstetric procedures have been reported (57–59).

Management of aneurysms found incidentally in pregnancy is not clear. Although some neurologists recommend clipping of aneurysms larger than 7 mm, there are not enough data regarding risks and benefits to make standard recommendations during pregnancy (60).

The management of AVMs in pregnancy is less clear than that of aneurysms (61). Despite the significant risk of rebleeding in the same pregnancy, which may be as high as 25% to 30%, and reports of successful surgery during pregnancy (62,63), surgical excision of the vascular malformation often is delayed until after childbirth (35,45). In some cases, this may reflect the lower incidence of surgically curable lesions compared with aneurysms and the greater technical difficulty of the operation (63). Neurosurgery may be technically easier when the hemodynamic changes associated with pregnancy have resolved (45). Retrospective evaluations of the efficacy of intrapartum excision of AVMs have not shown benefits (1). However, these studies are hampered by small numbers and variation in operative technique. More data are required to determine the proper timing of surgery for ruptured AVMs in pregnancy. No data are currently available regarding the use of embolization or radiosurgery in the pregnant patient.

The obstetric management of untreated AVMs and aneurysms is directed toward minimizing hemodynamic stress. Although many advocate elective cesarean section at 38 weeks of pregnancy to minimize cardiovascular complications of labor (45,64–66), no prospective data have been collected to support this approach. Retrospective series suggest that the complication rate is no higher in vaginal delivery with shortened second stage of labor, epidural anesthesia, and low forceps delivery, all of which minimize fluctuations in cardiac output and arterial blood pressure (1,24,27,28,67). When cesarean approach is chosen, some advocate general anesthesia to allow maximal control of arterial pressure (52), whereas others cite the risk of hypertension that occurs with induction and intubation and recommend regional anesthesia (65,66,68,69). Disadvantages of the latter approach include hypotension, which can attend sympathetic block (69). Oxytocic agents and amniotomy have been used safely to induce labor in patients with untreated vascular lesions (43,70), but their avoidance generally is recommended. Recommendations regarding future pregnancies in patients known to harbor AVMs are unclear. Although one study suggests that first hemorrhage rates are similar in pregnant and nonpregnant states (12), patients who have already suffered AVM rupture may be at higher risk.

Some anesthetic and neurosurgical modifications are necessary in pregnant women. Most problematic are the opposing needs to maintain fetal blood flow and limit bleeding in the neurosurgical field. The latter generally is accomplished in the nonpregnant patient with controlled hypotension; however, this carries a risk of fetal asphyxia in pregnancy. Hypotensive agents used with good outcome have included combinations of vasodilators, opiods, and sympathomimetic antagonists; many different approaches are recommended on the basis of one or two cases with good outcome, but there is no way to compare these approaches (52,71). Although nitroprusside is used successfully, it crosses the placenta and gets metabolized to cyanogen, which is potentially toxic to the fetus (53). Fetal heart monitoring is essential to avoid the risk of hypotension with use of nitroprusside. Loss of fetal heart rate variability or tachycardia or bradycardia indicate fetal distress and the need to reverse hypotension immediately and provide maternal oxygen (43,53,56,67,71). Hypothermia is not associated with any apparent excess fetal morbidity (25,71).

An approach to the management of patients with subarachnoid hemorrhage in pregnancy is summarized in Fig. 6.5. The major considerations are the obstetric condition of the patient and whether the patient is a candidate for surgery. The latter is based on the patient's neurologic grade and the neurosurgical accessibility of the vascular lesion. The literature suggests that many patients with AVMs are judged inoperable during pregnancy. Currently available data does not prove an advantage of cesarean section over modified vaginal delivery, and for the former, of regional over general anesthesia. This decision is made individually, influ-

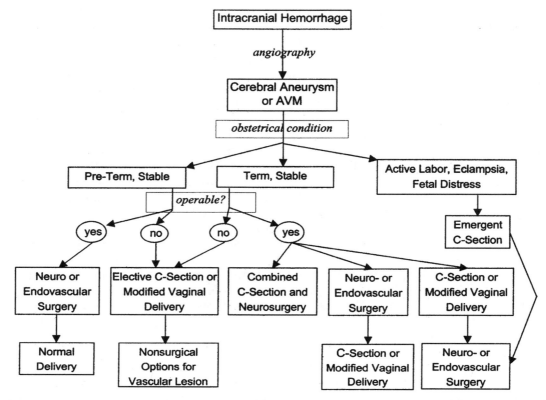

Fig. 6.5. Approach to the management of subarachnoid hemorrhage in pregnancy. See text for details.

enced by a patient's history of previous successful vaginal delivery and the preferences of the obstetrician. Similarly, stable patients at term with an operable vascular lesion have been managed successfully by any of the three approaches shown in Fig. 6.5.

Prognosis

Despite the best therapy, the mortality and morbidity of subarachnoid hemorrhage in pregnancy is high. For aneurysmal rupture, maternal mortality is 13% to 35% and fetal mortality is 7% to 25% (1,20,26,43,44). Following subarachnoid hemorrhage due to AVM, maternal mortality is 8% to 28% and fetal mortality is 9% to 18% (1,12,20,26,44, 45).

INTRACEREBRAL HEMORRHAGE

Etiology

The majority of intracerebral hemorrhages in pregnancy can be attributed to pregnancy-related hypertensive disorders. Eclampsia, discussed in more detail in Chapter 4, is usually associated with petechial or patchy, multifocal intracerebral hemorrhage, often disproportionately small in relation to neurologic deficits and often localized posteriorly (14,25,72). The presence and severity of intracerebral hemorrhage is increased in fatal cases of eclampsia (73). Intracerebral hemorrhage also contributes substantively to maternal mortality in atypical eclampsia expressed as HELLP syndrome (*h*emolysis, *e*levated *l*iver enzymes and *l*ow *p*latelets) in which, in one series, it was associated with 45% of maternal deaths (74).

Hypertensive intracerebral hemorrhage, whether in pregnant women or in chronically hypertensive individuals, typically occurs in the basal ganglia, thalamus, cerebellum, or pons (3,75). A similar underlying vascular pathology, fibrinoid necrosis of the small penetrating arteries, has been described in both patient populations as well. Microaneurysms, however, have not been described in pregnant women with hypertension (75).

Other causes (Table 6.1) of intracerebral hemorrhage include AVMs that may produce primary intracerebral as well as subarachnoid hemorrhage (14). Other vascular malformations, such as cavernous malformations, less commonly produce intracerebral hemorrhage. The endocrine changes of pregnancy are felt to increase the bleeding risk of these lesions and also cause their growth during this time (4,33). Primary ischemic strokes, especially those associated with cerebral venous thrombosis and cerebral embolism, may be associated with varying degrees of hemorrhagic transformation. Two commonly abused substances, cocaine and alcohol, are associated with intracerebral hemorrhage. The prevalence of drug abuse is high in women of reproductive age, and not all women alter their drug-use pattern during pregnancy. In different populations, cocaine was used by 8% to 17% of pregnant woman (76) and has been associated with both intracerebral hemorrhage and aneurysmal subarachnoid hemorrhage in pregnancy (8,14,36,53,77,78). Methamphetamine abuse also has been implicated in cerebral hemorrhage, including at least one pregnant women (79). Other uncommon causes of intracerebral hemorrhage in pregnancy include metastatic choriocarcinoma (50,80), Moyamoya disease (58,81–84), sarcoid (14), Kaposi's sarcoma (60), occult carotid-cavernous fistula (85), vasculitis (14,40), and various bleeding diatheses including disseminated intravascular coagulation and sickle-cell anemia (5). After evaluation, the cause may remain obscure in up to 20% of patients (4,14).

Clinical Presentation

The clinical presentation of intracerebral hemorrhage is typical of stroke, with a fairly abrupt onset of neurologic deficit, perhaps progressive over 1 to 2 hours, with symptoms referable to the site of hemorrhage. Headache, nausea, and vomiting are common accompaniments.

Diagnosis

Noncontrast CT scan is the most sensitive means of diagnosing ICH acutely. Diagnosis of the underlying etiology is made by the clinical setting; laboratory tests are helpful to rule out bleeding diatheses, infection, and drug intoxication; and imaging studies to exclude a structural etiology (contrast CT scan, MRI, or angiography) (51).

Management

Treatment is generally supportive, with blood pressure control and agents to limit ICH as discussed above. Surgical evacuation of intracerebral hemorrhage is controversial in any setting, including pregnancy, and generally is reserved for life-threatening hemorrhage with elevated intracranial pressure and herniation. If neurosurgically indicated, surgical evacuation can be performed in pregnancy (35,86). If a vascular lesion prone to rebleeding is discovered to be the cause of the cerebral hemorrhage, the discussion of neurosurgical and obstetric management discussed under subarachnoid hemorrhage applies (Fig. 6.5). As discussed under subarachnoid hemorrhage, there is no documented advantage of cesarean section over modified vaginal delivery in limiting the hemodynamic stress associated with delivery in patients who have had an intracerebral hemorrhage. Again, close blood pressure monitoring is required to avoid hemorrhage extension (if blood pressure remains elevated) and to avoid ischemic complications to mother and fetus (if blood pressure is allowed to drop too low). These competing concerns apply especially to Moyamoya disease, with its propensity to cause cerebral infarction as well as hemorrhage (58,84).

REFERENCES

1. Dias M, Sekhar L. Intracranial hemorrhage from aneurysms and arteriovenous malformations during pregnancy and the puerperium. *Neurosurgery* 1990;27: 855–866.
2. Maymon R, Fejgin M. Intracranial hemorrhage during pregnancy and puerperium. *Obstet Gynecol Surv* 1990; 45:157–159.
3. Simolke G, Cox S, Cunningham F. Cerebrovascular accidents complicating pregnancy and the puerperium. *Obstet Gynecol* 1991;78:37–42.
4. Sharshar T, Lamy C, Mas JL, Stroke in pregnancy study group. Incidence and causes of stroke associated with pregnancy and puerperium. A study in public hospitals of Ile de France. *Stroke* 1995;26:930–936.
5. Barno A, Freeman D. Maternal deaths due to spontaneous subarachnoid hemorrhage. *Am J Obstet Gynecol* 1976;125:384–392.
6. Dorfman S. Maternal mortality in New York City, 1981–1983. *Obstet Gynecol* 1990;76:317–493.
7. Sachs B, Brown D, Driscoll S, et al. Maternal mortality in Massachusetts. *NEJM* 1987;316:667–672.
8. Witlin AG, Mattar F, Sibai BM. Postpartum stroke: a twenty-year experience. *Am J Obstet Gynecol* 2000; 183:83–88.
9. Witlin AG, Friedman SA, Egerman RS, et al. Cerebrovascular disorders complicating pregnancy—beyond eclampsia. *Am J Obstet Gynecol* 1997;176:1139–1148.
10. Sameshima H, Nagaya K. Intracranial haemorrhage as a cause of maternal mortality during 1991–1992 in Japan: a report of the Confidential Inquiry into Maternal Deaths Research Group in Japan. *Br J Obstet Gynaecol* 1999;106:1171–1176.
11. Wong C, Giuliani M, Haley E. Cerebrovascular disease and stroke in women. *Cardiology* 1990;77:80–90.
12. Horton J, Chambers W, Lyons S, et al. Pregnancy and the risk of hemorrhage from cerebral arteriovenous malformations. *Neurosurgery* 1990;27:867–872.
13. Wiebers D, Whisnant J. The incidence of stroke among pregnant women in Rochester, Minn, 1955 through 1979. *JAMA* 1985;254:3055–3057.
14. Kittner SJ, Stern BJ, Feeser BR, et al. Pregnancy and the risk of stroke. *New Engl J Med* 1996;335:768–774.
15. Bevan H, Sharma K, Bradley W. Stroke in young adults. *Stroke* 1990;21:382–386.
16. Toffol GJ, Biller J, Adams HP. Nontraumatic intracerebral hemorrhage in young adults. *Arch Neurol* 1987;44: 483–485.
17. Nencini P, Inzitari D, Baruffi M, et al. Incidence of stroke in young adults in Florence, Italy. *Stroke* 1988; 19:977–981.
18. de la Monte S, Moore G, Monk M, et al. Risk factors for the development and rupture of intracranial berry aneurysms. *Am J Med* 1985;78:957–964.
19. Barrett J, Van Hooydonk J, Boehm F. Pregnancy-related rupture of arterial aneurysms. *Obstet Gynecol Surv* 1982;37:557–565.
20. Amias AG. Cerebral vascular disease in pregnancy. I. Haemorrhage. *J Obstet Gynaecol Br Commonw* 1970; 77:100–120.
21. Langer DJ, Lasner TM, Hurst RW, et al. Hypertension, small size, and deep venous drainage are associated with risk of hemorrhagic presentation of cerebral arteriovenous malformations. *Neurosurgery* 1998;42: 481–486.
22. Pedersen H, Finster M. Anesthetic risk in the pregnant surgical patient. *Anesthesiology* 1979;51:439–451.
23. Mashini I, Albazzaz S, Fadel H, et al. Serial noninvasive evaluation of cardiovascular hemodyanmics during pregnancy. *Am J Obstet Gynecol* 1987;156:1208–1213.
24. Metcalfe J, McAnulty J, Ueland K. Cardiovascular physiology. *Clin Obstet Gynecol* 1981;24:693–709.
25. Donaldson J. *Cerebrovascular disease. Neurology of pregnancy.* London: W.B. Saunders Co, 1989:137–184.
26. Robinson J, Hall C, Sedzimir C. Subarachnoid hemorrhage in pregnancy. *J Neurosurgery* 1972;36:27–33.
27. Hunt H, Schifrin B, Suzuki K. Ruptured berry aneurysms and pregnancy. *Obstet Gynecol* 1974;43: 827–836.
28. Williams KP, Wilson S. Evaluation of cerebral perfusion pressure changes in laboring women: effects of epidural anesthesia. *Ultrasound Obstet Gynecol* 1999;14: 393–396.
29. Blackburn S, Loper D. *Maternal, fetal and neonatal physiology. a clinical perspective.* Philadelphia: W.B. Saunders Co, 1992.
30. Bean W, Cogswell R, Dexter M, et al. Vascular changes of the skin in pregnancy: vascular spiders and palmar erythema. *Surg Gynecol Obstet* 1949;88:739–752.
31. Letterman G, Schuster M, Barter R, et al. Hemangiomas of pregnancy. *S Med J* 1957;50:594–599.
32. Elliott J, Rankin R, Inwood M, et al. An arteriovenous malformation in pregnancy: A case report and review of the literature. *Am J Obstet Gynecol* 1985;152:85–88.
33. Pozzati E, Acciarri N, Tognetti F, et al. Growth, subsequent bleeding, and de novo appearance of cerebral cavernous angiomas. *Neurosurgery* 1996;38:662–669.
34. Manallo-Estrella P, Barker AE. Histopathologic findings in human aortic media associated with pregnancy. *Arch Pathol* 1967;83:336–341.
35. Tuttleman R, Gleicher N. Central nervous system hemorrhage complicating pregnancy. *Obstet Gynecol* 1981; 58:651–656.
36. Henderson C, Torbey M. Rupture of intracranial aneurysm associated with cocaine use during pregnancy. *Am J Perinatol* 1988;5:142–143.
37. Heron JR, Hutchinson EC, Boyd WN, et al. Pregnancy, subarachnoid haemorrhage, and the intravascular coagulation syndrome. *J Neurol Neurosurg Psychiatry* 1974; 37:521–525.
38. Carmel P, Swift D. Spontaneous intracranial hemorrhage occurring during pregnancy. In: Kaufman H, ed. *Intracerebral hematomas.* New York: Raven Press, Ltd, 1992:117–125.
39. Oohara K, Yamazaki T, Kanou H, et al. Infective endocarditis complicated by mycotic cerebral aneurysm: two case reports of women in the peripartum period. *Eur J Cardiothorac Surg* 1998;14:533–535.
40. Ursell MR, Marras CL, Farb R, et al. Recurrent intracranial hemorrhage due to postpartum cerebral angiopathy. *Stroke* 1998;29:1995–1998.
41. Powell S, Rijhsinghani A. Ruptured bacterial intracranial aneurysm in pregnancy. A case report. *J Reprod Med* 1997;42:455–458.
42. Dagi TF, Maccabe JJ. Metastatic trophoblastic disease

presenting as a subarachnoid hemorrhage: report of two cases and review of the literature. *Surg Neurol* 1980;14: 175–184.

43. Minielly R, Yuzpe A, Drake C. Subarachnoid hemorrhage secondary to ruptured cerebral aneurysm in pregnancy. *Obstet Gynecol* 1979;53:64–70.

44. Robinson J, Hall C, Sedzimir C. Arteriovenous malformations, aneurysms, and pregnancy. *J Neurosurg* 1974; 41:63–70.

45. Sadasivan B, Malik G, Lee C, Ausman J. Vascular malformations and pregnancy. *Surg Neurol* 1990;33.

46. Verweij R, Wijdicks E, van Gijn J. Warning headache prior to rupture of an intracranial aneurysm. *Arch Neurol* 1988;45:1019–1020.

47. Gianotta S, Daniels J, Golde S, Zelman V, Bayat A. Ruptured intracranial aneurysms during pregnancy. A report of four cases. *J Reprod Med* 1986;31:139–147.

48. Graf CJ, Perret GE, Torner JC. Bleeding from cerebral arteriovenous malformations as part of their natural history. *J Neurosurg* 1983;58:331–337.

49. Brown R, Wiebers D, Forbes G, et al. The natural history of unruptured intracranial arteriovenous malformations. *J Neurosurg* 1988;68:352–357.

50. Kotsenas AL, Roth TC, Hershey BL, Yi JK. Imaging neurologic complications of pregnancy and the puerperium. *Acad Radiol* 1999;6:243–252.

51. Shojaku H, Seto H, Kakishita M, Yokoyama M, Ito J. Use of MR angiography in a pregnant patient with thalamic AVM. *Radiat Med* 1996;14:159–161.

52. Levy DM, Jaspan T. Anaesthesia for caesarean section in a patient with recent subarachnoid haemorrhage and severe pre-eclampsia. *Anaesthesia* 1999;54:994–998.

53. Gill TE, Mani S, Dessables DR. Anesthetic management of cerebral aneurysm clipping during pregnancy: a case report. *AANA J* 1993;61:282–286.

54. Tonks AM. Nimodipine levels in breast milk. *Aust N Z J Surg* 1995;65:693–694.

55. Donaldson J. Neurologic emergencies in pregnancy. *Obstet Gynecol Clin* 1991;18:199–212.

56. Newman B, Lam A. Induced hypotension for clipping of a cerebral aneurysm during pregnancy: A case report and brief review. *Anesth Analg* 1986;65.

57. Lennon R, Sundt T, Gronert G. Combined cesarean section and clipping of intracerebral aneurysm. *Anesthesiology* 1984;60:240–242.

58. Sun JC, Yakimov M, al-Badaw I, Honey CR. Hemorrhagic moyamoya disease during pregnancy. *Can J Neurol Sci* 2000;27:73–76.

59. D'Haese J, Christiaens F, D'Haens J, Camu F. Combined cesarean section and clipping of a ruptured cerebral aneurysm: a case report. *J Neurosurg Anesthesiol* 1997;9:341–345.

60. Stern B. Cerebrovascular disease and pregnancy. In: Goldstein P, Stern B, eds. *Neurological disorders of pregnancy.* Mount Kisco: Futura Pub, 1992:51–84.

61. Lanzino G, Jensen ME, Cappelletto B, Kassel INF. Arteriovenous malformations that rupture during pregnancy: a management dilemma. *Acta Neurochir (Wien)* 1994;126:102–106.

62. Matsuki A, Oyama T. Operation under hypothermia in a pregnant woman with an intracranial arteriovenous malformation. *Can Anaesth Soc J* 1972;19:184–191.

63. Finnerty JJ, Chisholm DA, Chapple H, Login IS, Pinkerton JV. Cerebral arteriovenous malformation in pregnancy: Presentation and neurologic, obstetric and ethical significance. *Am J Obstet Gynecol* 1999;181: 296–303.

64. Laidler J, Jackson I, Redfern N. The management of Caesarean section in a patient with an intracranial arteriovenous malformation. *Anaesthesia* 1989;44: 490–491.

65. Yih PS, Cheong KF. Anaesthesia for caesarean section in a patient with an intracranial arteriovenous malformation. *Anaesth Intensive Care* 1999;27:66–68.

66. Sharma SK, Herrera ER, Sidawi JE, Leveno KJ. The pregnant patient with an intracranial arteriovenous malformation. Cesarean or vaginal delivery using regional or general anesthesia? *Reg Anesth* 1995;20:455–458.

67. Holcomb W, Petrie R. Cerebrovascular emergencies in pregnancy. *Clin Obstet Gynecol* 1990;33:467–472.

68. Eldridge AJ, Kipling M, Smith JW. Anaesthetic management of a woman who became paraplegic at 22 weeks gestation after a spontaneous spinal cord haemorrhage secondary to a presumed arteriovenous malformation. *Brit J Anaesth* 1998;81:976–978.

69. Kee WD, Gomersall CD. Extradural anaesthesia for caesarean section in a patient with moyamoya disease. *Br J Anaesth* 1996;77:550–552.

70. Young D, Leveno K, Whalley P. Induced delivery prior to surgery for ruptured cerebral aneurysm. *Obstet Gynecol* 1983;61:749–752.

71. van Buul BJ, Nijhuis JG, Slappendel R, et al. General anesthesia for surgical repair of intracranial. *Am J Perinatol* 1993;10:183–186.

72. Drislane FW, Wang AM. Multifocal cerebral hemorrhage in eclampsia and severe pre-eclampsia. *J Neurol* 1997;244:194–198.

73. Mas JL, Lamy C. Stroke in pregnancy and the puerperium. *J Neurol* 1998;245:305–313.

74. Isler CM, Rinehart BK, Terrone DA, Martin RW, Magann EF, Martin JN. Maternal mortality associated with HELLP (hemolysis, elevated liver enzymes, and low platelets) syndrome. *Am J Obstet Gynecol* 1999;181: 924–928.

75. Richards A, Graham D, Bullock R. Clinicopathological study of neurological complications due to hypertensive disorders of pregnancy. *J Neurol Neurosurg Psychiatry* 1988;51:416–421.

76. Evans A, Gillogley K. Drug use in pregnancy: obstetric perspectives. *Clin Perinatol* 1991;18:23–30.

77. Mercado A, Johnson G, Calver D, Sokol R. Cocaine, pregnancy, and post partum intracerebral hemorrhage. *Obstet Gynecol* 1989;73:467–468.

78. Iriye BK, Asrat T, Adashek JA, et al. Intraventricular haemorrhage and maternal brain death associated with antepartum cocaine abuse. *Br J Obstet Gynaecol* 1995; 102:68–69.

79. Perez JA, Arsura EL, Strategos S. Methamphetamine-related stroke: four cases. *J Emer Med* 1999;17: 469–471.

80. Seigle J, Caputy A, Manz H. Multiple oncotic intracranial aneurysms and cardiac metastases from choriocarcinoma: case report and review of the literature. *Neurosurgery* 1987;20:39–42.

81. Enomoto H, Goto H. Moyamoya disease presenting as intracerebral hemorrhage during pregnancy: Case report and review of the literature. *Neurosurgery* 1987; 20:33–35.

82. Terai Y, Seiki Y, Goto M, et al. Moyamoya disease presenting as intracerebral hemorrhage at 32 weeks of ges-

tation; a case report and review of the literature. *Adv Obstet Gynecol* 1996;48:20–25.

83. Amin-Hanjani S, Kuhn M, Sloane N, et al. Moyamoya disease in pregnancy: a case report. *Am J Obstet Gynecol* 1993;169:395–396.

84. Komiyama M, Yasui T, Kitano S, et al. Moyamoya disease and pregnancy: Case report and review of the literature. *Neurosurgery* 1998;43:360–369.

85. Lin T, Chang C, Wai Y. Spontaneous intracerebral hematoma from occult carotid-cavernous fistula during pregnancy and puerperium. *J Neurosurg* 1992;76: 714–717.

86. Reece E, Chervenak F, Coultrip L, et al. The perinatal management of pregnancy complicated by massive intracerebral hemorrhage. *Am J Perinatol* 1984;1: 266–267.

Neurological Complications of Pregnancy, Second Edition, edited by Brian Hainline and Orrin Devinsky. Lippincott Williams & Wilkins, Philadelphia © 2002.

7

Maternal Head Trauma

Meheroz H. Rabadi and Barry D. Jordan

Department of Neurorehabilitation, Burke Rehabilitation Hospital, White Plains, New York, U.S.A.

Clinical management of maternal head trauma during pregnancy requires a detailed and expeditious diagnostic evaluation that will dictate the proper medical, surgical, and obstetric management, therefore minimizing potential maternal and fetal morbidity and mortality. Although fetal head trauma either in the prenatal period or at the time of delivery represents another aspect of head trauma during pregnancy, a detailed discussion of fetal head trauma during pregnancy is beyond the scope of this chapter.

EPIDEMIOLOGY

Traumatic brain injury (TBI) represents a major public health concern in the United States. According to Sosin, there were 1.5 million mild to moderate brain injuries (loss of consciousness without hospitalization) in 1991 in the United States (1). The annual death rate from TBI approximates 30 per 100,000 population and accounts for 44% of the injury death rate worldwide (2). Depending on the methodologic approaches and the catchment area, the incidence of TBI ranges from 152 to 430 cases per 100,000 per year (2). Head trauma primarily afflicts young males. Other major risk factors for head injury include motor-vehicle accidents and alcohol use. Alcohol ingestion is related to brain injury as a causative factor and complicates diagnosis, delays recovery, and impedes survival (3).

Despite the extensive literature addressing the epidemiology of head trauma, the epidemiology of TBI complicating pregnancy is poorly delineated. Considering that head trauma afflicts young adults and adults between the ages of 15 and 44, one might expect maternal head trauma to represent a significant public health problem. However, support of this hypothesis is lacking. Attention concerning trauma and pregnant women has focused on blunt abdominal trauma during motor-vehicle accidents.

Injury rates among women are influenced by increased automobile usage and alcohol intake. Injuries can occur at home or in the workplace. The causes of accidental deaths among women of childbearing age include motor-vehicle accidents, falls, fires and burns, drowning, firearms, and poisonings. The accident rate for pregnant women during the gestational period approximates 7% and appears to be equally distributed throughout the three trimesters (3).

CLASSIFICATION OF HEAD INJURY

Head injuries are classified into two major categories: closed (nonmissile) and open (missile) head injuries. The spectrum of traumatic brain injury is outlined in Table 7.1.

Closed (Nonmissile) Head Injury

Closed head injuries are classified into two general types: diffuse and focal. Focal or post-traumatic intracranial mass lesions include subdural hematomas (SDH), epidural hematomas (EDH), cerebral contusions (CCs), and intracerebral hematomas (ICH).

TABLE 7.1. *Spectrum of traumatic brain injuries*

(A) Nonmissile (closed) head injury
  Focal
    1. Subdural hematoma
    2. Epidural hematoma
    3. Intracerebral hematoma
    4. Cerebral contusion
  Diffuse
    1. Cerebral concussion (nonstructural)
       a. Mild
       b. Classic
    2. Diffuse axonal injury (structural)
       a. Mild
       b. Moderate
       c. Severe
(B) Missile (open) head injury
    1. Depressed
    2. Penetrating
    3. Perforating

Diffuse posttraumatic brain injuries are not associated with focal intracranial lesions and represent a continuum of progressively more severe brain dysfunction caused by increasing amounts of acceleration damage to the brain. In general, diffuse brain injury is classified according to whether structural or anatomic disruption occurs. Structural diffuse brain injury (diffuse axonal injury, or DAI) is the most severe because axonal disruption occurs. Nonstructural diffuse brain lesions (mild concussion and classic cerebral concussion syndromes) are typically less severe than structural brain lesions because the anatomic integrity of the central nervous system is maintained.

Cerebral Concussion

Cerebral concussion can be defined as a clinical syndrome characterized by immediate and transient impairment of neurologic function secondary to mechanical forces that does result in focal brain injury or DAI injury. In the clinical literature, concussion often is referred to as mild TBI. The clinical manifestations of concussion or mild TBI include unconsciousness or other neurologic symptoms such as disorientation, amnesia, dizziness, or disequilibrium. According to Gennarelli (4) the term "concussion" should

not be applied to traumatic head injuries that result in unconsciousness longer than 6 hours. Furthermore, for all practical purposes, cerebral concussion represents physiologic and neurologic dysfunction without substantial anatomic disruption. Nonfocal traumatic brain injury that results in coma longer than 6 hours should be classified as DAI because it is presumed that structural or axonal injury has occurred.

Cerebral concussions are divided into two major categories: the mild cerebral concussion and the classic cerebral concussion (4) (Table 7.2). In the mild cerebral concussion syndrome, consciousness is preserved after head trauma, but there is a transient disturbance of neurologic function. The classic cerebral concussion is characterized by loss of consciousness secondary to cerebral trauma and therefore is more severe than the mild concussion syndromes. Invariably, the classic cerebral concussion syndrome is accompanied by some degree of retrograde and posttraumatic amnesia. Usually the duration of unconsciousness correlates directly with the severity of the cerebral concussion. Unconsciousness occurs at the moment of impact and, by definition, does not exceed 6 hours.

Diffuse Axonal Injury

DAI represents a diffuse TBI associated with prolonged traumatic coma longer than 6 hours that is not secondary to a mass lesion or ischemia (4). DAI can be classified into three categories—mild, moderate, and severe—on the basis of the severity and duration of coma

TABLE 7.2. *Nonstructural (physiologic) diffuse brain injury*

Characteristic cerebral concussion	Mild	Classic
Loss of consciousness	None	Immediate
Duration of unconsciousness	None	Less than 6 hours
Decerebrate posturing	None	None
Posttraumatic amnesia	Minutes	Minutes to hours
Memory deficit	None	Minimal
Motor deficit	None	None

TABLE 7.3. *Diffuse axonal injury (structural diffuse brain injury)*

Characteristic	Mild	Moderate	Severe
Loss of consciousness	Immediate	Immediate	Days to weeks
Duration of unconsciousness	6–24 hours	Longer than 24 hours	
Decerebrate posturing	Rare	Occasional	Present
Posttraumatic amnesia	Hours	Days	Weeks
Memory deficit	Mild to moderate	Mild to moderate	Severe
Motor deficit	None	Mild	Severe

(4) (Table 7.3). Mild DAI is associated with coma lasting 6 to 24 hours. Approximately 30% of patients with mild DAI present with decerebrate or decorticate posturing, but they rapidly lose these signs and by 24 hours are then able to follow commands. In mild DAI there is a mild to moderate memory deficit and usually no motor deficit. Posttraumatic amnesia can last hours.

Moderate DAI is defined as coma lasting more than 24 hours without prominent, long-lasting brainstem signs (4). This is the most common type of DAI. Most cases of moderate DAI are caused by vehicular accidents and are commonly associated with basilar skull fractures. In moderate DAI, when patients awaken from coma, they are confused and experience long periods of posttraumatic and retrograde amnesia. Permanent deficits of intellectual, cognitive, memory, and personality function may be mild to severe (4).

Severe DAI has been described in the neurosurgical literature as a diffuse white-matter shearing injury. This category represents the most devastating form of diffuse brain injury and is associated with severe mechanical disruption of axons in both cerebral hemispheres, the diencephalon, and the brainstem. Severe DAI occurs almost exclusively in vehicular accidents (4). Patients with severe DAI are immediately unconscious and may remain unconscious for days to weeks. Severe DAI is differentiated from moderate DAI by the presence and persistence of abnormal brainstem signs, such as decerebrate posturing (4). Patients also may display autonomic dysfunction characterized by hypertension, hyperhydrosis, and hyperpyrexia.

Subdural Hematoma

SDHs occur when the bridging veins between the brain and the dural venous sinuses are ruptured. After an impact injury to the calvarium, the brain typically accelerates so the veins that bridge the subdural space are stretched; if stretching is severe enough, the veins are torn and venous blood escapes into the subdural space. The clinical presentation and the course are determined by the severity of the impact injury of the brain and the rate at which the SDH expands. SDH associated with parenchymal brain injury at impact tends to be the most severe. The clinical presentation is partially dependent on the rate of hemorrhaging into the subdural space. Acute SDHs, which expand more rapidly than chronic SDHs, present as rapidly enlarging mass lesions. Most patients present with hemiparesis, pupillary abnormalities (anisocoria), or both (5).

Epidural Hematoma

EDHs are caused by meningeal artery rupture. Meningeal arteries run between the skull and the dura and are usually embedded in the grooves of the skull. Unlike SDHs, EDHs do not typically result from acceleration–deceleration but from direct skull trauma. A skull fracture across a long groove of the skull or the inward bending of the calvarium causes dural detachment from the inner table of the skull, forming the EDH. The middle meningeal artery, the largest meningeal artery, runs across the floor of the middle cranial fossa and branches widely up the side of the skull. Middle meningeal artery is the most commonly traumatized meningeal artery and the most frequent source of EDH.

The classic clinical presentation of an EDH is immediate loss of consciousness at the time of impact with a subsequent period of lucid recovery. The patient then develops neurologic symptoms such as headache and increased lethargy. According to Bruno (6), only one-third of patients with EDH present in this manner. Another third do not experience unconsciousness until some time after the injury, and the other third display persistent loss of consciousness after impact.

Cerebral Contusion

CCs are heterogeneous areas of necrosis, infarction, hemorrhage, or edema within the brain parenchyma. Cerebral contusions can occur at the site of impact or at distant points. Coup lesions are at the site of impact, and contrecoup lesions are at distant sites from the point of impact. Coup lesions are usually produced by the deformation and bending inward of calvarium at the point of impact. Contrecoup lesions result primarily from impact deceleration of the brain against the bony surfaces of the skull. This type of injury can be encountered when a patient strikes her head on a stationary object or the floor so that the brain forcefully strikes the abruptly decelerated skull. CCs most frequently occur in the frontal and temporal poles of the cerebral hemispheres as they strike the irregular floor of the frontal and middle fossa.

Intracerebral Hematomas

ICHs are hemorrhagic areas within the brain parenchyma. The clinical presentation of these typically well-defined homogenous collections of blood depends on the location, size, and subsequent growth of the ICH. Intracerebral hematomas can result from depressed skull fracture, penetrating wounds, or acceleration–deceleration injuries.

Open (Missile) Head Injury

Open or missile head injuries are classified as depressed, penetrating, or perforating. A depressed head injury (depressed skull fracture) is defined as an outer table of fractured segment that lies below the inner table of the surrounding intact skull. Depressed skull fractures can be further classified as closed or compound. These distinctions are made on the basis of the absence (closed) or presence (compound) of a scalp laceration. In depressed injuries, the missile fails to penetrate the skull but injures (contuses) the underlying brain parenchyma. Penetrating head injuries are distinguished from perforating head injuries because a missile such as a bullet that penetrates the skull does not exit the skull as in perforating injuries. The pathologic clinical presentation of these injuries depends on the path of the missile in the brain.

SEQUELAE OF HEAD INJURY

Postconcussion Syndrome

After an episode of mild TBI or concussion, patients can exhibit persistent neurologic complaints that may include headache, dizziness, vertigo, irritability, inability to concentrate, impaired memory, and fatigue. This constellation of symptoms is characteristic of postconcussion syndrome (PCS). Patients exhibiting PCS usually have a normal neurologic examination; however, detailed neuropsychological testing may reveal subtle cognitive impairments (7, 8, 9). The exact duration of PCS varies and depends on several factors, including degree of axonal injury, extraneural injuries, secondary motivation, and the psychological composition of the individual. The duration of PCS usually reflects the severity of the initial injury, but psychological and motivational factors, especially litigation, can influence the duration of PCS. PCS usually resolves within 1 month, but symptoms can persist longer. Rimel and colleagues (10) evaluated 424 patients 3 months after mild TBI and noted that 79% complained of persistent headaches and 59% described problems with memory. Their criteria for mild TBI were loss of consciousness of 20 minutes or less, a GCS score of 13 to 15, and hospitalization not exceeding 48 hours.

Posttraumatic Seizures

Posttraumatic seizures (PTS) can be an immediate or delayed complication of head injury. During the acute period, seizures can precipitate adverse events secondary to elevations in intracranial pressure, blood pressure changes, reduced oxygen delivery, and excess neurotransmitter release. The occurrence of seizures also may be associated with accidental injury, psychological effects, and loss of driving privileges.

Seizures during the first week after head injury are referred to as early seizures and after the first week are referred to as late seizures (12). Of PTS, 70% to 80% occur within the first 2 years after injury (12). The incidence of seizures following penetrating injuries is about 50% in patients followed for 15 years (12). In civilian head injury studies that followed high-risk patients up to 36 months, the incidence of early PTS varied between 4% and 25%, and the incidence of late PTS varied between 9% and 42% in untreated patients (12). In a population-based study of seizures after TBI of 4,541 children and adults from 1935 to 1984, the standardized incidence ratio for people with mild head injuries was 1.5, for moderate head injuries was 2.9, and for severe head injuries was 17.0. Thus, the severity of injury had a bearing on subsequent seizures (13).

The risk factors affecting the incidence of early and late seizures are different. Early seizures in adults often is associated with prolonged posttraumatic amnesia (greater than 24 hours), depressed skull fractures, or ICH. Most early seizures are focal in onset. Focal seizures are common with ICH and prolonged posttraumatic amnesia but not with depressed skull fracture. Half of patients with early epilepsy have the first seizure within 24 hours of injury; of these, 50% seize within 1 hour of injury. Seizures during the first hour after trauma are more common in children 16 years of age or younger and with depressed skull fractures. Seizures associated with intracranial hematoma seldom occur within the first hour but more often after 24 hours, and recurrent seizures are common. Seizures associated with depressed skull fractures often occur within the first hour and less often after 24 hours, and they are often single. The risk of developing late seizures (seizures 1 week after head injury) is significantly increased by the presence of acute hematoma, depressed skull fracture, and the development of early epilepsy (11). Most cases of late epilepsy occur within 1 year of injury (excluding cases in the first week). No consistent correlation between electroencephalographic abnormalities in the first year after head injury and the development of late epilepsy has been observed (11). In the absence of an acute hematoma, depressed skull fracture, or a history of early epilepsy, the risk is approximately 1% (11). Certain risk factors have been identified that place head-injured patients at increased risk for developing PTS (13,14). (See Table 7.4).

Scientific evidence supports the use of prophylactic anticonvulsants to prevent early, but not late, PTS. A large prospective, randomized, double-blind, placebo-controlled trial of 404 patients evaluated the efficacy of phenytoin administration in the prevention of early and late PTS and noted a significant reduction in the incidence of early PTS, but not late PTS (14). Manaka conducted a prospective, randomized, double-blind study of 126 patients receiving placebo or phenobarbital and found no significant reduction in late PTS in the active treatment group (15). Similarly, McQueen and associates conducted a prospective, randomized, double-blind study of 164 patients receiving phenytoin or placebo for the prevention of late PTS and failed to

TABLE 7.4. *Risk factors for posttraumatic seizures*

Glasgow Coma Scale (GCS) score <10
Cortical contusion
Depressed skull fracture
Subdural hematoma
Epidural hematoma
Intracerebral hematoma
Penetrating head wound
Seizure within 24 hours of injury
Duration of loss of consciousness
Posttraumatic amnesia
Dural tear/penetration

demonstrate a significant reduction in late PTS in the treatment group (16). Valproate appears to be equally as effective as phenytoin in the prevention of early PTS; however, there was a trend toward a higher mortality in patients treated with valproate (17). Phenytoin and carbamazepine are effective in preventing early, but not late, PTS, whereas valproate should not be routinely used in the prevention of early PTS (17).

Posttraumatic Hydrocephalus

Acute obstructive or delayed communicating hydrocephalus can complicate significant head trauma. Pathophysiology of acute obstructive hydrocephalus is a midventricular shift with occlusion to the cerebrospinal fluid (CSF) outflow, whereas delayed communicating hydrocephalus is the result of defective CSF absorption by clogged arachnoid villi by blood products. Posttraumatic hydrocephalus (PTH) is one of the factors responsible for slow progress or failure to progress in a rehabilitation setting. Risk factors for PTH include intraventricular or subarachnoid hemorrhages and meningitis. Marmarou and colleagues found that 20% of 75 patients with severe TBI had PTH and 44% had ventriculomegaly during the initial 3 months after injury (18). PTH presents as psychomotor slowing, intellectual deterioration, gait disturbances resembling gait apraxia, and incontinence (19). Progressive hydrocephalus may require shunting. In pregnant women, ventriculoperitoneal (VP) shunts with unidirectional flow valves can reduce the likelihood of increased intraperitoneal pressure causing shunt failure.

MANAGEMENT

Management of traumatic brain injury depends on the type and severity of injury. Initial management of the head-injured gravida focuses on maintaining ventilatory and circulatory function, cerebral blood flow, and normal physiologic functions of the mother and fetus, including monitoring maternal intracranial pressure (ICP). When indicated, expedi-

TABLE 7.5. *Principles of management of traumatic brain injury during pregnancy*

Maintain circulatory and ventilatory function
Provide expeditious surgical intervention
Control intracranial pressure
Maintain cerebral blood flow
Maintain normal physiologic functions

tious neurosurgical intervention should be implemented (Table 7.5). Protocols emphasizing early intubation, prompt resuscitation, rapid transportation to an appropriate trauma facility, early neuroradiologic investigations, and meticulous management in an intensive care unit can decrease mortality rate from severe TBI (20, 21). Guidelines for the management of severe TBI recently have been published (22).

Initial Evaluation

The general physical examination establishes the extent of multisystem trauma. Initial evaluation should assess vital signs and cardiovascular and pulmonary functions. In the absence of a heartbeat or breathing, cardiopulmonary resuscitation should be initiated. The physical examination also should include an obstetric examination, which should note the size of the uterus for estimations of pregnancy duration and fetal weight. Auscultation for fetal heart tones and palpation for fetal activity also should be conducted. A pelvic examination should determine whether there is effacement and dilation of the cervix. The pregnant patient beyond 20 weeks gestation also should be placed on the left side to prevent compression of the inferior vena cava from an enlarged uterus.

The neurologic examination determines the focality and severity of neurologic injury. The Glasgow Coma Scale (GCS) (Table 7.6) is the assessment scale used most widely to document the severity of TBI (23) and has a high degree of inter- and intrarater reliability (24, 25). This scale assesses motor response, verbal response, and eye opening and provides a practical means of monitoring changes in the level of consciousness. A fully oriented, alert

TABLE 7.6. *Glasgow coma scale*

Response	Score
Verbal	
None	1
Incomprehensible sounds	2
Inappropriate words	3
Confused	4
Oriented	5
Eye opening	
None	1
To pain	2
To speech	3
Spontaneously	4
Motor	
None	1
Abnormal extension	2
Abnormal flexion	3
Withdraws	4
Localizes	5
Obeys	6

patient who obeys commands receives a maximum score of 15. A mute, flaccid patient who exhibits no eye opening to any stimuli receives a minimum score of 3. Mild TBI falls between 13 and 15 on the scale. Anyone scoring 8 or less is comatose and has suffered a severe head injury.

According to data from the Traumatic Coma Data Bank (TCDB), outcome following TBI is closely related to initial GCS score. Among 746 patients with closed TBI, the mortality rate for those with an initial posttraumatic GCS of 3 was 78.4%. In patients with an initial GCS of 4 the mortality rate was 55.9%, and for those with a GCS score of 5 this rate was 40.2%. Of note, however, was the good outcome of 4.1%, 6.3%, and 12.2% among the three groups, respectively (26). In another large study of 46,977 head-injured patients, a sharp progressive increase in mortality was noted in patients who presented to the emergency room with GCS scores of 3 to 8 (27).

Once the severity of TBI is assessed, patients should be classified according to risk of neurologic deterioration. Table 7.7 classifies head injury into three risk groups: low, moderate, and high (28). This classification serves as a guideline to manage head-trauma victims. This is particularly important because unnecessary or overzealous evaluation of pregnant women with head trauma may present undue risk to the fetus. The neuroradiologic approach to the gravida with head trauma requires careful clinical decisions that balance the potential neurologic deterioration associated with an operable mass lesion and the potential side effects of radiation on the fetus. According to the classification scheme listed in Table 7.7, low-risk patients usually can be followed without neuroradiologic intervention. However, moderate- or high-risk patients should undergo appropriate neuroimaging, such as computed tomography (CT) or magnetic resonance imaging examination.

Routine laboratory studies in the head-trauma victim should include a complete blood cell count, biochemistry profile, and coagulation studies. Blood also should be drawn for typing and cross matching. If the patient is unconscious or exhibits chest wounds, arterial blood gas is tested to determine pH and pO_2. Systemic insults must be minimized in the head-trauma victim. Arterial hypoxemia (pO_2 less than 60mm Hg), arterial hypotension (systolic blood pressure less than 90 mm Hg), anemia (hematocrit less than 30%), and arterial hypercarbia (pCO_2 more than 45mm Hg) are associated with poor out-

TABLE 7.7. *Relative risk of significant intracranial injury after closed head injury*

Low risk	Moderate risk	High risk
Asymptomatic	Mental status alterations	Lethargy, depressed consciousness
Mild headache/dizziness	Severe progressive headache	Focal neurologic finding
Scalp injury	Alcohol, drug intoxication	Decreasing consciousness
No moderate- or high-risk factors	Posttraumatic seizures	
	Protracted vomiting	
	Less than 2 years old	
	Multiple trauma	
	Facial fractures	

TABLE 7.8. *Percentage of poor outcomes associated with systemic insults in head trauma*

Systemic insults	Poor outcome (%)[a]
Arterial hypoxemia (pO$_2$ <60 mm Hg)	59
Arterial hypotension (SBP <90 mm Hg)	65
Anemia (hematocrit <30%)	62
Arterial hypercarbia (pCO$_2$ >45 mm Hg)	78
No systemic insults	35

[a]Includes severe disability, vegetative state, and death.

comes, including severe disability, vegetative state, and death (28) (see Table 7.8).

Resuscitation of Blood Pressure and Oxygenation

Early postinjury hypoxia and hypotension greatly increase morbidity and mortality in TBI patients. According to the TCDB, hypoxemia and hypotension occurred in more than one-third of severe head-injury patients. The TCDB study demonstrated that prehospital hypotension (a single observation of a systolic blood pressure of less than 90 mm Hg) or hypoxia (apnea/cyanosis in the field or a PaO$_2$ less than 60 mm Hg by arterial blood gas analysis) were among the five most powerful predictors of outcome. These predictors were statistically independent of the other major predictors such as age, admission GCS score, admission GCS motor score, intracranial diagnosis, and pupillary status (29,30). Accordingly, hypotension and hypoxemia should be closely monitored and treated. Patients with a GCS less than 9 who are unable to maintain their airway or who remain hypoxemic despite supplemental oxygen require a secure airway, preferably by endotracheal intubation (22). The mean arterial blood pressures should be maintained above 90 mm Hg, through the infusion of fluids throughout the patient's course to attempt to maintain cerebral perfusion pressure (CPP) at more than 70 mm Hg (22).

Intracranial Pressure Monitoring

Brain swelling and elevated ICP develop in 40% of patients with severe TBI (31). High or uncontrolled ICP is one of the most common causes of death and neurologic disability after TBI (32,33). The main objective of ICP monitoring is to maintain adequate cerebral perfusion and oxygenation, and it is primarily a means for guiding therapy. ICP monitoring is not routinely indicated in patients with mild or moderate head injury and is reserved for those individuals with severe TBI or an abnormal head CT scan (revealing hematomas, contusions, edema, or compressed basal cisterns) (22). Comatose head-injury patients (GCS 3-8) with abnormal CT scans should undergo ICP monitoring. Comatose patients with normal CT scans have a much lower incidence of intracranial hypertension unless they have two or more of the following features at admission: age over 40, unilateral or bilateral motor posturing, or systolic blood pressure of less than 90 mm Hg. Treatment should be initiated at an ICP threshold of 20 to 25 mm Hg.

Maintenance of Cerebral Perfusion Pressure

CPP is defined as the mean arterial blood pressure (MAP) minus ICP (i.e., CPP = MAP − ICP) and is the physiologic variable that defines the pressure gradient driving cerebral blood flow (CBF) and metabolic delivery (22). Despite the importance of maintaining adequate CPP (34), there are insufficient data to support treatment standards or guidelines (22). Clinical opinion suggests that CPP should be maintained at a minimum of 70 mm HG.

Hyperventilation and the Management of Intracranial Pressure

Hyperventilation reduces CBF and therefore decreases ICP. Although hyperventilation results in respiratory alkalosis, it has little effect on the fetus. The use of prophylactic hyperventilation (paCO$_2$ less than 35 mm Hg) therapy in the absence of increased ICP during the first 24 hours after severe TBI should be avoided because it can compromise cerebral perfusion during a time when CBF is reduced

(22). Hyperventilation therapy is necessary for brief periods when there is acute neurologic deterioration, or for longer periods if there is intracranial hypertension refractory to sedation, paralysis, CSF drainage, and osmotic diuretics (22). Although aggressive hyperventilation, defined as arterial pCO_2 of 25 or less, has been the cornerstone in the management of severe TBI, aggressive hyperventilation runs the risk of causing cerebral ischemia by further reducing CBF without decreasing ICP. In the absence of increased ICP, chronic prolonged hyperventilation therapy should be avoided following severe TBI (22).

Mannitol and Management of Intracranial Pressure

The majority of available evidence indicates that steroids do not improve outcome or lower ICP in severely head-injured patients, and the routine use of steroids is not recommended for these purposes (35–41). Accordingly, mannitol routinely is used to reduce ICP in TBI patients with intracranial hypertension. Mannitol exerts a beneficial effect on ICP, CPP, CBF, brain metabolism, and short-term neurologic outcome (42). Mannitol causes an osmotic diuresis, withdrawing free water from the brain and thereby reducing intracranial pressure. Mannitol has an immediate plasma-expanding effect that reduces blood viscosity, increases CBF, and increases cerebral oxygen delivery. (43). However, mannitol's osmotic diuresis may cause volume deficits and hypotension. Therefore, hypovolemia should be avoided at all cost by adequate fluid replacement, and a Foley catheter should be used to measure urine output in these patients. Mannitol is excreted entirely in the urine, and a significant risk of acute renal failure (acute tubular necrosis) exists if mannitol is administered in large doses, particularly if serum osmolarity exceeds 320 mOsm (44). Patients are prone to renal failure if other potentially nephrotoxic drugs are administered simultaneously or in the presence of sepsis or preexisting renal disease (44). The use of mannitol should be restricted in pregnancy because it also results in the flow of free water from the fetus and amniotic fluid to the mother. Potential fetal side effects include severe dehydration, contraction of blood volume, cyanosis, and bradycardia.

Barbiturates and Management of Intracranial Pressure

High-dose barbiturate therapy may be considered in hemodynamically stable salvageable severe head-injury patients with intracranial hypertension refractory to maximal medical and surgical ICP-lowering therapy (22). Currently, it is estimated that 10% to 15% of patients admitted with severe head injury ultimately will manifest medically and surgically intractable elevated ICP with an associated mortality of 84% to 100% (45,46). Barbiturates exert their cerebral protective and ICP-lowering effects through several distinct mechanisms: alterations in vascular tone, suppression of metabolism, and inhibition of free radical-mediated lipid peroxidation (47). The most important effect may relate to coupling of CBF to regional metabolic demands such that the lower the metabolic requirements, the less the CBF and related cerebral blood volume with subsequent beneficial effects on ICP and global cerebral perfusion. Pentobarbital is the most commonly used barbiturate.

Neurosurgical Management

Focal traumatic lesions, such as subdural and epidural hematomas associated with mass effect, neurologic deterioration, or both, require surgical intervention. Intracranial mass lesions causing greater than 5 mm of midventricular shift should be evacuated immediately (48). If the midventricular shift is less than 5 mm, the patient should be observed closely with ICP monitoring. If ICP exceeds 25 mm Hg or neurologic deterioration is seen, the ICH should be evacuated (48). Other indications for neurosurgical intervention include depressed skull fractures, shunting for post-traumatic hydrocephalus, and ICP monitoring.

DISCUSSION

The risk of fetal death is directly associated with the severity of trauma. The most frequent cause of fetal death is maternal death. Other variables associated with fetal demise in pregnant woman experiencing general trauma include abdominal injury, increasing fluid requirements, maternal acidosis, and maternal hypoxia (49). Postmortem cesarean section is indicated in cases of recent maternal death or brain death. Several factors may influence the fetal outcome of postmortem cesarean section (50). In general, the sooner the delivery after death, the better the fetal outcome. Delivery performed within 5 minutes is associated with an excellent outcome, compared to a poor outcome if 20 minutes or more have elapsed. Maternal death from head injury without significant systemic insult results in a more favorable fetal outcome, compared to other causes of maternal death such as hemorrhagic shock, drowning, or smoke inhalation (50). The fetal outcome is also more favorable in pregnancy when the gestational period is greater than 28 weeks and the fetus weighs more than 1,000 g.

CONCLUSION

In general, the management of the brain-injured gravida should follow the standards, guidelines, and recommendations for the management of TBI (22), with special consideration of potential untoward effects on the fetus. Once the mother and fetus are assessed, the appropriate diagnostic and therapeutic maneuvers should be implemented.

REFERENCES

1. Sosin DM, Sniezek JE, Thurman DJ. Incidence of mild and moderate brain injury in the United States. 1991. *Brain Inj* 1996;10:47–54.
2. Kraus JF. Epidemiologic features of injuries to the central nervous system. In: Anderson DW, ed. *Neuroepidemiology: a tribute to Bruce Schoenberg.* Boca Raton: CRC Press, 1991:334–354.
3. Jackson CF. Accidental injury: the problem and the initiatives. In: Buchsbaum HJ, ed. *Trauma in pregnancy.* Philadelphia: WB Saunders Co., 1979:1–20.
4. Gennarelli TA. Cerebral concussion and diffuse brain injuries. In: Cooper PR, ed. *Head injury.* Baltimore: Williams & Wilkins, 1987:108–124.
5. Cooper PR. Posttraumatic intracranial mass lesions. In: Cooper PR, ed. *Head injury.* Baltimore: Williams & Wilkins, 1987:238–284.
6. Bruno LA. Focal intracranial hematoma. In: Torg JS, ed. *Athletic injuries to the head, neck and face.* Philadelphia: Lea and Febiger, 1982:105–121.
7. Cicerone KD, Kalmar K. Persistent postconcussion syndrome: the structure of subjective complains after traumatic brain injury. *J Head Trauma Rehab* 1995;10:1–17.
8. Alves W, Macciocchi SN, Barth JT. Postconcussion Syndrome after uncomplicated mild head injury. *J Head Trauma Rehab* 1993;8:48–59.
9. Mittenberg W, Burton DB. A survey of treatment for postconcussion syndrome. *Brain Inj* 1994;8:429–437.
10. Rimel RQ, Geordani R, Borth JT, et al. Disability caused by minor head injury. *J Neurosurg* 1981;9:221–228.
11. Jennett B. *Epilepsy after non-missile head injury.* Chicago: Year-Book Medical Publishers, 1975.
12. Yablon SA. Posttraumatic seizures. *Arch Phys Med Rehab* 1993;74:983–1001.
13. Annegers JF, Hauser WA, Coan SP, et al. *New Engl J Med* 1998;338:20–24.
14. Temkin NR, Dikmen SS, Wilensky AJ, et al. A randomized, double-blind study of phenytoin for the prevention of post-traumatic seizures. *N Engl J Med* 1990;323:497–502.
15. Manaka S. Cooperative prospective study on posttraumatic epilepsy: risk factors and the effect of prophylactic anticonvulsant. *Jpn J Psychiatry Neurol* 1992;46:311–315.
16. McQueen JK, Blackwood DHR, Harris P, et al. Low risk of late post-traumatic seizures following severe head injury: implications for clinical trials of prophylaxis. *J Neurol Neurosurg Psychiatry* 1983;46:899–904.
17. Temkin NR, Dikmen SS, Anderson GD, et al. Valproate therapy for prevention of posttraumatic seizures: a randomized trial. *J Neurosurg* 1999;91:593–600.
18. Marmarou A, Foda MAA, Bandoh K, et al. Posttraumatic ventriculomegaly: hydrocephalus or atrophy? A new approach for diagnosis using CSF dynamics. *J Neurosurg* 1996;85:1026–1035.
19. Doherty D. Posttraumatic hydrocephalus. *Phys Med Rehabil Clin North Am* 1992;3:389–405.
20. Shackford SR, Mackersie RC, Hoyt DB, et al. Impact of trauma system on outcome of severely injured patients. *Arch Surg* 1987;122:523–527.
21. Marshall LF, Gautille T, Klauber MR, et al. The outcome of severe closed head injury. *J Neurosurg* 1991;75:S28–S36.
22. Guidelines for the management of severe traumatic brain injury. *J Neurotrauma* 2000;17:449–553.
23. Teasdale G, Jennett B. Assessment of coma and impaired consciousness: a practical scale. *Lancet* 1974;1:81–84.
24. Braakman R, Avezaat CJ, Maas AT, et al. Interobserver agreement in assessment of motor response of Glasgow Coma Scale. *Cl Neurol Neurosurg* 1977;80:100–106.
25. Fielding K, Rowley G: Reliability of assessment by skilled observers using Glasgow Coma Scale. *Aust J Adv Nursing* 1990;7:13–21.
26. Marshall LF, Gautille T, Klauber MR, et al. The out-

come of severe closed head injury. *J Neurosurg* 1991; 75:S28–S36.

27. Gennarelli TA, Champion HR, Copes WS, et al. Comparison of mortality, morbidity and severity in 59,713 head-injured patients with 114,447 patients with extracranial injuries. *J Trauma* 1994;37:962–968.

28. Wilberger JE. Emergency care and initial evaluation. In: Cooper PR, ed. *Head injury*. 3rd ed. Baltimore: Williams & Wilkins, 1993:27–41.

29. Chesnut RM, Marshall LF, Klauber MR, et al. The role of secondary brain injury in determining outcome from severe head injury. *J Trauma* 1993;34:216–222.

30. Marmarou A, Anderson RL, Ward JD, et al. Impact of ICP instability and hypotension on outcome in patients with severe head trauma. *J Neurosurg* 1991;75: S159–S166.

31. Miller JD, Becker DP, Ward JD, et al. Significance of intracranial hypertension in severe head injury. *J Neurosurg* 1977;47:503–510.

32. Marshall LF, Smith RW, Shapiro HM. The outcome with aggressive treatment in severe head injuries. The significance of intracranial pressure monitoring. *J Neurosurg* 1979;50:20–25.

33. Narayan RK, Kishore PRS, Becker DP, et al. Intracranial pressure: to monitor or not to monitor. *J Neurosurg* 1982;56:650–659.

34. Rosner MJ, Daughton S. Cerebral perfusion pressure management in head injury. *J Trauma* 1990;30: 933–941.

35. Braakman R, Schouten HJA, Blaauw-van DM, et al. Mega-dose steroids in severe head injury. *J Neurosurg* 1983;58:326–330.

36. Cooper PR, Moody S, Clark WK, et al. Dexamethasone and severe head injury. A prospective double-blind study. *J Neurosurg* 1979;51:307–316.

37. Dearden NM, Gibson JS, McDowell DG, et al. Effect of high-dose dexamethasone on outcome from severe head injury. *J Neurosurg* 1986;64:81–88.

38. Giannotta SL, Weiss MH, Apuzzo MLJ, et al. High-dose glucocorticoids in the management of severe head injury. *Neurosurgery* 1984;15:497–501.

39. Grumme T, Baethmann A, Kolodziejczyk D, et al. Treatment of patients with severe head injury by triamcinolone: a prospective, controlled multicenter clinical trial of 396 cases. *Res Exp Med (Berl)* 1995;195: 217–229.

40. Gudeman SK, Miller JD, Becker DP. Failure of high-dose steroid therapy to influence intracranial pressure in patients with severe head injury. *J Neurosurg* 1979;51: 301–306.

41. Saul TG, Ducker TB, Salcman M, et al. Steroids in severe head injury. A prospective randomized clinical trial. *J Neurosurg* 1981;54:596–600.

42. Bullock R, Teasdale GM. Head injuries. In: Driscoll P, Skinner D, Earlam R, eds. *ABC of major trauma*. BMJ Medical Publishing, 1991.

43. Muizelaar JP, Lutz HA, Becker DP. Effect of mannitol on ICP and CBF and correlation with pressure autoregulation in severely head-injured patients. *J Neurosurg* 1984;61:700–706.

44. Feig PU, McCurdy DK. The hypertonic state. *N Engl J Med* 1997;297:1449.

45. Langfitt TW, Gennarelli TA. Can the outcome from head injury be improved? *J Neurosurg* 1982;56:19–25.

46. Miller JD, Butterworth JF, Gudeman SK, et al. Further experience for the management of severe head injury. *J Neurosurg* 1981;54:289–299.

47. Kassell NF, Hitchon PW, Gerk MK, et al. Alterations in cerebral blood flow, oxygen metabolism, and electrical activity produced by high-dose thiopental. *Neurosurgery* 1980;7:598–603.

48. Gudeman SK, Young HF, Miller JD, et al. Indications for operative treatment and operative technique in closed head injury. In: Becker DP, Gudeman SK, eds. *Textbook of head injury*. Philadelphia: WB Saunders Co., 1989:128–181.

49. Hoff WS, D'Anekui LF, Tinkoff GH, et al. Maternal predictors of fetal demise in trauma during pregnancy. *Surg Gynecol Obstet* 1991;192:175–180.

50. Buchsbaum HJ, Cruikshank DP. Postmortem cesarean section. In: Buchsbaum HJ, ed. *Trauma in pregnancy*. Philadelphia: WB Saunders Co., 1979:236–249.

Neurological Complications of Pregnancy, Second Edition, edited by Brian Hainline and Orrin Devinsky. Lippincott Williams & Wilkins, Philadelphia © 2002.

8

Critical Care Management of Neurologic Catastrophes

Adam S. Mednick and *Stephan A. Mayer

*Neurological Associates of New Haven, P.C., New Haven, Connecticut; and *Division of Critical Care Neurology, Neurological Institute, New York, New York, U.S.A.*

Critically ill pregnant patients with neurologic disorders may present with either primary neurologic conditions, such as dural sinus thrombosis and subarachnoid hemorrhage, or systemic disorders with secondary neurologic involvement, such as eclampsia. Approximately 0.5% of all pregnant women require intensive care unit (ICU) admission for complications related to pregnancy, and of these, the mortality rate may be as high as 20%.

GENERAL PRINCIPLES OF NEUROCRITICAL CARE

General principles of ICU care involving the pregnant patient are the same as those for nonpregnant patients. In the antepartum period, evaluation and treatment of the mother should take precedence over that of the fetus. Continuous monitoring of fetal vital signs in the ICU may be accomplished using nonstress testing, which assesses acceleration in fetal heart rate with fetal movement.

General Considerations

In the ICU, the initial evaluation of the pregnant patient should focus on rapid correction of mean arterial blood pressure (MAP) abnormalities, rehydration using intravenous (IV) crystalloid fluids, maintenance of adequate arterial oxygenation, treatment of infec-

tion, correction of coagulopathies and electrolyte disturbances, and avoidance of peripheral deep venous thrombosis. Intubation and mechanical ventilation may be required to protect a patient's airway if her level of consciousness becomes depressed. Insertion of a central venous or pulmonary artery catheter may be required to assess hemodynamic status and to guide treatment if cardiac or pulmonary dysfunction is present.

Management issues specific to neurocritical care include control of agitation and pain, maintenance of normal intracranial pressure (ICP) and cerebral perfusion pressure (CPP), management of seizures, and anticoagulation in cerebrovascular disorders. A comprehensive review of the neurologic management of critically ill patients is beyond the scope of this chapter; many excellent reviews are available to the interested reader (1–5).

Cardiovascular Management

Correction of systemic blood pressure abnormalities in the critically ill pregnant patient can be crucial, particularly in the setting of eclampsia and subarachnoid or intracerebral hemorrhage. Hypertension may be exacerbated by pain, agitation, and resisting or "fighting" the ventilator. Left untreated, hypertension may overwhelm normal cerebral autoregulatory mechanisms, leading to devel-

TABLE 8.1. *Selected short-acting vasoactive drugs for ICP management*

Agent	Pharmacology	Dosage range
Blood pressure reduction		
Labetalol	α_1 and β_1 blocker	2–3 mg/min
Nicardipine	Calcium channel blocker	5–15 mg/hr
Blood pressure elevation		
Dopamine	α_1 and β_1 agonist	5–30 µg/kg/min
Norepinephrine	α_1 and β_1 agonist	.03–0.6 µg/kg/min
Phenylephrine	α_1 agonist	2–10 µg/kg/min

opment or exacerbation of cerebral edema and intracranial hypertension. Overzealous treatment with antihypertensive medications may lead to hypotension, which is less well tolerated by the brain than hypertension. Too-rapid correction of systemic hypertension may also result in compromised uteroplacental blood flow.

In patients with abnormal intracranial compliance, hypotension can trigger reflexive compensatory cerebral vascular dilatation in response to inadequate CPP, which can lead to further elevation of ICP (plateau waves). Severe hypertension (MAP greater than 130 or CPP greater than 110 mm Hg) should be treated with parenterally administered antihypertensive medications (Table 8.1), and blood pressure should be monitored with a radial arterial catheter. In patients with elevated ICP, blood pressure management should be guided in terms of target CPP levels (calculated as MAP minus ICP), rather than mean or systolic blood pressures. The goal of antihypertensive therapy in the critically ill pregnant patient should focus generally on reducing MAP not to premorbid levels, but to levels at which impairment of both cerebral autoregu-

lation and uteroplacental blood flow are avoided.

Neurologic Assessment

Neurologic assessment in the ICU focuses on repeated, standardized examinations. Either focal ("lateralizing") or generalized neurologic abnormalities may occur. Focal abnormalities include aphasia, visual field deficits, and hemiparesis, whereas generalized abnormalities are manifested as changes in the level of consciousness, ranging from confusion to coma, diffuse hyperreflexia, bilateral clonus, and extensor plantar responses. Causes of focal abnormalities include ischemic stroke or intracerebral hemorrhage; generalized abnormalities, indicative of encephalopathy, may occur in the setting of metabolic derangements, hypertensive encephalopathy, postictal states, or generalized cerebral edema or ischemia. Intravenous sedation with fast-acting continuous infusion agents such as propofol and fentanyl (Table 8.2) is critical for treating agitation or delirium, pain, elevated ICP, seizures, withdrawal states, or combinations of these problems. When using these agents, it is essential to

TABLE 8.2. *Selected short-acting intravenous sedatives for neurocritical care*

Agent	Pharmacology	Dosage range
Morphine sulfate	Opioid (sedative hypnotic with analgesic properties)	2–5 mg IVP Q 1–4 hr
Fentanyl	Opioid (short acting, 100× more potent than morphine)	0.3–3.0 µg/kg/hr
Propofol	Alkylphenol (sedative–hypnotic, ultrashort-acting)	0.6–6 mg/kg/hr
Midazolam	Benzodiazepine (short-acting sedative–hypnotic)	0.05–0.1 mg/kg/hr

Dosages are approximate and should be titrated to the patient's level of agitation and ICP.
Combinations of agents may be more effective than the use of a single agent.

intermittently discontinue them on a regular basis (one to four times daily) to allow for accurate neurologic examinations and to assess the need for continued treatment.

Intracranial Pressure

Intracranial hypertension always results from increased intracranial volume, and all therapies for elevated ICP work by reducing intracranial volume. Intracranial mass lesions also can lead to brain-tissue displacement and herniation without necessarily causing increased ICP. Because CPP is calculated as MAP minus ICP, any condition that increases ICP may result in decreased CPP. A CPP of greater than 110 mm Hg may promote the development of either diffuse or focal cerebral edema, whereas a CPP of 70 mm Hg or less may lead to cerebral ischemia. In most neuro-ICUs, the goal is to maintain CPP greater than 70 mm Hg and ICP less than 20 mm Hg. To accurately estimate CPP, both the ICP and MAP pressure transducers must be positioned at head level. Stepwise protocols for treating elevated ICP in the ICU are shown in Tables 8.3 and 8.4.

Although studies have shown that the use of osmotic agents such as mannitol may promote fetal dehydration (6), these agents should not be withheld in the treatment of cerebral edema leading to ICP elevation or herniation. As an alternative, hypertonic saline (3% solution at 0.5 cc per kg per hr to 1.0 cc per kg per hr, or 30 mL boluses of 23.4% solution) may be used to treat cerebral edema, either alone or in conjunction with mannitol.

TABLE 8.3. *Emergency measures for ICP reduction in an unmonitored patient with clinical signs of herniation*

1. Elevate head of bed 15–30 degrees
2. Normal saline (0.9%) at 80–100 cc/hr (avoid hypotonic fluids)
3. Intubate and hyperventilate (target pCO_2 = 26–30 mm Hg)
4. Mannitol 20% 1–1.5 g/kg via rapid IV infusion
5. Foley catheter
6. CT scan and neurosurgical consultation

TABLE 8.4. *Stepwise treatment protocol for elevated ICP (>20 mm Hg for more than 10 minutes) in a monitored patient*

1. Consider repeat CT scanning and definitive surgical intervention
2. Sedation to attain a quiet, motionless state
3. CPP optimization (pressor infusion if less than 70 mm Hg, or BP lowering agents if more than 110 mm Hg)
4. Mannitol .25–1 g/kg IV (repeat every 1–6 hours as needed)
5. Hyperventilation to pCO_2 levels of 26–30 mm Hg
6. High-dose pentobarbital therapy (load with 15–20 mg/kg, then 1–4 mg/kg/hr)
7. Hypothermia (32–33°C)

ACUTE ISCHEMIC STROKE

Cerebrovascular disease is the third leading cause of death among women in the United States, with an estimated incidence of approximately 10 per 100,000. According to some reports, the risk of developing a stroke increases during pregnancy and the puerperium (7,8), a conclusion not shared by other studies (9,10). The incidence of arterial cerebrovascular occlusive disease is highest in the second and third trimesters of pregnancy as well as during the puerperium; venous occlusive disease, however, occurs more commonly in the third trimester of pregnancy as well as during the puerperium. Previous pregnancies also may confer an increased risk of stroke (11,12).

Stroke during pregnancy has many causes that can be divided into five broad categories (13) (Table 8.5). The majority of strokes during pregnancy involve abnormalities of the internal and middle cerebral arteries (14), due most commonly to embolic disease. Women with a preexisting history of hypertension, diabetes mellitus, or tobacco use may be predisposed to early development of atherosclerotic disease. The risk of cardioembolic stroke may be increased in pregnant women with a history of preexisting cardiac disease, including valvular abnormalities (mitral valve prolapse, rheumatic heart disease) and dysrhythmias (atrial fibrillation). In some women without such a history of cardiac disease, peripartum cardiomyopathy may develop, which occurs

TABLE 8.5. *Causes of ischemic stroke during pregnancy*

1. Large-vessel atherothrombotic disease
2. Small-vessel (lacunar) disease
3. Cardioembolism
   Atrial fibrillation
   Valvular disease
     Rheumatic heart disease
     Mitral valve prolapse
     Atrial fibrillation
     Prosthetic heart valve
   Peripartum cardiomyopathy
   Endocarditis
     Subacute bacterial
     Nonbacterial thrombotic
   Patent foramen ovale
4. Other etiologies
   Arterial dissection
   Fibromuscular dysplasia
   Vasculitis
   Moyamoya disease
   Sickle cell disease
   Hypercoagulopathy
     Proteins C and S deficiencies
     Antithrombin III deficiency
     Antiphospholipid antibody syndrome
     Disseminated intravascular coagulation
     Factor V Leiden
     Prothrombin gene mutation
5. Unknown etiology

typically in late pregnancy and causes congestive heart failure. Acquired free protein-S deficiency is extremely common, and many consider pregnancy a hypercoaguable state in and of itself (14).

Diagnostic evaluation and treatment of ischemic stroke in the pregnant patient is the same as that of the nonpregnant patient, with few exceptions. Using appropriate precautions, such as abdominal shielding during x-rays, computed tomography (CT) scan, and angiography, the risk of exposure of the fetus to radiation can be minimized. Magnetic resonance imaging (MRI) has not been shown to be associated with fetal abnormalities, although long-term studies addressing this issue are lacking. Other diagnostic studies include carotid and transcranial ultrasonography and echocardiography.

Avoidance of hypotension in the acute phase of ischemic stroke is extremely important. Blood pressure often is elevated immediately following a stroke to ensure adequate cerebral perfusion pressure, and it tends to return to baseline levels within 2 days to 2 weeks (15). In general, the use of antihypertensive medications should be avoided in the acute phase (less than 48 hrs), unless either the systolic pressure is greater than 220 mm Hg or the diastolic pressure is in excess of 110 mm Hg. If antihypertensive medications are needed, either labetalol or nicardipine is preferred, administered by continuous IV infusion, titrated to maintain either a systolic pressure of 160 mm Hg to 180 mm Hg or a diastolic pressure of 90 mm Hg to 110 mm Hg (Table 8.1).

Antiplatelet agents, such as aspirin, may be used during the second and third trimesters of pregnancy; their use during the first trimester is limited by concerns that they may cause congenital malformations (16). The optimal dosage during pregnancy is uncertain, although low-dose aspirin currently is favored (17,18).

Anticoagulation in the treatment of acute ischemic stroke during pregnancy is controversial because it may be associated with the development of uteroplacental hemorrhage. In contrast to warfarin, which is teratogenic, heparin probably is safe in most cases because it does not cross the placenta and it has a short half-life. Anticoagulation should be discontinued prior to delivery to minimize the risk of uteroplacental hemorrhage. In addition, consensus is lacking with respect to which form of heparin should be administered (unfractionated or low molecular weight) to pregnant stroke patients and which stroke subtypes should be treated with heparin, although most neurologists would probably favor heparin anticoagulation if either an embolic source or a basilar artery syndrome is suspected. No studies have examined the use of thrombolytic agents in the treatment of acute ischemic stroke during pregnancy. However, t-PA has been used successfully to treat pulmonary embolism without significant adverse effects (19).

SUBARACHNOID AND INTRACEREBRAL HEMORRHAGE

Nontraumatic intracranial hemorrhage accounts for up to 10% of maternal mortality during pregnancy (20,21). The most common

TABLE 8.6. *Common causes of nontraumatic intracranial hemorrhage in pregnancy*

Hemorrhagic conversion of ischemic stroke
Rupture of congenital vascular abnormality
    Berry aneurysm
    Arteriovenous malformation
Eclampsia
Coagulopathies
Anticoagulant therapy
Drugs
    Cocaine
    Phenylpropanolamine
Cerebral venous sinus thrombosis
Moyamoya disease

TABLE 8.7. *Modified Hunt & Hess grading scale for subarachnoid hemorrhage*

Grade	Description
I	Asymptomatic or mild headache, with normal neurologic examination
II	Moderate-to-severe headache with normal neurologic examination
III	Lethargy, confusion, or mild focal neurologic signs (except isolated cranial nerve deficit)
IV	Stupor
V	Coma

presentations are subarachnoid hemorrhage (SAH) caused by rupture of an intracranial aneurysm and intracerebral hemorrhage caused by an arteriovenous malformation (AVM) (Table 8.6). The risk of initial aneurysmal or AVM rupture increases during pregnancy, presumably as cardiovascular stresses increase as a result of hemodynamic and hormonal changes (22,23); the highest incidence of SAH appears to be in the third trimester (24). Pregnancy does not, in and of itself, increase the incidence of SAH (25,26). The risk of rebleeding from either an aneurysm or AVM is reportedly highest during delivery and the puerperium (27).

Subarachnoid Hemorrhage

The clinical presentation of pregnant patients with SAH is similar to that of nonpregnant patients. The most common initial complaint is severe headache of sudden onset, in association with symptoms of meningeal irritation, including nausea and vomiting, nuchal rigidity, and photophobia. Patients may experience a transient loss of consciousness immediately following SAH onset, followed by variable changes in level of consciousness and possibly focal neurologic deficits, the severity of which are graded using the modified Hunt & Hess grading scale (Table 8.7) (28).

Brain CT imaging usually is performed first on a patient suspected of having an SAH; if negative, a lumbar puncture to assess for the presence of red blood cells and xanthochro-

mia should be performed. The absence of xanthochromia shortly after the onset of headache does not disprove the presence of SAH because xanthochromia requires at least 6 to 12 hours to develop. Furthermore, similar abnormalities of the cerebrospinal fluid (CSF) may be seen in other disorders, such as eclampsia.

If SAH is diagnosed, a four-vessel contrast cerebral angiogram, rather than a magnetic resonance angiogram, should be performed without delay. A negative angiogram, seen in up to 20% of patients with SAH (29), does not disprove the presence of a small intracranial vascular abnormality that may not have been visualized because local thrombosis, arterial spasm, or poor technique (30). With the exception of perimesencephalic SAH, in which case repeat angiography is always negative (31), a follow-up angiogram should be performed after 2 weeks.

All patients with acute aneurysmal SAH should be treated with nimodipine, which is a calcium-channel blocker shown to decrease adverse outcomes associated with SAH-induced vasospasm, and fosphenytoin, an anticonvulsant medication. Hemodynamic parameters, including blood pressure, heart rate, and respiratory rate, are monitored closely. Intubation and mechanical ventilation may be indicated if an SAH patient shows evidence of cardiopulmonary distress (such as from SAH-induced neurogenic stunned myocardium or neurogenic pulmonary edema (32), which tends to occur more frequently in young women) or if she is unable to protect her airway as a result of decreased level of consciousness.

If a patient with SAH is stuporous or comatose and either the initial or follow-up brain CT scans show hydrocephalus, an external ventricular drain is placed emergently, and both ICP and CPP are monitored closely. The decision to insert a pulmonary artery catheter is based on the patient's hemodynamic status; indications include development of systemic hypotension, pulmonary edema, impaired cardiovascular function, renal failure, and adult respiratory distress syndrome.

The immediate goal in treating patients with SAH is to prevent rebleeding by either clipping or coiling of the aneurysm. The risk of rebleeding from a ruptured aneurysm is highest within the first 24 hrs following the initial bleed and the cumulative risk is 20% over the first 2 weeks. Current opinion favors early treatment of pregnant SAH patients at the time of initial presentation (22,25,26,33), rather than deferring such treatment until after delivery. Decisions regarding whether to treat with surgical clipping or Guglielmi detachable coil embolization must balance the risk of prolonged fetal exposure to general anesthesia associated with clipping against increased exposure to IV contrast agents associated with coiling.

Two specific perioperative protocols implemented during aneurysmal surgery are induction of hypotension and hypothermia, both of which are done to minimize the risk of aneurysmal rupture during surgery. In the pregnant patient, hypotension may cause fetal ischemia and thus should be done cautiously if at all, whereas fetal risk from hypothermia is uncertain.

In addition to treatment of the aneurysm, other therapies are aimed at minimizing secondary complications related to SAH. Generalized cerebral edema may develop in the acute stage and require treatment of increased ICP. Arterial vasospasm, which occurs in up to 70% of patients with aneurysmal SAH, typically begins approximately 3 days following the initial aneurysmal bleed and peaks in 7 to 10 days, followed by gradual resolution over the course of 2 to 3 weeks. Vasospasm can be a serious complication associated with high rates of maternal morbidity and mortality, particularly for those patients whose Hunt & Hess grades (Table 8.7) are III or more. Worsening of the initial neurologic examination or the development of new neurologic signs may indicate symptomatic vasospasm. The extent and severity of arterial vasospasm can be estimated by performing transcranial Doppler sonography, which measures blood-flow velocity.

Symptomatic vasospasm should be treated with hypertensive hypervolemic therapy, comprising pharmacologically induced hypertension with phenylephrine, dopamine, or norepinephrine, and hypervolemia (34). Pressors are titrated to achieve the MAP at which the new neurologic deficits are eliminated, with a maximum systolic blood pressure not exceeding 220 mm Hg. Hypervolemic therapy comprises increasing IV fluid rate, using isotonic saline at a rate between 125 to 150 cc per hour, and administering colloid fluids (5% albumisol, given as 250 cc boluses every 2 hours) to keep the central venous pressure (CVP) greater than 8 mm Hg and the pulmonary artery diastolic pressure greater than 14 mm Hg. The cardiovascular status of the patient must be monitored carefully for the development of fluid overload. A four-vessel contrast angiogram should be repeated immediately in all SAH patients who exhibit new neurologic deficits as a result of suspected symptomatic vasospasm. Should angiography reveal spasm, angioplasty and administration of local papaverine or verapamil are further treatment options (35,36).

Intracerebral Hemorrhage

Intracerebral hemorrhage in pregnancy often is caused by a ruptured AVM; other causes are listed in Table 8.6. The treatment of intracranial AVMs, like that of aneurysms, is divided into nonsurgical and surgical categories. Nonsurgical therapies include embolization and occlusion via neuroangiographic endovascular procedures as well as gamma-knife irradiation, whereas surgical intervention involves resection of the AVM; in many cases, embolization is done prior to surgical resection. General medical management strategies of AVM-associated hemorrhage is similar to that of aneurysmal hemorrhage except that nimodipine is not recommended because vasospasm does not usually develop following SAH from AVM rupture. Left untreated, AVMs can cause recurrent hemorrhages, seizures and epilepsy, severe headaches, and "steal" phenomena (37,38), in which blood is shunted preferentially to the AVM from nearby brain regions, thereby producing symptoms and signs of focal ischemia. Bleeding into a ventricle may lead to the development of hydrocephalus.

The decision to surgically treat an AVM in a pregnant patient is based on the stability of her neurologic examination and the estimated risk of early rebleeding. Immediate surgery is indicated for those patients who experience acute deterioration (39,40) or for those with dural AVMs, which have a high risk of rebleeding. Other risk factors for early AVM rebleeding include small size, exclusively deep venous drainage, high feeding artery pressures, and identification of a discrete feeding artery or intranidal aneurysm. Conservative nonsurgical therapy is recommended for neurologically stable patients, in whom every attempt is made to bring the pregnancy to term; in these patients, AVM treatment can be deferred. The risks of peri- and postoperative complications incurred to both the patient and her fetus (such as induced hypotension, which can cause fetal ischemia) must be balanced against those risks of delaying surgery until after delivery.

DURAL VENOUS SINUS THROMBOSIS

Dural venous sinus thrombosis (DVST) is a serious disorder that occurs in approximately 0.04% of pregnant women, most commonly either in the third trimester of pregnancy or during the puerperium (17,41–43). Risk factors that increase the possibility of developing DVST during pregnancy are listed in Table 8.8,

TABLE 8.8. *Risk factors for the development of DVST*

Infectious	Noninfectious
Sinusitis	Hypercoagulable states
Otitis media	Trauma
Meningitis	Malignancy
	Connective tissue disorders

of which hypercoagulability occurs most commonly. DVST usually develops between the second and third postpartum weeks (44), although it may develop at any time during pregnancy (45–47).

The pathophysiologic mechanisms thought to cause DVST have not been completely elucidated. A triad of abnormalities may be involved, including stasis of blood flow, damage to intracerebral vasculature, and hypercoagulability (48,49). Abnormalities of coagulation have been implicated because certain antepartum disorders, including deficiencies of antithrombin III, protein C and protein S, factor V Leiden mutation, and sickle cell disease, are more commonly associated with DVST (50–52). Anemia, sepsis, and dehydration may further exacerbate the hypercoagulable state induced by these coagulopathic disorders.

Neurologic manifestations of DVST depend on which sinus is involved; either diffuse or focal cerebral dysfunction may occur. Diffuse dysfunction, which is seen in DVST involving the superior sagittal sinus, presents as headache, bilateral papilledema, vomiting, and decline in level of consciousness and is caused by acute intracranial hypertension (AIH) secondary to diffuse cerebral edema. Focal neurologic dysfunction, such as hemiparesis, visual changes, and seizures, may be caused by intraparenchymal venous hemorrhage or ischemic venous infarct induced by propagation of a thrombus extending from the dural sinus into a cortical vein. Ophthalmodynia, chemosis, and proptosis are associated with DVST involving the cavernous sinus.

The diagnostic evaluation of patients with DVST should include assessment of coagulation and hematologic parameters. Complete blood cell count, platelets, prothrombin time, partial thromboplastin time, erythrocyte sedimentation rate, serum chemistries, urinalysis, and chest x-ray should be performed. Additional studies include antithrombin III, proteins C and S, factor V Leiden, prothrombin gene mutation, lupus anticoagulant, and anticardiolipin antibodies. CT of the skull and chest also may be helpful to rule out potential sources of infection. CSF studies are often abnormal and include increased protein levels when the CSF is under increased pressure, and increased red blood cells (53), which may occur as a result of intraventricular extension of an intraparenchymal hemorrhage.

CT in DVST most often shows hypodensities, indicative of venous infarction, adjacent to a dural sinus, with or without associated hemorrhage. In approximately 20% of patients with DVST, brain CT studies may be normal (1), under which circumstances MRI should be performed. MRI with MR venography is generally the imaging procedure of choice in patients suspected of having DVST. On MRI, thrombus in a dural sinus or vein appears as an absence of flow void because of obstruction of free flow of blood. In addition to both CT and MRI, cerebral angiography may be performed. The gold standard to diagnose DVST is contrast angiography, which may demonstrate nonfilling of affected dural sinus and veins during the venous phase. Over the last decade, the use of MR venography in the evaluation of DVST has increased rapidly and is now often used in lieu of contrast angiography (54,55), particularly given the concern of contrast exposure to the unborn fetus.

Dural venous sinus thrombosis is associated with the development of various neurologic complications, including intracerebral hemorrhage, seizures, and acute intracranial hypertension, thereby making diagnosis and treatment of pregnant patients with DVST an extremely challenging task. It is best performed in an ICU. Treatment will depend on which risk factors are identified, which neurologic complications occur, identification of other medical comorbidity, and whether the patient is ante- or postpartum.

If an infectious cause of DVST is identified, antibiotic therapy is warranted, the choice of which depends on identification of the offending microorganism and which dural sinus is infected. Superior sagittal sinus thrombosis most commonly is associated with infections caused by *Staphylococcus aureus,* β-hemolytic streptococci species, pneumococci, and *Klebsiella;* cavernous sinus thrombosis is most often associated with *Staphylococcus aureus* infections; and lateral sinus thrombosis is often in association with infections caused by either staphylococci or anaerobes.

Treatment of DVST with anticoagulation during pregnancy, using either heparin or warfarin, is controversial because of a lack of definitive studies (17). In addition, experience with either local or direct thrombolytic therapy, using tissue plasminogen activator, streptokinase, or urokinase, in DVST during pregnancy is lacking (56,57). Although neither heparin nor its derivatives cross the uteroplacental barrier, thereby minimizing potential risks to the fetus, its use in the treatment of DVST during pregnancy often is avoided because of its association with the development of potentially dangerous complications, such as maternal intracerebral hemorrhage, puerperal bleeding, and thrombocytopenia. Low molecular weight heparin in the treatment of DVST has not been shown to be effective (58), but it remains a treatment alternative.

The use of warfarin during pregnancy or puerperium is contraindicated. Because warfarin crosses the uteroplacental barrier, its use may increase the fetal risk of developing bleeding or congenital abnormalities (59). According to one study (60) in which the effects of maternal warfarin therapy on the fetus were assessed, approximately 20% of pregnancies resulted in spontaneous abortions, stillbirths, or congenital abnormalities. Warfarin is also contraindicated after the thirty-fourth week of pregnancy because it may lead to serious bleeding in both the mother and fetus during delivery and in the puerperium.

Seizures, which are common in DVST, are the result of focal irritation of brain tissue secondary to the effects of either ischemia or hemorrhage. Patients usually present with focal seizures that may then secondarily generalize. The decision to begin antiepileptic drugs (AEDs) in a pregnant patient with DVST should weigh the benefits of such treatment against the potential risks. In the first trimester of pregnancy, AEDs, particularly phenytoin, may be teratogenic. The use of certain anticonvulsant medications, such as phenobarbital, at the time of delivery may be contraindicated because of an increased risk of bleeding caused by impairment of vitamin K metabolism.

Intracranial hypertension may develop in a patient with DVST as a consequence of cerebral edema secondary to either increased CSF pressure or an intracranial focal mass lesion. Management of increased ICP is shown in Table 8.4.

GENERALIZED TONIC-CLONIC STATUS EPILEPTICUS

Status epilepticus (SE) is an emergent neurologic disorder that demands immediate medical intervention. SE is defined as either a continuous seizure lasting at least 10 minutes, or two or more seizures over 30 minutes with incomplete recovery of consciousness between seizures (61,62). Utilizing both clinical and electroencephalographic criteria (63), the term "status epilepticus" encompasses several seizure types, including generalized seizures (tonic-clonic, absence, myoclonic, tonic, clonic, or atonic) and partial seizures (either simple or complex), which may be broadly classified into either convulsive SE (cSE) or nonconvulsive SE (ncSE). Generalized convulsive SE in the pregnant patient is the topic of the following discussion.

Although approximately 60,000 new cases of SE are diagnosed annually in the United States, this condition is exceedingly rare during pregnancy (64–66). Pregnant women with a previous history of seizures may develop SE, whereas for others, SE may be the first manifestation of seizures. In women without a prior history of seizures, pregnancy does not appear to be a risk factor for the development of SE (67). Common causes of SE in pregnant women are listed in Table 8.9. In approximately 30% of cases of SE, no cause can be determined (68).

Despite fears amongst newly pregnant patients regarding the potential teratogenic effects of AEDs, which may lead to problems with medication compliance in the first trimester, the incidence of SE is actually highest in the latter half of pregnancy, particularly during the third trimester, or during labor (67). Hormonal changes, such as increased levels of progesterone and estrogen, may lower the seizure threshold (69). Alterations in medication pharmacokinetics, including increased renal clearance, increased maternal volumes of distribution, and increased hepatic metabolism, may lead to subtherapeutic serum levels of AEDs during pregnancy (70); however, the effects associated with such alterations may be offset by an increased free (unbound) fraction of the AED, resulting from decreased protein binding (71).

Convulsive SE always should be managed in an ICU. The keys to management of SE are recognition of the emergent nature of this disorder and prompt initiation of appropriate therapy; without such treatment, SE can become resistant to any such treatment subsequently implemented, resulting in higher maternal and fetal morbidity and mortality (72,73). Severe, and sometimes permanent, cerebral damage may begin in less than 2 hours following the onset of SE and can occur in up to half of patients following termination of SE (68, 74).

TABLE 8.9. *Common causes of status epilepticus in pregnancy*

Subtherapeutic levels of antiepileptic medications
Infection
   Meningitis
   Encephalitis
Medication toxicity
Illicit drugs
Ethanol withdrawal
Eclampsia
Intracerebral hemorrhage
Head trauma
Brain tumor
Cardiac arrest

In the early part of the twentieth century, termination of pregnancy in a woman with SE was considered standard practice (64,75). Following introduction of AEDs, effective control of SE often was achieved without termination of pregnancy; many such pregnancies then could be carried to term, often with delivery of a healthy infant. Management and treatment of the pregnant patient in SE should be the same as that for nonpregnant patients. In deciding on the choice of AED, despite the concerns of teratogenicity, treatment of the mother always must take precedence over that of the fetus. Although any of the AEDs used in the treatment of SE may potentially harm the fetus, the effects of SE itself on the fetus, including hypoxemia, hypotension, and acidosis, are probably much more harmful and can threaten the well-being of the mother as well (74,75). Only if SE cannot be brought under control despite optimal therapy with medications should termination of pregnancy be considered; fortunately, this is rare.

Following established protocols (61,76,77, 78), attention should first be given to airway and adequate ventilation. Although intubation may be avoided initially, it may become necessary to maintain adequate oxygenation when aspiration, hypoxemia, or pulmonary edema occurs or to circumvent suppression of respiratory drive resulting from AEDs such as the benzodiazepines and phenobarbital. Laboratory studies should include glucose, electrolytes, calcium, magnesium, creatine phosphokinase (to assess for rhabdomyolysis), and arterial blood gases. Continuous electrocardiographic and blood pressure monitoring also should be implemented. Additional studies also may include urine toxicology screen, CSF analysis, and imaging studies of the brain. Continuous electroencephalographic (cEEG) monitoring during SE (79), although not always available, is essential for detecting subtle ncSE or purely electrographic seizures after cSE is terminated, and for differentiating true epileptiform seizures from nonepileptiform pseudoseizures. Treatment is aimed at both stopping SE and managing the secondary complications of cSE. Fever and metabolic derangements, such as acidosis, dehydration, electrolyte abnormalities, and hypo- or hyperglycemia, should be treated promptly (78).

During SE, AEDs always are administered parenterally because gastrointestinal absorption is unreliable. Following cessation of SE and stabilization of the patient, AEDs then may be given enterally, through either a nasoduodenal or nasogastric tube. Treatment of SE first begins with 0.1 mg per kg of lorazepam (80,81), given in repeated 2 mg IV boluses slowly over 2 to 5 minutes; alternatively, 10 mg to 20 mg of diazepam may be given slowly over 2 minutes. Because SE can recur following administration of benzodiazepines, a second-line IV drug, usually fosphenytoin, then should be administered as a bolus of 15 to 20 mg per kg phenytoin equivalents (PE), at a rate not exceeding 150 mg PE per minute (78).

If SE continues despite the use of first- and second-line medications, it is labeled as refractory (rSE), and a third-line IV drug then is added. Although phenobarbital often is used following phenytoin, we prefer to use IV valproic acid (82–84), given as a 30 to 60 mg per kg loading dose followed by standard maintenance dosages because it is less sedating and causes fewer hemodynamic alterations. Phenobarbital is administered at a dose of 15 to 20 mg per kg, infused at 50 mg per minute, followed by a maintenance dosage of 1 to 3 mg per kg per day, in divided doses. If SE is refractory to the initial bolus of phenobarbital, additional boluses of 5 to 10 mg per kg may be used, regardless of serum drug levels.

For the remaining cases of rSE that do not respond effectively to the medications just described, continuously infused anesthetic medications may become necessary, usually either midazolam (a benzodiazepine), propofol (a sedative-hypnotic), or pentobarbital (a barbiturate), in conjunction with cEEG monitoring. Both midazolam and pentobarbital are pregnancy D category drugs, and as such are considered unsafe during pregnancy, whereas propofol is a category B drug. However, given the emergent nature of cSE, neurologic treatment of the mother always must take precedence over obstetric concerns. Both midazolam and propofol have the advantage of rapid onset of action and of rapid clearance when compared to pentobarbital. Midazolam is administered as an initial slow IV bolus of 0.2 mg per kg, followed by continuous infusion of 1 to 10 µg per kg per minute. Propofol is given as a bolus of 1 to 2 mg per kg, followed by continuous infusion of 2 to 10 mg per kg per hour.

Pentobarbital is often the only AED that will terminate severe rSE (85). The standard dosage is 10 to 20 mg per kg followed by continuous infusion at 1 to 4 mg per kg per hour, titrated to achieve a burst suppression pattern on cEEG (86). Pentobarbital is continued for 24 hours, followed by reassessment of the patient. Pentobarbital may cause marked cardiac suppression and hypotension, necessitating the use of inotropic drugs, such as dopamine or phenylephrine.

ECLAMPSIA

Eclampsia, a pregnancy-induced systemic disorder unique to humans, can include systemic hypertension, proteinuria, peripheral edema, and neurologic manifestations related to hypertensive encephalopathy. Other associated complications may include pulmonary edema, oliguric renal failure, hepatic failure, thrombocytopenia, and disseminated intravascular coagulation (HELLP syndrome) (87, 88). Apart from seizures, other neurologic manifestations of eclampsia include encephalopathy, cortical blindness, and stupor or coma related to diffuse cerebral edema (89). Risk factors for the development of eclampsia include primigravidas, extremes in maternal age, multiple pregnancies, and poor maternal nutritional status (90,92). In the United States, eclampsia complicates approximately 0.05% of all pregnancies (87) and maternal mortality rates range from less than 1% (92,93) to 12% (94). Eclampsia-induced neurologic disorders account for approximately 40% of all maternal deaths (91).

The underlying pathophysiological mechanisms responsible for the development of eclampsia are poorly understood. Through a cascade of events, endothelial dysfunction occurs, which leads to endothelial proliferation and fibrinoid necrosis of small arteries and arterioles (95,96), the end-result of which is multiorgan microvascular vasospasm and thrombotic occlusion (87). Endothelial dysfunction of the cerebral arterioles, in the presence of systemic hypertension, can lead to disruption of the blood–brain barrier and the development of vasogenic edema with predominant involvement of the arterial border zones.

No laboratory or imaging abnormalities are pathognomonic for eclampsia. CSF pressure usually is increased, and the protein level may be mildly to moderately elevated (97). Moderately increased red blood cells (RBCs) in the CSF are common early in the course of eclampsia (98); however, the presence of more than 5,000 RBCs per mm^3, particularly if xanthochromia is present, may indicate either subarachnoid hemorrhage or cerebral intraparenchymal hemorrhage with intraventricular extension (4). EEG, which is often abnormal in the majority of patients with eclampsia (87,99,100), may reveal diffuse or focal slowing, epileptiform discharges, or electrographic seizures (with or without clinical accompaniment). CT and MRI abnormalities include focal or diffuse edema (involving white matter more than gray), sulcal effacement, and ventricular or cisternal compression; these abnormalities, which do not enhance following administration of contrast, usually are situated in watershed and periventricular areas, predominantly in the cortical and subcortical regions of the occipital lobes, and in the deep gray matter (101–104). These abnormalities can be completely reversible (Figure 8.1). Cerebral angiography may demonstrate diffuse vasospasm, involving both large- and medium-sized cerebral arteries (105-107).

Following initial general management, the definitive treatment of eclampsia is termination of pregnancy and delivery of a viable fetus. There is considerable debate regarding the circumstances under which termination of

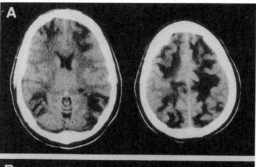

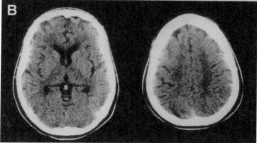

Fig. 8.1. **A:** Severe generalized cerebral edema with extensive bilateral lucencies involving the arterial borderzone regions in a 34-year-old woman with coma and elevated intracranial pressure due to eclampsia. **B:** Dramatic improvement was evident 28 days later, at which time she was profoundly disoriented but able to follow commands, with dysarthria, pseudobulbar effect, and bibrachial paresis. She eventually made a near-complete recovery.

pregnancy should be accomplished, and when. Most studies advocate the immediate termination of pregnancy if one or more of the following occur (90,108,109): rapid onset of eclampsia, patient exhibits worsening neurologic deficits, development of fetal distress, or multiorgan dysfunction. In the absence of any of these signs, a trial of antihypertensive therapy may be warranted in an effort to allow the pregnancy to progress to term (90).

Prompt treatment of systemic hypertension may lead to resolution of hypertensive encephalopathy, prevention of intracerebral hemorrhage, avoidance of both acute renal failure and congestive heart failure, and prevention of potentially life-threatening ventricular dysrhythmias. However, too rapid correction of systemic hypertension may result in

inadequate CPP, thereby placing the brain at risk for the development of diffuse ischemia (110,111). Control of severe systemic hypertension in patient with eclampsia is best done using intravenously administered parenteral antihypertensive agents, such as labetalol or nicardipine, which allow precise control of the blood pressure (Table 8.1). Hydralazine, diazoxide, and sodium nitroprusside all have been recommended for the treatment of hypertension in eclampsia, but they are difficult to titrate and may increase ICP as a result of direct vasodilatory effects on the cerebral vessels. Angiotensin-converting enzyme inhibitors (e.g., IV enalaprilat) are contraindicated because they may lead to fetal renal impairment. The goal of treatment should be to decrease the MAP to approximately premorbid levels and the cerebral perfusion pressure to 70 to 100 mm Hg.

Eclamptic seizures, which occur before the onset of labor in the majority of patients, usually begin focally and then may generalize secondarily. Neurologists and obstetricians have long differed with respect to treatment of seizures in eclampsia. Neurologists often first use benzodiazepines and phenytoin in the treatment of eclamptic seizures (90,91, 112,113), whereas obstetricians usually initiate therapy with magnesium sulfate (88, 114–117). The use of magnesium sulfate is frowned on by neurologists (112,113) because uncertainties regarding the cause of eclamptic seizures; however, recent studies have demonstrated the superiority of magnesium sulfate acutely (see Chapter 4). We recommend magnesium sulfate predelivery, and phenytoin and IV blood pressure medications postdelivery, as needed.

Increased ICP in eclampsia is most often a consequence of either cerebral edema or focal mass lesions and should be suspected in a patient with eclampsia who experiences neurologic deterioration or whose CT shows hydrocephalus, ventricular entrapment, or cisternal effacement. Management of increased ICP in the pregnant patient should be the same as that for nonpregnant patients, as shown in Table 8.4.

REFERENCES

1. Mayer SA, Dennis LJ. Management of increased intracranial pressure. *Neurologist* 1998;4:2–12.
2. Mayer SA, Coplin WM, Raps EC. Cerebral edema, intracranial pressure, and herniation syndromes. *J Stroke Cerebrovasc Dis* 1999;8:183–191.
3. Ropper AH. *Neurological and neurosurgical intensive care.* New York: Raven Press, 1993.
4. Wijdicks EFM. *The clinical practice of critical care neurology.* New York: Lippincott-Raven, 1997.
5. Bingaman WE, Frank JI. Malignant cerebral edema and intracranial hypertension. *Neurol Clin* 1995;13:479–509.
6. Knepper LE, Giuliani MJ. Cerebrovascular disease in women. *Cardiology* 1995;86:339–348.
7. Wiebers DO. Ischemic cerebrovascular complications of pregnancy. *Arch Neurol* 1985;42:1106–1113.
8. Simolke GA, Cox SM, Cunningham G. Cerebrovascular accidents complicating pregnancy and the puerperium. *Obstet Gynecol* 1991;78:37–42.
9. Awada A, Rajeh SA, Duarte R, et al. Stroke and pregnancy. *Int J Gynecol Obstet* 1995;48:157–161.
10. Kittner SJ, Stern BJ, Feeser BR, et al. Pregnancy and the risk of stroke. *N Engl J Med* 1996;335:768–774.
11. Qureshi AI, Giles WH, Croft JB, et al. Number of pregnancies and risk for stroke and stroke subtypes. *Arch Neurol* 1997;54:203–206.
12. Lamy C, Hamon JB, Coste J, et al. Ischemic stroke in young women: risk of recurrence during subsequent pregnancies. *Neurology* 2000;55:269–274.
13. Adams HP, Bendixen BH, Kappelle LJ, et al. Classification of subtype of acute ischemic stroke. Definitions for use in a multicenter clinical trial. TOAST. Trial of Org 10172 in Acute Stroke Treatment. *Stroke* 1993;24:35–41.
14. Walton J. Cerebrovascular disease. In: Donaldson JO, ed. *Neurology of pregnancy. Major problems in neurology.* Vol. 19. Philadelphia: WB Saunders Co; 1989:137–183.
15. Wallace JD, Levy LL. Blood pressure after stroke. *JAMA* 1981;246:2177–2180.
16. Hertz-Picciotto I, Hopenhayen-Rich C, Golub M, et al. The risks and benefits of taking aspirin during pregnancy. *Epidemiol Rev* 1990;12:108–148.
17. Wilterdink JL, Easton JD. Cerebral ischemia. In: Devinsky O, Feldmann E, Hainline B, eds. *Neurological complications of pregnancy.* New York: Raven Press, 1994;1–11.
18. Mas J-L, Lamy C. Stroke in pregnancy and the puerperium. *J Neurol* 1998;245:305–313.
19. Nishimura K, Kawaguchi M, Shimokawa M, et al. Treatment of pulmonary embolism during cesarean section with recombinant tissue plasminogen activator. *Anesthesiology* 1998;89:1027.
20. Barnes JE, Abbott KH. Cerebral complications incurred during pregnancy and the puerperium. *Am J Obstet Gynecol* 1961;82:192–207.
21. Barno A, Freeman DW. Maternal deaths due to spontaneous subarachnoid hemorrhage. *Am J Obstet Gynecol* 1976;125:384–392.
22. Robinson JL, Hall CJ, Sedzimir CB. Subarachnoid hemorrhage in pregnancy. *J Neurosurg* 1972;36:27–33.
23. Barrett JM, Van Hooydonk JE, Boehm FH. Pregnancy-related rupture of arterial aneurysms. *Obstet Gynecol Surv* 1982;37:557–566.
24. Wilterdink JL, Feldmann E. Cerebral hemorrhage. In: Devinsky O, Feldmann E, Hainline B, eds. *Neurological complications of pregnancy.* New York: Raven Press, 1994;13–23.
25. Wiebers DO. Subarachnoid hemorrhage in pregnancy. *Semin Neurol* 1988;8:226–229.
26. Dias MS, Sekhar LN. Intracranial hemorrhage from aneurysms and arteriovenous malformations during pregnancy and the puerperium. *Neurosurgery* 1990;27:855–866.
27. Robinson JL, Hall CS, Sedzimir CB. Arteriovenous malformations, aneurysms, and pregnancy. *J Neurosurg* 1974;41:63–70.
28. Hunt WE, Hess RM. Surgical risk as related to time of intervention in the repair of intracranial aneurysms. *J Neurosurg* 1968;28:14–20.
29. Giannotta SL, Daniels JD, Golde SH, et al. Ruptured intracranial aneurysms during pregnancy. *J Reprod Med* 1986;31:139–147.
30. Iwanaga H, Wakai S, Ochiai C, et al. Ruptured cerebral aneurysm missed by initial angiographic study. *Neurosurgery* 1990;27:45–51.
31. Schwartz TH, Solomon RA. Perimesencephalic nonaneurysmal subarachnoid hemorrhage: review of the literature. *Neurosurgery* 1996;39:433–440.
32. Mayer SA, Swarup R. Neurogenic cardiac injury after subarachnoid hemorrhage. *Curr Opin Anesth* 1996;9:356–361.
33. Solomon RA, Fink, ME, Lennihan L. Early aneurysm surgery and prophylactic hypervolemic hypertensive therapy for the treatment of aneurysmal subarachnoid hemorrhage. *Neurosurgery* 1988;23:699–704.
34. Klebanoff LM, Fink ME, Lennihan L, et al. Management of cerebral vasospasm in the 1990s. *Clin Neuropharmacol* 1995;18:127–137.
35. Firlik KS, Kaufmann AM, Firlik AD, et al. Intra-arterial papaverine for the treatment of cerebral vasospasm following aneurysmal subarachnoid hemorrhage. *Surg Neurol* 1999;51:66–74.
36. Katoh H, Shima K, Shimizu A, et al. Clinical evaluation of the effect of percutaneous transluminal angioplasty and intra-arterial papaverine infusion for the treatment of vasospasm following aneurysmal subarachnoid hemorrhage. *Neurol Res* 1999;21:195–203.
37. Dias MS. Neurovascular emergencies in pregnancy. *Clin Obstet Gynecol* 1994;37:337–354.
38. Finnerty JJ, Chisholm CA, Chapple H, et al. Cerebral arteriovenous malformation in pregnancy: presentation and neurologic, obstetric, and ethical significance. *Am J Obstet Gynecol* 1999;181:296–303.
39. Sadasivan B, Malik GM, Lee C, et al. Vascular malformations and pregnancy. *Surg Neurol* 1990;33:305–313.
40. Lanzino G, Jensen ME, Cappelletto B, et al. Arteriovenous malformations that rupture during pregnancy: a management dilemma. *Acta Neurochir (Wien)* 1994;126:102–106.
41. Ameri A, Bousser M-G. Cerebral venous thrombosis. *Neurol Clin* 1992;10:87–111.
42. Lanska DJ, Kryscio RJ. Peripartum stroke and intracranial venous thrombosis in the national hospital discharge survey. *Obstet Gynecol* 1997;89:413–418.
43. Villringer A, Einhaupl KM. Dural sinus and cerebral venous thrombosis. *New Horiz* 1997;5:332–341.

44. Donaldson JO. *Neurology of pregnancy. Major problems in neurology.* Vol 19. Philadelphia: WB Saunders Co, 1989;137–183.

45. Fishman RA, Cowen D, Silbermann M. Intracranial venous thrombosis during the first trimester of pregnancy. *Neurology* 1957;7:217–220.

46. Stevens H, Ammerman HH. Intracranial venous thrombosis in early pregnancy. *Am J Obstet Gynecol* 1959;78:104–108.

47. Lavin PJM, Bone I, Lamb JT, et al. Intracranial venous thrombosis in the first trimester of pregnancy. *J Neurol Neurosurg Psychiatry* 1978;41:726–729.

48. Younker D, Jones MM, Adenwala J, et al. Maternal cortical vein thrombosis and the obstetric anesthesiologist. *Anesth Analg* 1986;65:1007–1012.

49. Kendall D. Thrombosis of intracranial veins. *Brain* 1948;71:386–402.

50. Roos KL, Pascuzzi RM, Kuharik MA, et al. Postpartum intracranial venous thrombosis associated with dysfunctional protein C and deficiency of protein S. *Obstet Gynecol* 1990;76:492–494.

51. Hallak M, Senderowicz J, Cassel A, et al. Activated protein C resistance (factor V Leiden) associated with thrombosis in pregnancy. *Am J Obstet Gynecol* 1997; 176:889–893.

52. Lockwood CJ. Heritable coagulopathies in pregnancy. *Obstet Gynecol Surv* 1999;54:754–765.

53. Bousser MG. Cerebral venous thrombosis: diagnosis and management. *J Neurol* 2000;247:252–258.

54. Vogl TJ, Bergman C, Villringer A, et al. Dural sinus thrombosis; value of venous MR angiography for diagnosis and follow-up. *AJR Am J Roentgenol* 1994; 162:1191–1198.

55. Wang AM. MRA of venous sinus thrombosis. *Clin Neurosci* 1997;4:158–164.

56. Barbour LA. Current concepts of anticoagulant therapy in pregnancy. *Obstet Gynecol Clin North Am* 1997; 24:499–521.

57. Turrentine MA, Braems G, Ramirez MM. Use of thrombolytics for the treatment of thromboembolic disease during pregnancy. *Obstet Gynecol Surv* 1995; 50:534–541.

58. de Bruijn SF, Stam J. Randomized, placebo-controlled trial of anticoagulant treatment with low-molecular-weight heparin for cerebral sinus thrombosis. *Stroke* 1999;30:484–488.

59. Ramin SM, Ramin KD, Gilstrap LG. Anticoagulants and thrombolytics during pregnancy. *Semin Perinatol* 1997;21:149–153.

60. Hall JG, Pauli RM, Wilson KM. Maternal and fetal sequelae of anticoagulation in pregnancy. *Am J Med* 1980;68:122–140.

61. Treatment of convulsive status epilepticus: recommendations of the epilepsy foundation of America's working group on status epilepticus. *JAMA* 1993;270: 854–859.

62. Lowenstein DH, Bleck T, MacDonald RL. It's time to revise the definition of status epilepticus. *Epilepsia* 1999;40:120–122.

63. Gastaut H. Classification of status epilepticus. *Adv Neurol* 1983;34:15–35.

64. Klein MD, Goodfriend MJ, Shey IA. Status epilepticus and pregnancy: case report. *Am J Obstet Gynecol* 1956;72:188–190.

65. Knight AH, Rhind EG. Epilepsy and pregnancy: a study of 153 pregnancies in 59 patients. *Epilepsia* 1975;16:99–110.

66. Bardy AH. Incidence of seizures during pregnancy, labor and puerperium in epileptic women: a prospective study. *Acta Neurol Scand* 1987;75:356–360.

67. Licht EA, Sankar R. Status epilepticus during pregnancy. *J Reprod Med* 1999;44;4:370–372.

68. Uthman BM, Wilder BJ. Emergency management of seizures: an overview. *Epilepsia* 1989;30:S33–S37.

69. Mattson RH, Cramer JA. Epilepsy, sex hormones, and anticonvulsant drugs. *Epilepsia* 1985;26:S40–S51.

70. Levy RH, Yerby MS. Effects of pregnancy on anticonvulsant drug utilization. *Epilepsia* 1985;26:S52–S57.

71. Yerby MS, Friel PN, McCormick K, et al. Pharmacokinetics of anticonvulsants in pregnancy: alterations in plasma protein binding. *Epilepsy Res* 1990;5:223–228.

72. Celesia GG. Modern concepts of status epilepticus. *JAMA* 1976;235:1571–1574.

73. Towne AR, Pellock JM, Ko D, et al. Determinants of mortality in status epilepticus. *Epilepsia* 1994;35: 27–34.

74. Donaldson JO. Neurologic emergencies in pregnancy. *Obstet Gynecol Clin North Am* 1991;18:199–212.

75. Goodwin JF, Lawson CW. Status epilepticus complicating pregnancy. *BMJ* 1947;2:332–333.

76. Dalessio DJ. Current concepts: seizure disorders and pregnancy. *N Engl J Med* 1985;1312:559–563.

77. Jagoda A, Riggio S. Emergency department approach to managing seizures in pregnancy. *Ann Emerg Med* 1991;20:80–85.

78. Lowenstein DH, Alldredge BK. Current concepts: status epilepticus. *N Engl J Med* 1998;338:970–976.

79. Treiman DM, Walton NY, Kendrick C. A progressive sequence of electroencephalographic changes during generalized convulsive status epilepticus. *Epilepsy Res* 1990;5:49–60.

80. Leppik IE, Derivan AT, Homan RW, et al. Double-blind study of lorazepam and diazepam in status epilepticus. *JAMA* 1983;249:1452–1454.

81. Treiman DM, Meyers PD, Walton NY, et al. A comparison of four treatments for generalized convulsive status epilepticus. *N Engl J Med* 1998;339:792–798.

82. Naritoku DK, Mueed S. Intravenous loading of valproate for epilepsy. *Clin Neuropharmacol* 1999;2: 102–106.

83. Venkataraman V, Wheless JW. Safety of rapid intravenous infusion of valproate loading doses in epilepsy patients. *Epilepsy Res* 1999;35:147–153.

84. Sinha S. Naritoku DK. Intravenous valproate is well tolerated in unstable patients with status epilepticus. *Neurology* 2000;55:722–724.

85. Rashkin MC, Youngs C, Penovich P. Pentobarbital treatment of refractory status epilepticus. *Neurology* 1987;37:500–503.

86. Krishnamurthy KB, Drislane FW. Depth of EEG suppression and outcome in barbiturate anesthetic treatment for refractory status epilepticus. *Epilepsia* 1999; 40:759–762.

87. Sibai BM. Eclampsia. In: Goldstein PJ, Stern BJ, eds. *Neurological disorders of pregnancy.* 2nd ed. New York: Futura Publishing Co., 1992;1–24.

88. American College of Obstetricians and Gynecologists. Hypertension in pregnancy. ACOG Technical Bulletin 219. *Int J Gynaecol Obstet* 1996;53:175–183.

89. Sibai BM, Spinnato JA, Watson DL, et al. Eclampsia.

IV. Neurological findings and future outcomes. *Am J Obstet Gynecol* 1985;152:184–192.

90. Donaldson JO. Eclampsia. In: Walton J, ed. *Neurology of pregnancy. Major Problems in Neurology.* Vol. 19. Philadelphia: WB Saunders Co., 1989:269–310.

91. Kaplan PW. Neurological issues in eclampsia. *Rev Neurol (Paris)* 1999;155:335–341.

92. López-Llera M. Complicated eclampsia: fifteen years' experience in a referral medical center. *Am J Obstet Gynecol* 1982;142:28–35.

93. Pritchard JA, Cunningham FG, Pritchard SA. The Parkland Memorial Hospital protocol for treatment of eclampsia: evaluation of 245 cases. *Am J Obstet Gynecol* 1984;148:951–963.

94. Sibai BM. Eclampsia. VI. Maternal-perinatal outcome in 254 consecutive cases. *Am J Obstet Gynecol* 1990; 163:1049–1055.

95. Roberts JM, Taylor RN, Musci TJ, et al. Preeclampsia: an endothelial cell disorder. *Am J Obstet Gynecol* 1989;161:1200–1204.

96. Roberts JM, Taylor RN, Goldfien A. Clinical and biochemical evidence of endothelial cell dysfunction in the pregnancy syndrome preeclampsia. *Am J Hypertens* 1991;4:700–708.

97. Morrison JC, Whybrew DW, Wiser WL, et al. Enzyme levels in the serum and cerebrospinal fluid in eclampsia. *Am J Obstet Gynecol* 1971;110:619–624.

98. Fish SA, Morrison JC, Bucovaz ET, et al. Cerebral spinal fluid studies in eclampsia. *Am J Obstet Gynecol* 1972;112:502–512.

99. Sibai BM, Spinnato JA, Watson DL, et al. Effect of magnesium sulfate on electroencephalographic findings in preeclampsia-eclampsia. *Obstet Gynecol* 1984; 64:261–266.

100. Thomas SV, Somanathan N, Radhakumari R. Interictal EEG changes in eclampsia. *Electroencephalogr Clin Neurophysiol* 1995;94:271–275.

101. Colosimo C, Fileni A, Moschini M, et al. CT findings in eclampsia. *Neuroradiology* 1985;27:313–317.

102. Naheedy MH, Biller J, Schiffer M, et al. Toxemia of pregnancy: cerebral CT findings. *J Comput Assist Tomogr* 1985;9:497–501.

103. Crawford S, Varner MW, Digre KB, et al. Cranial magnetic resonance imaging in eclampsia. *Obstet Gynecol* 1987;70:474–477.

104. Vandenplas O, Dive A, Dooms G, et al. Magnetic resonance evaluation of severe neurological disorders in eclampsia. *Neuroradiology* 1990;32:47–49.

105. Will AD, Lewis KL, Hinshaw DB, et al. Cerebral vasoconstriction in toxemia. *Neurology* 1987;37:1555–1557.

106. Lewis LK, Hinshaw DB, Will AD, et al. CT and angiographic correlation of severe neurological disease in toxemia of pregnancy. *Neuroradiology* 1988;30: 59–64.

107. Trommer BL, Homer D, Mikhael MA. Cerebral vasospasm and eclampsia. *Stroke* 1988;19:326–329.

108. Dildy GA, Cotton DB. Management of severe preeclampsia and eclampsia. *Crit Care Clin* 1991;7: 829–850.

109. Sibai BM. Treatment of hypertension in pregnant women. *N Engl J Med* 1996;335:257–265.

110. Graham DI. Ischaemic brain damage of cerebral perfusion failure type after treatment of severe hypertension. *BMJ* 1975;4:739.

111. Ledingham JG, Rajagopalan B. Cerebral complications in the treatment of accelerated hypertension. *Q J Med* 1979;189:25–41.

112. Donaldson JO. Eclampsia. In: Devinsky O, Feldman E, Hainline B, eds. *Neurological complications of pregnancy.* New York: Raven Press, 1994:25–33.

113. Kaplan PW, Lesser RP, Fisher RS, et al. No, magnesium sulfate should not be used in treating eclamptic seizures. *Arch Neurol* 1988;45:1361–1364.

114. Dinsdale HB. Does magnesium sulfate treat eclamptic seizures? Yes. *Arch Neurol* 1988;45:1360–1361.

115. Sibai BM. Magnesium sulfate is the ideal anticonvulsant in preeclampsia-eclampsia. *Am J Obstet Gynecol* 1990;162:1141–1145.

116. Lazard EM. A preliminary report on the intravenous use of magnesium sulphate in puerperal eclampsia. 1925. *Am J Obstet Gynecol* 1996;174:1390–1391.

117. Pritchard JA. The use of the magnesium ion in the management of eclamptic toxemias. *Surg Gynecol Obstet* 1955;100:131–140.

Neurological Complications of Pregnancy, Second
Edition, edited by Brian Hainline and Orrin Devinsky.
Lippincott Williams & Wilkins, Philadelphia © 2002.

9

Neurologic Aspects of Rheumatologic Disorders

Lisa R. Sammaritano

*Department of Internal Medicine, Weill Medical College of Cornell University, and Division of
Rheumatology, Hospital for Special Surgery, New York, New York, U.S.A.*

Rheumatologic disorders are multisystem diseases characterized by inflammation, usually in the absence of known infection. The pathogenic mechanisms responsible for tissue injury are immunologic. Alterations in both humoral and cellular immune responses are seen, and most disorders are characterized by the presence of autoantibodies, which may be involved in tissue damage. Antibodies may cause inflammation either by cytotoxic mechanisms or by immune complex-mediated processes. Clinical manifestations vary according to the site of tissue inflammation. Most rheumatologic diseases affect the nervous system to varying extents, often resulting in severe complications.

Studies of pregnancy-induced effects on the maternal immune response demonstrate an altered maternal recognition of foreign tissue to permit fetal survival. Cell-mediated immunity generally is depressed, as reflected by abnormal lymphocyte stimulation and other functional tests, decreased T-cell to B-cell ratios, and decreased lymphocyte–monocyte ratios (1). Although the number of immunoglobulin-secreting cells increases, inflammatory responses decrease overall. Pregnancy-specific proteins modulate the immune response by suppressing lymphocyte function and include α-fetoprotein, α_2-globulins, β_1-globulins, and placental corticosteroids. Finally, particular cytokines (primarily Th2 profile), partially regulated by sex hormones, may be critical in sustaining pregnancy, including interleukin-1, interleukin-3, tumor necrosis factor alpha, in-

terferon gamma, and granulocyte-macrophage colony-stimulating factor (2). Abnormal production and/or metabolism of cytokines are thought to be important in rheumatic illness.

Maternal shifts in immune function may affect an underlying autoimmune disorder. Conversely, presence of underlying immune dysregulation may affect pregnancy outcome, both maternal and fetal. Transplacental passage of autoantibody may directly cause fetal inflammation, and fetal outcome may be impaired in the setting of severe maternal illness (3).

Neurologic complications in pregnant patients with rheumatologic disorders may be related to the underlying disease, to normal pregnancy, or to pregnancy-induced complications. New-onset neurologic disease in pregnancy may be difficult to diagnose, especially if the rheumatologic disorder is also of new onset.

Rheumatologic disorders include a broad range of diseases (Table 9.1). Collagen vascular diseases are multisystem diseases accompanied by inflammation in a number of organ systems, although one organ system may predominate. The vasculitis syndromes are also rheumatologic disorders, but with inflammation limited to blood vessels. Finally, sarcoidosis and thrombotic thrombocytopenic purpura are included here although they are not classically considered rheumatologic disorders. Multisystem diseases of unknown etiology, they often are included in the differential of rheumatologic diseases. They may have significant neurologic complications.

TABLE 9.1. *Summary of general and neurologic manifestations of rheumatologic disorders*

Disease	Common clinical manifestations	Neurologic manifestations	Commonly used therapies
Systemic lupus erythematosus	Rash, arthritis, serositis, nephritis, cytopenia, neurologic involvement, systemic symptoms	Psychoaffective disorders Cerebrovascular syndromes Seizures Transverse myelitis Peripheral neuropathy	NSAID Corticosteroid Hydroxychloroquine Cyclophosphamide Azathioprine
Rheumatoid arthritis	Symmetric polyarthritis, especially small joints Nodules, scleritis, pulmonary disease	Peripheral neuropathy Entrapment neuropathy Atlantoaxial disease Rare CNS, meningitis	Aspirin, NSAID Hydroxychloroquine Sulfasalazine Gold Penicillamine Methotrexate Azathioprine Infliximab Etanercept
Systemic sclerosis	Sclerodermatous skin changes, pulmonary disease, renal crisis with hypertension, gastrointestinal dysmotility, cardiac dysrhythmias	Uncommon: Trigeminal neuropathy Other cranial neuropathy Peripheral neuropathy	Penicillamine Angiotensin-converting enzyme inhibitors Calcium channel blockers
Sjögren's syndrome	Keratoconjunctivitis sicca, xerostomia	Cranial neuropathy Peripheral neuropathy CNS, psychiatric	Corticosteroid
Polymyositis/ dermatomyositis	Inflammatory myopathy, pulmonary disease, cardiac arrythmia, congestive heart failure	Rare	Corticosteroid Methotrexate Immunoglobulin
Behçet's disease	Oral ulcerations, genital ulcerations, iritis. Also skin rash, arthritis, thrombophlebitis, neurologic	Cranial neuropathy Wide spectrum CNS involvement including paresis, seizure, other focal deficit	Corticosteroid Azathioprine Other immunosuppressives

Vasculitis syndromes
Polyarteritis nodosa
	Vasculitis: small/medium arteritis with renal, gastrointestinal, cardiac muscle, and neurologic involvement	Peripheral neuropathy
		Cerebrovascular syndromes including:
		  Subarachnoid hemorrhage
		  Seizure
		  Focal deficits
			Corticosteroid
			Cyclophosphamide
			Other immunosuppressives

Primary angiitis of CNS	Limited to CNS, no systemic involvement	Headache, confusion Cerebrovascular syndromes Focal deficits Seizure	Corticosteroid Cyclophosphamide Other immunosuppressives
Takayasu's arteritis	Granulomatous arteritis of aorta and branches, vascular insufficiency	Cerebral ischemia including seizure, CVA, syncope	Corticosteroid Cyclophosphamide Other immunosuppressives
Wegener's granulomatosis	Granulomatous vasculitis of upper and lower respiratory tract, glomerulonephritis	Cranial neuropathy Peripheral neuropathy CNS less common: Headache, focal deficits, subarachnoid hemorrhage	Corticosteroid Cyclophosphamide Other immunosuppressives
Sarcoidosis	Multisystem, granulomatosis disorder, pulmonary involvement characteristic. Also eye, cardiac, gastrointestinal inflammation; arthritis	Cranial neuropathy (facial nerve) Meningitis Encephalitis, masses Seizure	Corticosteroid Methotrexate Other immunosuppressives
Thrombotic thrombocytopenic purpura	Thrombocytopenic purpura, microangiopathic hemolytic anemia, neurologic symptoms, renal disease, fever	Confusion Headache, aphasia Paresis and other focal deficits Seizure	Plasma infusion and/or plasma exchange Antiplatelet therapy ? corticosteroid

NSAID, nonsteroidal antiinflammatory drug; CNS, central nervous system; CVA, cerebrovascular accident.

COLLAGEN VASCULAR DISEASES

Systemic Lupus Erythematosus

Systemic lupus erythematosus (SLE) is a multisystem autoimmune disorder characterized by a wide range of organ involvement, the presence of characteristic autoantibodies, and a broad spectrum of clinical disease severity. Affecting up to 1 in 700 women ages 15 to 64, the ratio of female to male prevalence is 9 to 1 (4). Onset is most frequent during the reproductive years.

Although symptoms vary widely among individuals, common clinical manifestations include arthritis, skin rash, lymphadenopathy, nephritis, serositis, neuropsychiatric illness, hemocytopenias, and fever or other systemic symptoms. Vasculitis may be a prominent manifestation. Antinuclear antibodies are present in most patients, and antidouble-stranded DNA antibodies are relatively specific. Antiphospholipid antibodies (associated with a clinical syndrome of thrombosis, thrombocytopenia, and recurrent fetal loss) are seen in up to 30% of SLE patients. Antibodies to SS-A/Ro and SS-B/La ribosomal particles, present in about 30% of patients, confer a risk for development of neonatal lupus. Antibody to Sm antigen is a specific but not sensitive finding.

Neurologic Manifestations

The neuropsychiatric manifestations of SLE are diverse, ranging from recently recognized mild cognitive deficits (5) to psychosis and coma. A standardized nomenclature system for neuropyschiatric lupus (NPSLE) syndromes has been developed to aid in improved diagnostic agreement (6).

Neurologic disease is the second leading cause of death in SLE (7). In Estes' and Christian's (8) landmark prospective series of 150 patients, 59% had evidence of neuropsychiatric disease on follow-up, including seizures, organic brain syndromes, psychosis, hemiparesis, cerebellar signs, and peripheral neuropathy. Defining precise etiology of neurologic dysfunction is often complex: up to two-thirds of serious CNS events in SLE are due at least in part to the presence of superimposed complications, including focal vascular abnormalities, fever, metabolic imbalance, severe hypertension, or drug toxicity (9).

Pathophysiology of the primary process in central nervous system (CNS) lupus is not clear; suggested pathogenetic mechanisms include cerebral vessel vasculitis (10,11), immune complex deposition in the choroid plexus (12), and presence of circulating brain-reactive antibodies (13,14). Immune complexes have been demonstrated in the choroid

plexus of patients with neuropsychiatric disease (12) and antibodies to neuronal antigens are present in cerebrospinal fluid (CSF) of patients with SLE (13). An association between lupus psychosis and serum anti-ribosomal P protein antibodies also suggests autoantibody-mediated pathogenicity (14).

Although medium- to large-vessel cerebral vasculitis is clearly uncommon in SLE, microinfarction (with vascular hyalinization, endothelial proliferation, thrombosis, and capillary wall thickening) is frequent and suggests evidence of small-vessel vasculitis (10,11) or *in situ* thrombosis. In autopsy studies of patients with clinically defined neuropsychiatric disease, anatomic CNS lesions were found in 50%, with embolic branch infarct and CNS infection being the most common (15). No patient demonstrated active CNS vasculitis at the time of death; however, cardiac embolic disease and thrombotic thrombocytopenic purpura (TTP) were frequently noted.

Antiphospholipid antibodies (aPL) are a significant factor in the pathogenesis of neurologic disease in SLE. In recent studies, the two greatest risk factors for development of NPSLE are presence of aPL and history of previous NPSLE (16,17). aPL are a group of related autoantibodies directed against phospholipid-binding protein–phospholipid complexes and are seen in about 30% of patients with SLE and less than 2% of normal controls (18). A primary antiphospholipid syndrome (aPL in the absence of SLE) has been defined as well (19). Although infections or drugs may induce antiphospholipid antibodies, in general, only the autoimmune antibodies show an association with clinical complications (20). The syndrome includes both arterial and venous thrombosis, recurrent miscarriage, and thrombocytopenia (21,22). Other manifestations include valvular heart disease with Libman-Sacks endocarditis, livedo reticularis, and neurologic complications distinct from stroke.

The most common neurologic manifestations associated with aPL are cerebral infarction and transient ischemic attack. Strokes are often multiple and may progress to multiinfarct dementia (22). Other neurologic conditions have been noted, including chorea and transverse myelitis (23–25). Chorea gravidarum may be more common in aPL-positive patients. In one large series of aPL-positive patients evaluated for the presence of neurologic disease, CNS disease occurred in 35%; most common were encephalopathy, multiple cerebral infarctions, migraine, and visual abnormalities including amaurosis fugax and ischemic optic neuropathy (25).

General treatment of SLE manifestations depends on severity of disease and specific organ involvement. Minor disease often is managed with aspirin, nonsteroidal anti-inflammatory agents, or antimalarial medications. The mainstay of therapy for more severe disease is corticosteroid, used for significant renal, CNS, and hematologic manifestations. Corticosteroid for acute flare commonly is administered as high-dose "pulse" intravenous methylprednisolone, usually 1 g per day for 3 consecutive days. Cytotoxic therapy, (including cyclophosphamide and azathioprine), plasmapheresis, and intravenous gammaglobulin, are used for severe or steroid-resistant disease.

Treatment of CNS lupus is not clearly defined. Cerebrovascular events in association with aPL generally require anticoagulation therapy. Superimposed metabolic or other medical problems require appropriately directed management. Although very high doses of corticosteroids have been used for organic brain syndromes or functional psychosis, it is not clear that these doses of corticosteroid are beneficial. In reviewing effect of corticosteroid therapy in 28 patients with SLE and neuropsychiatric disease, Sergent and colleagues (26) found 12 patients to have major complications of corticosteroid therapy, including death in five, without clear benefit. Anecdotal success with cyclophosphamide in NPSLE is promising, but no controlled trials are published to date (27).

Overall prognosis in SLE has improved dramatically. Early estimates of mortality in SLE were 50% at 5 years; more recent studies find a 90% survival at 5 years (7,28). This is largely the result of earlier diagnosis, more sophisticated diagnostic methods, and more aggressive therapies. The course for many patients has become that of a chronic disease with intermittent exacerbation. As outcome has improved, the option of pregnancy for these patients has improved as well.

Pregnancy and Systemic Lupus Erythematosus

Initial reports (29) of pregnancy in SLE patients described an almost certain deterioration in clinical status with frequent exacerbation, especially in the postpartum period. Therapeutic abortion often was suggested. Several factors have dramatically modified this view: recognition of the mild end of the SLE disease spectrum, identification of specific risk factors for poor outcome in pregnancy, distinction of SLE activity from pregnancy-induced complications, and aggressive obstetric care. Many SLE patients can undergo successful pregnancy without significant deterioration in their clinical status and with good fetal outcome.

Normal pregnancy is accompanied by numerous physiologic changes that may mimic SLE or other rheumatic disease manifestations. Increased blood flow to the skin may cause prominent facial flushing, and hyperpigmentation in the malar area (chloasma gravidarum) can mimic a lupus rash. Dilutional anemia and mild thrombocytopenia may mimic SLE-related signs. Increased production of fibrinogen and other proteins causes elevation of the erythrocyte sedimentation rate, rendering it less useful as a gauge of systemic inflammation. Bland joint effusions and diffuse arthralgias, common in pregnancy, may be confused with active arthritis (30).

Pregnancy-induced hypertension (PIH) may be particularly difficult to differentiate from active SLE. Prominent symptoms of PIH include hypertension, proteinuria, renal insufficiency, edema, thrombocytopenia, and liver enzyme abnormalities, all of which may be seen in SLE. In eclampsia, seizures and other neurologic complications may ensue, which may be confused with CNS lupus. Signs suggestive of active SLE include inflammatory arthritis, inflammatory rash, fever, lymphadenopathy, hematuria, leukopenia, and presence of anti-DNA antibody (30) (Table 9.2).

Estimates of risk of flare in SLE pregnancy vary greatly, ranging from 8% to 74% (31–38). This is likely the result of several factors. In general, risk of flare in the nonpregnant lupus patient is difficult to assess because of imprecise definition of flare and unpredictable disease course. Flare scales to rate level of disease activity objectively are commonly used (39), but during pregnancy many of the clinical and serologic parameters become less useful. Lack of appropriate control populations is a frequent problem. Although there have been many attempts to address the question of SLE flare in pregnancy, there is no firm agreement as yet. The most recent study, by Ruiz-Irastorza (31) demonstrated higher flare rates in pregnant lupus patients compared both to nonpregnant controls and to the patients themselves after pregnancy. Flares were most frequent in the second and third trimesters and in the puerperium.

In addition to rate of global exacerbation, consideration of specific organ system involvement is important in assessing significance of flare symptoms. In Lockshin's series of SLE pregnancies, he found thrombocytopenia, proteinuria, and hypocomplementemia to be the most common abnormalities. If interpreted as SLE-related, flare rate was 25%; if interpreted as due to pregnancy itself, preeclampsia, or antiphospholipid antibody, rate of flare dropped to 13% (32). In the Hopkins Lupus Pregnancy Center series (33), flare was twice as common in pregnant as in nonpregnant patients and occurred in 60% of pregnancies. Most common flare manifestations in this group were constitutional symptoms, renal involvement, and involvement of skin or joints.

Despite continued controversy concerning risk of exacerbation, there is agreement on several key observations. First, inactive disease at the time of conception (and for the 6 months preceding pregnancy) is associated with a lower chance of disease exacerbation (34,35). Second, renal insufficiency and hypertension may worsen during pregnancy and may predispose to pregnancy complications (35–37). Finally, fetal outcome is related more to presence of renal involvement and aPL than to occurrence of lupus flare (32).

The presence of renal insufficiency is an important risk factor for poor fetal outcome and serious renal deterioration during pregnancy (40–42). Precise renal histology is less impor-

TABLE 9.2. *Differentiation of active SLE from normal pregnancy and/or pregnancy-induced hypertension*

Nonspecific signs and symptoms[a]	Specific signs and symptoms[b]
Malar erythema, palmar erythema	Inflammatory malar rash, cutaneous vasculitis
Bland joint effusion	Inflammatory arthritis
Edema	Lymphadenopathy
Seizures	Hematuria, erythrocyte casts
Hypertension	Elevated anti-double-stranded DNA antibody
Elevated erythrocyte sedimentation rate	Low CH50/Ba ratio[c]
Anemia	
Thrombocytopenia	
Proteinuria	
Disseminated intravascular coagulation (DIC)	
Alternations in C3, C4 levels	

[a]Signs and symptoms that may be seen in association with active SLE but *also* with pregnancy alone and/or pregnancy-induced hypertension.
[b]Signs and symptoms that may be seen in association with active SLE and are *not* expected as a manifestation of pregnancy alone or pregnancy-induced hypertension.
[c]Research observation (ref. 45) not generally used in clinical setting.

tant than the presence of clinical renal dysfunction (42). Although exacerbation of renal disease may occur in 40% of cases, severe or permanent renal deterioration develops in about 10% to 20%. The physiologic stress of pregnancy in patients with quiescent renal disease may accelerate this process, especially in those with initial serum creatinine greater than 1.6 mg per dL. Onset of worsening renal function in the latter half of pregnancy, especially when associated with hypertension and edema, must be differentiated from superimposed PIH. Other indications of SLE flare are helpful in making this distinction, including clinical signs of active SLE, rising anti-double–stranded DNA antibody, and presence of erythrocyte casts. Use of complement levels in defining flare in pregnancy is controversial because pregnancy itself may induce activation of the classical complement pathway (43,44). Buyon and associates (45) found ongoing activation of the alternative complement pathway (low CH50/Ba ratio) to differentiate pregnant SLE patients with flare from those with pre-eclampsia.

Neurologic Disease in SLE Pregnancy

Neurologic events during the course of pregnancy are unusual (46–48). Incidence of neurologic disease in pregnant SLE patients may be increased in the setting of superimposed conditions. Eclampsia, associated with seizures, is more common in SLE patients (30), and it is often difficult to differentiate between late pregnancy seizures due to eclampsia and those due to active SLE. Chorea gravidarum may be increased in patients with aPL (23). Finally, a generalized state of hypercoagulability accompanies pregnancy, and although an additive risk for aPL-related thrombosis is not definite, an increased risk for thrombotic complications, including stroke, in the pregnant aPL patient seems likely (49).

Neurologic complications are regularly reported in small numbers in most series of lupus pregnancies (32,33,36–38). In Lockshin's series (32), he noted only one patient with neurologic symptoms (seizures) during pregnancy, attributed to eclampsia rather than SLE itself. In the Hopkins series (33), overall rate of flare was 60%, but only 4% of flares involved neurologic disease. Mintz and colleagues (37) counted 8 of 55 exacerbations in 102 SLE pregnancies to involve the CNS. Not all involved focal findings or were definitely attributable to SLE; complications included postpartum generalized seizures, chorea, transient memory loss, and headache. Higher rates of both maternal morbidity and maternal mortality for pregnant SLE patients with a history of prior CNS involvement have been described (36).

Isolated cases of unusual neurologic involvement during pregnancy have been reported. Suzuki and associates (50) described a young woman diagnosed with SLE at 14 weeks gestation who went on to develop severe necrotizing cerebral and systemic vasculitis unresponsive to steroid therapy, with eventual death. Transverse myelitis occurring in a patient with established but otherwise inactive lupus and positive aPL at 16 weeks of gestation has been reported (48). Cerebral infarction in patients with antiphospholipid syndrome (APS) ostpartum with discontinuation of aspirin therapy is reported in several patients (51). Finally, Devic's neuromyelitis optica, rarely reported in SLE, has been described in a pregnant SLE patient in her fourth month of pregnancy who presented with transverse myelitis and optic neuropathy. Treatment with plasmapheresis and corticosteroid produced improvement in symptoms. A postpartum recurrence subsequently was treated successfully with cyclophosphamide (52).

Pregnancy Outcome

Systemic lupus erythematosus clearly affects overall reproductive potential. Fertility in SLE generally is not impaired, although use of cyclophosphamide may lead to premature ovarian failure. Although the fertility rate is normal, the rate of miscarriage and fetal loss approaches 40% in women with SLE, due largely to the presence of aPL.

Antiphospholipid antibodies traditionally include the biologic false-positive serologic test for syphilis, the lupus anticoagulant (LAC), and antibodies to cardiolipin (aCL), but LAC and aCL seem to have greatest value in predicting clinical events (30). Lupus anticoagulant is measured in a functional clotting assay and causes prolongation of clotting time, which is not corrected on mixing with normal plasma (53). Anticardiolipin antibodies are detected in an immunoassay using cardiolipin as antigen (54).

The mechanism for aPL pathogenicity is not clear and may involve several mechanisms (55–60). The serum protein $beta_2$-Glycoprotein I (β_2GPI), which demonstrates *in vitro* anticoagulant properties, is a requirement for the binding of autoimmune aCL to cardiolipin in the standard ELISA. β_2GPI bound to phospholipid produces an epitope against which most autoimmune aCL are directed (55). Interference with the natural anticoagulant function of β_2GPI may result in thrombosis. Autoantibodies to other phospholipid-binding proteins (e.g., prothrombin) have been demonstrated as well (56). Additional suggested factors include a decrease in prostacyclin production (57), interference with protein C activation (58,59), and a decrease in functional tissue plasminogen activator (60).

Lupus anticoagulant and aCL are strongly associated with recurrent fetal loss; rates of loss in untreated aPL pregnancies may approach 80% (61,62). Two factors strongly influence this risk: presence of high titer immunoglobulin G (IgG), aCL and a history of prior fetal loss (63). Lupus anticoagulant and aCL coexist about 70% to 80% of the time, depending on the coagulation assay used (64). Presence of anti-β_2GPI antibodies may predict risk as well, but these rarely are seen in the absence of more traditional aCL (65,66).

Obstetric complications associated with the presence of aPL include fetal distress, usually related to placental insufficiency, and fetal death (62,67). Mid-trimester loss is considered characteristic; however, up to one half of losses may be in the first trimester and may reflect defects in implantation (68). Preeclampsia is common (69,70), and many pregnancies, even when successful, are preterm (71). The major risks to the neonate are those associated with prematurity. Antiphospholipid antibodies may enter the fetal circulation but rarely cause thrombosis in the neonate (71).

SLE also may influence neonatal outcome by more direct effects on the fetus. The risk of positive antinuclear antibodies in the offspring of women with SLE is about 10%, and the risk of clinical SLE is about 1% (72). Neonatal lupus erythematosus (NLE), a syndrome distinct from SLE, is uncommon and reflects inflammation in the fetus due to transplacental passage of autoantibody. This syndrome is seen almost exclusively in offspring of women who have antibodies to the SS-A/Ro and SS-B/La antigens. Clinical manifestations include photosensitive rash, thrombocytopenia, liver function abnormalities, and, rarely, irreversible congenital heart block (73). With the exception of heart block, all other manifestations disappear with the clearance of maternal antibody at about 4 to 6 months. Risk of any manifestation of NLE for the neonate of an anti-Ro positive woman is about 25%, and risk of congenital heart block is less than 3% (74).

Management and Therapy

Optimal management of the pregnant patient with SLE involves a prepregnancy evaluation for level of disease activity, medication use, review of renal function, and assessment of autoantibody status, including aPL and anti-SS-A/Ro. On the basis of these data, medications can be modified, plans can be made for therapy, or a decision can be made to postpone pregnancy until the disease is better controlled. Once the patient is pregnant, appropriate laboratory monitoring of renal and hematologic parameters is accompanied by obstetric monitoring. Intensive fetal monitoring is critical, usually with antepartum fetal heart rate testing (nonstress test) or umbilical artery waveform determinations.

Medical therapy for lupus activity in pregnancy is based on evidence of active SLE.

Prophylactic corticosteroid generally is not given, although all rheumatic disease patients on chronic corticosteroid therapy should receive stress-dose steroid at the time of delivery, especially if by cesarean section. Prophylactic treatment in women with aPL and previous fetal loss markedly improves pregnancy outcome, from 25% to 75% (49, 75–81). In the absence of prior pregnancy loss, it is not clear that treatment is necessary, although most aPL-positive patients are treated with low-dose (80 to 100 mg) aspirin daily, given the low risk of side effects. Standard therapy for the patient with antiphospholipid syndrome, based on several recent controlled trials, is low-dose aspirin and prophylactic (low-dose) heparin (79–81). High-dose corticosteroid increases risk of both maternal and fetal morbidity and generally is not used for aPL indications alone. Treatment for refractory cases often includes intravenous gammaglobulin, although controlled studies do not yet support this approach (82).

Treatment of neurologic complications during pregnancy is generally high-dose corticosteroid if the symptoms are believed to represent active SLE rather than antiphospholipid or PIH-related events. Experts disagree as to whether it is permissible for an APS patient with a history of stroke or severe thrombosis to undertake pregnancy. Several reports describe successful pregnancies in such patients treated with aggressive anticoagulation (83). Patients with a history of thrombotic stroke (or other significant thrombosis) should receive therapeutic (anticoagulant doses) of heparin throughout pregnancy and the postpartum period. Low-molecular weight heparins increasingly are used for both greater consistency in level of anticoagulation and the lower risk of side effects. Therapeutic efficacy may be monitored with serial levels of activated Factor X (84).

Summary

Pregnancy in SLE may be completed successfully in many patients despite the increased risk of maternal and neonatal morbidity. Exacerbation of disease, including neurologic manifestations, is still controversial. Neurologic symptoms may result from SLE flare, aPL in the absence of SLE flare, or superimposed preeclampsia–eclampsia. Risk of complications is increased by several factors: activity of disease at conception, current renal function, presence of aPL, and presence of anti-SS-A/Ro and SS-B/La antibodies. Prophylactic corticosteroid therapy generally is not given. Antiphospholipid antibody in the presence of a history of fetal loss or documented previous thrombosis is treated with anticoagulant therapy.

Rheumatoid Arthritis

Rheumatoid arthritis (RA) is a chronic, systemic inflammatory disorder characterized by prominent joint involvement. The etiology remains obscure, although infectious causes have been proposed. Women are affected two to three times more often than men are, and overall prevalence is estimated at 0.3% to 1.5%. Genetic susceptibility is associated with the presence of specific HLA-DR4 alleles. The pattern of joint involvement is usually symmetrical and characteristically involves small joints of the hands and feet. However, larger joints commonly are involved, and cervical spine disease is frequent. Extraarticular manifestations emphasize the systemic nature of the disease and include low-grade fever and fatigue, rheumatoid nodules, vasculitis, neuropathy, pericarditis, pulmonary disease, and scleritis. Anemia of chronic disease is common, and about 80% of patients are positive for rheumatoid factor (IgM antibody directed against IgG). A smaller percentage may have other autoantibodies, including antinuclear antibodies and anti-SS-A/Ro and SS-B/La antibodies (85).

Diagnostic criteria for RA are primarily clinical and include morning stiffness, arthritis of three or more joint areas, arthritis of hand joints, symmetric arthritis, rheumatoid nodules, serum rheumatoid factor, and typical radiologic changes (86). Presence of four of the seven criteria is needed for diagnosis.

Neurologic Manifestations

Several broad categories of neurologic involvement in RA are seen, including cerebral vasculitis and pachymeningitis, peripheral neuropathy, and, most commonly, compressive or entrapment neuropathies secondary to cervical spine or peripheral articular disease (87). Nodulosis may occur rarely in the CNS, with rheumatoid nodules involving the leptomeninges and even the choroid plexus (88,89). Pachymeningitis of the thoracic and lumbar cord have been reported as well (90,91). Cerebral vasculitis rarely has been reported (92,93).

Peripheral neuropathy is usually a mild distal sensory neuropathy or mononeuritis multiplex (87). Compressive neuropathy may be secondary to arthritis in the cervical vertebrae or the peripheral joints. Cervical myelopathy as a result of narrowing of the cervical canal may be caused by atlantoaxial subluxation or subluxation at lower levels of the cervical spine. Twenty percent of patients with RA have radiologic evidence of atlantoaxial subluxation on lateral flexion views of the cervical spine (94), although clinical evidence of cervical myelopathy is less common and is usually associated with long-standing, seropositive erosive disease (95). Pain in the cervical spine may be absent, and presenting symptoms may include only weakness or sensory changes.

Peripheral entrapment neuropathies, a common neurologic complication of RA, include carpal tunnel syndrome, tarsal tunnel syndrome, ulnar nerve entrapment, and posterior interosseous nerve entrapment. Carpal tunnel syndrome (entrapment of the median nerve in the carpal canal) is the most common entrapment neuropathy in RA, and evidence of median nerve compression on electrophysiology studies may be found in up to two-thirds of patients with early RA (96). Ulnar nerve compression occurs most commonly at the elbow secondary to compression at the cubital fossa, with synovitis extending extraarticulary (87). Tarsal tunnel syndrome (compression of the posterior tibial nerve beneath the flexor retinaculum distal to the medial malleolus) is caused by rheumatoid tenosynovitis affecting these tendon sheaths. The radial or posterior interosseous nerve is sometimes compressed at the elbow as it passes anterior to the lateral epicondyle, and the resulting loss of finger extension with preserved wrist extension may be confused with extensor tendon rupture.

Pregnancy and Rheumatoid Arthritis

The effect of pregnancy on RA is usually positive: up to 73% of patients experience some degree of clinical remission of symptoms during pregnancy, even in the absence of usual medications (3,97,98). Cecere and Persellin (97) analyzed 308 pregnancies in patients with RA for change in their underlying disease. Amelioration in symptoms was detected in about 50% of patients in the first trimester, in an additional 14% in the second trimester, and in a further 6% in the third trimester. Improvement persisted throughout the course of the pregnancy. A prospective study of 140 women with RA during pregnancy, however, has demonstrated significant variability in degree of response, with only 16% of patients attaining complete remission (99).

Regardless of the degree of improvement experienced during gestation, almost all patients relapse following delivery by the end of 8 months postpartum, most of these within the first 6 weeks (3,97,98). Although this suggests that pregnancy-related hormones initiate and maintain remission, breastfeeding does not appear to change the timing of relapse (98). Recent work suggests that persistence of active disease during pregnancy may relate to a similarity between maternal and fetal human leukocyte antigen (HLA-DQ system) (100).

The effect of pregnancy on the development of RA is controversial. Pregnancy itself and use of oral contraceptives at any time may reduce the risk of disease onset. An increased risk of disease onset is noted in the postpartum period (101). A large case-control study (102) found a decreased risk of development of RA in women who had at some point been pregnant. The earlier the first pregnancy, the lower the risk of subsequent development of RA. In addition, oral contraceptive use (independent of dose or duration of use) is associated with a lower relative risk of developing RA (103).

Neurologic Disease in a Pregnancy with Rheumatoid Arthritis

The effect of gestation on the extraarticular manifestations of RA is not known, although one report (98) does suggest regression of lymphadenopathy and subcutaneous nodules in some patients beginning in the first trimester. Alteration in neurologic disease during pregnancy has not been well documented, but several areas of concern exist. Because an increased incidence of carpal tunnel syndrome is noted during normal pregnancy, pregnancy edema may cause further impingement of a nerve already compressed by synovial tissue. Cervical spine arthritis with atlantoaxial instability dictates careful management of the unconscious patient under general anesthesia because manipulation of the unstable spine may produce spinal cord compression. Severe cricoarytenoid involvement also may be a relative contraindication to intubation with general anesthesia.

Pregnancy Outcome

Fertility and parity are not clearly decreased in patients with RA (104), and no conclusive increase in fetal morbidity or mortality has been demonstrated. Fetal growth retardation has been described in severe RA with associated vasculitis (105).

Management and Therapy

Common medications for treatment of RA include aspirin; nonsteroidal antiinflammatory drugs; and remittive agents, which include hydroxychloroquine, azulfidine, methotrexate, azathioprine, leflunomide, and gold. Use of newer agents has revolutionized treatment of RA. Biologic therapies, the tumor necrosis factor inhibitors infliximab and etan-

ercept, now are commonly used. Pregnancy data are not available for the biologic therapies. Corticosteroid may be used for resistant disease, and prednisone and methylprednisolone are considered safe for use in pregnancy. Fluorinated steroids, such as dexamethasone, traverse the placenta and are not recommended for routine use. Most other medications generally are stopped because of concerns regarding safety. Treatment of neurologic problems during pregnancy varies according to the underlying etiology. Rheumatoid meningitis or neuropathy due to active vasculitis should be treated with corticosteroids. Entrapment neuropathies generally benefit from appropriate splinting, although injection or surgical decompression may be required.

Summary

RA is a systemic disease affecting primarily joints but with significant extraarticular manifestations. The most common neurologic complications result from entrapment neuropathies or cervical spine disease, although peripheral neuropathy does occur and CNS disease (although rare) has been reported. Pregnancy in RA usually is accompanied by a clinical remission, followed by a postpartum exacerbation. Extraarticular manifestations including neurologic complications have not been well studied during pregnancy, but they seem uncommon. Risk of developing RA may be higher in the immediate postpartum period, although parity may exert an overall protective effect. Most patients do not require medications during the course of pregnancy. Neonatal outcome is probably normal.

Systemic Sclerosis

Systemic sclerosis, or scleroderma, is a disease of connective tissue characterized by fibrosis in the skin and other organ systems. Although there may be an early inflammatory component, the hallmark of the disease is skin thickening caused by excessive accumulation of connective tissue. Proliferative changes in vessels lead to Raynaud's phenomenon and other obliterative vascular disease. Systemic sclerosis is divided into two major categories: diffuse cutaneous disease and limited cutaneous disease. The CREST syndrome (*c*alcinosis, *R*aynaud's phenomenon, *e*sophageal hypomotility, *s*clerodactyly, and *t*elangiectasia) generally represents limited disease, although pulmonary hypertension may arise. Women are affected three times as often as men (106). Etiology is unknown, but recent data suggest a persistent microchimerism that occurs following pregnancy, with long-term persistence of fetal cells in the maternal system. Women with scleroderma exhibit a more pronounced form of fetal microchimerism than do controls, possibly provoking a graft-versus-host reaction that leads to progressive fibrosis (107).

Onset of systemic sclerosis generally begins between ages 30 and 50 years. Clinical features include skin thickening and subcutaneous calcinosis. Raynaud's phenomenon occurs in more than 95% of patients and may lead to digital ischemic necrosis. Esophageal dysfunction eventually develops in more than 90% of patients and represents the most common internal manifestation of disease. Hypomotility of both small and large intestines is common. Pulmonary fibrosis and myocardial vascular spasm and fibrosis are serious complications. Renal involvement is an important manifestation of systemic sclerosis and a major cause of death. Of patients with diffuse disease, 20% develop scleroderma renal crisis, characterized by the abrupt onset of malignant hypertension with rapidly progressive renal insufficiency (106).

Neurologic Manifestations of Systemic Sclerosis

Neurologic manifestations are distinctly uncommon in systemic sclerosis, and CNS events are particularly rare. Of 125 patients with systemic sclerosis followed for a mean of 31 months, only 5.6% developed definite neurologic manifestations (108), which included carpal tunnel syndrome, trigeminal

neuralgia, mononeuritis multiplex, and peripheral sensory neuropathy. Cerebral arteritis has been described rarely (109) as have cutaneous vasculitis and mononeuritis multiplex (110). One patient with established scleroderma and prominent Raynaud's phenomenon has been reported to have transient global ischemia, possibly as a result of vasospasm (111).

Trigeminal sensory neuropathy is the most commonly reported nerve disorder. Polyneuropathy, mononeuritis multiplex, and entrapment syndromes are probably less common. While abnormal cutaneous sensory thresholds have been demonstrated in up to 50% of patients with limited and diffuse systemic sclerosis, most patients are asymptomatic (112).

Pregnancy and Systemic Sclerosis

Because systemic sclerosis often affects women in later reproductive years, pregnancy during established disease is less common than with SLE or RA, and the course of pregnancy in these patients is not well defined. In a combined analysis of early studies, about one-third of patients reported pregnancy-related aggravation of their disease (113); 10% died of pregnancy-related complications, mainly hypertension, renal failure, and cardiovascular complications. Importantly, these series included a number of cases described prior to advances in management.

In contrast, a retrospective case-control study (114) found no difference in the rates of accelerated hypertension or renal failure in parous versus nulliparous scleroderma patients, suggesting that pregnancy may not adversely affect disease course. Incidence of hypertension, preeclampsia, or proteinuria was no different in pregnancies after diagnosis as compared with pregnancies prior to diagnosis of disease.

In Steen's prospective studies of 91 pregnancies in 59 patients with systemic sclerosis, maternal outcome was generally good. Raynaud's phenomenon improved during pregnancy, whereas esophageal reflux became worse. There were three cases of renal crisis during pregnancy, all in women with early diffuse disease. Four women had five healthy infants while taking angiotensin-converting enzyme (ACE) inhibitors (115,116).

Neurologic Disease in Systemic Sclerosis Pregnancy

Little is known about primary neurologic complications of scleroderma in pregnancy. Any overall increased risk of renal hypertensive disease is of concern, however, because accelerated hypertension and renal failure may predispose to associated secondary neurologic complications. Pregnancy-related edema may worsen existing clinical or subclinical entrapment neuropathies.

Pregnancy Outcome

Scleroderma patients have been reported to have both decreased fertility and decreased parity when compared with control populations. Early case-control studies showed twice the rate of spontaneous abortion and three times the rate of infertility compared to controls as well as a significant incidence of intrauterine growth retardation and preterm births that occurred with equal frequency before and after the diagnosis of systemic sclerosis (113). Recent prospective data, however, show no increase in frequency of miscarriage except in those with longstanding diffuse scleroderma. Preterm births occurred in 29% pregnancies, but neonatal survival was good (115,117). Controlled ovarian hyperstimulation with *in vitro* fertilization and surrogacy has been suggested as an option for those patients with longstanding advanced disease (118).

Management and Therapy

Treatment of pregnant patients with systemic sclerosis involves careful monitoring of renal function and treatment of hypertension. In general, ACE inhibitors should be stopped because of the risk of fetal renal toxicity. Other antihypertensives may be substituted.

For true scleroderma renal crisis, however, a life-threatening complication, ACE inhibitors may be the only effective therapy. Penicillamine, sometimes used to treat early disease, should be discontinued. Entrapment neuropathies arising during pregnancy may be treated with splinting or injection.

Summary

Systemic sclerosis, a collagen vascular disease characterized by fibrosis, generally responds poorly to therapy. Because onset is often after peak reproductive years, complications of pregnancy are not frequent. Increased risk of infertility is controversial. Preterm delivery occurs in about one-third of pregnancies. Neurologic manifestations are uncommon and usually involve peripheral or entrapment neuropathies. Accelerated hypertension and renal insufficiency are the most significant disease complications during pregnancy and, when severe, may produce secondary neurologic complications such as encephalopathy.

Sjögren's Syndrome

Sjögren's syndrome is a chronic inflammatory disorder characterized by the presence of the sicca syndrome, a decrease in lacrimal and salivary gland secretion that results in xerophthalmia and xerostomia. The glandular insufficiency is the result of lymphocyte infiltration. The syndrome may be primary (unassociated with other collagen vascular disease) or secondary, most often in patients with RA. More than 90% of patients are women, and mean age at onset is 50 years (119).

Characteristic symptoms include dry eyes, dry mouth, and parotid gland enlargement. Other manifestations include skin or vaginal dryness, renal tubular acidosis, pulmonary syndromes, and neurologic disease. Raynaud's phenomenon occurs in 20% of patients. Anti-SS-A/Ro and anti-SS-B/La antibodies occur in a high percentage of patients with primary Sjogren's syndrome. Other laboratory findings may include anemia, leukopenia, positive antinuclear antibody test (ANA), rheumatoid factor, and cryoglobulins. The risk of developing malignant lymphoma is increased.

Neurologic Manifestations

Neurologic complications in Sjögren's syndrome are seen in up to one-fourth of patients and include both peripheral and CNS events. In a series of 40 patients with neuropsychiatric Sjögren's syndrome, 25 patients had psychiatric abnormalities (affective disturbance was most common) and 27 had neurologic abnormalities, both CNS (16 patients) and peripheral (19 patients). Most CNS events involved the brain alone rather than the spinal cord; abnormal CSF was found in 16 of 20 patients evaluated. Peripheral abnormalities included entrapment neuropathies and other cranial and sensory-motor neuropathies (120). A neurologic presentation that may mimic multiple sclerosis has been described (121).

Pregnancy and Sjögren's Syndrome

Sjögren's syndrome is often secondary to RA and other autoimmune diseases, and little is known about the interaction of pregnancy with the primary syndrome. Fetal and neonatal outcome have been evaluated in patients with primary Sjögren's syndrome, and study results differ (122,123). One study suggested that pregnancies in patients with primary syndrome may have an increased risk of fetal loss, unrelated to presence of aCL or anti-Ro and La antibodies (122). Fetal growth retardation is uncommon. Further studies may answer the question of whether pregnancy affects CNS and other clinical manifestations of Sjögren's.

Management and Therapy

The most common management issue during pregnancy is evaluation for presence of anti-SS-A/Ro and anti-SS-B/La antibodies to assess risk of NLE discussed above. Risk of NLE appears to be related to antibody rather than underlying diagnosis (74). Severe neurologic involvement during pregnancy may be treated with corticosteroids. Immunosuppressives (other than azathioprine) should not be used. Entrapment neuropathies may improve with splinting or injection.

Summary

Primary Sjogren's syndrome is characterized by lymphocytic infiltration of exocrine glands, with prominent eye and mouth dryness. Other serious complications may be seen, including neurologic manifestations, which include a multiple sclerosis-like syndrome, other CNS abnormalities, psychiatric disorders, and peripheral neuropathies. Impact of pregnancy on this disorder, if any, is not yet defined.

Polymyositis and Dermatomyositis

Polymyositis and dermatomyositis (PM/DM) are chronic inflammatory muscle diseases. A characteristic rash distinguishes dermatomyositis from polymyositis. As with most collagen vascular disorders, a female predominance is noted. Onset is usually in the fifth or sixth decade, although it may develop at any age.

The major clinical manifestation is symmetric proximal muscle weakness with histologic findings of inflammation and myofiber damage and electrophysiologic evidence of myopathy. In severe cases, muscles involved in swallowing may be affected, and the cardiorespiratory system may be involved. Pulmonary fibrosis as well as ventilatory insufficiency resulting from muscle weakness is seen. Cardiac manifestations include heart block and dysrhythmias and, less commonly, myocarditis and congestive heart failure. Soft-tissue calcification may occur, most commonly in childhood cases.

Serologic findings include ANA, Jo-1 antibody, and other antibodies directed against transfer RNA synthetases. Treatment is high-dose corticosteroid and, for severe or resistant cases, immunosuppressive agents. Later age onset of dermatomyositis may reflect a paraneoplastic syndrome (124).

Neurologic Manifestations

CNS involvement only rarely has been reported. Symptoms of weakness are almost always related to pure myositis both histologically and on electrodiagnostic testing. Subarachnoid hemorrhage believed due to CNS vasculitis has been reported in a single patient (125).

Pregnancy and Polymyositis/Dermatomyositis

A small number of cases of PM/DM have been reported in pregnancy (126–132). Time of disease onset seems to have a marked effect on pregnancy outcome. Acute onset may occur during pregnancy or in the postpartum period. Disease presenting during pregnancy may be acute and severe and often improves after delivery. Associated rhabdomyolysis and myoglobinuria have been reported (128,129). Response to steroid therapy is usually prompt. Recurrence of exacerbation in subsequent pregnancies is not certain (130). Neonatal outcome is worst for patients with new-onset disease, with about 50% survival. Maternal death, even in these cases, is rare. Onset in the postpartum period is less common (131,132). Patients with established diagnoses who are in remission prior to conception have roughly a 25% risk of exacerbation during pregnancy. Fetal outcome in these patients is better, with 20% rate fetal loss.

Neurologic Disease in Polymyositis/Dermatomyositis Pregnancy

One case has been reported (127) of a patient with PM/DM and severe exacerbation of disease in the postpartum period with hemiplegia and death.

Management and Therapy

As with SLE, timing of pregnancy in relation to disease onset or exacerbation has a significant effect on pregnancy outcome. Prepregnancy evaluation of patients with known PM/DM for assessing disease activity is prudent. No evidence supports prophylactic corticosteroid treatment of patients in remission. Prompt diagnosis and therapy with corticosteroids may improve prognosis.

Summary

Polymyositis and dermatomyositis are chronic inflammatory diseases of muscle, characterized primarily by muscle weakness. Neurologic involvement is extremely rare. Pregnancy experience is limited by small numbers, but review of available cases suggests significant worsening of pregnancy outcome in patients with disease diagnosed during pregnancy; this is less so in patients with flare of established disease during pregnancy.

Behçet's Disease

Behçet's disease is a multisystem disorder of unknown etiology characterized by the triad of recurrent oral ulcerations, recurrent genital ulcerations, and iritis. The disease is most frequent in the Middle East and Japan. Other manifestations, which may be variable, include skin lesions, arthritis, vascular disease including migratory thrombophlebitis, gastrointestinal disease, epididymitis, hemorrhagic pneumonitis, and glomerulonephritis. Neurologic complications are common. Serologic studies are generally negative, although cryoglobulins may be demonstrated and acute phase reactants tend to be abnormal during periods of exacerbation (133).

Neurologic Manifestations

Neurologic complications of Behçet's are variable. A large prospective study (134) evaluated 323 patients with Behçet's disease for neurologic involvement. Of the 323 patients, 46 had headache or neurologic symptoms and signs. Twenty-three patients had headache alone, all with normal computerized tomography (CT) studies. Fourteen patients had headache in association with other neurologic findings, and six had neurologic symptoms other than headache. The most frequent presentation in these patients were pyramidal signs and headache; less common were cerebellar signs, sensory changes, pseudobulbar signs, and intracranial hypertension. Diagnoses included cerebral hemispheric lesions, superior sagittal sinus thrombosis, aseptic meningitis, brainstem syndromes, spinal cord involvement, and peripheral neuropathy. There was a predominantly male prevalence for the more severe manifestations, and uveitis was more common among patients with neurologic manifestations. Neurologic disease may be the most frequent cause of death in patients with Behçet's disease (133).

Pregnancy and Behçet's Disease

Review of the literature on Behçet's disease and pregnancy reveals contradictory reports of pregnancy's effect on disease activity (135–141). Individual case reports document both exacerbations and remissions of disease. In one family, a mother and two daughters had severe and prolonged exacerbation of disease during pregnancies (135). One daughter experienced similar symptoms while taking oral contraceptives, and the mother's symptoms remitted with menopause. In another case (136), a woman with mild manifestations developed severe oral and genital ulcers and iridocyclitis by week 25 of gestation. Postpartum chronic uveitis occurred with visual loss. In contrast, other case reports (137,138) describe dramatic amelioration of all symptoms during pregnancy, with exacerbation in the postpartum period. The effect of pregnancy may well be variable: one report of 27 prospectively followed pregnancies identified remission in nine pregnancies and exacerbation in 18. Exacerbations reported during pregnancy included oral and genital ulcerations and arthritis (139). A recent series of 61 pregnancies in 23 women, however, reported a disease flare in only two of the 23 women (140).

Few neurologic complications have been reported. One patient suffered a cerebral venous thrombosis at 31 weeks of gestation. She presented with progressive right-sided headache, photophobia and visual change (141).

Pregnancy Outcome

Fetal outcome is generally good, although, rarely, infants with pustulo-necrotic skin lesions and other manifestations have been reported (142). Lesions healed with scarring by 8 weeks.

Management and Therapy

Patients with Behçet's disease generally are treated with corticosteroids and, for severe manifestations, immunosuppressive medications, including azathioprine. Neurologic disease during pregnancy may require both corticosteroids and azathioprine. Other immunosuppressives are contraindicated during pregnancy. Prepregnancy counseling should include the possible risk of exacerbation related to pregnancy and the need to discontinue teratogenic medications.

Summary

Recurrent oral and genital ulcerations and uveitis characterize Behçet's disease. Other prominent manifestations include neurologic and vascular complications. Pregnancy's effect on the course of underlying disease is probably variable, with remission and exacerbation of skin lesions and ulcerations reported. Pregnancy in Behçet's disease does not seem to represent a major risk to the mother or fetus. Fetal outcome is generally good, and initial therapy during pregnancy, if required, should be corticosteroids.

VASCULITIS SYNDROMES

The vasculitis syndromes include a number of disorders characterized by inflammation involving blood vessels. The resulting damage leads to compromise of the vessel lumen with ischemic tissue changes (133). Although vasculitis may be a prominent feature of a number of rheumatic diseases, especially SLE, the vasculitis syndromes described here are primary. There is limited information on pregnancy outcome in these patients because most of the primary vasculitides occur in older individuals and are more common in males (143).

Polyarteritis Nodosa

The arteritis seen in polyarteritis nodosa (PAN) classically involves small and medium arteries, is segmental in nature, and shows a predilection for arterial bifurcations that may form small aneurysms. Edema, fibrinoid necrosis, and polymorphonuclear cell infiltration characterize acute lesions. These progress to chronic lesions, with mononuclear cell infiltration, granulation tissue, and, finally, scarring with intimal thickening and perivascular fibrosis. Acute and chronic changes may coexist within the same vessel. Common organs involved include kidney, gastrointestinal tract, heart, muscle, and nervous system. Lung involvement in PAN is uncommon.

Peak incidence is in the fifth and sixth decades, and the ratio of males to females is about 2 to 1. Early symptoms may be nonspecific. Common presentations include abdominal pain, hypertension, renal insufficiency or failure, and polyneuritis. Laboratory testing may show a leukocytosis, elevated sedimentation rate, and anemia. Serologic tests for antinuclear antibodies are characteristically negative. A high percentage of patients are positive for hepatitis B surface antigen (144). Diagnosis is made on the basis of histopathology and occasionally classical angiographic findings of typical aneurysms at arterial bifurcations and segmental narrowing ("beading") of small- and medium-sized arteries. Treatment is with high-dose corticosteroids and immunosuppressive therapy, usually oral cyclophosphamide (133).

Neurologic Manifestations

Peripheral neuropathy is a common manifestation of PAN, affecting 60% to 70% of patients (87). Mononeuropathy, multiple mono-

neuropathy, and polyneuropathy are all seen. CNS manifestations, less common than peripheral involvement, are usually a later manifestation (145). A review of 114 patients with PAN found 60 patients with CNS manifestations, although only six had CNS symptoms at time of diagnosis (146). Patients with intraabdominal aneurysms were more likely to have CNS disease. Cerebral thrombosis or hemorrhage may result in focal neurologic deficits, seizure, visual disturbance, vertigo, and coma.

Pregnancy and Polyarteritis Nodosa

Pregnancy in association with PAN is relatively uncommon due to the older mean age at onset and the male predominance of the disease. For the pregnant patient, time of onset of disease impacts on both maternal and fetal outcome. Initial presentation of PAN during pregnancy results in significant maternal mortality, with better fetal than maternal outcome (147,148). Whether pregnancy actually affects the course of PAN is unclear.

In cases of PAN reported in pregnancy, the disease had its onset during pregnancy or in the immediate postpartum period more than half of the time. Few patients who present during pregnancy have been diagnosed and treated at the time of onset. Of seven cases reported with onset during pregnancy, all seven patients died by postpartum day 42, with diagnosis made at autopsy for six of the seven cases (147). Outcome is significantly better for patients with established disease who are in clinical remission at the time of pregnancy. Preeclampsia with malignant hypertension and acute renal failure have been reported in a case of stable PAN, with dramatic improvement after delivery (149).

Although onset of PAN during pregnancy carries a significant risk of maternal mortality, a role for therapeutic abortion, suggested by some as a reasonable alternative, is not clear (150). PAN is a rapidly fatal disease without appropriate therapy, and it is likely that the high maternal mortality seen reflects at least partly the difficulty in diagnosis, especially when hypertension and renal insufficiency may be interpreted as resulting from preeclampsia.

Neurologic Manifestations of PAN in Pregnancy

The spectrum of neurologic complications in PAN during pregnancy has not been reported to vary from that occurring overall. Reed and Smith (148) reported a patient with an acute febrile illness with abdominal pain in the first trimester of pregnancy. She subsequently developed blurred vision from retinal edema and optic atrophy. PAN was diagnosed on skin biopsy, but although diagnosed antemortem, she failed to respond to high-dose corticosteroids and died after spontaneous abortion.

Pregnancy Outcome

Fetal outcome has been surprisingly good, probably because most reported cases of PAN with onset during pregnancy have been in the third trimester or immediate postpartum period. In one series, eight of 12 pregnancies (two with therapeutic abortions) produced viable neonates (147). Three infants have been reported with transient cutaneous vasculitis (151).

Management and Therapy

The effect of pregnancy on PAN is not clear because a number of cases reported were not diagnosed until postmortem. Those cases in remission prior to pregnancy report a low rate of exacerbation. Neurologic disease is treated as any other serious manifestation of active vasculitis—with high-dose corticosteroids. If required, corticosteroid therapy may be maintained or initiated during pregnancy. Immunosuppressive therapy with cyclophosphamide is contraindicated because of the risk of teratogenicity.

Summary

Polyarteritis nodosa is a systemic vasculitis that is often fatal if not treated aggressively.

Neurologic complications most commonly include peripheral neuropathy, especially mononeuritis multiplex. CNS manifestations are seen frequently but later in the course of disease. Effect of pregnancy on PAN is unclear, although maternal mortality has been 100% in the limited number of patients who present initially with their disease during pregnancy. Fetal outcome is surprisingly good. Neurologic complications during pregnancy are likely rare, although optimal therapy for these manifestations, cyclophosphamide, is considered to be prohibited during pregnancy because of the risk of teratogenicity.

Churg-Strauss Syndrome

Closely related to PAN, Churg-Strauss Syndrome (CSS) also is termed *allergic granulomatosis and angiitis*. Bronchial asthma and eosinophilia in addition to vasculitis involving one or more extrapulmonary sites characterize CSS. Biopsy often shows blood vessels with extravascular eosinophils. Mean age at onset is 47 years. Neurologic manifestations are similar to those reported in PAN; however, overall prognosis is better (133).

The first report of successful pregnancy in a patient with CSS was in 1993 (152). A 33-year-old woman with a 1-year history of CSS presented with mononeuritis multiplex, cutaneous vasculitis and pleuritis at the twenty-fourth week of pregnancy. Treated with high-dose corticosteroid, she ultimately delivered a healthy infant with mild intrauterine growth retardation. Numbers are small, but it is likely that maternal mortality rate in CSS pregnancy is less than that seen with PAN (153). A successful twin pregnancy has been reported after treatment with corticosteroid and cyclophosphamide (154). Exacerbation induced by pregnancy is suggested by one case with relapse of disease in four successive pregnancies, which was fatal in the fourth pregnancy despite aggressive treatment of fulminant vasculitis and cardiac disease (155).

Primary Angiitis of the Central Nervous System

Primary angiitis of the central nervous system (PACNS) is an uncommon vasculitis characterized by involvement limited to the vessels of the CNS, without other systemic signs or symptoms. Early manifestations of disease generally include severe headache and altered mental function, with progression to multifocal neurologic deficits. The most common pattern on histopathology is involvement of small vessels with a mononuclear cell infiltrate and various degrees of granuloma formation. However, any size vessel may be involved (156).

Neurologic Manifestations

Focal neurologic deficits are found in less than 25% of patients at presentation. Focal deficits subsequently develop in more than 90% of patients during the disease course and eventually multiple focal deficits develop in more than 80% of patients (156). Systemic symptoms are characteristically absent.

In a large series of 48 patients with PACNS (157), headache was the most common presenting symptom, and a combination of focal and diffuse deficits was found in 79% of patients. Five patients had involvement of the spinal cord only. Laboratory results were variable. Although the average erythrocyte sedimentation rate (ESR) was 44 mm per hour, the ESR was normal in 12 of 35 patients. CSF analysis showed elevated protein levels in 70% of cases, with a lymphocytic pleocytosis in 68%. Electroencephalogram was abnormal in 81% of patients in whom it was performed, with the most common abnormality being diffuse slowing. Of patients, 65% underwent cerebral angiography, and results were abnormal in 71%, with characteristic changes including widespread irregular areas of narrowing and dilatation. Histopathology on leptomeningeal biopsy was diagnostic in the remainder of the cases.

Pregnancy and Primary Angiitis of the Central Nervous System

Several reports document development of PACNS in pregnancy and the postpartum period. Farine and associates (158) reported the first case in pregnancy, a 28-year-old woman admitted in labor with acute severe bitemporal headache. An angiogram done 12 days postpartum for continued symptoms showed multiple areas of segmental narrowing. Of eight cases reported by Calabrese and Mallek (157), two involved onset of symptoms in the puerperium. One 32-year-old patient developed severe headache followed by visual symptoms, seizure, and hemiparesis. CT examination showed right parietooccipital infarct. The second patient, a 26-year-old woman, developed headache and hemiparesis several days postpartum in association with hypertension. These patients were treated with corticosteroid and oral cyclophosphamide with complete resolution of symptoms. Fetal outcome was normal.

Isolated angiitis of the CNS has presented as intracranial hemorrhage during cesarean section and during the postpartum (159,160).

Hypertension-induced vasospasm in the puerperium may mimic PACNS. A clear example is Garner and colleague's report of a 35-year-old woman with severe headache 9 days postpartum associated with blood pressure elevation to 160/90 and left parietal symptoms. Angiogram showed widespread irregularities with areas of narrowing and dilatation consistent with vasculitis. The hypertension was treated, and the angiogram repeated 9 days later showed complete normalization. The authors suggest that some pregnancy or postpartum cases of PACNS may represent hypertension-induced changes rather than true vasculitis (161).

Management and Therapy

Usual treatment of PACNS is high-dose corticosteroid and immunosuppressive medication, usually cyclophosphamide, which has dramatically improved prognosis (157). Azathioprine is a reasonable alternative immuno-suppressive during pregnancy.

Summary

PACNS is a rare disorder with isolated vasculitis affecting the CNS. It may be more common in pregnancy and the puerperium. The role of pregnancy-induced hypertension with vasospastic changes is not clear but needs to be considered in the differential diagnosis of this syndrome. Although no systemic symptoms are present, abnormalities often are found on analysis of CSF and angiography. Definitive diagnosis, however, is based on leptomeningeal biopsy.

Takayasu's Arteritis

Takayasu's arteritis is a chronic inflammatory condition affecting primarily young females, with involvement of large vessels, usually the aorta and its main branches. It is a rare disease with incidence estimated at 2.6 per million per year worldwide, but is more common in Asia. Etiology is not known. Histopathology shows granulomatous arteritis with active inflammation and changes confined to the media and adventitia. Sclerosing arteritis is a later finding, although inflammatory and stenotic phases may coexist.

Features at presentation vary, depending on the duration of the disease. Most patients present with vascular insufficiency of the upper extremity, usually arm claudication or numbness. Multiple vascular bruits and absent or reduced pulses are common. An early inflammatory phase with prominent systemic symptoms such as fever, malaise, and weight loss often occurs prior to diagnosis. Other symptoms include arthralgia, skin involvement with small-vessel vasculitis, hypertension, cardiac involvement including coronary artery disease, aortic insufficiency, myocarditis, and pulmonary artery involvement with mild to moderate pulmonary hypertension. Diagnosis usually is made on the basis of angiogram or tissue histopathology, if available (162).

Neurologic Manifestations

Neurologic complications in Takayasu's arteritis are primarily the result of cerebral ischemia secondary to the involvement of the carotid and/or vertebrobasilar systems. Dizziness, syncope, headache, blindness, diplopia, hemiparesis and paraparesis, cerebellar symptoms, seizures, and memory deficits all have been reported, presumably secondary to ischemia (87). Stroke, seizure, or syncope may be the initial manifestation of the disease (145). Of patients, 30% note some disturbance of vision, including blurring, diplopia, or amaurosis fugax, but retinopathy is less common. Stroke is an important cause of death in patients who die from their disease.

Pregnancy and Takayasu's Arteritis

Despite the significant vascular abnormalities, pregnancy in patients with Takayasu's arteritis generally has a good outcome if appropriate antihypertensive therapy is administered. Aggressive hemodynamic monitoring is critical for labor and delivery (163). Preeclampsia is significantly increased as a result of chronic hypertension. A large series, reported by Wong and colleagues (164), included a total of 30 pregnancies in 13 patients. Eleven pregnancies were prior to disease onset and were uneventful. In the other 19 pregnancies, four terminated in abortions—three spontaneous and one elective. Of the remaining 15 pregnancies, 11 were complicated by preeclampsia. No case of eclampsia was seen. More than half of the patients were first diagnosed during their pregnancy. No major obstetric problems were noted other than hypertension. Pharmacologic therapy for hypertension was required in half of the pregnancies.

To detect effect of pregnancy itself on course of disease and disease manifestations, Matsumara and associates prospectively followed 22 pregnancies in 18 patients and measured C-reactive protein and blood pressure measurements before, during, and after pregnancy and concluded that inflammatory activity and hemodynamics actually improve during pregnancy, possibly secondary to hormonal changes (165).

Neurologic Disease in Takayasu's Arteritis Pregnancy

Risk of neurologic complications appears greatest around the time of delivery. Tomioka and associates reported a young woman with a history of Takayasu's arteritis and cerebral hemorrhage during normal vaginal delivery (166). Blood pressure was managed successfully by monitoring central aortic blood pressure at the thoracic aorta during a subsequent uncomplicated delivery. Even more extensive monitoring has been suggested: a patient with pulseless upper extremities, history of cerebrovascular disease, and severe bilateral carotid artery stenoses was additionally monitored with processed electroencephalography to detect cerebral ischemia during cesarean section (167). Surgery was uncomplicated.

Although numbers are small, pregnancy-related exacerbation of hypertension and risks of preeclampsia–eclampsia probably increase the risk of neurologic events, including stroke or seizure. Anesthesia management at the time of labor and delivery is critical. Both hypertension and hypotension should be avoided in Takayasu's arteritis due to vessel changes with marked variation in regional blood flow and, potentially, in organ perfusion. Epidural anesthesia may affect blood pressure. Aggressive hemodynamic monitoring is important (163).

Pregnancy Outcome

Fetal outcome is generally good, although infants frequently may show evidence of intrauterine growth retardation related to severity of hypertension, extent of abdominal aorta and renal artery involvement, and onset of preeclampsia. Changes in placental blood flow may influence outcome (164).

Management and Therapy

In general, active Takayasu's arteritis is treated with high-dose corticosteroid, al-

though benefit is controversial (155). Chronic disease may require vascular surgery intervention even during the pregnancy itself. A report describes placement of wall stent following angioplasty of abdominal aortic stenosis immediately following emergency cesarean section for toxemia at 27 weeks (168). Usual management during pregnancy includes corticosteroid, if indicated; careful monitoring and treatment of hypertension; and aggressive hemodynamic and pharmacologic management in the peripartum period.

Summary

Takayasu's arteritis, a granulomatous large-vessel vasculitis, often is diagnosed after active inflammation has produced vascular insufficiency and occlusion. Neurologic complications are common and usually are caused by cerebrovascular insufficiency or hemorrhage. Pregnancy, often complicated by preeclampsia, is best managed with frequent monitoring of blood pressure and aggressive treatment. In patients with significant occlusive disease, central aortic pressure monitoring may be necessary. Fetal outcome, generally good, is notable for a high rate of intrauterine growth retardation.

Wegener's Granulomatosis

Wegener's granulomatosis is characterized by granulomatous vasculitis of the upper and lower respiratory tracts with glomerulonephritis. Vessels involved may include both small arteries and small veins. The ratio of males to females is 2 to 1, and usual age of onset is in the fourth and fifth decades (133).

Common signs and symptoms include pulmonary infiltrates (71%), sinusitis (67%), arthralgia or arthritis (44%), fever (34%), cough (34%), and otitis (25%). Renal failure occurs in 11% of patients (169).

Neurologic Manifestations

Involvement of the nervous system occurs in up to 22% of patients with Wegener's granulomatosis (169). Nervous system involvement may involve granulomatous lesions of the CNS or vasculitis of the central or peripheral nervous systems. Infection of the CNS also may occur with immunosuppressive therapy and must be differentiated from active vasculitis (87). CNS disease usually develops in the setting of active sinusitis, otitis, or pulmonary disease. Aphasia and subarachnoid hemorrhage have been reported (145). Of 88 patients with neurologic involvement secondary to Wegener's granulomatosis, cranial nerve and peripheral nerve involvement was most common, especially optic nerve involvement and hearing loss (169–171).

Pregnancy and Wegener's Granulomatosis

The spectrum of clinical manifestations of Wegener's granulomatosis appears to be similar in the pregnant and nonpregnant patient. It has been suggested that Wegener's granulomatosis occurring during pregnancy may have a more aggressive course. Twenty-one pregnancies in 18 patients with Wegener's granulomatosis and pregnancy now have been reported (172). Twelve of the 18 reported patients initially were diagnosed with Wegener's during the course of the affected pregnancy (including postpartum diagnoses). Nine cases of disease exacerbation during pregnancy occurred, all antepartum, with two relapses during second pregnancies. Two maternal deaths have been reported.

Cases with new diagnosis during pregnancy have had variable presentations (173–177), including new-onset tracheal stenosis during pregnancy (177). Diagnosis in the first trimester presents a particularly difficult problem. Palit and Clague (174) reported a woman who presented with arthritis, hemoptysis, dyspnea, and other symptoms at week 7 of pregnancy. Because of concerns regarding teratogenicity of cyclophosphamide, she terminated pregnancy. Another patient with a previous diagnosis of Wegener's who relapsed during the first trimester was treated unsuccessfully with corticosteroid and suffered a spontaneous abortion at 5 months, followed by increased disease activity with new pulmonary involvement treated with oral cyclophosphamide (178). Finally, a patient with arthralgia, cutaneous lesions, hemoptysis, renal insufficiency, and nasal symptoms at 17 weeks of pregnancy was diagnosed on nasal biopsy and was treated with oral cyclophosphamide, corticosteroid, and hemodialysis during the second and third trimesters, with delivery of a healthy male infant at 33 weeks gestation (175).

Neurologic Manifestations in Wegener's Granulomatosis Pregnancy

Neurologic involvement during pregnancy has been reported infrequently but appears severe. Milford and Bellini reported a patient who presented with nasal obstruction, epistaxis, and arthralgia in gestational week 21. Biopsy of mucosal and cutaneous lesions confirmed the diagnosis of Wegener's granulomatosis. Several days after institution of prednisone and azathioprine, the patient developed a left lower quadrantic field deficit, became unresponsive, and died. CT scan showed bilateral intracerebral hematomas in the right frontoparietal and left occipital regions (170).

Management and Therapy

Usual treatment of Wegener's granulomatosis involves both high-dose corticosteroid and immunosuppressive medication, usually oral cyclophosphamide. Cyclophosphamide is relatively contraindicated during pregnancy, especially during the first trimester because of the risk of teratogenicity. Ideally, pregnancy should be planned during a period of remission. For patients with active disease presenting during pregnancy, alternative therapy with corticosteroid alone or with azathioprine should be considered. A small number of patients with active disease in the late second or third trimesters have been treated successfully with cyclophosphamide with good neonatal outcome (174,179). In at least one severe case, aggressive therapy has included empiric intravenous immunoglobulin and plasma exchange to avoid use of cyclophosphamide (175 same as earlier). Neurologic complications, unless resulting from infection, should be treated in the same way as other manifestations of active vasculitis.

Summary

Wegener's granulomatosis, a granulomatous vasculitis, classically affects the upper and lower respiratory tracts as well as the kidney, but may affect the central or peripheral nervous systems. Cases occurring in pregnancy are rare. Treatment with corticosteroid and immunosuppressive therapy has improved prognosis significantly.

SARCOIDOSIS

Sarcoidosis is a multisystem granulomatous disorder of unknown etiology. Affecting women more often than men, its peak incidence is in the third and fourth decades. Infection or allergic reaction with an exaggerated immune response is suspected. The classic histologic feature is the sarcoid granuloma, a tightly packed collection of macrophages and epithelioid cells that fuse to form multinucleated Langerhan's cells.

The clinical presentation of sarcoidosis varies. Most patients are asymptomatic, with bilateral hilar adenopathy found on routine chest radiograph. Of patients, 20% to 30% present with respiratory symptoms of cough or shortness of breath; 25% present with systemic symptoms of fever, fatigue, and weight loss; and a small percent (less than 10%) present with arthritis. The acute arthritis usually is seen as part of Lofgren's syndrome, defined by the triad of arthritis, erythema nodosum, and bilateral hilar adenopathy, which tends to be self-limited with a good prognosis.

Although pulmonary manifestations predominate, many other organ systems may be involved in systemic sarcoidosis. The pulmonary involvement ranges from isolated bilateral hilar adenopathy to severe restrictive fibrotic disease and is classified as Stage 0

through IV. Eye involvement is common, typically anterior or posterior uveitis. Cardiac manifestations include arrhythmia secondary to myocardial granuloma. Arthritis may be severe, and both acute and chronic arthropathies are seen. The acute arthritis often is associated with Lofgren's syndrome. The chronic arthritis may produce an erosive-deforming picture similar to that seen with RA. Treatment of significant disease requires corticosteroid (180).

Neurologic Manifestations

Neurologic complications, although well described, affect only 5% of patients with sarcoidosis. Neurologic disease may be the presenting manifestation, and a significant number of these patients may have a normal chest radiograph (181). The most common neurologic abnormality is facial nerve palsy, although other cranial nerves may be affected. CNS involvement tends to occur in early acute sarcoidosis. Manifestations reported include aseptic meningitis, basilar obstructive pachymeningitis, single or multiple sarcoid masses in the brain, and diffuse encephalopathy (181,182). Seizures in neurosarcoidosis are associated with a more severe and progressive course. Krumholz and associates evaluated 79 patients with neurosarcoid; 15% of these had seizures. These patients were more likely to have intracranial mass lesions, encephalopathy, vasculopathy, or hydrocephalus. Two of the 13 patients with seizures died (183).

Pregnancy and Sarcoidosis

The effect of pregnancy on sarcoidosis is not clearly established and may be variable (184–186). Amelioration of disease during pregnancy, with increased risk postpartum, has been suggested (184). Agha and associates (185) identified variable disease courses in 18 sarcoidosis patients during pregnancy: no effect was seen in nine patients, improvement was noted in six patients, and a deleterious effect was seen in three patients. In another series of 15 pregnant patients with sarcoidosis, ten women had stable disease with prepregnancy resolution of chest radiograph abnormalities, and they experienced no recurrence during pregnancy (186). One patient with an abnormal but improving chest radiograph continued to improve during pregnancy, and two patients, both with Stage II disease, had disease progression. Two patients had fatal courses during pregnancy; both of these had Stage IV, severe restrictive disease prior to conception.

Most reports suggest that patients with inactive and mild disease do not worsen during pregnancy. Patients with severe restrictive lung disease or other severe manifestations may worsen with the physical stress of pregnancy. Neurologic complications during pregnancy have not been specifically reported. It is not known whether patients with neurosarcoid worsen during pregnancy, and this may depend on severity and activity of disease. Poor maternal outcome overall has been associated with advanced maternal age, chronic disease with insidious onset, pulmonary fibrosis on chest radiography, and requirement for other drugs in addition to corticosteroid (186).

Pregnancy Outcome

Fetal survival is generally good. In a recent review, no increased risk of fetal loss, obstetric complications, or congenital abnormalities associated with mothers with sarcoidosis were found (187). Haynes de Regt (186) did find an increased rate of cesarean section (40%) in patients, as well as a significant number of infants weighing less than 2,500 g (27%).

Management and Therapy

Asymptomatic hilar adenopathy or mild disease need not be treated. When treatment is necessary, corticosteroid most commonly is used. Severe neurologic disease generally requires high-dose corticosteroid. Some patients have steroid-resistant disease or require

addition of other immunosuppressives as corticosteroid sparing agents. Peripartum care requires careful observation, especially if staging on chest radiograph examination is other than Stage I, or other organ system involvement is present.

Summary

Sarcoidosis is a granulomatous disease primarily affecting the lungs. Patients are often asymptomatic. Other organ involvement includes skin, eye, joint, heart, gastrointestinal tract, and nervous system. Neurosarcoid is uncommon and may affect both central and peripheral nervous systems. CNS sarcoid may involve focal lesions, diffuse encephalopathy, or aseptic meningitis. Cranial neuropathy is common, and peripheral neuropathy is associated with longstanding chronic disease. Pregnancy may have an ameliorating effect in some cases. Patients with severe, longstanding disease generally have a poorer maternal prognosis.

THROMBOTIC THROMBOCYTOPENIC PURPURA

Thrombotic thrombocytopenic purpura (TTP) is a rare syndrome characterized by the pentad of thrombocytopenic purpura, microangiopathic hemolytic anemia, neurologic symptoms, renal disease, and fever (188). A related syndrome, hemolytic-uremic syndrome (HUS), is a TTP-like variant that affects primarily the kidneys and has less prominent neurologic manifestations. Current data suggest the presence of unusually large von Willebrand multimers as the most likely underlying abnormality (189,190). Characteristic microvascular hyaline occlusions are seen on biopsy of affected organs, although the diagnosis most often is made clinically. Although TTP may arise at any age, peak incidence is in the third decade; the ratio of females to males is 2 to 1. TTP usually develops spontaneously, but reports of associations with antecedent infection, drug use, pregnancy, or autoimmune disease suggest that these may play a role in precipitating disease (188). HUS may be more common among users of oral contraceptives and in the postpartum period (191).

An association of TTP with SLE has been suggested, although the clinical manifestations of TTP may be found in SLE alone as a manifestation of severe disease flare. Ridolfi and Bell (188) identified nine patients in the TTP literature with either clinical SLE or autoimmune serologies. Meyers and colleagues (192) also described a patient with known SLE who subsequently developed TTP. A review of postmortem studies of 50 SLE patients found some patients with CNS disease to have significant clinical and histopathologic evidence of TTP, implicating this as a cause of lupus-related CNS disease (15).

A summary of features of more than 250 patients with TTP found the most common chief complaints to be weakness, headache, dizziness, confusion, and dysarthria (188). Organ system manifestations included neurologic (84% of patients), renal (76%), fever (59%), microangiopathic hemolytic anemia (91%), and purpura or other bleeding (83%). Skin was the major site of hemorrhage. Hematuria was the most common renal abnormality, with 45% of patients having serum creatinine levels greater than 2.0 mg per dL, and 11.5% of patients with acute renal failure. Anemia was prominent, and 38% of patients had serum hemoglobin levels less than 6.5. Platelet counts of less than 20,000 were found in 56% of patients. Cardiac manifestations included congestive heart failure and sudden death.

Neurologic Manifestations

Of patients, 84% have neurologic symptoms at some point in their disease course. Neurologic symptoms involve primarily the CNS and are the presenting complaint in 54% of cases. Specific manifestations include confusion, paresis, dysphasia, headache, coma, seizures, altered mental state, parasthesias, and visual problems. Symptoms may be transient and are often recurrent (188).

Pregnancy and TTP

A large number of cases of TTP have occurred in pregnancy or the postpartum setting, and an association with pregnancy has been suggested (193-197). This is especially true of HUS, which commonly is reported in the postpartum period. Up to 70 cases of TTP have been reported in pregnant or postpartum women (194). Of 25 pregnant patients with TTP reported by Ridolfi and Bell, the majority were in their third trimester, with three cases appearing in the postpartum period, four during the first trimester, and six during the second trimester. Ten of these patients died, and their overall response was no different than that of other patients with TTP (188).

These numbers are small, and, although it is not clear that pregnancy increases the risk of TTP, some case reports are compelling. Wiznitzer and colleagues (195) reported two sisters with classic TTP developing during late pregnancy. The second sister developed TTP in the setting of *Escherichia coli* urosepsis. The authors suggest that a genetic predisposition with one or more inciting events, in this case pregnancy and infection, may trigger the disease. TTP diagnosed during pregnancy has a high chance of relapse during later pregnancies (196).

Prognosis of TTP in pregnancy has been poor for both mother and child, although many cases were reported prior to institution of current therapy with plasma infusion and plasma exchange. Of 70 cases reviewed by Rozdzinski and colleagues (194), 38 mothers and 22 children survived, but only 14 mother–child pairs survived. Although TTP does not reliably remit postpartum, Natelson and White (197) reported a case of TTP, diagnosed at 13 weeks, which was unresponsive to usual therapy, including plasma exchange. Their patient underwent a therapeutic termination of pregnancy with complete resolution of her disease.

A recent series of patients with TTP during pregnancy, diagnosed and followed since inception of plasma exchange therapy, suggests significant but improved mortality rates: 18% maternal mortality, 30% fetal mortality, and 45% maternal morbidity (198).

As with other diseases complicating pregnancy, TTP may be difficult to distinguish from pregnancy-induced hypertension (PIH) syndromes because both may involve microangiopathic anemia, thrombocytopenia, and neurologic complications. Although both TTP and PIH may have evidence of microangiopathy and thrombocytopenia, these are more marked in TTP. Similarly, neurologic dysfunction is more common in TTP, as is fever, which is not expected in PIH. Hypertension, characteristic of PIH, is less common in TTP (193). Delay or error in diagnosis may affect outcome because the current treatment of choice for TTP involves plasma infusion and plasma exchange. Immediate delivery is not clearly indicated, as it is for severe preeclampsia–eclampsia.

Neurologic Manifestations in TTP Pregnancy

There is no evidence of a difference in disease course in pregnant patients with TTP as compared to those with TTP in the absence of pregnancy. However, diagnosis may be difficult because of the similar presentation of preeclampsia–eclampsia. Neurologic manifestations probably do not differ in pregnancy-associated TTP. In Egerman and colleague's series of 11 patients with TTP or HUS in pregnancy, five patients had neurologic symptoms, most commonly blurred vision with confusion and/or headache (198).

Pregnancy Outcome

Reports of fetal survival with maternal TTP are largely limited to those cases presenting in the third trimester, often with preterm delivery. When TTP presents in the first trimester, fetal death is the usual result; severe maternal anemia and thrombi formation in the placenta may be responsible (199). No cases of neonatal TTP have been reported.

Management and Therapy

Initial reports of treatment for TTP included corticosteroid, antiplatelet agents, splenectomy, and immunosuppressive agents. Only with the institution of plasma infusion and plasma exchange did the survival rate for TTP increase to 80% to 90% (188). Management during pregnancy is directed at treating the underlying disease. No evidence supports termination of pregnancy as an alternative therapy, although in at least one case report (197) this has apparently prompted remission of disease.

Summary

TTP is characterized by a pentad of thrombocytopenic purpura, microangiopathic hemolytic anemia, fever, renal disease, and neurologic complications. Neurologic manifestations occur in most patients and range from headache to paresis, aphasia, and coma. Although TTP may be more common in pregnancy, no evidence exists to suggest that the clinical course in these patients differs. Treatment is plasma therapy, plasma exchange, or both, and possibly antiplatelet agents.

MEDICATION USE IN PREGNANCY

A number of medications are used routinely to treat rheumatologic disorders, depending on the precise diagnosis and the severity of disease. These include aspirin, nonsteroidal anti-inflammatory drugs, antimalarials (such as hydroxychloroquine), gold, corticosteroid, and immunosuppressive medications such as azathioprine, methotrexate, leflunomide, mycophenolate mofetil, and cyclophosphamide. Newer biologic agents for RA include etanercept and infliximab. It is often not possible to discontinue all medications during pregnancy. In addition, if symptoms worsen, treatment may need to be initiated during pregnancy. Concerns during pregnancy include risk of inducing fetal malformation and contribution to pregnancy complications such as hypertension, diabetes, or preeclampsia.

A summary of medications used in treatment of rheumatic diseases is shown in Table 9.3. Because of greater experience in pregnancy, aspirin is preferred to the relatively newer nonsteroidal anti-inflammatory drugs. Prednisone and prednisolone are considered relatively safe in pregnancy because of their 90% metabolism by placental 11-β-dehydrogenase. Animal studies have suggested an increased risk of cleft palate, which has not been seen in humans (200). Other corticosteroid medications are not metabolized in this way, and unless corticosteroid effect on the fetus is desired (for cardiac inflammation in NLE or to promote lung maturity), these should not be used. Corticosteroids may increase risk for developing gestational diabetes, hypertension, and premature rupture of membranes. Data on safety of hydroxychloroquine are encouraging but not conclusive

TABLE 9.3. *Common medications for rheumatic disease: potential fetal effects*

Drug	Potential effects
Aspirin	Placental transfer occurs.
	Generally safe.
	Increased risk of bleeding, prolongation of labor, premature closure of ductus arteriosus. (Discontinue 1–2 weeks prior to delivery if possible.)
NSAID	No long-term studies; safety has not been established. Indomethacin near term has significant risk of premature closure of ductus arteriosus.
Hydroxychloroquine	Placental transfer occurs.
	Animal studies: accumulation in fetal uveal tract, inner ear. Safety has not been established in human pregnancy. Case reports suggest no adverse outcome, but possible risk of ocular- and ototoxicity.
Corticosteroid	Placental transfer depends on preparation.
	Animal studies: increased risk of cleft palate, low birthweight.
	Prednisone, prednisolone: largely metabolized by placental enzymes.
	Considered safe in pregnancy in low to moderate doses.
	Dexamethasone and betamethasone: should be used only when fetal corticosteroid effect desired (high degree of placental transfer). May lead to adrenal insufficiency in the neonate.
Gold	Placental transfer occurs.
	Animal studies: demonstrate teratogenicity.
	Small number of human pregnancies reported. Safety in pregnancy cannot be established.
Sulfasalazine	Placental transfer occurs.
	Safety has not been established in human pregnancy, but used in some patients with inflammatory bowel disease with folate supplementation.
Penicillamine	Placental transfer occurs.
	Animal studies: teratogenic in large doses.
	Safety not established in human pregnancy and has been associated with cutis laxa (rare connective tissue disorder) in neonate.
Azathioprine	Placental transfer limited by placental metabolism.
	Animal studies: toxic at high doses.
	Probably safe in human pregnancy but some risk of neonatal immunosuppression.
	Does not commonly cause sterility.
Methotrexate	Placental transfer occurs.
	Lethal in dose-dependent fashion.
	Probably not safe in human pregnancy: may cause fetal malformation including cranial ossification defects.
	Does not commonly induce sterility.
	Fetal anomalies rare if discontinued 1 year prior to conception.
Cyclophosphamide	Placental transfer occurs.
	Animal studies: teratogenic.
	Unsafe in human pregnancy with high rate of malformations, especially if administered in first trimester.
	May cause sterility.
	Fetal anomalies uncommon if discontinued 1 year prior to conception.

(201,202); theoretical risks include retinal toxicity and ototoxicity. Gold, penicillamine, and sulfasalazine have not been established as safe for use in pregnancy and generally are discontinued. Immunosuppressive medications generally are stopped, but if necessary, azathioprine may be continued with relatively low risk to the fetus. Methotrexate and cyclophosphamide should not be administered during pregnancy because they are teratogenic (203).

Postpartum use of medication in the breast-feeding mother should follow similar guidelines. Some medications may become more concentrated in breast milk, so caution should be used. Generally, corticosteroids and aspirin may be administered, and other drug use is discouraged.

REFERENCES

1. Branch DW. Physiologic adaptations of pregnancy. *Am J Reprod Immunol* 1992;28:120–122.
2. Hill JA. Cytokines considered critical in pregnancy. *Am J Reprod Immunol* 1992;28:123–125.
3. Johnson MJ. Obstetric complications and rheumatic disease. *Rheum Dis Clin North Am* 1997;23:169–182.
4. Fessel WJ. Systemic lupus erythematosus in the community. *Arch Intern Med* 1974;134:1027–1035.
5. Hanley JG, Fisk JD Sherwood G, et al. Cognitive impairments in patients with systemic lupus erythematosus. *J Rheumatol* 1992;19:562–567.
6. Anonymous. The American College of Rheumatology nomenclature and case definitions for neuropsychiatric lupus syndromes. *Arthritis Rheum* 1999;42: 599–608.
7. Rosner S, Ginzler EM, Diamond HS, et al. A multicenter study of outcome in systemic lupus erythematosus. II: Causes of death. *Arthritis Rheum* 1982; 25:612–619.
8. Estes D, Christian CL. The natural history of systemic lupus erythematosus by prospective analysis. *Medicine* 1971;50:85–95.
9. Kaell AT, Shetty M, Lee BCP, et al. The diversity of neurologic events in systemic lupus erythematosus. *Arch Neurol* 1986;43: 273–276.
10. Ellis SG, Verity MA. Central nervous system involvement in systemic lupus erythematosus: a review of neuropathologic findings in 57 cases, 1955–1977. *Semin Arthritis Rheum* 1979;8:212–221.
11. Adelman DC, Saltiel E, Klinenberg JR. The neuropsychiatric manifestations of systemic lupus erythematosus: an overview. *Semin Arthritis Rheum* 1986;15: 185–199.
12. Schwartz MM, Roberts JL. Membranous and vascular choroidopathy: two patterns of immune deposits in systemic lupus erythematosus. *Clin Immunol Immunopathol* 1983;29:369–380.
13. Bluestein HG, Williams GW, Steinberg AD. Cerebrospinal fluid antibodies to neuronal cells: association with neuropsychiatric manifestations of systemic lupus erythematosus. *Am J Med* 1981;70:240–246.
14. Bonfa E, Golombek SJ, Kaufman LD, et al. Associations between lupus psychosis and antiribosomal P protein antibodies. *N Engl J Med* 1987;317:265–271.
15. Devinsky O, Petito CK, Alonso DR. Clinical and neuropathological findings in systemic lupus erythematosus: the role of vasculitis, heart emboli, and thrombotic thrombocytopenic purpura. *Ann Neurol* 1988;23: 380–384.
16. Futrell N, Schultz LR, Millikan C. Central nervous system disease in patients with systemic lupus erythematosus. *Neurology* 1992;42:1649–1661.
17. Karassa FB, Ionnadis JP, Boki KA, et al. Predictors of clinical outcome in patients with neuropsychiatric manifestations of systemic lupus erythematosus. *Am J Med* 2000;109:628–634.
18. Amigo MC, Khamashta MA. Antiphospholipid (Hughes) syndrome in systemic lupus erythematosus. *Rheum Dis Clin North Am* 2000;26:331–349.
19. Alarcon-Segovia D, Sanchez-Guerrero J. Primary antiphospholipid syndrome. *J Rheumatol* 1989;16: 482–488.
20. Sammaritano LR. Drug-induced antiphospholipid antibodies. In: Khamashta MA, ed. *Hughes syndrome: antiphospholipid syndrome.* London: Springer, 2000: 144–154.
21. Harris EN, Gharavi AE, Hughes GR. Antiphospholipid antibodies. *Clin Rheum Dis* 1985;11:591–609.
22. Harris EN, Gharavi AE, Asherson RA, et al. Cerebral infarction in systemic lupus: association with anticardiolipin antibodies. *Clin Exp Rheumatol* 1984;2: 47–51.
23. Asherson RA, Derkson RH, Harris EN, et al. Chorea in systemic lupus erythematosus and "lupus-like" disease: association with antiphospholipid antibodies. *Semin Arthritis Rheum* 1987;16:253–257.
24. Lavalle C, Pizzaro S, Drenkard C, et al. Transverse myelitis: a manifestation of systemic lupus erythematosus strongly associated with antiphospholipid antibodies. *J Rheumatol* 1990;17:34–37.
25. Briley DP, Coull BM, Goodnight SH. Neurological disease associated with antiphospholipid antibodies. *Ann Neurol* 1989;25:221–227.
26. Sergent JS, Lockshin MD, Klempner MS, et al. Central nervous system disease in systemic lupus erythematosus: therapy and prognosis. *Am J Med* 1975;58: 644–654.
27. Takada K, Illei GG, Boumpas DT. Cyclophosphamide for the treatment of systemic lupus erythematosus. *Lupus* 2001;10:154–161.
28. Ward MM, Pyun E, Studenski S. Long-term survival in systemic lupus erythematosus: patient characteristics associated with poorer outcomes. *Arthritis Rheum* 1995;274–287.
29. Ellis FA, Bereston ES. Lupus erythematosus associated with pregnancy and menopause. *AMA Arch Dermatol Syph* 1952;65:170–177.
30. Lockshin MD, Sammaritano LR, Schwartzman S. Lupus pregnancy. In: Lahita RG, ed. *Systemic lupus erythematosus.* 3rd ed. San Diego: Academic Press 1999: 507–536.
31. Ruiz-Irastorza G, Lima F, Alves J, et al. Increased rate

of lupus flare during pregnancy and the puerperium: a prospective study of 78 pregnancies. *Br J Rheumatol* 1996;35:133–138.

32. Lockshin MD. Pregnancy does not cause systemic lupus erythematosus to worsen. *Arthritis Rheum* 1989; 32:665–670.

33. Petri M, Howard D, Repke J. Frequency of lupus flare in pregnancy. *Arthritis Rheum* 1991;34:1538–1545.

34. Tozman EC, Urowitz MB, Gladman DD. Systemic lupus erythematosus and pregnancy. *J Rheumatol* 1980; 7:624–632.

35. Zulman JI, Talal N, Hoffman GS, et al. Problems associated with management of pregnancies in patients with systemic lupus erythematosus. *J Rheumatol* 1980;7:37–49.

36. Gimovsky ML, Montoro M, Paul RH. Pregnancy outcome in women with systemic lupus erythematosus. *Obstet Gynecol* 1984;63:686–692.

37. Mintz G, Niz J, Gutierrez G, et al. Prospective study of pregnancy in systemic lupus erythematosus: results of a multidisciplinary approach. *J Rheumatol* 1986;13: 732–739.

38. Nossent HC, Swaak TJ. Systemic lupus erythematosus. VI: Analysis of the interrelationship with pregnancy. *J Rheumatol* 1990;17:771–776.

39. Liang MH, Sochen SA, Larson MG, et al. Reliability and validity of six systems for the clinical assessment of disease activity in systemic lupus erythematosus. *Arthritis Rheum* 1989;32:1107–1118.

40. Imbasciati E, Surian M, Bottino S, et al. Lupus nephropathy and pregnancy: a study of 26 pregnancies in patients with systemic lupus erythematosus and nephritis. *Nephron* 1984;36:46–51.

41. Bobrie G, Liote F, Houllier P, et al. Pregnancy in lupus nephritis and related disorders. *Am J Kidney Dis* 1987; 4:339–343.

42. Devoe LD, Loy GL, Spargo BH. Renal histology and pregnancy performance in systemic lupus erythematosus. *Clin Exper Hypertens B* 1983; 2:325–340.

43. Hopkinson ND, Powell RJ. Classical complement activation induced by pregnancy: implications for management of connective tissue disease. *J Clin Pathol* 1992;45:66–67.

44. Lockshin MD, Harpel PC, Druzin ML, et al. Lupus pregnancy. II: Unusual pattern of hypocomplementemia and thrombocytopenia in the pregnant patient. *Arthritis Rheum* 1985;28:58–65.

45. Buyon JP, Tamerius J, Ordorica S, et al. Activation of the alternative complement pathway accompanies disease flares in systemic lupus erythematosus during pregnancy. *Arthritis Rheum* 1992;35:55–61.

46. Kuzis CS, Druzin ML, Lambert RE. Case report: a patient with severe CNS lupus during pregnancy. *Ann Med Interne (Paris)* 1996;147:274–277.

47. Wolf RE, McBeath JG. Chorea gravidarum in systemic lupus erythematosus. *J Rheumatol* 1985;12: 992–997.

48. Marabani M, Zoma A, Hadley D, et al. Transverse myelitis occurring during pregnancy in a patient with systemic lupus erythematosus. *Ann Rheum Dis* 1989; 48:160–162.

49. Sammaritano LR. Update on the management of the pregnant patient with antiphospholipid antibody. *Curr Rheumatol Rep* 2001;3:213–221.

50. Suzuki Y, Kitagawa Y, Matsuoka Y, et al. Severe cerebral and systemic necrotizing vasculitis developing during pregnancy in a case of systemic lupus erythematosus. *J Rheumatol* 1990;17:1408–1411.

51. Le Thi Huong D, Wechsler B, Edelman P, et al. Postpartum cerebral infarction associated with aspirin withdrawal in the antiphospholipid syndrome. *J Rheumatol* 1993;20:1229–1232.

52. Bonnet F, Mercie P, Morlat P, et al. Devic's neuromyelitis optica during pregnancy in a patient with systemic lupus erythematosus. *Lupus* 1999;8: 244–247.

53. Pengo V, Thiagarajan P, Shapiro S, et al. Immunological specificity and mechanism of action of IgG lupus anticoagulants. *Blood* 1987;70:69–76.

54. Harris EN, Gharavi AE, Boey ML, et al. Anticardiolipin antibodies: detection by radioimmunoassay and association with thrombosis in systemic lupus erythematosus. *Lancet* 1983;2:1211–1214.

55. MacNeil HP, Simpson RJ, Chesterman CV, et al. Antiphospholipid antibodies are directed against a complex antigen that includes a lipid-binding inhibitor of coagulation: B2-glycoprotein I (apolipoprotein H). *Proc Nat Acad Sci USA* 1990;87:4120–4124.

56. Galli M. Should we include anti-prothrombin antibodies in the screening for the antiphospholipid syndrome? *J Autoimmun* 2000;15:101–106.

57. Carreras LO, Vermylon JG. Lupus anticoagulant and thrombosis: possible role of inhibition of prostacyclin formation. *Thromb Haemost* 1982;42:38–40.

58. Cariou R, Tobelen G, Soria C, et al. Inhibition of protein C activation by endothelial cells in the presence of lupus anticoagulant. *N Engl J Med* 1986;314:1193–1194.

59. Moreb J, Kitchens CS. Acquired functional protein S deficiency, cerebral venous thrombosis, and coumarin skin necrosis in association with antiphospholipid syndrome: report of 2 cases. *Am J Med* 1989;87:207–210.

60. Tsakiris DA, Marbet GA, Makris PE, et al. Impaired fibrinolysis as an essential contribution to thrombosis in patients with lupus anticoagulant. *Thromb Haemost* 1989;61:175–177.

61. Triplett DA. Antiphospholipid antibodies and recurrent pregnancy loss. *Am J Reprod Immunol* 1989;20: 52–67.

62. Lockshin MD, Druzin ML, Goei S, et al. Antibody to cardiolipin as a predictor of fetal distress or death in pregnant patients with systemic lupus erythematosus. *N Engl J Med* 1985;313:152–156.

63. Lockshin MD, Druzin ML, Qamar T. Prednisone does not prevent recurrent fetal death in women with antiphospholipid antibody. *Am J Obstet Gynecol* 1989; 160:439–443.

64. Lo SCL, Oldmeadow MJ, Howard MA, et al. Comparison of laboratory tests used for identification of the lupus anticoagulant. *Am J Hematol* 1989;30:213–220.

65. Lee RM, Emlen W, Scott JR, et al. Anti-b2-Glycoprotein I antibodies in women with recurrent spontaneous abortion, unexplained fetal death, and antiphospholipid syndrome. *Am J Obstet Gynecol* 1999;181:642–648.

66. Franklin RD, Hollier N, Kutteh WH. Beta-2 Glycoprotein I as a marker of antiphospholipid syndrome in women with recurrent pregnancy loss. *Fertil Steril* 2000;73:531–535.

67. Branch DW, Scott JR, Kochenour NK, et al. Obstetric complications associated with the lupus anticoagulant. *N Engl J Med* 1985;313:1322–1326.

68. Sthoeger ZM, Mozes E, Tartakovsky B. Anti-cardi-olipin antibodies induce pregnancy failure by impairing embryonic implantation. *Proc Nat Acad Sci USA* 1993;90:6464–6467.

69. Branch DW, Andres R, Digre KB, et al. The association of antiphospholipid antibodies with severe pre-eclampsia. *Obstet Gynecol* 1989;73: 541–545.

70. Arun Rao A, Anantha Krishna NC. Anticardiolipin antibodies in eclampsia. *Int J Gynecol Obstet* 1992;38: 37–40.

71. Navarro F, Dona-Naranjo MA, Villanueva I. Neonatal antiphospholipid syndrome. *J Rheumatol* 1997;24: 1240–1241.

72. Block SR, Winfield JB, Lockshin MD, et al. Studies of twins with systemic lupus erythematosus. A review of the literature and presentation of 12 additional sets. *Am J Med* 1975;59:533–552.

73. Buyon JP. Complete heart block and antibodies to the SSA/Ro-SSB/La antigen systems. *Clin Aspects Autoimmunity* 1990;4:8–17.

74. Lockshin MD, Bonfa E, Elkon K, et al. Neonatal risk to newborns of mothers with systemic lupus erythematosus. *Arthritis Rheum* 1988;31:697–702.

75. Englert HJ, Derue GM, Loizous S, et al. Pregnancy and lupus: prognostic indicators and responses to treatment. *Q J Med* 1988;66:125–136.

76. Silveira LH, Hubble CL, Jara LJ. Prevention of anti-cardiolipin antibody-related pregnancy losses with prednisone and aspirin. *Am J Med* 1992;93:403–409.

77. Rosove MN, Tabsh K, Wasserstrum N, et al. Heparin therapy for pregnant women with lupus anticoagulant or anticardiolipin antibodies. *Obstet Gynecol* 1990;75: 630–634.

78. Cowchock FS, Reece EE, Balaban D, et al. Repeated fetal losses associated with antiphospholipid antibodies: a collaborative randomized trial comparing prednisone with low-dose heparin treatment. *Am J Obstet Gynecol* 1992;166:1318–1323.

79. Kutteh WH. Antiphospholipid antibody-associated recurrent pregnancy loss: treatment with heparin and low-dose aspirin is superior to low-dose aspirin alone. *Am J Obstet Gynecol* 1996;174:1584–1589.

80. Kutteh WH, Ermel LD. A clinical trial for the treatment of antiphospholipid antibody-associated recurrent pregnancy loss with lower dose heparin and aspirin. *Am J Reprod Immunol* 1996;35:402–406.

81. Rai R, Cohen H, Dave M, et al. Randomized controlled trial of aspirin and aspirin plus heparin in pregnant women with recurrent miscarriage associated with phospholipid antibodies (or antiphospholipid antibodies). *BMJ* 1997;314:253–259.

82. Branch DW, Peaceman AM, Druzin M, et al. A multicenter placebo-controlled study of intravenous immunoglobulin treatment of antiphospholipid syndrome during pregnancy. The Pregnancy Loss Study Group. *Am J Obstet Gynecol* 2000;182:122–127.

83. Langevitz P, Livneh A, Dulitzki M, et al. Outcome of pregnancy in three patients with primary antiphospholipid syndrome after stroke. *Sem Arthritis Rheum* 1998;28:26–30.

84. Inbar O, Blank M, Faden D, et al. Prevention of fetal loss in experimental antiphospholipid syndrome by low-molecular weight heparin. *Am J Obstet Gynecol* 1993;169:423–426.

85. Harris ED Jr. Rheumatoid arthritis: clinical aspects. In: Kelly WN, Harris ED Jr, Ruddy S, et al, eds. *Textbook of rheumatology.* Philadelphia: WB Saunders Co, 1997;898–932.

86. Arnett FC, Edworthy SM, Black DA, et al. The American Rheumatism Association 1987 revised criteria of the classification of rheumatoid arthritis. *Arthritis Rheum* 1988;31:315–324.

87. Cohen SB, Hurd ER. Neurological complications of connective tissue and other "collagen vascular" diseases. *Semin Arthritis Rheum* 1981;11:190–212.

88. Maher JA. Dural nodules in rheumatoid arthritis: report of a case. *Arch Pathol* 1954;58: 354–359.

89. Kim RC, Collins GH, Parisi JE. Rheumatoid nodule formation within the choroid plexus: report of a second case. *Arch Pathol Lab Med* 1982;106:83–84.

90. Hauge T, Magnes B, Loken AC, et al. Treatment of rheumatoid pachymeningitis involving the entire thoracic region. *Scand J Rheumatol* 1978;7:209–211.

91. Markenson JA, McDougal JS, Tsairis P, et al. Rheumatoid meningitis: a localized immune process. *Ann Intern Med* 1979;90:786–789.

92. Skowronski T, Gatter RA. Cerebral vasculitis associated with rheumatoid disease: a case report. *J Rheumatol* 1974;1:473.

93. Ramos M, Mandybur TI. Cerebral vasculitis in rheumatoid arthritis. *Arch Neurol* 1975;32:271–275.

94. Winfield J, Cooke D, Brook AS, et al. A prospective study of the radiological changes in the cervical spine in early rheumatoid disease. *Ann Rheum Dis* 1981;40: 109–114.

95. Matthews JA. Atlanto-axial subluxation in rheumatoid arthritis. *Ann Rheum Dis* 1969;28:260–266.

96. Chamberlain MA, Bruckner FE. Rheumatoid neuropathy: clinical and electrophysiological features. *Ann Rheum Dis* 1970;29:609–616.

97. Cecere FA, Persellin RH. The interaction of pregnancy and the rheumatic diseases. *Clin Rheum Dis* 1981;7: 747–768.

98. Ostensen M, Husby G. A prospective study of the effect of pregnancy on rheumatoid arthritis and ankylosing spondylitis. *Arthritis Rheum* 1983;26:1155–1159.

99. Barrett JH, Brennan P, Fiddler M, et al. Does rheumatoid arthritis remit during pregnancy and relapse postpartum? Results from a nationwide study in the United Kingdom preformed prospectively from late pregnancy. *Arthritis Rheum* 1999;42:1219–1227.

100. Nelson JL, Hughes KA, Smith AG, et al. Maternal-fetal disparity for HLA class II allo-antigens and the pregnancy-induced amelioration of rheumatoid arthritis. *New Engl J Med* 1993;329:500–501.

101. Silman A, Kay A, Brennan P. Timing of pregnancy in relation to the onset of rheumatoid arthritis. *Arthritis Rheum* 1992;35:152–155.

102. Hazes JM, Dijkmans BA, Vandenbroucke JP, et al. Pregnancy and the risk of developing rheumatoid arthritis. *Arthritis Rheum* 1990;33:1770–1775.

103. Hazes JM, Dijkmans BA, Vandenbroucke JP, et al. Reduction of the risk of rheumatoid arthritis among women who take oral contraceptives. *Arthritis Rheum* 1990;33:173–179.

104. Nelson JL, Ostenson M. Pregnancy and rheumatoid arthritis. *Rheum Dis Clin N Am* 1997;23:195–212.

105. Duhring JL. Pregnancy, rheumatoid arthritis, and intrauterine growth retardation. *Am J Obstet Gynecol* 1970;108:325–327.

106. Seibold JR. Scleroderma. In: Kelly WN, Harris ED Jr, Ruddy S, et al, eds. *Textbook of rheumatology.* Philadelphia: WB Saunders Co, 1997:1133–1162.

107. Bianchi DW. Fetomaternal cell trafficking: a new cause of disease? *Am J Med Genetics* 2000;91:22–28.

108. Lee P, Bruni J, Sukenik S. Neurological manifestations in systemic sclerosis (scleroderma). *J Rheumatol* 1984;11:480–483.

109. Estey E. Cerebral arteritis in scleroderma. *Stroke* 1979;10:595–597.

110. Oddis CV, Eisenbeis CH, Reidbord HE, et al. Vasculitis in systemic sclerosis: association with Sjogren's syndrome and the CREST syndrome variant. *J Rheumatol* 1987;14:942–948.

111. Nishida A, Kaiya H, Vematsu M, et al. Transient global ischemia and Raynaud's phenomenon in scleroderma. *Acta Neurol Scand* 1990;81:550–552.

112. Schady W, Sheard A, Hassell A, et al. Peripheral nerve dysfunction in scleroderma. *Q J Med* 1991;80: 661–675.

113. Maynon R, Jejgin M. Scleroderma in pregnancy. *Obstet Gynecol Surv* 1989;44:530–534.

114. Steen VD, Conte C, Day N, Ramsey-Goldman R, Medsger TA. Pregnancy in women with systemic sclerosis. *Arthritis Rheum* 1989;32:151–157.

115. Steen VD. Pregnancy in women with systemic sclerosis. *Obstet Gynecol* 1999;94:15–20.

116. Steen VD, Medsger TA Jr. Fertility and pregnancy outcome in women with systemic sclerosis. *Arthritis Rheum* 1999;42:763–768.

117. Silman AJ, Black C. Increased incidence of spontaneous abortion and infertility in women with scleroderma before disease onset: a controlled study. *Ann Rheum Dis* 1988;47:441–444.

118. Tsirigotis M, Lammiman D, Craft IL. Induction of ovulation and systemic sclerosis: a case for surrogacy. *J Assist Reprod Genetics* 1993;10:529–531.

119. Fox RI. Sjogren's syndrome. In: Kelly WN, Harris ED Jr, Ruddy S, eds. *Textbook of rheumatology.* Philadelphia: WB Saunders Co, 1997:955–968.

120. Malinow KW, Molina R, Gordon B, et al. Neuropsychiatric manifestations in primary Sjogren's syndrome. *Ann Intern Med* 1985;103:344–349.

121. Alexander EL. Primary Sjogren's syndrome with central nervous system disease mimicking multiple sclerosis. *Ann Intern Med* 1986;104:323–330.

122. Julkunen H, Kaaja R, Kurki P, et al. Fetal outcome in women with primary Sjogren's syndrome: a retrospective case-control study. *Clin Exp Rheum* 1995;13: 65–71.

123. Skopouli FN, Papanikolaou S, Malamov-Mitsi V, et al. Obstetric and gynecological profile in patients with primary Sjogren's syndrome. *Ann Rheum Dis* 1994;53: 569–573.

124. Wortmann RL. Inflammatory diseases of muscle and other myopathies. In: Kelly WN, Harris ED Jr, Ruddy S, et al, eds. *Textbook of rheumatology.* Philadelphia: WB Saunders Co, 1997:1177–1206.

125. Gotoff SP, Smith RD, Sugar O. Dermatomyositis with cerebral vasculitis in a patient with agammaglobulinemia. *Am J Dis Child* 1972;123:53–56.

126. Gutierrez G, Dagnino R, Mintz G. Polymyositis/dermatomyositis and pregnancy. *Arthritis Rheum* 1984; 27:291–294.

127. England MJ, Perlmann T, Veriava Y. Dermatomyositis in pregnancy: a case report. *J Reprod Med* 1986;31: 633–635.

128. Ditzian-Kadanoff R, Reinhard JD, Thomas C, et al. Polymyositis with myoglobinuria in pregnancy: a report and review of the literature. *J Rheumatol* 1988; 15:513–514.

129. Kofteridis DP, Malliotakis PI, Sotsiou F, et al. Acute onset of dermatomyositis presenting in pregnancy with rhabdomyelosis and fetal loss. *Scand J Rheumatol* 1999;28:192–194.

130. Papapetropoulos T, Kanella-Kopoulou N, Tsibri E, et al. Polymyositis and pregnancy: report of a case with three pregnancies (letter). *J Neurol Neoursurg Psych* 1998;64:406.

131. Kanah H, Izumi T, Seishima M, et al. A case of dermatomyositis that developed after delivery: the involvement of pregnancy in the induction of dermatomyositis. *Br J Dermatol* 1999;141:897–900.

132. Steiner I, Auerbuch-Heller L, Abramsky O, et al. Postpartum idiopathic polymyositis. *Lancet* 1992;339:256.

133. Valente RM, Hall S, O'Duffy JD, et al. Vasculitis and related disorders. In: Kelly WN, Harris ED Jr, Ruddy S, et al, eds. *Textbook of rheumatology.* Philadelphia: WB Saunders Co, 1997:1079–1122.

134. Serdaroglu P, Yazici H, Ozdemir C, et al. Neurologic involvement in Behçet's syndrome: a prospective study. *Arch Neurol* 1989;46:265–269.

135. Madkour M, Kudwah A. Behçet's disease [Letter]. *BMJ* 1978;11:1786

136. Hurt WG, Cooke CL, Jordan WP, et al. Behçet's syndrome associated with pregnancy. *Obstet Gynecol* 1979;53:315–335.

137. Larsson LG, Baum J. Behçet's syndrome in pregnancy and after the delivery [Letter]. *J Rheumatol* 1987;14: 183.

138. Hamza M, Elleuch M, Zrib A. Behçet's disease and pregnancy. *Ann Rheum Dis* 1988;47:350.

139. Bang D, Chun YS, Haam IB, et al. The influence of pregnancy on Behçet's disease. *Yonsei Med J* 1997;38: 437–443.

140. Marsal S, Falga C, Simeon CP, et al. Behçet's disease and pregnancy relationship study. *Br J Rheumatol* 1997;36:234–238

141. Wechsler B, Genereau T, Biousse V, et al. Pregnancy complicated by cerebral venous thrombosis in Behçet's disease. *Am J Obstet Gynecol* 1995;173: 1627–1629.

142. Stark AC, Bhakta B, Chamberlain MA, et al. Life-threatening transient neonatal Behçet's disease. *Br J Rheumatol* 1997;36:700–702.

143. Ramsey-Goldman R. The effect of pregnancy on the vasculitides. *Scand J Rheumatol* 1998;107:116–117.

144. Sergent JS, Lockshin MD, Christian CL. Vasculitis with hepatitis B antigenemia: long term observation in nine patients. *Medicine (Baltimore)* 1976;55:1–18.

145. Sigal LH. The neurologic presentation of vasculitis and rheumatologic syndromes: a review. *Medicine (Baltimore)* 1987;66:157–180.

146. Ford RG, Siekert RG. Central nervous system manifestations of periarteritis nodosa. *Neurology* 1965;15: 114–129.

147. Owen J, Hauth JC. Polyarteritis nodosa in pregnancy: a case report and brief literature review. *Am J Obstet Gynecol* 1989;160:606–607.

148. Reed NR, Smith MT. Periarteritis nodosa in preg-

nancy: report of a case and review of the literature. *Obstet Gynecol* 1990;55:381–385.

149. Aya AG, Hoffet M, Mangin R, et al. Severe preeclampsia superimposed on polyarteritis nodosa. *Am J Obstet Gynecol* 1996;174:1659–1660.

150. Nagey DA, Fortier KJ, Linden J. Pregnancy complicated by periarteritis nodosa: induced abortion as an alternative. *Am J Obstet Gynecol* 1983;147:103–105.

151. Stone MS, Olsen RR, Weismann DN, et al. Cutaneous vasculitis in the newborn of a mother with cutaneous polyarteritis nodosa. *J Am Acad Dermatol* 1993;28: 101–105.

152. Debby A, Tanay A, Zakut H. Allergic granulomatosis and angiitis (Churg-Strauss vasculitis) in pregnancy. *Int Arch Allergy Immunol* 1993;102:307–308.

153. Ogasawara M, Kajiura S, Inagaki H, et al. Successful pregnancy in a Churg-Strauss syndrome patient with a history of intrauterine fetal death. *Int Arch Allergy Immunol* 1995;108:200–202.

154. Barry C, Davis S, Garrard P, et al. Churg-Strauss disease: deterioration in a twin pregnancy. Successful outcome following treatment with corticosteroids and cyclophosphamide. *Br J Obstet Gynecol* 1997;104:746–747.

155. Connolly JO, Lanham JG, Partridge MR. Fulminant pregnancy-related Churg-Strauss syndrome. *Br J Rheumatol* 1994;33:776–777.

156. Cupps TR, Moore PM, Fauci AS. Isolated angiitis of the central nervous system: prospective diagnostic and therapeutic experience. *Am J Med* 1983;74:97–105.

157. Calabrese LH, Mallek JA. Primary angiitis of central nervous system: report of 8 new cases, review of the literature, and proposal for diagnostic criteria. *Medicine (Baltimore)* 1987;67:20–39.

158. Farine D, Andreyko J, Lysikiewicz A, et al. Isolated angiitis of brain in pregnancy and puerperium. *Obstet Gynecol* 1984; 63:586–588.

159. Yasuda Y, Matsuda I, Kang Y, et al. Isolated angiitis of the central nervous system first presenting as intracranial hemorrhage during cesarean section. *Int Med* 1993;32:745–748.

160. Ursell NR, Marras CL, Farb R, et al. Recurrent intracranial hemorrhage due to post-partum cerebral angiopathy: implications for management. *Stroke* 1998; 29:1995–1998.

161. Garner BF, Burns P, Bunning RD, et al. Acute blood pressure elevation can mimic arteriographic appearance of cerebral vasculitis (a postpartum case with relative hypertension). *J Rheumatol* 1990;17:93–97.

162. Hall S, Buchbinder R. Takayasu's arteritis. *Rheum Dis Clin North Am* 1990;16:411–422.

163. Crofts SL, Wilson E. Epidural analgesia for labor in Takayasu's arteritis: case report. *Br J Obstet Gynaecol* 1991;98:408–409.

164. Wong VCW, Wang RYC, Tse TF. Pregnancy and Takayasu's arteritis. *Am J Med* 1983;75: 597–601.

165. Matsumara A, Morwaki R, Numaro F. Pregnancy in Takayasu arteritis from the view of internal medicine. *Heart Vessels* 1992;7:120–124.

166. Tomioka N, Hirose K, Abe E, et al. Indications for peripartum aortic pressure monitoring in Takayasu's disease. A patient with a past history of intrapartum cerebral hemorrhage. *Jpn Heart J* 1998;39:255–260.

167. Clark AG, al-Qatari M. Anesthesia for Caeserean section in Takayasu's disease. *Can J Anaesthes* 1998; 45:377–379.

168. Wang YM, Mak GY, Lai KN, et al. Treatment of Takayasu's aortitis with percutaneous transluminal angioplasty and wall stent—a case report. *Angiology* 1998;49:945–949.

169. Fauci AS, Haynes BF, Katz P, et al. Wegener's granulomatosis: prospective clinical and therapeutic experience with 85 patients for 21 years. *Ann Intern Med* 1983;98:76–85.

170. Milford CA, Bellini M. Wegener's granulomatosis arising in pregnancy. *J Laryngol Otol* 1986;100: 475–476.

171. Sahn EE, Sahn SH. Wegener's granulomatosis with aphasia. *Arch Intern Med* 1976;136:87–89.

172. Harber MA, Tso A, Taheri S, et al. Wegener's granulomatosis in pregnancy—the therapeutic dilemma. *Nephrol Dial Transplant* 1999;14:1789–1791.

173. Talbot SF, Main DE, Levison AI. Wegener's granulomatosis: first report of a case with onset during pregnancy. *Arthritis Rheum* 1984;27:109–112.

174. Palit J, Clague RB. Wegener's granulomatosis presenting during first trimester of pregnancy. *Br J Rheumatol* 1990;29:389–390.

175. Fields CL, Ossorio MA, Roy TM, et al. Wegener's granulomatosis complicated by pregnancy: a case report. *J Reprod Med* 1991;36:463–466.

176. Habib A, MacKay K, Abrons HL. Wegener's granulomatosis complicating pregnancy: presentation of two patients and review of the literature. *Clin Nephrol* 1996;46:332–336.

177. Pauzner R, Mayan H, Hershko E, et al. Exacerbation of Wegener's granulomatosis during pregnancy: report of a case with tracheal stenosis and literature review. *J Rheumatol* 1994;21:1153–1156.

178. Kumar A, Mohan A, Gupta R, et al. Relapse of Wegener's granulomatosis in the first trimester of pregnancy: a case report. *Br J Rheumatol* 1998;37: 331–333.

179. Luisiri P, Lance NJ, Curran JJ. Wegener's granulomatosis in pregnancy. *Arthritis Rheum* 1997;40: 1354–1360.

180. Barnard J, Newman LS. Sarcoidosis: immunology, rheumatic involvement, and therapeutics. *Curr Opinion Rheum* 2001;13:84–91.

181. Stern BJ, Krumholz A, Johns C, et al. Sarcoidosis and its neurological manifestations. *Arch Neurol* 1985;42: 909–917.

182. Zajjicek JP. Neurosarcoidosis. *Curr Opinion Neurol* 2000;13:323–325.

183. Krumholz A, Stern BJ, Stern EG. Clinical implications of seizures in neurosarcoidosis. *Arch Neurol* 1991;48: 842–844.

184. Mayock RL, Sullivan RD, Greening RR, et al. Sarcoidosis and pregnancy. *JAMA* 1957;164:158–163.

185. Agha FP, Vade A, Amendola MA, et al. Effects of pregnancy on sarcoidosis. *Surg Gynecol Obstet* 1992; 155:817–822.

186. Haynes de Regt R. Sarcoidosis and pregnancy. *Obstet Gynecol* 1987;70:369–372.

187. Selroos O. Sarcoidosis and pregnancy: a review with results of a retrospective survey. *J Intern Med* 1990; 227:221–224.

188. Ridolfi RL, Bell WR. Thrombotic thrombocytopenic purpura: report of 25 cases and review of the literature. *Medicine* 1981;60:413–428.

189. Moake JL, Rudy CK, Troll JH, et al. Unusually large

plasma factor. VIII: von Willebrand factor multimers in chronic relapsing thrombotic thrombocytopenic purpura. *N Engl J Med* 1982;307:1432–1435.

190. Furlan M, Robles R, Galbusera M, et al. Von Willebrand factor—cleaving protease in thrombocytopenic purpura and the hemolytic uremic syndrome. *N Eng J Med* 1998;339:1578–1584.

191. Schoolwerth AC, Sandler RS, Klahi S, et al. Nephrosclerosis postpartum and in women taking oral contraceptives. *Arch Intern Med* 1976;135:178–184.

192. Meyers JJ, Wakem CJ, Ball ED, et al. Thrombotic thrombocytopenic purpura: combined treatment with plasmapheresis and antiplatelet agents. *Ann Intern Med* 1980;92:149–155.

193. Miller JM, Pastoric JG 2nd. Thrombotic thrombocytopenic purpura and hemolytic uremic syndrome in pregnancy. *Clin Obstet Gynecol* 1991;34:64–71.

194. Rozdzinski E, Hertenstein B, Schmeiser T, et al. Thrombotic thrombocytopenic purpura in early pregnancy with maternal and fetal survival. *Ann Hematol* 1992;64:245–248.

195. Wiznitzer A, Mazor M, Leiberman JR, et al. Familial occurrence of thrombotic thrombocytopenic purpura in two sisters during pregnancy. *Am J Obstet Gynecol* 1992;166:20–21.

196. Ezra Y, Rose M, Eldor A. Therapy and prevention of thrombocytopenic purpura during pregnancy: a clinical study of 16 pregnancies. *Am J Hematol* 1996; 51:1–6.

197. Natelson FA, White D. Recurrent thrombocytopenic purpura in early pregnancy: effect of uterine evaluation. *Obstet Gynecol* 1985;66:545.

198. Egerman RS, Witlin AG, Friedman SA, et al. Thrombotic thrombocytopenic purpura and hemolytic uremic syndrome in pregnancy: review of 11 cases. *Am J Obstet Gynecol* 1996;175:950–956.

199. Van de Kerchove F. TTP mimicking toxemia. *Am J Obstet Gynecol* 1984;150:320–324.

200. Janssen NM, Genta MS. The effects of immunosuppressives and anti-inflammatory medicines on fertility, pregnancy, and lactation. *Arch Int Med* 2000;160: 610–619.

201. Roubenoff R, Hoyt J, Petri M, et al. Effects of anti-inflammatory and immunosuppressive drugs on pregnancy and fertility. *Semin Arthritis Rheum* 1988;18:88.

202. Parke AL. Antimalarial drugs, systemic lupus erythematosus and pregnancy. *J Rheumatol* 1988;15:607.

203. Rudolph JE, Schweizer RT, Bartus SA. Pregnancy in renal transplant patients. *Transplantation* 1979;27: 26.

Neurological Complications of Pregnancy, Second Edition, edited by Brian Hainline and Orrin Devinsky. Lippincott Williams & Wilkins, Philadelphia © 2002.

10

Multiple Sclerosis

Stuart D. Cook

Department of Neurosciences, UMDNJ, New Jersey Medical School, Newark, New Jersey, U.S.A.

Multiple sclerosis (MS) is an acquired inflammatory demyelinating disorder of the central nervous system with clinical manifestations reflecting the varied distribution of lesions within the neuraxis. MS primarily affects young adults, with a mean age of onset of about 30 years and approximately 2 to 1 ratio of females to males. Consequently, women of childbearing age are a major target group for the disease.

Although the etiology and pathogenesis of MS are unknown, accumulating evidence supports the hypothesis that one or more environmental agents, probably infectious in nature, triggers an autoimmune process in a genetically susceptible host. Epidemiologic clues abound as to environmental triggers, with changing incidence rates in disparate geographic areas, controversial reports of epidemics, and an unusual worldwide disease distribution. Mean annual incidence in the United States is approximately 4 per 100,000 population, with an estimated 250,000 to 350,000 individuals currently afflicted with the disease.

Signs and symptoms reflect the multifocal location of white matter lesions in the brain and spinal cord; paresis, spasticity, tremors, incoordination, paresthesias, pain, sphincteric disturbances, visual loss, nystagmus, diplopia, dysarthria, and cognitive changes are common manifestations as the disease progresses. Early in the course, diagnosis may be difficult. With a monosymptomatic presentation, focal structural and mass occupying le-

sions must be considered. B_{12} deficiency, vasculitides, the anticardiolipin syndrome, infections (Lyme disease, human immunodeficiency virus, human T-cell lymphotropic virus type I, syphilis), sarcoidosis, spinocerebellar degenerations, the leukodystrophies, and lymphomas also can mimic MS. With the passage of time, the typical fluctuations with or without progression in patient disability and dissemination of lesions limited to the central nervous system simplify diagnosis.

No laboratory test is pathognomonic for MS; however, white matter lesions on magnetic resonance imaging (MRI) of the brain and spinal cord, abnormal evoked potentials (visual, auditory, and somatosensory), and the characteristic cerebrospinal fluid abnormalities (increased IgG and oligoclonal banding) typically are seen in 90% or more of patients.

The prognosis in MS is quite varied and may be unpredictable in any given patient. Some individuals have a subclinical course, the diagnosis being considered only after an incidental MRI scan or at autopsy. A few have a fulminating course with early disability. Most have an intermediate course characterized by remissions and exacerbations with deterioration over time. Insidious progression without frank remissions also can be seen in some patients. Regardless of clinical course, MRI studies indicate that MS is a more active and aggressive disease than previously appreciated. Follow-up MRI and pathological studies show that disease activity is much more common than indicated by the patients' symptoms or the neurologists' findings. MS not only causes physical disability but also has major psychosocial and economic impact on the individual, family members, and society.

For many years no effective therapy was available to alter the natural history of MS, and approximately 50% of patients required the use of an assistive device for ambulation 15 years after onset of symptoms (1). Over the past decade, significant progress has been made in the development of palliative, although not curative, treatments. At present, several human proteins or derivatives thereof are available that decrease attack rate, slow the rate of deterioration in neural functioning, and decrease MRI activity. These include the beta interferons: IFN-β1b (Betaseron), IFN-β1a (Avonex, Rebif), and glatiramer acetate (Copaxone) (2–8).

Although approved primarily for relapsing-remitting types of MS, beta interferons may be effective as well in inflammatory forms of secondary-progressive MS (9,10). Recently, mitoxantrone (Novantrone), an immunosuppressive drug used to treat certain types of cancer, also has proved to be effective in progressive forms of MS, decreasing relapses, slowing deterioration, and inhibiting new MRI lesions from appearing (11). A number of other immunosuppressive and immuno-modulating regimens, although not yet approved by the Food and Drug Administration, have had beneficial effects on clinical course or MRI activity in some, but not all, controlled studies. These include intravenous gamma globulin (12–14), azathioprine (15), methotrexate (16), cladribine (17), cyclophosphamide (18), and total lymphoid irradiation (19). Because of risk–benefit considerations, preference is given to using protein therapies before using the more invasive and probably riskier immunosuppressants.

Currently, corticosteroids are used to treat acute exacerbations of MS, although dosage, route of administration, and duration of therapy remain controversial. It is also important to relieve symptoms, prevent complications, and enhance patient quality of life. As the precise mechanism of tissue injury becomes known, it can be anticipated that more effective and safer therapies will become available to treat the unfortunate individuals who suffer both emotionally and physically from this disease.

HISTORICAL PERSPECTIVE: MULTIPLE SCLEROSIS AND PREGNANCY

A common question posed to a neurologist by a young female patient recently diagnosed as having MS is, "What effect will pregnancy have on my disease?" The answer to this question has changed considerably in recent years.

Prior to 1950, based on case reports and small, less rigorously controlled series than in recent years, pregnancy and the puerperium were generally thought to have an adverse effect on MS; some authorities even recommended termination of pregnancy to prevent disease progression. In 1950 Tillman reviewed the records of 52 patients in whom multiple sclerosis preceded pregnancy, obtained from the Sloane Hospital and New York Neurological Institute (20,21). He noted 28 exacerbations in 70 pregnancies in this group of patients, 22 of which occurred in the postpartum year. During 30 other pregnancies, there was no evident deterioration. Tillman concluded that there was "no gross difference in behavior of the disease" among single MS patients, those married but never pregnant, or patients who had MS onset after or before pregnancy. Two years later McAlpine and Compston reviewed 33 pregnancies in 24 patients. They and others (22,23) also concluded that the relapse rate in pregnant MS patients did not differ significantly from the relapse rate generally seen in nonpregnant MS patients. Over the past 50 years, there have been a number of well-controlled retrospective studies and reviews as well as some prospective studies that have generally supported the concept that pregnancy and the puerperium do not have an overall long-term adverse effect on MS, although the relapse rate in the postpartum period is relatively high as compared with the relapse rate during pregnancy. The purpose of this chapter is to review these contemporary studies and to attempt to reach a consensus on the relationship between pregnancy and MS.

RETROSPECTIVE CONTROLLED STUDIES: EFFECT OF PREGNANCY ON MS

Between 1966 and 1991, six major retrospective studies were carried out in which comparative data could be obtained to determine MS attack rates or progression of disability using the MS patient as her own control before, during, and after pregnancy or comparing pregnant MS patients to nonpregnant MS controls (23–28). However, such studies, even when well controlled, are apt to be less informative than prospective studies because of the likelihood of methodologic deficiencies, including: less rigorous definitions and confirmation of endpoints when data are examined in hindsight; potential biases in patient recall; poor experimental designs. For example, rapidly progressive or severely disabled patients may be less apt to become pregnant or, after pregnancy, may be lost to follow-up. Both possibilities could bias results against showing deterioration in pregnant patients when compared with nonpregnant controls. Patients with mild forms of MS may not be followed longitudinally as often as patients with more active disease, especially in tertiary MS referral centers. Retrospective interviews might be misleading because of impaired patient memory or preferential recall of a relapse related to a major personal landmark, such as pregnancy or childbirth. The latter could lead to a false conclusion that a higher relapse rate is related to pregnancy or its aftermath. In addition, several studies have shown a higher relapse rate in younger MS patients with disease of short duration—circumstances that might be more closely linked to women of childbearing age. In this regard, most recent studies have adjusted relapse rates by age and duration when comparing pregnant MS patients to nonpregnant controls.

Gestational Exacerbations

Most retrospective studies have shown fewer exacerbations during pregnancy than in nongestational periods. In 1994, by meta-analysis we found that in the six major published studies for which appropriate control data were available (23–28), a significantly lower relapse rate was seen during the 9 months of pregnancy as compared with non-pregnant periods in the same patients (p of 0.0001) or all female patients (p less than 0.03) (29). On the basis of this retrospective data, it appears that pregnancy is a period of relatively decreased MS clinical activity.

Several of these retrospective studies also compared relapse rates by trimester of pregnancy; however, by meta-analysis no predilection for attacks of MS to occur in any trimester of pregnancy was found (24,28,29).

Postpartum Exacerbations

We also compared relapse rates in the 3-month postpartum period to the nonpregnant period in the same patients. The mean relative risk of relapse in the postpartum period was 3.9 (range 1.3 to 11) compared to the same patients when not pregnant, and 5.4 compared to all nonpregnant patients (29). By meta-analysis, these differences were highly significant (p less than 0.0001). In contrast, only one of three studies showed a significantly higher exacerbation rate in the 3 to 6 months postpartum when compared with nonpregnancy, and meta-analysis showed no increased risk in this postdelivery period (23,24,28,29).

When analysis of relapse rates was carried out comparing the 3-month postpartum period to the 9 months of pregnancy in the same patients, even more dramatic differences were observed. The six retrospective studies (23-28) each showed a significantly higher risk of MS exacerbation in the 3-month postpartum period as compared with pregnancy, with risk rates ranging from 2.2 to 18.4 (mean 7.0, p less than 0.0001) (29).

Several studies have compared relapse rates occurring in the initial 3 months postdelivery with the subsequent 3 months (23,24, 28). Of 119 total relapses occurring in the 6 months postpartum, 77 took place in the initial 3 months, whereas 42 occurred in the subsequent 3 months (p equals 0.001) (29).

In summary, these retrospective studies indicate that there is a high risk of relapse in the first 3 months postpartum as compared to pregnant or nonpregnant periods. This risk does not appear to extend into the 3- to 6-month postpartum period when compared to other nonpregnant intervals. It should be noted that it is likely the risk of MS exacerbations post partum may be much lower in patients treated with interferons or Copaxone.

Pregnancy and Puerperium Combined

We then compared relapse rates in the pregnancy year (pregnancy and the 3 months postpartum) to relapse rates in nonpregnant periods in the same and other MS patients (29). In the six studies (23-28) in which relapse risk in the pregnancy year was compared to the relapse risk in the same patients when not pregnant, a significant increase in risk ratio was found in the pregnancy year in four studies (25–28) and in the nonpregnant year in one study (24); no significant difference was noted in the other study (23). However, by meta-analysis (29), a significantly increased mean relapse risk ratio (1.6) in the pregnancy year was found as compared to the same patients when not pregnant (p less than 0.0001). When the relapse rate in the pregnancy year was compared to all nonpregnant controls, mean annual relapse rates of 0.37 and 0.19, respectively, were found with a mean risk ratio of 2.0 (p less than 0.0001).

We conclude that in retrospective studies the risk for relapse of MS in the pregnancy year might be increased compared to nonpregnant periods. However, it should be pointed out that there is no evidence that pregnancy increases the lifetime relapse rate in MS. It is also likely this increased risk will not be found in patients started on drug therapy immediately post partum.

Postpuerperal Year

Two retrospective studies determined the relapse rate of MS in the postpuerperal year. Ghezzi and Caputo (27) found a lower annualized relapse rate of 0.16 per patient from 3 to 15 months postpartum as compared to 0.22 in the same patients during gestation and compared to 0.29 in nonpregnant controls. Korn-Lubetzki and colleagues (28) found a low mean annual relapse rate of 0.14 in the 6 to 18 months postdelivery (similar to the 0.13 rate during pregnancy), compared to 0.29 in the same patients in all nonpregnant years and 0.28 in nonpregnant controls.

We conclude that because of the limited number of patients, further studies are needed to determine if the postpuerperal year is truly a time of decreased risk for clinical exacerbations of MS.

Long-Term Sequelae of Pregnancy on Multiple Sclerosis

Although relapse rates are of great concern, the critical issue is whether pregnancy-related relapses are more severe than in nonpregnant periods and whether they lead to more rapid and permanent neurologic deterioration. Unfortunately, little data are available on the severity of relapses during pregnancy and its aftermath based on retrospective studies.

Poser and Poser mailed questionnaires to 189 female MS patients from Lower Saxony and 450 women registered in a multicenter study in Germany, inquiring about gynecologic and obstetric histories (30). Patients then were stratified as to pregnancy status. As a measure of MS progression, they calculated a progression index obtained by dividing DSS (a disability status scale) by duration of MS in years. No difference in MS progression indices was found on comparison of women never pregnant, those pregnant only before onset of the disease, and those pregnant during the disease. Further analysis of prognosis revealed no significant difference with respect to the number of pregnancies during the disease. Although Poser and Poser failed to show an adverse effect of pregnancy in MS patients, the sensitivity of the progression index as a measure of rate of decline in MS has not been determined.

In 1986, Thompson and associates (31) reported the results of a clinic-based review of medical records from 178 women with MS. Women were stratified according to the number of completed pregnancies and timing of pregnancy relative to onset of MS. No differences in age-duration–adjusted DSS scores were found on comparison of women with no pregnancies, one pregnancy, or two or more pregnancies.

Subsequently, Weinshenker and colleagues (32) carried out a retrospective population-based survey of 185 women from Middlesex County, Ontario. Because their study was population based, Weinshenker and colleagues were better able to follow up certain subsets of MS patients who might be lost to tertiary referral centers—that is, those with minimal or severe disabilities. No association was noted between disability and total number of term pregnancies, timing of pregnancy relative to onset of MS, or disability in patients who had experienced either onset or worsening of MS in relation to a pregnancy. The mean number of pregnancies both before and after onset of MS was no different among groups stratified by disability. Weinshenker and associates believed the lack of close association between attack frequency and disability was the likely explanation for the inability to show a worse prognosis in pregnant MS patients despite the high postpartum relapse rate.

In the most recent retrospective but longitudinal study, Verdru and colleagues (33) studied 200 patients with MS to determine if pregnancy after the onset of MS influenced long-term disability. They used as their endpoint time between disease onset and wheelchair dependence. A significantly longer time to require a wheelchair was found in those women becoming pregnant post MS onset. Of course, it could be argued that women with aggressive MS might be more apt to avoid pregnancy or have more difficulty becoming pregnant. In summary, retrospective studies fail to indicate a long-term risk of worsening in previously pregnant MS patients, even in those who had experienced pregnancy-related relapses.

PROSPECTIVE STUDIES: EFFECT OF PREGNANCY ON MS

The ideal way to assess the impact of pregnancy on MS would be to carry out a prospective controlled study on female patients determining the number of relapses, disability status, and number of lesions revealed by MRI scans at regular intervals each year prepregnancy, during gestation, in the postpartum period, and long term thereafter. In addition to using the same patient as her own control in nonpregnant periods, other nonpregnant patients, matched for age, duration, and disability could be similarly monitored.

Controlled prospective studies offer the advantage of more precisely defined and evaluatable endpoints and less investigator or patient bias. Fortunately, over the past 10 years, a number of prospective investigations have been carried out to assess the effect of pregnancy on the course of MS, including frequency of exacerbations, rate of deterioration, and MRI disease activity.

Gestational Exacerbations

Several clinical and one MRI study have prospectively examined the rate of exacerbations during the 9 months of pregnancy in MS patients. A decrease in exacerbation rates during pregnancy was found by Duquette and Girard (34) and by Roullet and associates (35). Similar results were found by Confavreux and associates (36) in the most definitive such study involving 254 women from 12 European centers, with the lowest exacerbation rate being noted during the third trimester. A decrease in exacerbation rate in the third trimester, but not other trimesters, was also reported by Sadovnick and associates (37). Although not studying exacerbation rates, Runmarker and Andersen (38) found a lower risk of an MS onset bout during the 8 months preceding delivery than in nonpregnant periods. In addition to clinical evidence of decreased relapse rates during pregnancy, a decrease in the number of active MRI lesions was found in the second half of pregnancy in two MS patients who had periodic MRIs preceding, during, and after pregnancy by van Walderveen and associates (39). In contrast to these results, Worthington and colleagues (40) and Roullet and associates (35) in small studies found no decrease in exacerbations during pregnancy as compared with a prepregnancy baseline.

Postpartum Exacerbations

Three prospective studies have shown no increase in relapse rate in the postpartum period as compared with nonpregnancy periods in the same or control patients. Sadovnick and associates (37) identified 42 relapses during 58 pregnancies, which were uniform throughout the entire pregnancy and 6-month postpartum period. In their frequent MRI study spanning pregnancy and the postpartum period, van Walderveen and colleagues (39) found a return to prepregnancy MRI disease activity in the early months postpartum. However, only two patients were so studied. Runmarker and Andersen (38) studied women prospectively and found no higher risk of an MS bout onset in the 8 months postpartum as compared with nonpregnancy periods. In considering their result, it should be pointed out that most studies have found the greatest risk of postpartum MS attacks to be predominantly in the 3 months post-delivery, not 8 months, so that a potential effect on the former period could be lost by considering the latter time frame.

However, consistent with results from retrospective studies, several groups (34–36,40) have found relapse rates to be increased up to 1.7 to 1.9 times higher than expected in the 3 to 6 months postpartum (34–36,40). In the latter study, exacerbations also were found to be below expected values for the 6 to 24 months postpartum, similar to the findings of Ghezzi and Caputo (27) and Korn-Lubetzki (28) in retrospective studies, suggesting the possibility of a subsequent (greater than 3 or 6 months) postpartum reduced risk of MS flareups as if these had been moved forward in time.

Based on consideration of retrospective and prospective studies, it appears likely that the postpartum 3 months is a period of increased risk for MS exacerbations, and that after 3 to 6 months postpartum there may be a decreased exacerbation risk for up to 24 months thereafter.

Unsuccessful attempts have been made to correlate the high rate of exacerbations in the postpartum period to a number of variables, including the physical and emotional stress of childbirth and caring for the newborn, sleep deprivation, type and dose of anesthesia, breastfeeding, and other socioeconomic factors. In one such study, Poser and Poser (30) retrospectively determined that the proportion of patients with clinical worsening after childbirth was not higher for nursing than nonnursing mothers. In fact, using an index of progression (DSS/disease duration), they found that nursing mothers appeared to have a more benign prognosis than nonnursing mothers. Similarly, in their prospective multicenter trial, Confavreux and colleagues (36) also noted no apparent acceleration in disability associated with breastfeeding, and, in fact, exacerbations were significantly less in these mothers. To assess the effect of stress on deterioration, Poser and Poser compared mothers with sufficient help to those lacking help. Again, no statistical difference in mean progression index was found. However, because of the relatively small number of patients, the retrospective nature of the study, and the unproven sensitivity of the progression index, their data are not sufficient to exclude physical or emotional strain as aggravating factors in postpartum relapses.

Bader and associates (41), in a combined retrospective and prospective study of 20 women having a combined 32 pregnancies, attempted to correlate relapse rate in the puerperium to type and amount of anesthetic agent used. Nine relapses were documented in the postpartum period. No apparent difference was noted in relapse rate of patients receiving local, epidural, or general anesthesia. A similar conclusion was reached by Confavreux and associates (36), who noted no increase in exacerbation rates or progression of disability in women who received epidural analgesia.

Pregnancy and Puerperium Combined

Three prospective studies (35–37) have addressed the risk of relapses in the pregnancy year (pregnancy and 3 months postpartum) compared to nonpregnancy controls. No increased risk was found in two (36,37), but there was increased risk noted in the third (35). In these prospective studies, insufficient data are available to adequately assess severity of relapses in the pregnancy year (gestation and postpartum 3 months) as compared to other periods.

Long-Term Sequelae

In a small prospective study, Birk and associates (42) followed eight women through pregnancy and the postpartum period. Six of eight women experienced relapses within 7 weeks of delivery. Expanded Disability Status Score (EDSS) declined from 2.4 at 35 weeks of gestation to 2.8 at 6 weeks postpartum and 3.4 at 6 months postdelivery. Thus, in this small study, a disturbing deterioration in the 3 months postpartum persisted or worsened over the next 3 months. In contrast, five other prospective studies on long-term sequelae of pregnancy on subsequent MS course have been carried out with follow-up periods ranging from 12 months to 10 years or more. No deleterious effect of pregnancy on subsequent neurologic disability was found in any of these studies, which is consistent with the findings in retrospective studies.

POSSIBLE EXPLANATIONS FOR A PROTECTIVE EFFECT OF PREGNANCY IN MS

Numerous hypothesis have been put forward to explain the protective effect of gestation and the adverse effect of the 3-month postpartum period on MS clinical and MRI exacerbation rates (43–48). These include physiologic and biochemical changes that oc-

cur during pregnancy and that reverse postgestationally, particularly those suppressing the immune response thought to be pivotal in MS lesion genesis. Suppression of the immune response could be considered to be advantageous by preventing rejection of the fetus, with its different antigenic structure, by the pregnant mother. Several publications have thoroughly addressed the nature of these factors (43–48). In brief, there is a shift in T-helper cells and secreted cytokines from a Th1 proinflammatory to a Th2 antiinflammatory profile. In addition, a variety of hormones (estrogens, cortisol, cortisol-releasing hormone, progesterone, androgens, calcitriol, human chorionic gonadotropin), pregnancy-associated proteins (alpha fetoprotein, early pregnancy factor, human placental lactogen, alpha-2 pregnancy-associated glycoprotein, pregnancy-associated plasma protein, heat shock protein), and blocking antibodies are released during pregnancy that might affect the immune response, inflammation, or the patency of the blood–brain barrier so as to decrease MS disease activity. Clearly, further studies are needed to determine the factors responsible for changes in disease activity that occur during pregnancy and reverse in the postpartum period.

TREATMENT OF DISEASE ACTIVITY IN PREGNANCY AND THE POSTPARTUM PERIOD

Although relapses are significantly reduced during pregnancy, they still occur and can occasionally be severe. No controlled studies have been carried out specifically addressing the treatment of relapses during pregnancy. Consequently, therapy for gestational relapses is similar to that for relapses in general, except that special consideration must be given to avoiding fetal injury. As a rule, we do not treat mild exacerbations. More severe relapses are treated with corticosteroids. We prefer short-term, high-dose regimens whenever possible, in contradistinction to therapy during nonpregnant periods when this regimen may be followed by a more protracted, tapered course of corticosteroids. Obviously, immunosuppression should be avoided during pregnancy because of potential fetal injury, and patients are advised not to become pregnant while taking these or other drugs that can cause fetal harm (48). In the unlikely event of recurrent severe relapses during pregnancy, the possibility of utilizing therapies thought to have minimal risk for fetal damage or miscarriage, such as Copaxone or intravenous gamma globulin, could be considered (48). Symptomatic therapy of pregnant MS patients follows similar guidelines. Unnecessary and potentially fetal-toxic treatments should be avoided.

Treatment for the postpartum patient is the same as for the nonpregnant patient. Drugs toxic to the child should be avoided in nursing mothers. In the nonbreastfeeding patient starting therapy, particularly with a beta interferon, copolymer 1 or other medication should begin as soon as possible postpartum in an attempt to minimize the risk of a severe relapse in this high-risk period.

Effect of Multiple Sclerosis on Pregnancy

MS does not change a woman's fertility rate and is thought to have little, if any, impact on the course or outcome of pregnancy. Specifically, MS has not been shown to have a deleterious influence on the incidence of toxemia or on the rate of miscarriages, prematurity, infant mortality, or congenital malformations. However, some MS patients are more likely to experience constipation or urinary tract infections than normal pregnant women because of the pressure of a gravid uterus on a neurogenic bowel or bladder.

Delivery is not more complicated in MS patients, and the mode of delivery is decided strictly on obstetric criteria. Epidural, regional, or general anesthesia is preferred to spinal anesthesia, although no convincing deleterious effect of spinal anesthesia has been demonstrated. MS patients who recently have received long-term corticosteroid therapy or who are on low-dose corticosteroid therapy at the time of delivery may have relative adrenal insufficiency and should be given

supplemental corticosteroids. Hydrocortisone 100 mg intramuscularly or intravenously, or the equivalent, administered every 8 hours for 24 hours, is an appropriate regimen unless postpartum complications necessitate a longer course of treatment.

The postpartum period is often a physically and emotionally stressful period and a time of increased disease activity. Because of functional impairment, some patients may have difficulty caring for their babies. For example, in one study, 30% of patients could not adequately care for the newborn child because of limb weakness or gait disturbances. There is no contraindication to breastfeeding unless patients require drugs excreted in breast milk deemed toxic to the baby.

CONCLUSIONS

On the basis of all available evidence, gestation is a period of decreased risk for a relapse of MS, whereas the 3 months postpartum is a period of high risk. However, the lifetime risk rate does not appear to change because of pregnancy, and on the basis of current retrospective and prospective studies, long-term disability is not higher in pregnant women, even in women who experienced relapses during the pregnancy year.

MS has little or no effect on the course of pregnancy or delivery although patients with severe MS may have difficulty fully caring for their newborns. The decision to become pregnant should be made by the patient after being appropriately informed about the risks involved.

REFERENCES

1. Confavreux C, Aimard G, Devic M. Course and prognosis of multiple sclerosis assessed by the computerized data processing of 349 patients. *Brain* 1980;103: 281–300.
2. The IFNβ Multiple Sclerosis Study Group. Interferon beta-1b is effective in relapsing-remitting multiple sclerosis. Clinical results of a multicenter, randomized, double-blind, placebo-controlled trial. *Neurology* 1993;43: 655–661.
3. Paty DW, Li DKB, the University of British Columbia MS/MRI Analysis Group. Interferon beta-1b effective in relapsing-remitting multiple sclerosis. MRI analysis results of a multicenter, randomized, double-blind,

placebo-controlled trial. *Neurology* 1993;43:662–667.

4. Jacobs LD, Cookfair DL, Rudick RA, et al. Intramuscular interferon beta-1a for disease progression in relapsing multiple sclerosis. The Multiple Sclerosis Collaborative Research Group (MSCRG). *Ann Neurol* 1996;39:285–294.

5. Jacobs LD, Beck RW, Simon JH, et al. Intramuscular interferon beta-1a therapy initiated during a first demyelinating event in multiple sclerosis. *N Engl J Med* 2000; 343:898–904.

6. PRISMS Study Group. Randomised double-blind placebo-controlled study of interferon beta-1a in relapsing/remitting multiple sclerosis. *Lancet* 1998;352: 1498–1504.

7. Johnson KP, Brooks BR, Cohen JA, et al. Copolymer 1 reduces relapse rate and improves disability in relapsing-remitting multiple sclerosis: results of a phase III multicenter, double-blind placebo-controlled trial. *Neurology* 1995;45:1268–1276.

8. Johnson KP, Brooks BR, Cohen JA, et al. Extended use of glatiramer acetate (Copaxone) is well tolerated and maintains its clinical effects on multiple sclerosis relapse rate and degree of disability. *Neurology* 1998;50: 701–708.

9. European Study Group on interferon beta-1b in secondary progressive MS. Placebo controlled multicentre randomised trial of interferon beta-1b in treatment of secondary progressive multiple sclerosis. *Lancet* 1998; 352:1491–1497.

10. Miller DH, Molyneux PD, Barker GJ, et al. Effect of interferon β-1b on magnetic resonance imaging outcomes in secondary progressive multiple sclerosis: results of a European multicenter, randomized, double-blind, placebo-controlled trial. *Ann Neurol* 1999;46: 850–859.

11. Hartung HP, Gonsette R and the MIMS-Study Group. Mitoxantrone in progressive multiple sclerosis: a placebo-controller, randomized, observer-blind phase III trial: clinical results and three-year follow-up. *Neurology* 1991;52:A290

12. Fazekas F, Deisenhammer F, Strasser-Fuchs S, et al. Randomised placebo-controlled trial of monthly intravenous immunoglobulin therapy in relapsing-remitting multiple sclerosis. *Lancet* 1997;349:589–593.

13. Achiron A, Gabbay U, Gilad R, et al. Intravenous immunoglobulin treatment in multiple sclerosis: effect on relapses. *Neurology* 1998;50:398–402.

14. Sorensen PS, Wanscher B, Jensen CV, et al. Intravenous immunoglobulin G reduces MRI activity in relapsing multiple sclerosis. *Neurology* 1998;50:1273–1281.

15. Yudkin PL, Ellison GW, Ghezzi A, et al. Overview of azathioprine treatment in multiple sclerosis. *Lancet* 1991;338:1051–1055.

16. Goodkin DE, Rudick RA, Medendorp SV, et al. Low-dose (7.5 mg) oral methotrexate reduces the rate of progression in chronic progressive multiple sclerosis. *Ann Neurol* 1995;37:30–41.

17. Rice GPA, Cladribine Study Group. Cladribine and chronic progressive multiple sclerosis: the results of a multicenter trial. *Neurology* 1997;48:1730.

18. Hauser SL, Dawson DM, Lehrich JR, et al. Intensive immunosuppression in progressive multiple sclerosis. A randomized, three-arm study of high-dose intravenous cyclophosphamide, plasma exchange, and ACTH. *N Engl J Med* 1983;308:173–180.

19. Cook SD, Devereux C, Troiano R, et al. Modified Total Lymphoid Irradiation and Low Dose Corticosteroids in Progressive Multiple Sclerosis. *Journal of Neurological Sciences* 1997;152:172–181.

20. Tillman AJB. The effect of pregnancy on multiple sclerosis and its management. *Res Publ Assoc Res Nerv Ment Dis* 1950;8:548–582.

21. Birk K, Rudick R. Pregnancy and multiple sclerosis. *Arch Neurol* 1986;43:719–726.

22. McAlpine D, Compston N. Some aspects of the natural history of disseminated sclerosis. *Q J Med* 1952; 21:135–167.

23. Frith JA, McLeod JG. Pregnancy and multiple sclerosis. *J Neurol Neurosurg Psychiatry* 1988;51:495–498.

24. Bernardi S, Grasso MG, Bertollini R, et al. The influence of pregnancy on relapses in multiple sclerosis: a cohort study. *Acta Neurol Scand* 1991;84:403–406.

25. Millar JHD, Allison RS, Cheesman EA, et al. Pregnancy as a factor influencing relapse in disseminated sclerosis. *Brain* 1959;82:417–426.

26. Schapira K, Poskanzer DC, Newell DJ, et al. Marriage, pregnancy and multiple sclerosis. *Brain* 1966;89: 419–428.

27. Ghezzi A, Caputo D. Pregnancy: a factor influencing the course of multiple sclerosis? *Eur Neurol* 1981;20: 115–117.

28. Korn-Lubetzki I, Khana E, Cooper G, et al. Activity of multiple sclerosis during pregnancy and puerperium. *Ann Neurol* 1984;16:229–231.

29. Cook SD, Troiano R, Bansil S, et al. Multiple sclerosis and pregnancy. In: Devinsky O, Feldmann E, Hainline B, eds. *Neurological complications of pregnancy.* New York: Raven Press, 1994:83–95.

30. Poser S, Poser W. Multiple sclerosis and gestation. *Neurology* 1983;33:1422–1427.

31. Thompson DS, Nelson IM, Burns A, et al. The effects of pregnancy on multiple sclerosis: a retrospective study. *Neurology* 1986;36:1097–1099.

32. Weinshenker BG, Hader W, Carriere W, et al. The influence of pregnancy on disability from multiple sclerosis: a population-based study in Middlesex County, Ontario. *Neurology* 1989;39:1438–1440.

33. Verdru P, Theys P, D'Hooghe MB, et al. Pregnancy and multiple sclerosis: the influence on long term disability. *Clin Neurol Neurosurg* 1994;96:38–41.

34. Duquette P, Girard M. Hormonal factors in susceptibility to multiple sclerosis. *Curr Opin Neurol Neurosurg* 1993;6:195–201.

35. Roullet E, Verdier-Taillefer MH, Amarenco P, et al. Pregnancy and multiple sclerosis: a longitudinal study of 125 remittent patients. *J Neurol Neurosurg Psychiatry* 1993;56:1062–1065.

36. Confavreux C, Hutchinson M, Hours MM, et al. Pregnancy in Multiple Sclerosis Group. Rate of pregnancy-related relapse in multiple sclerosis. *N Engl J Med* 1998;339:285–291.

37. Sadovnick AD, Eisen K, Hashimoto SA, et al. Pregnancy and multiple sclerosis: a prospective study. *Arch Neurol* 1994;51:1120–1124.

38. Runmarker B, Andersen O. Prognostic factors in a multiple sclerosis incidence cohort with twenty-five years of follow-up. *Brain* 1993;116:117–113

39. van Walderveen MA, Tas MW, Barkhof F, et al. Magnetic resonance evaluation of disease activity during pregnancy in multiple sclerosis. *Neurology* 1994;44:327–329.

40. Worthington J, Jones R, Crawford M, et al. Pregnancy and multiple sclerosis—a 3-year prospective study. *J Neurol* 1994;241:228–233.
41. Bader AM, Hunt CO, Datta S, et al. Anesthesia for the obstetric patient with multiple sclerosis. *J Clin Anesth* 1988;1:21–24.
42. Birk K, Ford C, Smeltzer S, et al. The clinical course of multiple sclerosis during pregnancy and the puerperium. *Arch Neurol* 1990;47:738–742.
43. Whitaker JN. Effects of pregnancy and delivery on disease activity in multiple sclerosis. *New Engl J Med* 1998;339:339–340.
44. Abramsky O, Brenner T, Mizrachi R, et al. Alpha-feto-protein suppresses experimental allergic encephalomyelitis. *J Neuroimmunol* 1982;2:1–7.
45. James WH. Pregnancy, the puerperium, hormones and multiple sclerosis. *Brain* 1995;118:1617–1618.
46. Schwartz GG. Hypothesis: calcitriol mediates pregnancy's protective effect on multiple sclerosis. *Arch Neurol* 1993;50:455.
47. Koch CA, Robyn JA, Pacak K. How do levels of (endogenous) glucocorticoids, interleukin-10, and interleukin-12 relate to multiple sclerosis relapse before, during and after pregnancy? *Clin Endocrinol (Oxf)* 1999;50:818–819.
48. Damek DM, Shuster EA. Pregnancy and multiple sclerosis. Mayo Clinic Proceedings 1997;72:977–989.

Neurological Complications of Pregnancy, Second Edition, edited by Brian Hainline and Orrin Devinsky. Lippincott Williams & Wilkins, Philadelphia © 2002.

11

Infections

Richard T. Johnson

Department of Neurology, Johns Hopkins Hospital, and Departments of Neurology, Microbiology, and Neuroscience, Johns Hopkins University School of Medicine, Bloomberg School of Public Health, Baltimore, Maryland, U.S.A.

Infections during pregnancy may have varied effects on the pregnant woman and on the fetus or neonate. The average pregnancy is complicated by a number of infections, but the majority are trivial upper-respiratory infections, urinary tract infections, or skin blemishes. A few infections, such as coccidioidomycosis and malaria, can have more dire consequences in the pregnant than in the nonpregnant woman. However, some infections, such as those caused by *Toxoplasma gondii*, parvovirus B19, and cytomegalovirus (CMV), may cause minimal signs in the pregnant woman yet have profound effects on fetal survival or postnatal development. Therefore, this chapter is divided into two sections to address complications in the pregnant woman, including systemic or placental effects leading to abortion and stillbirth, and the effects of infections on the nervous system development of the fetus or neonate (Table 11.1).

EFFECTS ON THE MOTHER

Immune Responses During Pregnancy

Some specific and innate immune responses are altered during pregnancy because the maternal immune system must adapt to an array of foreign antigens of the fetus and placenta (1,2). This tolerance is achieved by two groups of mechanisms. The first are structural safeguards against fetal and placental rejection and include the anatomic separation of maternal and fetal blood circulation and the masking of surface alloantigens on the trophoblastic cells. The second group of mechanisms are modifications of the maternal cell-mediated immune responses that are normally crucial in allograft rejection. This is accomplished by the production by the fetus of immunosuppressant agents or cells that enter the maternal circulation, such as fetal suppressor T cells, alpha-fetoprotein, and lymphokines

TABLE 11.1. *Organisms that pose an increased risk during pregnancy*

	Increased severity of maternal illness	Fetal infection causing neurologic deficits
Bacteria	*Mycobacterium tuberculosis*	*Treponema pallidum*
	Listeria monocytogenes	
	Brucella melitensis	
Fungi	*Coccidiodoides immitis*	
Parasites	Plasmodia (particularly *P. falciparum*)	*Toxoplasma gondii*
Viruses	Influenza viruses	Rubella virus
	Hepatitis E	Parvovirus B19
	Varicella-zoster virus (chicken pox only)	Cytomegalovirus
	Polioviruses	Herpes simplex viruses
		Human T-cell lymphotropic virus, type 1
		Human immunodeficiency virus

from stimulated fetal lymphocytes. In the placenta, the syncytial trophoblasts produce hormones that are present in high local concentration that may play some immunosuppressant roles, such as progesterone, estrogens, chorionic gonadotropin, and cortisol-binding globulin. The maternal immune response is altered by an increased synthesis of adrenal corticosteroids and other soluble factors and of blocking antibodies, increased presence of suppressor cells, and diminished T cells with larger numbers of B cells in the peripheral blood (3). In contrast, the innate immune system is activated by pregnancy and may compensate so that clinical severity of most infections is not seen (2,4).

The structure of the placenta that separates maternal and fetal blood also deters the movement of infectious agents from the maternal to the fetal circulation. Conversely, the immune suppression may enhance the dissemination of infectious agents. Because cell-mediated immune responses that are central in graft rejection are suppressed by pregnancy, the infections that cause greater risk to the mother and fetus are intracellular organisms (Table 11.1).

Specific Infections That Cause Increased Maternal Morbidity

Most extracellular bacterial infections are cleared by humoral immune mechanisms. Therefore, pneumococcal or meningococcal meningitis do not appear to carry a higher mortality or morbidity rate in the pregnant woman. However, obligate intracellular bacteria do. Pregnancy does not appear to increase the rate of reactivation of *Mycobacterium tuberculosis*, but tuberculosis infection, when it does occur, may be more severe, and tuberculous meningitis during pregnancy appears to carry higher mortality and morbidity rates (5). *Listeria monocytogenes* also poses an increased risk during pregnancy, including listeria meningitis in addition to intrauterine infection with abortions or neonatal infection. In a large outbreak of listeriosis in California in 1985, 65% of cases occurred in pregnant

women or their offspring with many fetal or neonatal deaths and high rates of neonatal meningitis (6). *Brucella melitensis* increases rates of abortion, prematurity, and fetal death (7). Medical lore maintains that leprosy presents more often during pregnancy, but careful studies are lacking.

Spirochetal diseases, such as syphilis and Lyme disease, do not appear to have altered clinical courses during pregnancy. The threats to the developing fetus are discussed below. Coccidioidomycosis is the only deep mycosis that is predisposed to disseminate because of the pregnant state, and during the second half of pregnancy it may lead to fatal disease (8). Transmission to the fetus or newborn is rare.

The intracellular parasite that has the most adverse affect on maternal health is malaria. Pregnancy increases the level of parasitemia, and during pregnancy much higher rates of maternal mortality and morbidity are seen as well as increased rates of abortion, stillbirth, prematurity, and low birthweight (9). With more frequent recreational and business travel of pregnant women as well as the increasing number of immigrants entering the United States from malaria-infested areas, treatment of malaria in the pregnant woman is becoming an increasing problem (10). Falciparum malaria poses the greatest problem because it sequesters in the brain causing cerebral malaria and in the placenta causing fetal distress. Many strains of falciparum are chloroquine resistant; therefore, in Asia and Africa where these strains are prevalent, severe malaria, particularly cerebral malaria, must be treated with intravenous quinine. Quinine induces abortion, but the drug-induced release of insulin may be more injurious to the fetus than the oxytocic effect (11). Congenital malaria is rare; the infected placenta and toxic medications are the major threats to the fetus. In contrast, the other important parasitic infection of pregnancy, toxoplasmosis, usually is asymptomatic or causes a mild infectious mononucleosis-like disease in the pregnant woman (12); however, it is a major cause of congenital neurologic infection.

In theory, viruses should show greater virulence in pregnancy with the suppression of cell-mediated immune responses, but few do. Neuroinvasiveness is not appreciably altered because viral meningitis and encephalitis are not recognized to be increased in frequency or severity in pregnancy. However, paralytic disease was more frequent and widespread in pregnant women during poliovirus epidemics (13). Some nonneurologic viral infections are intensified with pregnancy; smallpox showed high rates of mortality in pregnant women and also high rates of abortion thought to be the result of placental infection. Life-threatening pneumonia is a complication of influenza and chickenpox during pregnancy. Women who contract hepatitis E in the third trimester of pregnancy have a high probability of fulminant fatal course (14).

Treatment and Prevention

The treatment and prevention of neurologic infections must be modified during pregnancy. Some antibiotics, such as the aminoglycides and tetracyclines, are contradicted during pregnancy. Both mefloquin and quinine, used for prophylaxis or treatment of chloroquine-resistant strains of malaria, may be toxic to the fetus, but their use may be required nevertheless (15). Pyrimethamine, important in the treatment of toxoplasmosis in the mother, has, in animal studies, been implicated as a teratogen (1).

The official recommendation is that all killed vaccines, including postexposure rabies vaccines, are safe during pregnancy, but no live vaccines should be given. The live vaccine of greatest concern is the attenuated oral polio vaccine because immunized children can spread these viruses to pregnant mothers and neighbors with whom they come in contact. During a poliomyelitis outbreak in Finland, pregnant women were advised to take the live alternated vaccine. No vaccine-related paralysis was seen, and the oral polio vaccine during early pregnancy seemed to have no harmful effects on fetal development (16).

EFFECTS ON THE FETUS AND NEONATE

Spirochetes

Treponema pallidum is the classic infectious agent known to cross the placenta and cause fetal death, neonatal malformations, or chronic neurologic disease. As the incidence of syphilis increases and prenatal care falters, congenital syphilis has become a greater problem. There is no evidence that pregnancy alters either the clinical manifestations or the clinical course of syphilis. The fetal risk is based on the stage of maternal infection and the stage of pregnancy. To cross the placenta, the treponemes must be circulating in the maternal blood; thus untreated primary and secondary syphilis pose the greatest threat to the fetus. In these circumstances, more than half of the fetuses will be born prematurely or will be stillbirths. The remainder will be infected with or without the stigmata of congenital syphilis. Time of gestation is also important because the treponemes cannot normally pass the Langhans cell layer of the placenta. This layer, however, atrophies in the fourth month of gestation, so most fetal infection occurs after mid gestation. Therefore, serologic testing and treatment during routine prenatal care during the first half of pregnancy can prevent most fetal infection. This explains why such a high correlation exists between congenital syphilis and poor prenatal care (17).

The infected infant may have clinical signs of syphilis (early congenital syphilis) or only subtle stigmata or no clinical signs in the neonatal period (late congenital syphilis). Early congenital syphilis is characterized by hepatosplenomegaly, generalized lymphadenopathy, persistent rhinitis, and bony and dental stigmata. Neurologic disease primarily is seen in late congenital syphilis. Late congenital syphilis may occur in a child who has no stigmata or in whom abnormalities such as Hutchinson's triad (abnormal teeth, interstitial keratitis, eighth nerve deafness) or the more subtle frontal bossing may have been missed. Chronic neurosyphilis now is rarely seen, but it follows a time course remarkably similar to neurosyphilis in adults. There may be an acute aseptic meningitis during the first year of life, "childhood" strokes due to meningovascular syphilis occur during the early years of life, "juvenile" paresis most frequently develops between 8 and 12 years of age, and "adolescent" tabes makes its appearance in the late teens.

Interest continues in the possibility that Lyme disease may cause analogous congenital complications. Maternal to fetal transmission of *Borrelia burgdorferi* has been documented (18). A follow-up of individual patients infected during various trimesters showed a number of adverse outcomes, but congenital neurologic disease resulting from maternal infection has not been established (19). In an epidemiologic study comparing an endemic and a nonendemic area, no difference was found between the geographic areas and no association of congenital malformations was correlated with the presence of detectable antibody in cord blood (20). Pregnancy is not an indication for more aggressive therapy of Lyme disease (21).

Toxoplasmosis

Toxoplasmosis is a relatively benign infection in immunocompetent adults that occurs either without symptoms or with a mild lymphadenopathy, myalgias, and fatigue often without recognizable fever. Intensity of the disease is not accentuated in immunocompetent women who are pregnant. About 20% of women in the United States are immune, and the risk of infection during a pregnancy is about 0.1% (12). Fetal infection only occurs during the parasitemia of primary infection, and less than half of the primary maternal infections result in fetal infection. Fetal infection during early pregnancy is less frequent, but it leads to the most severe disease. Infection in late pregnancy is more likely to cause fetal infection, but the sequelae of infection are less severe. Of neonates infected with *Toxoplasma gondii,* only a small percentage present the classical triad of congenital toxoplas-

mosis with hydrocephalus, chorioretinitis, and intracranial calcification. Others may appear perfectly normal at birth and have the delayed onset of either systemic disease with lymphadenopathy or purely neurologic disease with encephalitis, seizures, retardation, hydrocephalus, or ocular lesions with visual impairment. The majority infected during late gestation have only chorioretinitis or learning disabilities (22).

Prevention of toxoplasmosis includes the recommendations that pregnant women should not eat raw meat or raw eggs and they should avoid cat feces. More important is to counsel them on the handling of meat and eggs during cooking and the importance of washing their hands after food processing. Maternal screening for antibody remains controversial (22,23).

Rubella

Rubella virus was the first recognized viral teratogen (Table 11.2). In 1941 Gregg in Australia reported 67 children with congenital cataracts; half also had microphthalmia and congenital heart disease, and many had low birthweights. He associated these abnormalities with the maternal history of German measles in the early months of pregnancy (24). In the aftermath of the same epidemic, microcephaly, deafness, and mental retardation also were recognized as consequences of maternal rubella.

The risk of both infection and severity of disease is related to the time of maternal rubella. Following maternal infection during the first 12 weeks of gestation, more than 80% of fetuses are infected and virtually all have congenital lesions. Between the thirteenth and the sixteenth weeks of gestation, more than 50% of fetuses are infected, but of this group, less than 35% have clinical findings consisting largely of hearing loss. Between 16 weeks and the end of the second trimester, only about 25% of fetuses are infected, and this rarely leads to any deficit (25).

The mechanism of virus-induced lesions is not well understood, but it has been observed

TABLE 11.2. *Viral infections of the nervous system in the human fetus or neonate*

Virus	Time of infection	Neurologic disease
Major importance		
Rubella	First trimester	Chronic encephalitis, microcephaly, retardation, diplegia, visual and auditory deficits
	Later gestation	Hearing loss and minor retardation
Cytomegalovirus	During gestation	Silent infection with minor mental and auditory deficits; cytomegalic inclusion disease with microcephaly, retardation, and motor, visual, and auditory deficits
Human immunodeficiency virus	During gestation and intrapartum	Chronic encephalopathy with acquired microcephaly, diplegia, and basal ganglia calcification
Herpes simplex virus	During parturition	Severe encephalitis
Minor importance		
Herpes simplex virus	During gestation	Encephalitis with congenital microcephaly
Varicella-zoster virus	First half of gestation	Cicatricial scar, limb hypoplasia, and encephalomyelitis
Parvovirus B19	During gestation	Hydrops fetalis with central nervous system infection
Coxsackie, group B viruses, and echoviruses	Neonatal (?late gestation)	Encephalitis associated with myocarditis
Polioviruses	Late gestation	Congenital or neonatal paralytic poliomyelitis
Influenza virus	First trimester	Possible relation to varied malformations, including neural tube defects and hydrocephalus
Lymphocytic choriomeningitis virus	?	Hydrocephalus (?)
BK virus	?	Hydrocephalus, microcephaly (?)
Arboviruses		
Venezuelan equine encephalitis virus	Late gestation	Congenital or neonatal encephalitis
Cache Valley virus	?	Hydrocephalus and microcephaly
Tenshaw virus		
Human T lymphotropic virus-1	?	Hydrocephalus (?)

Modified from Johnson RT. *Viral infections of the nervous system,* 2nd ed. Lippincott-Raven, 1998, with permission.

that rubella virus in cell culture leads to inhibition of mitosis. In neonates born with rubella virus infection, focal areas of noncytopathic virus infection can be found in tissues. This inhibition of mitosis might explain not only the low birthweight of infants, but the patchy nature of infection might explain the presence of microphthalmia in one eye with normal ocular development in the other (26).

The congenital rubella syndrome seen at birth is one of cataracts, microphthalmia, cardiac malformations, deafness, spastic diplegia, and chorioretinitis. In the neonatal period, relatively acute meningoencephalitis also may develop in addition to the hepatosplenomegaly, lymphadenopathy, and pneumonitis (Table 11.3). After later gestational infections,

deafness and mild retardation usually are detected as the child matures. Of children with the congenital rubella syndrome, 80% have neurologic deficits, yet long-term studies show the outcomes of these to be less severe than anticipated. Hearing loss and ocular problems are common and children may remain small in stature, but many show good socioeconomic adjustment (27).

Prevention can be accomplished only by immunization of women prior to their childbearing years. Once virus infection has occurred, no known treatment will clear the virus or modify the infection. A registry was kept of pregnant women who became inadvertent vaccinees; from this study no cases of congenital rubella have been found in more than 200 live deliveries, and birth defects

TABLE 11.3. *Abnormalities in congenital rubella virus infections*

| | Evident in neonatal period | | May not be evident until months or years later |
	Common	Rare	
Central nervous system	Encephalitis, enlarged anterior fontanelle	Microcephaly	Mental retardation, language abnormalities, motor deficits, autism
Eye	Pigmentary retinopathy, cataract, microphthalmia	Glaucoma, cloudy cornea, iris hypoplasia	Pigmentary retinopathy
Ear	Sensorineural deafness	—	Sensorineural hearing deficits
Skeletomuscular	Low birthweight, postnatal growth retardation, bone radiolucencies, micrognathia	Dermal erythropoiesis	High palate, pes cavus, talipes equinovarus, finger abnormalities, dental abnormalities
Hematological	Hepatosplenomegaly, thrombocytopenia, leukopenia, adenopathy	Hepatitis, immunological dyscrasias, hemolytic anemia, hypoplastic anemia	—
Cardiovascular–pulmonary	Pulmonary arterial hypoplasia, patent ductus arteriosus, coarctation of aortic isthmus	Septal defects, interstitial pneumonitis, myocardial necrosis	—
Other	Undescended testes	Genitourinary malformations	Diabetes mellitus, growth hormone deficiency, hypothyroidism

From Johnson RT. *Viral infections of the nervous system,* 2nd ed. Lippincott-Raven, 1998, with permission.

have not been higher than those found in pregnancies without immunization (28).

Other RNA Viruses

Infants of mothers infected late in gestation have been reported with acute neonatal infections with measles, paralytic poliomyelitis, and acute encephalitis due to Western equine encephalitis virus (26). Enteroviruses can cause severe disease in the first 3 to 5 days of life, but these infections are thought to be acquired in the immediate postnatal period. None of these infections has been associated with malformations or chronic central nervous system infection similar to rubella infections.

There have been solitary reports suggesting the possible relationship of influenza to congenital progressive neurologic disease (29), lymphocytic choriomeningitis virus to congenital hydrocephalus (30), and an unidentified agent related to animal pestiviruses to microcephaly (31).

Parvovirus B19

Parvovirus B19 is the cause of erythema infectiosum of children. Infection during pregnancy may be a nonspecific illness or asymptomatic, but fetal infection can cause hydrops fetalis and abortion or stillbirth (22). The fetal brain is infected with multinucleated giant cells and pervascular calcifications (32). Only rare cases of congenital malformation in liveborn infants have been reported (33), presumably because the virulence of this small DNA virus in the fetus seldom allows survival.

Cytomegalovirus

CMV is a common fetal infection. Serologic evidence of congenital infection, determined by human immunoglobulin M antibodies in cord blood, is found in 1% of all infants. However, only 5% of these infected infants have cytomegalic inclusion disease. An additional 20% may have a "silent infection" with hearing loss or mild retardation detected later.

CMV is the most important known single cause of mental retardation.

In the pregnant woman, CMV infection frequently is activated without symptoms. Primary infections in adults are usually silent, although a few may have infectious mononucleosis-like symptoms. Fetal infection can occur with either primary or reactivated maternal infections, but during primary infection chance of fetal infection is higher (about 50%) and neurologic damage is greater.

Cytomegalic inclusion disease is characterized by microcephaly, and a quarter of the children show intracranial calcifications. Severe hematologic and hepatic dysfunction may be present initially, but these resolve, leaving the lasting damage restricted to the nervous system with subsequent seizures and mental retardation. Children often suffer from deafness. The chorioretinitis may lead to severe visual impairment. Only 15% of the survivors of neonatal cytomegalic inclusion disease have subsequent normal development (Table 11.4).

More than 95% of infants with congenital infection are normal at birth and do not show the acute signs of classic cytomegalic inclusion disease. These children subsequently may show mild degrees of microcephaly and deafness. In case-controlled population studies, a tendency for hearing loss and lower intelligent quotients are present in children with evidence of otherwise asymptomatic congenital CMV infection (34).

Potential vaccines against CMV continue to be explored. Two antiviral drugs, ganciclovir and foscarnet, have proven to be effective in immune-deficient patients with CMV retinitis. The efficacy or safety of the drugs in neonatal cytomegalic inclusion disease is yet to be determined.

Other Herpesviruses

Herpes simplex virus (HSV), type 2, is an important cause of neonatal infection causing a severe, often fatal, encephalitis. With the increased incidence of genital herpes infection in recent decades, the frequency of this formerly very rare neonatal encephalitis has increased to approximately 1 in 3,500 live births. The majority of mothers have a history of recurrent genital herpes or of lesions on their sex partners. Some, but certainly not all,

TABLE 11.4. *Abnormalities in congenital cytomegalovirus infections*

	Cytomegalic inclusion disease in neonatal period		Silent congenital infection (late appearance)
	Common	Rare	
Central nervous system	Microcephaly, periventricular calcification, severe psychomotor retardation, seizures	Hydrocephalus	Microcephaly, low intelligence
Eye	Chorioretinitis, strabismus, optic atrophy	Microphthalmia, cataract, retinalnecrosis, optic disc malformations	Chorioretinitis
Ear	Sensorineural deafness		Sensorineural deafness
Skeletomuscular	Low birthweight, indirect inguinal hernia	Clubfoot, dislocations of hips, diastasis recti	—
Hematological	Hepatosplenomegaly, thrombocytopenia, hyperbilirubinemia	Hemolytic anemia	—
Cardiovascular–pulmonary	Pneumonitis	Cardiovascular anomalies (but no consistent pattern)	—
Other	—	Biliary atresia, gastrointestinal ulcerations	—

From Johnson RT. *Viral infections of the nervous system*, 2nd ed. Lippincott-Raven, 1998, with permission.

have evidence of genital herpes infection at the time they present in labor. Clinically, the infants are normal at birth but have a high rate of prematurity. The development of disease within a few days after birth suggests that infection occurs during passage through the birth canal. Those with generalized disease may show disseminated skin lesions, respiratory distress, and clinical evidence of hepatic and adrenal necrosis as well as encephalitis. In 35% of these infants, findings are limited to encephalitis and retinitis (35).

A randomized study compared acyclovir and vidarabine for the treatment of neonatal HSV and found no significant difference between the two treatments. In patients receiving treatment, those who had disseminated disease showed a mortality rate of 57%, whereas in those with only encephalitis, the mortality rate was 15%. However, sequelae were frequent among those survivors of encephalitis (36).

Prevention of the disease by cesarean section of women with evidence of infection has been advocated, but because about one-third of pregnant women are seropositive at risk of reactivation and an additional 10% have a risk of contracting primary herpes genitalis from their seropositive partners, this could lead to an unacceptably high rate of cesarean sections (37). In a decision analysis based on physical examination at labor, weekly screening of pregnant women for virus shedding, use of serologic methods, and forms of rapid diagnostic tests at labor, it was concluded that given current available data and technology, physical examination at labor is the optimal strategy if the primary goal is to minimize the ratio of excess cesarean sections to cases of neonatal HSV infection averted (38).

HSV-1 also can cause neonatal diffuse encephalitis, but it is more commonly associated with the focal encephalitis seen in older children. Herpes simplex viruses also, in rare occasions, can cause intrauterine infections with primary maternal infection during the first 20 weeks of gestation. This can lead to microcephaly with marked brain atrophy, calcification, and retinitis. These severely retarded babies have recurrences of herpetic lesions on their skin after birth (39). This is a very rare disease, presumably because most infections of the placenta or fetus during early gestation lead to abortion.

Varicella-zoster virus infection of the fetus only occurs when the mother has chickenpox—not when the mother has herpes zoster. Chickenpox during the last 3 weeks of gestation can lead to the delivery of a baby with classical chickenpox or to, on occasion, a child with zoster. These do not pose serious problems, however. Approximately 2% of children born of mothers who have had chickenpox in the early period of gestation have been born with cicatricial lesions in a zosteriform pattern and hypoplasia of the corresponding limb (40). These children also have evidence of ocular and diffuse brain disease. This syndrome is sufficiently rare that it does not warrant consideration of therapeutic abortion (40,41).

Retroviruses

During the last decade, two retroviruses, human T lymphotropic virus-1 (HTLV-1) and human immune deficiency virus (HIV) have been associated with perinatal infection and subsequent neurologic disease. HTLV-1 is the cause of acute T-cell leukemia and chronic spastic paraparesis (known as tropical spastic paraparesis [TSP] and in Japan as HTLV-1-associated myelopathy [HAM]). TSP/HAM develops, however, only in about 1 in 300 infected persons. The virus is acquired most commonly from breast milk of infected mothers, but it also can be acquired through sexual relations and by transfusion of contaminated blood. The neurologic syndrome of TSP/HAM does not develop until midlife and is a chronic disabling disorder. The patients usually maintain the functional use of their upper extremities and do not suffer cognitive deficits. The rate of myelopathy following transmission by transfusion appears to be higher and seems to have a shorter incubation period. Despite the low incidence of disease following infection, blood supplies are now tested for HTLV-1. The low rates of infection-related disease, however, do not appear to justify routine prenatal testing, although it is recommended that women who have infected family members or are known to be seropositive themselves should be discouraged from breastfeeding.

HIV causes more consistent and serious neurologic diseases in both adults and infants. Perinatal infection with HIV is becoming an increasing problem in the United States, with the higher rate of infection among intravenous drug users and their sex partners, the majority of whom are members of the black and Hispanic communities. In Africa and Asia, where heterosexual transmission is the major mode of transmission of HIV infection, more than 3 million women of childbearing age are already infected. There is no evidence, as was originally thought, that pregnancy accelerates the onset of acquired immunodeficiency syndrome (AIDS) in the infected woman.

Transmission to the fetus or neonate from the infected mother is not universal. It occurs in somewhere between 15% and 50% of cases; the true incidence probably is approximately 25%. Women who have lower CD4 cell counts and lower levels of antibody to GP 120 (glycoprotein 120) may be more likely to transmit the virus. The virus can infect the fetus in utero as judged by the finding of virus in fetal tissue and documented viremia at birth. The virus also can infect the neonate intrapartum, presumably by maternal blood contact with mucous membranes or damaged skin or possibly by the transfusion of maternal blood with disruption of placental barriers. Finally, the virus can infect the neonate postpartum via breast milk as documented by mothers infected by postpartum transfusion transmitting the virus to a nursing infant. Although infection by all three modes have been documented, the relative frequency of each is uncertain.

Infected infants usually appear normal at birth. About 50% to 90% of those infected have some developmental delay, and about half develop symptoms in the first year, with a high incidence of progressive encephalopathy and early death. In other infected children, immunodeficiency and neurologic disease develop with a median age of onset of 6 years (Table 11.5). The reasons for this apparent bimodal distribution of disease are unknown; it may depend on the mode or timing of infection, as seen with other viruses. Children with acute encephalopathy usually have a normal head size at birth, but there is developmental microcephaly, loss of motor milestones with weakness and pyramidal tract signs, and a variety of other findings (such as ataxia, cortical blindness, myoclonic jerking, and occasionally epilepsy). Children with late-onset disease may show insidious loss of cognitive and

TABLE 11.5. *Abnormalities in congenital human immunodeficiency virus infections*

	Evident in neonatal period	Appears in subsequent months to years	
		Common	Rare
Central nervous system	0	Acquired microencephaly, progressive encephalopathy, basal ganglia calcification	Ataxia, movement disorders, myoclonus, seizures, opportunistic infections
Skeletomuscular	HIV dysmorphism (?)	—	—
Hematological	0	Generalized lymphadenopathy, hepatosplenomegaly	Thrombocytopenia, hepatitis, lymphomas
Cardiovascular–pulmonary	0	Interstitial pneumonitis	Cardiomyopathy
Other	0	Failure to thrive, chronic diarrhea, bacterial infections, oral candidiasis	Nephropathy, parotitis

From Johnson RT. *Viral infections of the nervous system,* 2nd ed. Lippincott-Raven, 1998, with permission.

motor skills similar to the adult AIDS dementia. Vascular changes and mineralization within the brain are much more frequent in children than in adults. Opportunistic infections are much less common in the infants with HIV encephalopathy (42,43).

Neonatal diagnosis is difficult because maternal antibodies are present at birth, and serologic diagnosis is delayed until 15 months of age when there is a decline of maternal HIV antibody and evidence of persistence or new generation of antibody by the child. By this time, children with rapidly progressing disease already have developed the disease and a number have died. Therefore, new reliable methods of diagnosis are being sought, including the more widespread use and standardization of polymerase chain reactions for diagnosis of infection in the neonate.

Azidothymidine (AZT) is licensed for use in children and appears to slow neurologic disease progression. Randomized trials of antiretroviral therapies have shown substantial reduction of maternal-to-child transmission when given in late gestation and at delivery to mother or infant. Cesarean sections and avoidance of breastfeeding also have reduced transmission from women not taking antiviral drugs (44). Some advocate universal HIV testing of pregnant women; certainly all women in high-risk groups should be tested. They then can be advised of risks and options and can be monitored so that antiviral treatment may be started at appropriate times.

Worldwide, about 600,000 infants are infected each year (45). In addition to the millions of children worldwide who will develop AIDS in the next decade and require prolonged hospitalization and medical care before their death, there will be twice as many children who will be orphaned by AIDS-associated deaths of their parents. The AIDS orphans already constitute an enormous social and economic problem in sub-Saharan Africa and will soon present increasing problems in Asia.

REFERENCES

1. Levin ML, Horn J, Eldred L, et al. Infections of the nervous system during pregnancy. In: Goldstein PJ, Stern BJ, eds. *Neurological disorders of pregnancy*, 2nd ed. Mount Kisco: Futura Publishing, 1992:125–163.
2. Sacks G, Sargent I, Redman C. An innate view of human pregnancy. *Immunol Today* 1999;20:114–118.
3. Gall SA. Maternal adjustments in the immune system in normal pregnancy. *Clin Obstet Gynecol* 1983;26: 521–536.
4. Nahmias AJ, Kourtis AP. The great balancing acts. The pregnant woman, placenta, fetus, and infectious agents. *Clin Perinatol* 1997;24:497–521.
5. Kingdom JC, Kennedy DH. Tuberculous meningitis in pregnancy. *Br J Obstet Gynaecol* 1989;96:233–235.
6. Linnan MJ, Mascola L, Lou XD, et al. Epidemic listeriosis associated with Mexican-style cheese. *N Engl J Med* 1988;319:823–828.
7. Gotuzzo E, Carrillo C. Brucella. In: Gorbach SL, Bartlett JG, Blacklow NR. *Infectious Diseases,* 2nd ed. Philadelphia: WB Saunders 1998:1837–1845.
8. Ampel NM, Wieden MA, Galgiani JN. Coccidioidomycocis: clinical update. *Rev Infect Dis* 1989;11:897–911.
9. Nair LS, Nair AS. Effects of malaria infection on pregnancy. *Indian J Marlariol* 1993;30:207–214.
10. Subramanian D, Moise KJ Jr, White AC Jr. Imported malaria in pregnancy: report of four cases and review of management. *Clin Infect Dis* 1992;15:408–413.
11. Looareesuwan S, Phillips RE, White NJ, et al. Quinine and severe falciparum malaria in late pregnancy. *Lancet* 1985;2:4–7.
12. Evengard B, Lilja G, Capraru T, et al. A retrospective study of seroconversion against Toxoplasma gondii during 3,000 pregnancies in Stockholm. *Scand J Infect Dis* 1999;31:2,127–129.
13. Weinstein L, Aycock WL, Feemster RF. The relation of sex, pregnancy and menstruation to susceptibility in poliomyelitis. *N Engl J Med* 1951;245:54–58.
14. Michielsen PP, Van Damme P. Viral hepatitis and pregnancy. *Acta Gastroenterol Belg* 1999;62:21–29.
15. Nosten F, Vincenti M, Simpson J, et al. The effects of mefloquine treatment in pregnancy. *Clin Infect Dis* 1999;28:808–815.
16. Harjulehto T, Hovi T, Aro T, et al. Congenital malformations and oral poliovirus vaccination during pregnancy. *Lancet* 1989;1:771–772.
17. Fiumara NJ, Fleming WL, Downing JG, et al. The incidence of prenatal syphilis at the Boston city hospital. *N Engl J Med* 1952;247:48–52.
18. Schlesinger PA, Duray PH, Burke BA, et al. Maternal-fetal transmission of the Lyme disease spirochete, *Borrelia burgdorferi. Ann Intern Med* 1985;103:67–68.
19. Markowitz LE, Steere AC, Benach JL, et al. Lyme disease during pregnancy. *JAMA* 1986;255:3394–3396.
20. Williams CL, Benach JL, Curran AS, et al. Lyme disease during pregnancy: a cord blood serosurvey. *Ann N Y Acad Sci* 1988;539:504–506.
21. Silver HM. Lyme disease during pregnancy. *Infect Dis Clin North Am* 1997;11:93–97.
22. Ager LS. Toxoplasmosis and parvovirus B19. *Infect Dis Clin North Am* 1997;11:55–75.
23. Hall SM. Congenital toxoplasmosis. *BMJ* 1992;305: 291–297.

24. Gregg NM. Congenital cataract following German measles in mother. *Trans Ophthal Soc Austral* 1941;3: 35–46.

25. Miller E, Cradock-Watson JE, Pollock TM. Consequences of confirmed maternal rubella at successive stages of pregnancy. *Lancet* 1982;2:781–784.

26. Johnson RT. *Viral infections of the nervous system,* 2nd ed. Philadelphia: Lippincott-Raven, 1998.

27. MacFarlane DW, Boyd RD, Dodrill CB, et al. Intrauterine rubella, head size, and intellect. *Pediatrics* 1975; 55:797–801.

28. Centers for Disease Control and Prevention. Current trends. Rubella vaccination during pregnancy—United States, 1971–1988. *MMWR Morb Mortal Wkly Rep* 1989;38:289–294.

29. Tentsov YY, Zuev VA, Rzhaninova AA, et al. Influenza virus genetic sequences in the blood of children with congenital pathology of the CNS. *Arch Virol* 1989; 108:301–306.

30. Ackermann P, Körver G, Turss R, et al. [Prenatal infection with the virus of lymphocytic choriomeningitis: report of two cases (author's transl)]. *Dtsch Med Wochenschr* 1974;99:629–632.

31. Potts BJ, Sever JL, Tzan NR, et al. Possible role of pestiviruses in microcephaly. *Lancet* 1987;1:972–973.

32. Isumi H, Nunoue T, Nishida A, et al. Fetal brain infection with human parvovirus B19. *Pediatr Neurol* 1999;21:661–663.

33. Eis-Hubinger AM, Dieck D, Schild R, et al. Parvovirus B19 infection in pregnancy. *Intervirology* 1998;41: 178–184.

34. Alford CA, Stagno S, Pass RF, et al. Congenital and perinatal cytomegalovirus infections. *Rev Infect Dis* 1990;12:S745.

35. Whitley R, Arvin A, Prober C, et al. Predictors of morbidity and mortality in neonates with herpes simplex virus infections. *N Engl J Med* 1991;324:450–454.

36. Whitley R, Arvin A, Prober C, et al. A controlled trial comparing vidarabine with acyclovir in neonatal herpes simplex virus infection. *N Engl J Med* 1991;324:444–449.

37. Kulhanjian JA, Soroush V, Au DS, et al. Identification of women at unsuspected risk of primary infection with herpes simplex virus type 2 during pregnancy. *N Engl J Med* 1992;326:916–20.

38. Libman MD, Dascal A, Kramer MS, et al. Strategies for the prevention of neonatal infection with herpes simplex virus: a decision analysis. *Rev Infect Dis* 1991;13: 1093–1104.

39. Whitley RJ. Neonatal herpes simplex virus infections. *J Med Virol* 1993;1:13–21.

40. Paryani SG, Arvin AM. Intrauterine infection with varicella-zoster virus after maternal varicella. *N Engl J Med* 1986;314:1542–1546.

41. Pastuszak AL, Levy M, Schick B, et al. Outcome after maternal varicella infection in the first 20 weeks of pregnancy. *N Engl J Med* 1994;330:901–905.

42. Epstein LG, Sharer LR, Oleske JM, et al. Neurologic manifestations of human immunodeficiency virus infection in children. *Pediatrics* 1986;78:678–687.

43. Belman AL, Diamond G, Dickson D, et al. Pediatric acquired immunodeficiency syndrome. Neurologic syndromes. *Am J Dis Child* 1988;142:29–35.

44. Stringer JS, Vermund SH. Prevention of mother-to-child transmission of HIV-1. *Curr Opin Obstet Gynecol* 1999;11:427–434.

45. Fowler MG, Simonds RJ, Roongpisuthipong A. Update on perinatal HIV transmission. *Pediatr Clin North Am* 2000;47:21–38.

Neurological Complications of Pregnancy, Second Edition, edited by Brian Hainline and Orrin Devinsky. Lippincott Williams & Wilkins, Philadelphia © 2002.

12

Nervous System Neoplasms

Martin Goldstein and *Lisa M. DeAngelis

*Department of Neurology, New York Hospital/Cornell Medical Center; and
Department of Neurology, Memorial Sloan-Kettering Cancer Center, New York, New York, U.S.A.

Brain tumor coincident with pregnancy is one of many neurologic diseases that may occur during pregnancy (1). Despite speculation regarding the pathogenic connections between pregnancy and brain tumors, the relative rarity of brain tumors coincident with pregnancy and the difficulty of performing studies in this population forces us to rely primarily on anecdotal reports to infer pathophysiologic and epidemiologic relationships. A detailed understanding of the occurrence of central nervous system (CNS) neoplasms during pregnancy remains to be elucidated.

The majority of brain tumors tend to occur in older individuals, and for women, usually after the childbearing years. However, some neoplasms occur primarily in young women and some are associated specifically with pregnancy, such as choriocarcinoma. In the general population, intracranial and spinal tumors are relatively rare, and the presentation of these tumors during pregnancy is even less common. Although brain tumors in pregnant patients are fortunately rare, when they do occur they pose specific diagnostic and therapeutic problems for the physician.

EPIDEMIOLOGY

Most types of CNS neoplasms have been reported in pregnant women, and the range of tumor types is similar to those that occur in nonpregnant women of similar age (Table 12.1). There is no greater overall incidence of primary brain and spinal tumors in pregnant women than in age-matched nonpregnant women (2). However, accurate epidemiology of brain tumors in pregnancy is difficult to obtain because data are frequently not reported. Nevertheless, a review of the literature provides informative cases.

In 1961, Barnes and Abbott recorded four fatal cases of intracranial brain tumors, all of which were malignant, diagnosed during pregnancy (3). A 1986 population-based review of a tumor registry from East Germany recorded all CNS neoplasms from 1961 as well as data regarding pregnancy at diagnosis. The study revealed that between 1961 and 1979, 17 pregnant women were diagnosed with malignant brain tumors yielding a frequency of 3.6 per 10^6 live births. However, the same authors reported that the number of meningiomas, acoustic neuromas, and primary malignant intracranial neoplasms diagnosed during pregnancy were less than expected when compared with general population prevalences; the ratio of observed to expected malignant primary tumors associated with pregnancy was 0.38 (4). The authors hypothesized that women with subclinical brain tumors become pregnant less often secondary to ill-defined fertility-reducing effects of a brain tumor (e.g., decreased libido, early spontaneous abortion).

From a literature review, Roelvink and colleagues collected 223 cases of pregnancy-related brain tumors from 86 separate reports.

TABLE 12.1. *Brain tumors in pregnancy*
(n = 195)

Tumor	Number (%)
Glioma	62 (32)
Meningioma	57 (29)
Acoustic neuroma	30 (15)
Cerebellar astrocytoma	12 (6)
Medulloblastoma	6
Plexus papilloma	5
Ependymoma	3
Pinealoma	1
Other	19

Modified from Roelvink NCA, Kamphorst W, van Alphen HA, et al. Pregnancy-related primary brain and spinal tumors. *Arch Neurol* 1987;44:209–215, with permission.

The authors concluded that the relative frequency of brain tumors of different types occurring in pregnancy was, in fact, equal to their respective frequencies in age-matched nonpregnant women (Table 12.1) (5).

Using statistics from the mid- to late 1980s on the number of live births per year, number of cancers diagnosed in women aged 15 to 45 years, and the proportion of these cancers likely to be brain tumors, Simon determined that in the United States approximately 90 women per year would have a brain tumor diagnosed during a pregnancy. Although a reasonable estimate, it is based on several assumptions. For example, this calculation ignores the impact a brain tumor may have on reproductive potential (6). In another study, Isla and associates reported seven women with brain tumors coincident with pregnancy in a series of 126,413 pregnancies reviewed from 1983 to 1995 at La Paz Hospital in Madrid (7).

In one of the most ambitious efforts to characterize coincident brain tumor and pregnancy, Tewari and associates conducted a review of cases from 1978 through 1998 at five separate California hospitals to better define the epidemiology of pregnancy-associated malignant brain tumors (8). A total of 312,645 births occurred in the five hospitals during the study period. Patients who had been diagnosed with a malignant brain tumor antenatally or within 6 weeks postpartum were iden-

tified via tumor registries. In all, ten women were found to have a malignant brain tumor during pregnancy (8 women) or postpartum (2 women), yielding a "malignant-brain-tumor-complicating-pregnancy" rate of 3.2×10^{-5}. All the women diagnosed antenatally with a malignant brain tumor developed a neurologic crisis during pregnancy. Median age was 24 (range of ages 19 to 37 years), and parity ranged from 0 to more than 2. Six of these patients were first seen during the second trimester and two were seen during the third trimester, all with rapidly escalating neurologic complaints. Intractable nausea and vomiting were most common, but severe headache, gait disturbance, seizure disorder, urinary incontinence, memory loss, and paralysis also were observed. In six instances, a catastrophic neurologic event prompted premature pregnancy termination (8).

PREGNANCY AND BRAIN TUMOR PATHOPHYSIOLOGY

There are conflicting opinions regarding the effect of pregnancy on brain tumor pathophysiology. Some investigators believe that pregnancy has little effect on brain tumors despite many anecdotal reports of symptom aggravation secondary to tumor enlargement. Others note that while pregnancy is not a specific risk factor for development of a particular type of intracranial neoplasm, it nevertheless can affect tumor growth by producing or exacerbating neurologic symptoms.

In 1938 Cushing and Eisenhardt were the first to describe a relationship between pregnancy and worsening neurologic symptoms in women with meningiomas (9). A comprehensive case-control study was performed using the Swedish Fertility and Cancer Registries (10). Among women born between 1925 and 1975, 1,088 patients with meningiomas and 1,657 patients with gliomas were identified. For every woman diagnosed with a brain tumor, five age-matched controls were used as a control group. Analysis revealed ever-parous women at reduced risk of glioma compared with nulliparous women, although parity was unrelated to meningioma risk. Age at first birth was unrelated to both meningioma and glioma risk. These data suggest that neither hormonal- nor any other pregnancy-related physiologic changes play an important role in the development of brain tumors.

A number of theories have been advanced to account for pregnancy-associated brain tumor symptom exacerbation, including pregnancy-related immunologic tolerance, steroid hormone-mediated growth, hemodynamic instability, and water retention with consequent increased tumor swelling or surrounding brain edema. However, there is no simple pregnancy-related pathophysiology that explains the appearance of brain tumor symptoms. For example, efforts to tie neurologic symptoms in pregnant women with a previously quiescent brain tumor to pregnancy-related cerebrospinal fluid (CSF) pressure changes failed because it was recognized that intracranial pressure (ICP) remains normal throughout pregnancy until labor and delivery (11).

Nevertheless, there exist strong suggestions of a pregnancy-related hormonal impact on the pathophysiology of at least some brain tumors, especially meningiomas. Lee and associates found high levels of progesterone receptors in 14 of 17 meningiomas, one of two astrocytomas, and one neurilemoma studied (12). In the Isla and colleagues study from Spain, estrogen and progesterone receptors were studied in two cases—one meningioma and one astrocytoma—and were present in both (7).

Nomura and associates investigated the relationship between placenta growth factor and brain tumor angiogenesis (13). Primary brain (meningiomas, gliomas, schwannomas, pituitary adenomas, germinoma, and choriocarcinoma) and metastatic tumors were examined. Using a quantitative reverse transcriptase polymerase chain reaction, placenta growth factor was detected in approximately 64% of all brain tumors. For primary brain tumors, placenta growth factor messenger RNA (mRNA) was expressed in 100% of hypervascular tumors but in only 31% of hypovascular tumors. No metastatic hypervascular tumors

expressed placenta growth factor. Also, to determine the mechanism of placenta growth factor gene regulation, placenta growth factor mRNA level was assayed in different oxygen concentrations. It was found that decreased oxygen concentration was associated with increased placenta growth factor mRNA expression in glioma cell cultures. This suggests a mechanism for angiogenesis when tumor size exceeds existing vascular supply, resulting in decreased tumor oxygen tension. Therefore, primary brain tumors may be sensitive to circulating placenta growth factor during pregnancy, which may contribute to brain tumor angiogenesis and subsequent tumor growth.

BRAIN TUMORS

Clinical Features

Brain tumors produce both specific and nonspecific symptoms and signs. Nonspecific tumor symptoms include headache, which occurs in about half of patients, and the symptoms associated with increased ICP (e.g., nausea and vomiting), which is observed in 25% of patients. Nausea and vomiting may be easily confused with "morning sickness"; however, pregnancy-related nausea and vomiting is maximal in the first trimester and tends to remit, whereas tumor-related nausea and vomiting may appear at any time during pregnancy and does not improve with time. Constant daily headache should not be attributed to pregnancy, particularly in patients without a prior history of headache. The majority of patients with these symptoms as a result of brain tumor also have specific or lateralizing neurologic symptoms indicating a structural process. Lateralizing signs reflect tumor location and commonly include hemiparesis, sensory loss, visual field defects, and aphasia. The presence of these signs necessitates neuroimaging for evaluation. Seizures are a relatively common presenting symptom in patients with brain tumors, particularly low-grade gliomas and meningiomas. Seizures from brain tumors may be either generalized or focal; all generalized seizures have a focal onset even if not clinically apparent. This focality reflects the intracranial location of the underlying mass. Development of seizures during pregnancy, particularly in the second half of pregnancy, is more likely the result of eclampsia than brain tumor. However, focal seizures are rare with eclampsia; eclampsia-associated hypertension, proteinuria, edema, and generalized hyperreflexia are absent in patients with brain tumors. Therefore, any pregnant patient who has an isolated seizure warrants neuroradiologic investigation.

Diagnosis

All brain tumors, primary and metastatic, require neuroimaging by either computerized tomography (CT) or magnetic resonance imaging (MRI) for diagnosis. MR scan is the best method to establish the diagnosis of a brain tumor and should be the first test obtained in a patient with symptoms or signs suggestive of an intracranial mass. It is the most sensitive method available and is particularly advantageous in the pregnant patient because no ionizing radiation is involved. There is no known risk to humans using MR scans of less than 2.0 Tesla, which encompasses all commercially available scanners, and many patients have undergone cranial MRI without any ill effect on the fetus. CT scan also is accurate for the diagnosis of a brain tumor, but the scan may be negative in patients with a low-grade glioma. Posterior fossa and pituitary tumors are also difficult to delineate on CT. CT scans use conventional x-rays and, therefore, pregnant patients should have abdominal shielding during the examination. In spite of this potential concern, many women have had cranial CT scans at various stages of pregnancy without deleterious consequences. Therefore, physicians should not hesitate to use CT or MRI to assess worrisome symptoms in pregnant women (14) (see Chapter 1).

Both CT and MR scans performed to assess a potential brain tumor must be done with IV contrast (CT scan) or gadolinium (MR scan). Iodinated contrast agents for CT are physio-logically inert and harmless to the developing fetus; however, adequate maternal hydration should be maintained during contrast administration to prevent fetal dehydration or maternal renal insufficiency. Gadolinium is not associated with any fetal risks and is associated with only rare maternal complications. Malignant brain tumors, either primary or metastatic, usually appear as a contrast-enhancing mass lesion with edema extending throughout peritumoral white matter. Low-grade malignancies, such as an astrocytoma, typically do not enhance and are best appreciated on T2-weighted MR images. Meningiomas arise from the dural surface and are extraaxial, often causing compression of underlying brain tissue but not invasion. Meningiomas may be isodense (CT scan) or isointense (MR scan) prior to contrast administration, but they have a prominent and usually homogeneous enhancement pattern after contrast. A necrotic center rarely may be evident in meningiomas, whereas this is commonly seen with malignant gliomas or metastatic lesions.

There are almost no data on positron emission tomography (PET) imaging of brain tumors in pregnant patients. A single case of ^{11}C methionine PET imaging in a woman after an abortion highlights potential imaging artifacts as a result of pregnancy (15). The patient was a 31-year-old woman with a seizure in the ninth week of pregnancy. CT demonstrated an abnormal mass lesion in the right frontal lobe, and a brain tumor was suspected. The patient requested that the pregnancy be terminated. Seven days after surgical abortion, methionine PET was performed. The scan showed high methionine uptake in the right frontal lobe mass as well as the pituitary, prompting suspicion that another tumor was present in the pituitary. The right frontal tumor was partially resected and pathologic examination showed an astrocytoma. Two months later, the authors performed a second methionine PET scan, which showed high uptake in the residual right frontal tumor but not in the pituitary. Results of other radiologic and physiologic studies of the pituitary were normal. These findings suggest that the transport of ^{11}C methionine into the pituitary gland may increase during pregnancy. Moreover, "pituitary gland of pregnancy" should be included in the differential diagnosis of pituitary adenomas in methionine PET scanning (16).

GLIAL NEOPLASMS

Glial tumors are the most common primary brain tumor both in the general population and in pregnant patients. Glial tumors arise from astrocytes or oligodendrocytes and give rise to tumors of varying malignancy. Astrocyte-derived tumors are graded pathologically according to the World Health Organization criteria using a three-tier system: astrocytoma, anaplastic astrocytoma, and glioblastoma multiforme. Oligodendrogliomas are divided into low-grade tumors and the uncommon anaplastic oligodendroglioma. The pathologic grade of glial tumors is one of the most important prognostic factors for patients and also determines their treatment (17).

Management decisions in pregnant patients with gliomas are difficult. With low-grade tumors it may be possible to defer all treatment until after delivery, whereas higher-grade lesions often require surgical resection and immediate therapy. If feasible, delivery of the baby should precede subsequent treatment with radiotherapy since radiotherapy may cause congenital defects (18). However, if delivery is not possible, radiotherapy can be administered with reasonable safety, resulting in less than 0.10 Gy exposure to the fetus (19). Chemotherapy may lead to fetal malformations and always is deferred until after delivery. Steroids may be used when necessary.

LOW-GRADE GLIOMAS

Astrocytomas and oligodendrogliomas frequently present with seizures in a previously neurologically normal patient. They are identified on CT or MR scan as a nonenhancing mass that is hypodense on CT and hyperintense on T2-weighted MR scan. If feasible, surgical extirpation or subtotal resection is the treatment of choice. If the lesion cannot be removed, stereotactic biopsy is performed for diagnosis. Although surgery can be performed during pregnancy, urgent treatment of a low-grade glioma is almost never necessary. Frequently these lesions have been present for many years before diagnosis and may persist for many more without producing neurologic disability. For this reason, diagnosis and treatment often can be delayed safely until after completion of pregnancy to eliminate even the minor risk that craniotomy poses to the fetus.

After surgery, additional treatment may include cranial radiotherapy (RT) or chemotherapy for the oligodendroglioma (20,21). The best timing for adjuvant RT has not been established, but adjuvant RT does benefit those patients with progressive neurologic signs or increased seizure frequency (22). Even if resection or biopsy has been undertaken during a pregnancy and adjuvant therapy is deemed appropriate for the patient, it can be deferred until completion of the pregnancy. The overall prognosis for astrocytomas is quite good, with approximately 50% surviving 5 years. Oligodendrogliomas can have a median survival as long as 16 years (21). Young women with an oligodendroglioma may desire pregnancy. Although each patient's condition must be evaluated individually, there is no *a priori* reason that such patients cannot successfully conceive and complete a pregnancy.

HIGH-GRADE GLIOMAS

Anaplastic astrocytoma, anaplastic oligodendroglioma, and glioblastoma multiforme are highly malignant and aggressive neoplasms that require prompt diagnosis and treatment. They almost always appear as single ring-enhancing lesions on CT or MR scan. When a lesion of this type is identified, the patient should undergo prompt surgery for the purpose of removing as much tumor as possible. Complete resection often can be achieved and is the surgical goal (23). If the tumor involves the midline, is bilateral, or is restricted to deep structures, diagnostic biopsy is performed (Fig. 12.1). Surgery should not be delayed until completion of pregnancy unless the patient is near term and delivery can be accomplished by induction or cesarean section.

Cranial RT (about 6,000 cGy to the tumor) and chemotherapy (usually with a nitrosourea or temozolomide) follow surgery in all patients with a malignant glioma (24,25). Despite maximal treatment, prognosis for these tumors remains poor. Median survival is 1 year for a glioblastoma multiforme and 3 years for an anaplastic astrocytoma; however, a pregnant woman is likely to do better because of her young age, which is a strong prognostic variable (17). The timing of RT and chemotherapy often is dictated by the stage of the pregnancy because these therapies pose significant risks to the unborn child. If the patient already has

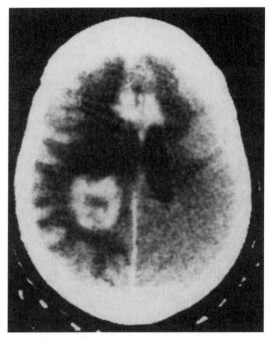

Fig. 12.1. A contrast-enhanced CT scan of a woman with a multifocal malignant glioma. Note the extensive edema throughout the right hemisphere. She was in her first trimester of pregnancy. A therapeutic abortion was performed to facilitate immediate cranial RT and chemotherapy.

delivered, adjuvant therapy usually begins within a few weeks of surgery. If a woman is early in her pregnancy, termination should be offered because the potential hazards to the fetus are greatest in the first trimester, and completion of the pregnancy would impose a lengthy delay in therapy even if a complete resection has been achieved. For patients in the second and third trimester, treatment decisions must be tailored to the individual. For example, a neurologically normal patient with a complete resection of an anaplastic astrocytoma may defer RT for 1 to 2 months to allow adequate maturation of the child for an early delivery. Alternatively, a woman with a midline glioblastoma multiforme who only had a biopsy should not wait 2 to 4 months for RT. This patient may be treated with cranial RT using abdominal shielding and a treatment regimen designed to minimize fetal exposure. Because chemotherapy of any type has only a modest impact on survival, it should be deferred until after delivery. Delay of a few months in the initiation of chemotherapy would not reduce its potential benefit.

MENINGIOMAS

Meningiomas are mesenchymal tumors that arise from the membranous coverings of the brain and spinal cord (26). They are commonly located over the surface of the brain, at the skull base, near the optic nerve, adjacent to the cavernous sinus, or on the sphenoid wing. Depending on its location, a meningioma may produce symptoms identical to parenchymal brain tumors, such as hemiparesis or seizures, but also may lead to headache, diplopia, visual loss, or cranial neuropathies in the absence of other segmental signs. The vast majority of meningiomas are histologically benign lesions, although atypical and malignant variants occasionally are seen. Despite their benign pathologic appearance, some have an aggressive course because of frequent recurrences.

Meningiomas are slow growing and may be present for years before producing symptoms.

They are a frequent autopsy finding in patients who never had neurologic difficulties. Sixty percent of meningiomas occur in women. Although the percentage of meningiomas is no greater in pregnant women than in nonpregnant women of the same age, pregnancy can have a dramatic effect on a preexisting, even if clinically silent, meningioma (Fig. 12.2). There are numerous examples of patients who develop neurologic symptoms and signs with pregnancy which resolve after delivery and are subsequently attributed to a meningioma (27–30). In many of these cases, the meningioma was in the suprasellar, parasellar, or medial sphenoid wing region (31). In the Roelvink and associates series, meningiomas slightly increased in number during pregnancy, and 60% of intracranial meningiomas in pregnant women were basal meningiomas (5). Bickerstaff reported a dramatic patient who developed recurrent neurologic symptoms and mass effect (documented by arteriogram) with menses and successive pregnancies that remitted after completion of a menstrual cycle or delivery of a child (30). However, many women who have pregnancy-related growth of a meningioma have had prior uneventful pregnancies when the tumor likely was present.

Two mechanisms are thought to explain the rapid and occasionally temporary enlargement of a meningioma during pregnancy. First, fluid retention and increased blood volume during pregnancy may exacerbate tumor edema and enlarge a vascular tumor such as a meningioma; the increased total mass effect leads to neurologic symptoms.

Second, the predominance of meningiomas in females, their accelerated growth during the luteal phase of the menstrual cycle, the association with breast cancer, and reported expansion during pregnancy have led to a number of studies examining the potential role of sex steroids on meningioma growth. Meningioma cells contain cytosolic and nuclear sex steroid receptors (31,32). Up to 96% of

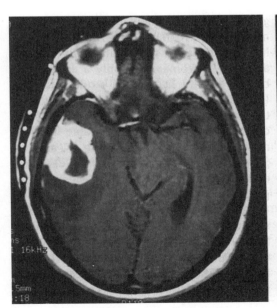 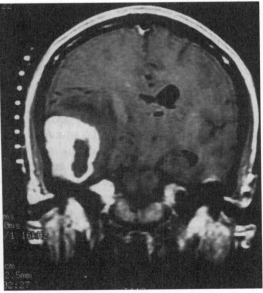

Fig. 12.2. A gadolinium-enhanced MR scan of a woman with a right temporal meningioma. Note the central necrosis, a very unusual feature of benign meningiomas. She became acutely symptomatic with intractable headaches, nausea, and vomiting within hours after a spontaneous abortion of her sixth pregnancy. This was completely resected and she is neurologically normal.

meningiomas have detectable high-affinity progesterone receptors. Progesterone levels correlate with CNS tumor symptoms, but the initial appearance of symptoms often is not until late pregnancy, suggesting that not only progesterone is involved.

Although it is generally agreed that the majority of meningiomas possess progesterone and androgen receptors, controversy exists regarding the frequency of estrogen receptors (ER) in meningiomas. Carroll and associates analyzed 34 meningiomas (via reverse transcriptase Southern blot analysis) for ER presence. Up to 68% of samples were positive for ER subunits (33). Other reports have placed the estimate of meningiomas with ERs at 33% to 38%. The presence and concentration of sex steroid receptors have no relationship to the sex or menopausal status of the patient with the neoplasm. Although these receptors may facilitate meningeal growth during gestation, the proportion of pregnant women harboring a meningioma experiencing these changes is unknown, but likely occurs in a minority of patients. Of course, additional unidentified factors may contribute to tumor expansion.

Although accelerated or even explosive growth of meningiomas during pregnancy is well known, unless serious neurologic impairment is present or imminent, treatment often can be delayed until after delivery, by which time tumor size and symptom severity may be reduced (2). Treatment of meningiomas is surgical. Complete resection can be achieved in approximately 30% of patients with meningiomas, but the probability of complete removal varies greatly with tumor location (34). Most patients can undergo a substantial subtotal resection, and only about 15% of patients have a limited resection or biopsy. Cure can be achieved with surgical extirpation. Residual disease after surgery will result in recurrence, but that may not occur for 5 to 10 years after the initial resection. Surgery can be performed safely in a pregnant patient, and it is unusual that early termination of pregnancy is necessary; however, craniotomy should be postponed until after delivery, if possible. The patient's neurologic status and the degree of mass effect or compression of critical structures (e.g., the optic nerve) determine the timing of surgery. RT usually is reserved for recurrent tumors, surgically inaccessible lesions, or the rare malignant variety (35). RT is almost never an emergency treatment for this tumor and can virtually always wait until the patient has completed her pregnancy.

ACOUSTIC NEUROMAS

Acoustic neuromas are benign neoplasms that arise from the vestibular portion of the eighth cranial nerve (36). They occur with increased incidence in patients with von Recklinghausen's disease, and bilateral acoustic neuromas constitute the specific diagnosis of central neurofibromatosis or neurofibromatosis type II. Acoustic neuromas have a peak onset at about age 40 to 45—beyond the childbearing years for most women. However, they are a relatively common intracranial neoplasm and account for 15% of brain tumors in pregnant women. The first symptoms typically are tinnitus and ipsilateral hearing loss, followed by ataxia and ipsilateral facial weakness.

Like meningiomas, pregnancy may affect the clinical presentation of an undiagnosed preexisting acoustic neuroma. There are several examples in the literature of patients developing neurologic symptoms, usually during the last trimester. In Allen and colleagues' series, 17% (6 of 36) of women with an acoustic neuroma developed symptoms or had exacerbation of symptoms during the last months of pregnancy (37). They reported a total of eight patients with acoustic neuromas symptomatic during pregnancy. Unlike patients with meningiomas, all but one of these women had persistence of their symptoms after delivery, some developing progressive neurologic impairment over the ensuing months to years after termination of the pregnancy. These patients were all seen in the pre-CT scan era, but their diagnosis was established pathologically in all cases. Four of the eight women had had earlier pregnancies, which were not associated with worsening of neurologic symptoms.

Fluid retention, with transient lesion expansion and hormonal effects, is a postulated mechanism for the apparent growth or enlargement of acoustic neuromas during pregnancy. ERs have been demonstrated in 44% to 100% of acoustic neuromas, but only a small number of tumors have been studied (38,39). Progesterone receptors were not found on the two acoustic neuromas studied (39). It does, however, appear reasonable that hormone-mediated tumor growth is at least partially responsible for the development of neurologic symptoms and signs during pregnancy.

Acoustic neuromas are usually treated surgically, and timing should be guided by the patient's neurologic status. A new therapeutic option for acoustic neuromas is the use of stereotactic radiosurgery (40). A single high dose (about 1,400 cGy) of radiation is administered as the sole treatment. The radiation is highly focused to reduce toxicity to the surrounding brain. Only tumors that are relatively small and not producing significant brainstem compression can be treated by this method. Patients with tumors of this size usually only have mild symptoms referable to the eighth nerve. Because this tumor is slow growing, a pregnant patient with a lesion eligible for radiosurgery usually can wait until delivery to receive treatment; the duration of pregnancy should not be shortened to expedite treatment.

PITUITARY TUMORS

Pituitary tumors are classified according to size (macroadenoma, when greater than or equal to 1cm, microadenoma when less than 1 cm) and by the secreted hormone (prolactin, growth hormone, corticotrophin, thyrotrophin, gonadotrophin, or a nonsecretory tumor) (41). Prolactinomas are the most common pituitary tumor, but nonprolactinomas also may produce a modest elevation of prolactin by disrupting the dopamine inhibitory pathway from the hypothalamus, which controls prolactin secretion. Pituitary tumors are common, identified in 8% to 13% of all autopsies, with some reports giving an incidence as high as 27% (41).

However, the majority of microadenomas remain asymptomatic.

Pituitary tumors have a complicated and important relationship to fertility and pregnancy. Patients frequently present to their obstetrician or gynecologist with amenorrhea, galactorrhea, and/or infertility caused by hyperprolactinemia (42). In addition, many women with pituitary tumors are managed by endocrinologists rather than neurologists (43). Neurologic symptoms, especially headaches and visual symptoms, are a consequence of pituitary proximity to the optic nerves and chiasm. Classically, a bitemporal hemianopia is observed as a result of optic chiasm compression, but a variety of visual defects can occur. Pituitary apoplexy caused by hemorrhage into or infarction of a tumor is rarely the presentation of a pituitary neoplasm (44).

The pituitary normally enlarges during pregnancy (11), and a previously asymptomatic pituitary tumor (e.g., adenoma) can enlarge, resulting in neurologic symptoms that may develop at any time throughout the 9-month gestation (45). In patients with microadenomas or presumed microadenomas measuring less than 1 cm, the risk of developing visual loss after as many as four full-term pregnancies is very small. However, six of eight women with larger tumors develop visual problems during pregnancy (43). Most symptoms are mild and progress at a subacute rate, allowing the physician time to intervene before the onset of serious irreversible neurologic deficits. Pregnancy-related pituitary apoplexy is extremely rare but not necessarily preceded by less serious symptoms.

Diagnosis of pituitary tumors has been greatly facilitated by MR scans. Microadenomas, optic nerve, and optic chiasm can be well defined on coronal MR images through the sella turcica. The high resolution of MR images not only facilitates diagnosis, but is an important tool for serial evaluation of the pregnant patient known to harbor a pituitary tumor because small changes may be appreciated on MR scan before symptoms develop.

Treatment of pituitary tumors may be surgical, medical, or a combination of both. Successful treatment of pituitary tumors is partially assessed by the uneventful completion of pregnancy as well as the incidence of subsequent desired pregnancies. Hammond and associates reported equal success rates (89% to 100%) of transsphenoidal resection or bromocriptine pharmacotherapy leading to pregnancy in previously infertile women with a prolactinoma (46). In patients with microadenomas, Samaan and colleagues found that surgery was significantly more successful, leading to pregnancy in 91% compared to 56% of patients treated with bromocriptine (47). However, this difference may have been due to poor compliance with bromocriptine because of side effects. The choice of surgery or dopamine agonists is based on individual patient considerations. The transsphenoidal approach results in successful removal or substantial subtotal resection in almost all patients. Surgery is associated with a very low morbidity and virtually no mortality when performed by a skilled surgeon. Unlike dopamine agonists, it is curative in many patients, although some with persistently elevated prolactin may require postoperative medication or radiotherapy. Nevertheless, many patients prefer medical treatment. Cabergoline is a dopamine agonist that inhibits prolactin secretion; it is the current medication of choice because of a more favorable side-effect profile than bromocriptine. It can shrink an adenoma and normalize serum prolactin, but if the medication is discontinued, prolactin levels again rise and the tumor may reappear on imaging studies. For those taking bromocriptine or cabergoline at the time of conception, the drug usually is stopped during pregnancy because of concerns regarding teratogenicity, particularly in the first trimester. However, it appears safe for the developing fetus if discontinued 4 to 6 weeks after conception once pregnancy is evident (48). The risk of microadenoma growth is 1% after stopping the drug, but 23% for patients with a macroadenoma. Once medication is stopped, if symptoms reappear or an adenoma is seen to be significantly enlarging during a pregnancy, bromocriptine can be re-

instituted safely and maintained throughout gestation (48,46). This is usually sufficient to shrink the tumor and resolve neurologic symptoms, and there have been no reports of adverse fetal effects of bromocriptine or cabergoline when used throughout pregnancy. Once pregnancy and lactation are over, the adenoma will regress spontaneously. Whether continued dopamine agonist or additional therapy is necessary should be reevaluated.

MEDULLOBLASTOMA

Medulloblastoma is a rare neoplasm in adults, and extraneural metastases are especially unusual. However, Belleza and colleagues recently described the eighth reported case of medulloblastoma discovered during pregnancy with subsequent metastases to muscle and lymph nodes (49).

BRAIN METASTASES

Systemic cancer is unusual in young women and is present rarely during pregnancy. No particular systemic neoplasm is associated with pregnancy except choriocarcinoma. There are, however, instructive isolated case reports of metastatic brain disease. For example, Chen and associates report a case of a 34-year-old pregnant woman with poorly differentiated lung carcinoma and brain metastasis (50). Left hemiparesis developed during the third trimester. She underwent excision of the metastatic brain tumor and received radiotherapy to the lung tumor and brain. The patient was still alive after a follow-up period of greater than 1 year. Delayed diagnosis may be the main problem in the management of metastatic lung cancer during pregnancy because of misinterpretation of respiratory symptoms (e.g., differentiation from a physiologic tachypnea of pregnancy) and physician reluctance to use radiologic imaging studies secondary to concerns over fetal safety.

Regardless of the primary malignancy, brain metastases may be treated with surgery, cranial irradiation, or chemotherapy. Resection usually is reserved for those patients with a single metastatic lesion or those who require urgent decompression for a mass obstructing the fourth ventricle. The use of cranial RT and chemotherapy is associated with risks to the developing fetus and is avoided during pregnancy unless the mother's life is in immediate danger. In patients with choriocarcinoma, these therapeutic restrictions do not apply (see below).

The prognosis for most patients with brain metastases is poor, with median survival averaging 6 months using cranial RT alone. However, surgery followed by RT significantly prolongs survival and improves the quality of life in patients with a single brain metastasis (51,52).

CHORIOCARCINOMA

Choriocarcinoma, or gestational trophoblastic disease (GTD), occurs only with pregnancy and is the most common systemic cancer associated with pregnancy (2). Choriocarcinoma can develop from trophoblastic tissue after a molar pregnancy, abortion, ectopic gestation, or term pregnancy. The incidence of choriocarcinoma after a term pregnancy is 1 in 50,000, and these patients accounted for 12% of all patients treated with trophoblastic disease at a large referral center (53). By rigorous definition, postpartum patients with choriocarcinoma are different from those described in this chapter because they have recently completed a pregnancy or do not harbor a viable fetus; however, they may present to their obstetrician, internist, or neurologist with neurologic symptoms as the first manifestation of their neoplasm.

Cerebral metastases are common (often associated with lung metastases), occurring in 14% to 28% of cases (53); approximately 3% to 20% of patients have metastatic brain disease at diagnosis (54,55). Patients may develop subacute neurologic signs identical to those associated with any space-occupying intracranial lesion. Tumor also can invade blood vessel walls or occlude an artery, leading to hemorrhage into a brain metastasis or ischemic infarct.

Diagnosis is aided by assay for serum beta-human chorionic gonadotropin (beta-HCG). Rising CSF:serum beta-HCG ratio traditionally has been regarded as indicative of brain metastases (11). However, Bakri and associates investigated the accuracy of using CSF:serum ratio of beta-HCG in detecting brain metastases from GTD (56). They studied ten subjects with GTD and known brain metastases. Synchronous lumbar puncture and venipuncture were performed for measurement of CSF and serum beta-HCG. CSF:serum ratios were calculated before starting multiagent chemotherapy and/or RT. Half of patients manifested CSF:serum beta-HCG at a ratio of greater than 1:60, and half had a ratio of less than 1:60. The authors concluded that CSF:serum beta-HCG ratio was not useful for diagnosis or surveillance of brain metastases in GTD.

Mortality of untreated choriocarcinoma with brain metastases is high. Survival is significantly improved by early diagnosis and treatment (57). GTD patients require a vigorous multimodality therapeutic plan, which always includes combination chemotherapy and frequently cranial RT (54,55,58). Early brain metastases in choriocarcinoma do not carry the same dismal prognosis as other systemic cancer brain metastases, and patients can experience a 50% to 80% cure rate, usually with nonsurgical treatment (54,55,58). Nevertheless, among the more than 50 cases of postterm choriocarcinoma with intracranial metastases reported, only four survivors have been recorded in the medical literature (59,60).

Schechter and colleagues recently evaluated the effect of multiple treatment and disease-related variables on the outcome of patients receiving whole-brain radiation therapy (WBRT) for metastatic GTD (61). Between November 1967 and December 1994, 21 patients were treated at Memorial Sloan-Kettering for GTD metastatic to the brain. All received WBRT at a median dose of 2,200 cGy (range 200 to 3,600 cGy). Five-year local control of initial brain metastases with more than 2,200 cGy was 91%, compared to 24% with less than 2,200 cGy ($p=0.05$). The 2- and 5-year survivals of the nine patients whose disease was controlled at extracranial sites were 100% and 83%, respectively, compared to 8% and 0%, respectively, for the 12 whose extracranial disease was not controlled ($p=0.0002$). One-third of patients with persistent or progressive extracranial disease later developed new sites of brain metastases, compared to 0% of patients whose extracranial disease was controlled ($p=0.05$). Eleven patients progressed at their initial site of brain metastasis or developed new intracranial lesions; six died secondary to brain metastases. The investigators concluded that (i) survival of patients with GTD metastatic to brain is excellent if extracranial disease can be controlled, (ii) total radiation dose is critical in achieving control of initial brain metastases, (iii) patients with uncontrolled extracranial disease are more likely to develop new brain metastases, and (iv) salvage of intracranial failures after WBRT is rare.

Recent case reports have described treatment-refractory gestational trophoblastic disease with brain metastases successfully responding to combination multiregimen chemotherapy (ifosfamide, carboplatin, and etoposide) and high-dose paclitaxel monotherapy (62,63).

SPINAL TUMORS

Spinal tumors are much less common than brain tumors, and the concurrence of pregnancy and a spinal tumor is extremely rare. In Roelvink and colleagues' review of brain and spinal tumors in pregnancy, they identified 28 cases of spinal tumors, representing only 12.5% of nervous system neoplasms presenting during pregnancy (5). Of spinal tumors, 61% were vertebral hemangiomas and 18% were meningiomas (Table 12.2) (5). In all series, hemangiomas represent the majority of spinal neoplasms in pregnant women (5,64).

Despite their relative rarity, it can be crucially important to diagnose spinal tumors antenatally. For example, Kawasaki and associates report two cases of acute onset of spinal cord compression following spinal anesthesia

TABLE 12.2. *Spinal tumors in pregnancy*
(n = 28)

Tumor	Number (%)
Vascular (hemangioma)	17 (61)
Meningioma	5 (18)
Ependymoma	3 (11)
Cerebellar astrocytoma	2 (7)
Glioma	1 (4)

Modified from Roelvink NCA, Kamphorst W, van Alphen HA, et al. Pregnancy-related primary brain and spinal tumors. *Arch Neurol* 1987;44:209–215, with permission.

for cesarean section (65). Complications occurred secondary to displacement and/or vascular engorgement due to lumbar puncture-induced fluid dynamic effects in the spinal canal.

Hemangiomas are present in up to 10% of the population in large autopsy series, but they rarely become symptomatic. They can involve the spine at any level, but those that become symptomatic in pregnancy are usually in the thoracic vertebrae (64,66,67). Enlargement of a preexisting hemangioma during pregnancy has been attributed to increased blood volume, enhanced vascular distention due to elevated progesterone levels, and promotion of endothelial growth by estrogen. An additional factor is elevated venous pressure from an enlarging uterus compressing the inferior vena cava, thereby shunting blood through the vertebral venous plexus. Meningiomas of the spine usually occur at the thoracic level and are subject to the same rapid growth during pregnancy as intracranial meningiomas, and for the same hypothesized reasons (69).

With either tumor, patients present with painless leg weakness and numbness, which can progress to paralysis and loss of sphincter function. Onset can be abrupt or subacute, and symptoms typically begin in the third trimester in more than 64% of patients. The remaining patients present in the second trimester. Back pain is not a common symptom, but thoracic back pain should not be confused with the common low back pain seen in pregnancy. Patients who present with a myelopathy need rapid diagnosis. Myelography, CT scans, and spinal MR scans all have been performed in pregnant patients without difficulty. At the present time, MR imaging is the method of choice because of its safety to the fetus and high degree of accuracy.

Spinal tumors with rapidly progressing symptoms require urgent intervention. Vertebral resection and intradural surgery are necessary to treat the hemangiomas and meningiomas typically seen in pregnant patients. These procedures have been performed successfully in pregnant women. Castel and colleagues advocated consideration of posterior fixation in cases of vertebral hemangioma to prevent perinatal vertebral collapse and consequent risk for spinal cord compression (70). After surgery, patients can continue gestation without difficulty, but spinal anesthesia during labor may not be appropriate, particularly if the dura has been opened.

GENERAL CONSIDERATIONS AND MANAGEMENT OF PREGNANT PATIENTS WITH INTRACRANIAL NEOPLASMS

Use of Anticonvulsants

Intracranial tumors of any type may be associated with seizures. Seizures as a result of brain tumors must be treated with anticonvulsants, often for prolonged periods and certainly throughout pregnancy. The choice of anticonvulsants in a pregnant woman is discussed in detail in Chapter 14 and applies to patients with intracranial lesions as well as to those with idiopathic epilepsy. Prophylactic anticonvulsants are ineffective in patients with primary and metastatic brain tumors and should be avoided in pregnant patients (71).

Use of Corticosteroids

Corticosteroids frequently are used in patients with brain tumors to reduce peritumoral edema and total mass effect. Theoretically, edema may be exacerbated by the fluid retention and increased intravascular volume asso-

ciated with pregnancy, but this has not been proven. Corticosteroids often produce prompt clinical improvement, which can last for weeks to months in the absence of additional therapy. In the pregnant patient, this short-term, immediate response often allows time to decide the fate of the fetus, permitting an early delivery or even termination if indicated. However, corticosteroids are never considered definitive therapy, and edema often will redevelop in a patient on a standing dose of corticosteroid. Prednisone is the corticosteroid of choice because it is metabolized before crossing the placenta (see Chapter 9). The initial dose is usually 100 mg per day, but this is empiric and often a lower or higher dose is necessary.

For most patients, the requirement for corticosteroids diminishes with the institution of definitive treatment. The majority can be tapered off corticosteroids completely whether they have a primary or secondary brain tumor, either malignant or benign. Sustained corticosteroid use is associated with hypertension, hyperglycemia, myopathy, insomnia, weight gain, osteoporosis, peptic ulcers, and psychiatric complications (72). Some toxicities (e.g., myopathy) cause increased disability in patients who already may be neurologically impaired secondary to their tumor; others are particularly worrisome in a pregnant patient (e.g., hypertension, diabetes, and increased weight). However, systemic corticosteroids may serve a dual purpose in the pregnant patient under consideration for early delivery to facilitate treatment of a brain tumor corticosteroids hasten pulmonary maturation in utero, thus reducing respiratory complications in the premature child (see Chapter 9).

Cranial Radiotherapy During Pregnancy

Cranial RT is an important treatment modality for every malignant and many benign nervous system tumors. However, in utero exposure to RT can have teratogenic and long-term medical effects on the developing fetus (73). Although every effort should be made to defer cranial RT until completion of pregnancy, there are some circumstances in which delay is not possible. Understanding the timing of risk to the fetus and careful treatment planning can minimize the potential toxicity of therapy.

The greatest risk of teratogenicity and fetal loss occurs when RT is administered during the first trimester. For this reason, abortion should be offered to women in the early stages of pregnancy who have a malignant brain tumor necessitating immediate treatment. If the pregnancy is to be carried to term, attempts should be made to delay RT until the patient is in the second or third trimester. Cranial RT during the later stages of pregnancy is not associated with an increased risk of birth defects, but does carry an increased risk of childhood leukemia. The risk is directly related to the total RT exposure, which is a factor of the dose administered to the mother and the port of administration. Fetal RT exposure is due to external scatter of the beam (which can be reduced by shielding of the mother's abdomen during treatment) and to internal scatter (which can be minimized by careful design of the fields and ports of RT, or avoidance of vertex fields). With careful planning using modern techniques, fetal exposure can be reduced to a reasonably safe level (19).

Labor and Delivery

The presence of raised ICP often is considered a contraindication to labor and vaginal delivery. CSF pressure has been measured in normal patients during labor. Hopkins and associates demonstrated that CSF pressure increases with each contraction to a maximum of 250 to 280 mm water and that the increase in pressure occurrs in response to an increase in arterial blood pressure (74). Fundal pressure, vaginal examination, and pain all tend to increase the CSF pressure further during contractions. Bearing down just prior to delivery cause a marked increase in CSF pressure, and the maximal pressure achieved could not be recorded on their scale. Marx and colleagues showed that uterine contractions were associated with a significant increase in CSF pres-

sure only when the patient experienced pain associated with the contraction (75). CSF pressures would increase from 110 to 390 mm water above normal with painful contractions. Bearing-down efforts during the first stage of labor produced an average rise in CSF pressure of 530 mm water above normal, comparable to elevations seen in men during straining. However, during the second stage of labor, when bearing down was accompanied with uterine contractions and discomfort, CSF pressure increased an average of 710 mm water above normal.

The prominent increase in CSF pressure seen during normal labor and delivery is not problematic for the healthy patient; however, such increases in ICP in a patient with an elevated baseline ICP can lead to brain herniation. Nevertheless, some patients with intracranial mass lesions can undergo vaginal delivery sucessfully (76–78). Each patient must be assessed individually, but most with pituitary tumors or meningiomas can undergo vaginal delivery because neither tumor type usually is associated with significant mass effect or edema. When a patient with an intracranial mass lesion is allowed to labor and deliver, every effort should be made to ensure that labor is pain free, and forceps delivery may be indicated to avoid pushing. Most patients with significant space-occupying mass lesions, however, will require cesarean section, and this may be done under general or extradural anesthesia.

MATERNAL HYDROCEPHALUS

Treatment of hydrocephalus with shunting procedures has dramatically improved the outcome of patients with hydrocephalus, regardless of etiology. Most modern shunts are ventriculoperitoneal (VP) because they have the lowest incidence of infection, although some patients still have ventriculoatrial, ventriculopleural, or lumboperitoneal shunts. The majority of patients with hydrocephalus present during childhood or young adulthood; the effective use of shunts has permitted these patients to lead productive lives and reproduce. Consequently, pregnant patients with a shunt are being seen with increasing frequency.

Fetal Considerations

Pregnancy in a patient with shunted hydrocephalus has potential implications for both fetus and mother. Maternal hydrocephalus may have a hereditary component when it accompanies a neural tube defect. Some neural tube defects are subtle, and these patients have an increased incidence (2% to 3%) of giving birth to a similarly affected child (79). Therefore, women with hydrocephalus and neural tube defects should be monitored throughout pregnancy for the presence of such a defect in their offspring. Alpha-fetoprotein should be measured by amniocentesis, and serial ultrasound examinations should be performed after the twentieth week of gestation to assess the status of the fetal ventricles. However, most women do not have a potentially heritable cause of hydrocephalus. Hydrocephalus as a result of prior infection or subarachnoid hemorrhage is not inherited, and congenital abnormalities such as aqueductal stenosis or the Dandy-Walker anomaly are usually sporadic events and do not carry increased risks for the offspring of such patients.

Maternal Considerations

Hydrocephalus presents with symptoms of increased intracranial pressure, headache, and nausea and vomiting that can be intermittent and relieved by simple analgesics in the early stages; ataxia and lethargy also can be seen, but frequently they do not occur immediately. Symptoms are often more prominent than signs, and although one looks for papilledema, ataxia, or sixth nerve paresis, examinations may be normal in the setting of markedly increased ICP. A CT or MR scan demonstrates enlarged ventricles, but if symptoms are significant and the scan is normal, a lumbar puncture is indicated to exclude other processes, such as pseudotumor cerebri.

Hydrocephalus can present for the first time in a pregnant patient, or symptoms can appear in a pregnant woman with a previously well functioning shunt (80,81). In a previously healthy patient, symptoms may appear at any time during pregnancy. Often the condition that leads to hydrocephalus has been present for years, and CSF dynamics were well compensated. Pregnancy increases blood volume and cardiac output. The patient with hydrocephalus has reduced brain compliance, and a small increase in blood volume can lead to a large incremental increase in ICP causing decompensation and symptoms.

The clinical situation is more straightforward in patients who already have a shunt in place and develop symptoms of increased ICP. CT or MR scan indicates the acute appearance of hydrocephalus in a previously decompressed patient. Common causes of shunt malfunction include shunt infection, usually with coagulase negative *Staphylococcus,* or shunt discontinuity with fracture, usually of the exterior tubing. Infection can be documented by culture of CSF taken from the shunt, and it can be treated with antibiotics; occasionally a shunt must be replaced to eradicate infection. Shunt integrity can be assessed with plain x-rays and must be repaired if interrupted. However, there are many situations in which shunt malfunction occurs without any clear identifiable cause. These patients frequently require shunt revision and typically have a prompt clinical improvement after shunt repair. A history of prior shunt revision may predict neurosurgical and obstetric complications in pregnant women (82). Women with CSF shunts can be particularly vulnerable to shunt malfunction during pregnancy and the postpartum period. These patients must be followed carefully, and ordinary symptoms such as headache or abdominal pain may be the harbinger of more serious problems.

If necessary, shunt placement or revision can be performed safely at any time during the course of a pregnancy. It is a relatively short and safe procedure, done under general anesthesia. Currently, all shunts are ventricu-

loperitoneal unless there is a contraindication to placement of the distal catheter into
the peritoneal cavity. Pregnancy is not a contraindication to a VP shunt, even if the patient is in the third trimester. Moreover, a
shunt is not a contraindication to labor and
vaginal delivery provided the patient has
normal ICP.

REFERENCES

1. Block F. Neurologic diseases and pregnancy. *Nerve-narzt* 1999;70:1062–1071.
2. Sawle GV, Ramsay MM. The neurology of pregnancy. *J Neurol Neurosurg Psychiatry* 1998;65:810–821.
3. Barnes JE, Abbott KH. Cerebral complications during pregnancy and the puerperium. *Am J Obstet Gynecol* 1961;82:192–207.
4. Haas JF, Janisch W, Staneczek W. Newly diagnosed primary intracranial neoplasms in pregnant women: a population-based assessment. *J Neurol Neurosurg Psychiatry* 1986;49:874–880.
5. Roelvink NC, Kamphorst W, van Alphen HA, et al. Pregnancy-related primary brain and spinal tumors. *Arch Neurol* 1987;44:209–215.
6. Simon RH. Brain tumors in pregnancy. *Semin Neurol* 1988;8:214–221.
7. Isla A, Alvarez F, Gonzalez A, et al. Brain tumor and pregnancy. *Obstet Gynecol* 1997;89:19–23.
8. Tewari KS, Cappuccini F, Asrat T, et al. Obstetric emergencies precipitated by malignant brain tumors. *Am J Obstet Gynecol* 2000;182:1215–1221.
9. Cushing H, Eisenhardt L. *Meningiomas: their classification, regional behavior, life history, and surgical end result.* Springfield, Illinois: Charles C. Thomas, 1938.
10. Lambe M, Coogan P, Baron J. Reproductive factors and the risk of brain tumors: a population-based study in Sweden. *Int J Cancer* 1997;72:389–393.
11. Halsey JH. Neurology of pregnancy. In: Rowland LP, ed. *Merritt's textbook of neurology.* Baltimore: Williams & Wilkins, 1995:962–966.
12. Lee LS, Chi CW, Chang TJ, et al. Steroid hormone receptors in meningiomas of Chinese patients. *Neurosurgery* 1989;25:541–545.
13. Nomura M, Yamagishi S, Harada S, et al. Placenta growth factor (PlGF) mRNA expression in brain tumors. *J Neurooncol* 1998;40:123–130.
14. Simon RH. Brain tumors in pregnancy. *Semin Neurol* 1988;8:214–221.
15. Hanakawa K, Ikeda H, Ishii K, et al. High uptake on 11C methionine PET scan in the pituitary gland of a patient with cerebral glioma after surgical abortion. *No To Shinkei* 1998;50:573–577.
16. Dalessio DJ. Neurologic diseases. In: Burrow GN, Ferris TF, eds. *Medical complications during pregnancy.* Philadelphia: WB Saunders Co., 1982:435–447.
17. DeAngelis LM: Brain tumors. *New Engl J Med* 2001; 344:114–123.
18. Brent RL. The effect of embryonic and fetal exposure to x-ray, microwaves, and ultrasound: counseling the pregnant and nonpregnant patient about these risks. *Semin Oncol* 1989;16:347–368.
19. Sneed PK, Albright NW, Wara WM, et al. Fetal dose es-

timates for radiotherapy of brain tumors during pregnancy. *Int J Radiat Oncol Biol Phys* 1995;32:823–830.
20. Mason WP, Krol GS, DeAngelis LM. Low-grade oligodendroglioma responds to chemotherapy. *Neurology* 1996;46:203–207.
21. Olson JD, Riedel E, DeAngelis LM. Long-term outcome of low-grade oligodendroglioma and mixed glioma. *Neurology* 2000;54:1442–1448.
22. Recht LD, Lew R, Smith TW. Suspected low-grade glioma: is deferring treatment safe? *Ann Neurol* 1992; 31:431–436.
23. Wood JR, Green SB, Shapiro WR. The prognostic importance of tumor size in malignant gliomas: a computed tomographic scan study by the Brain Tumor Cooperative Group. *J Clin Oncol* 1998;6:338–343.
24. Walker MD, Green SB, Byar DP, et al. Randomized comparisons of radiotherapy and nitrosoureas for the treatment of malignant glioma after surgery. *N Engl J Med* 1980;303:1323–1329.
25. DeAngelis LM, Burger PC, Green SB, et al. Malignant glioma: who benefits from adjuvant chemotherapy? *Ann Neurol* 1998;44:691–695.
26. Russell DS, Rubinstein LJ, eds. Tumours of the meninges and related tissues. In: *Pathology of tumours of the nervous system.* 5th ed. Baltimore: Williams & Wilkins, 1989:449–532.
27. Fox MW, Harms RW, David DH. Selected neurologic complications of pregnancy. *Mayo Clin Proc* 1990;65: 1595–618.
28. Wan WL, Geller JL, Feldon SE, et al. Visual loss caused by rapidly progressive intracranial meningiomas during pregnancy. *Ophthalmology* 1990;97:18–21.
29. DeGrood RM, Beemer WH, Fenner DE, et al. A large meningioma presenting as a neurologic emergency in late pregnancy. *Obstet Gynecol* 1987;69:439.
30. Bickerstaff ER, Small JM, Guest IA. The relapsing course of certain meningiomas in relation to pregnancy and menstruation. *J Neurol Neurosurg Psychiatry* 1958; 21:89.
31. Poisson M, Pertuiset BF, Hauw JJ, et al. Steroid hormone receptors in human meningiomas, gliomas and brain metastases. *J Neurooncol* 1983;1:179–189.
32. Moguilewsky M, Pertuiset BF, Verzat C, et al. Cytosolic and nuclear sex steroid receptors in meningioma. *Clin Neuropharmacol* 1984;7:375–381.
33. Carroll RS, Zhang J, Black PM. Expression of estrogen receptors alpha and beta in human meningiomas. *J Neurooncol* 1999;42:109–116.
34. Adegbite AB, Khan MI, Paine KWE, et al. The recurrence of intracranial meningiomas after surgical treatment. *J Neurosurg* 1983;58:51–56.
35. Carella RJ, Ransohoff J, Newall J. Role of radiation therapy in the management of meningioma. *Neurosurgery* 1982;10:332–339.
36. Russell DS, Rubinstein LJ, eds. The schwannomas. In: *Pathology of tumours of the nervous system.* 5th ed. Baltimore: Williams & Wilkins, 1989:537–560.
37. Allen J, Eldridge R, Koerber T. Acoustic neuroma in the last months of pregnancy. *Am J Obstet Gynecol* 1974; 119:516–520.
38. Kasantikul V, Brown WJ. Estrogen receptors in acoustic neurilemmomas. *Surg Neurol* 1980;15:105–109.
39. Martuza RL, MacLaughlin DT, Ojemann RG. Specific estradiol binding in schwannomas, meningiomas, and neurofibromas. *Neurosurgery* 1981;9:665.
40. Flickinger JC, Lunsford LD, Coffey RJ, et al. Radio-

surgery of acoustic neurinomas. *Cancer* 1991;67: 345–353.

41. Russell DS, Rubinstein LJ, eds. Secondary tumours of the nervous system. In: *Pathology of tumours of the nervous system*. 5th ed. Baltimore: Williams & Wilkins; 1989:809–854.

42. Leavens ME, McCutcheon IF, Samann NA. Management of pituitary adenomas. *Oncology* 1992;6:69–80.

43. Kupersmith MJ, Rosenberg C, Kleinberg D. Visual loss in pregnant women with pituitary adenomas. *Ann Intern Med* 1994;121:473–477.

44. Cardoso ER, Peterson EW. Pituitary apoplexy: a review. *Neurosurgery* 1984;14:363–373.

45. Magyar DM, Marshall JR. Pituitary tumors and pregnancy. *Am J Obstet Gynecol* 1978;132:739.

46. Hammond CB, Haney AF, Land MR, et al. The outcome of pregnancy in patients with treated and untreated prolactin-secreting pituitary tumors. *Am J Obstet Gynecol* 1983;147:148.

47. Samaan NA, Schultz PN, Leavens TA, et al. Pregnancy after treatment in patients with prolactinoma: operation versus bromocriptine. *Am J Obstet Gynecol* 1986;155: 1300–1305.

48. Molitch ME. Management of prolactinomas during pregnancy. *J Reprod Med* 1999;44:1121–1126.

49. Belleza G, Pietropaoli N, Sidoni A. Medulloblastoma during pregnancy. *Pathologica* 1997;89:301–303.

50. Chen KY, Wang HC, Shih JY, et al. Lung cancer in pregnancy: report of two cases. *J Formosan Med Assoc* 1998;97:573–576.

51. Patchell RA, Tibbs PA, Walsh JW, et al. A randomized trial of surgery in the treatment of single metastases to the brain. *N Engl J Med* 1990;322:494–500.

52. Patchell RA, Tibbs PA, Regine WF, et al. Postoperative radiotherapy in the treatment of single metastases to the brain. A randomized trial. *JAMA* 1998;280:1485–1489.

53. Olive DL, Lurain JR, Brewer JI. Choriocarcinoma associated with term gestation. *Am J Obstet Gynecol* 1984; 148:711.

54. Athanassiou A, Begent RH, Newlands ES, et al. Central nervous system metastases of choriocarcinoma. *Cancer* 1983;52:1728–1735.

55. Weed JC JR, Hunter VJ. Diagnosis and management of brain metastasis from gestational trophoblastic disease. *Oncology* 1991;5:48–51.

56. Bakri Y, al-Hawashim N, Berkowitz R. CSF/serum beta-hCG ratio in patients with brain metastases of gestational trophoblastic tumor. *J Reprod Med* 2000;45:94–96.

57. Sekl MJ, Newlands ES. Treatment of gestational trophoblastic disease. *Gen Diagn Pathol* 1997;142:159–171.

58. Rustin GJS, Newlands ES, Begent RHJ, et al. Weekly alternating etoposide, methotrexate, and actinomycin/vincristine and cyclophosphamide chemotherapy for the treatment of CNS metastases of choriocarcinoma. *J Clin Oncol* 1989;7:900–903.

59. Ishizuka T, Tomoda Y, Kaseki S, et al. Intracranial metastases of choriocarcinoma: a clinicopathologic study. *Cancer* 1983;52:1896–1903.

60. Rodabaugh KJ, Bernstein MR, Goldstein DP, et al. Natural history of post-term choriocarcinoma. *J Reprod Med* 1998;43:75–80.

61. Schechter NR, Mychalczak B, Jones W, et al. Prognosis of patients treated with whole-brain radiation therapy for metastatic gestational trophoblastic disease. *Gynecol Oncol* 1998;68:183–192.

62. van Besein K, Verschraegen C, Mehra R, et al. Complete remission of refractory gestational trophoblastic disease with brain metastases treated with multicycle ifosfamide, carboplatin, and etoposide (ICE) and stem cell rescue. *Gynecol Oncol* 1997;65:366–369.

63. Termrungruanglert W, Kudelka AP, Piamsomboon S, et al. Remission of refractory gestational trophoblastic disease with high-dose paclitaxel. *Anticancer Drugs* 1996;7:503–506.

64. Carmel PW. Neurologic surgery in pregnancy. In: Barber HR, Graberk EA, eds. *Surgical disease in pregnancy*. Philadelphia: WB Saunders Co, 1974:203–223.

65. Kawasaki K, Hoshino K, Takahashi M, et al. Complications of spinal anesthesia as the initial symptom in patients with spinal tumor—a report of two cases. *Masui* 1999;48:1340–1342.

66. Schwartz DA, Nair S, Hershey B, et al. Vertebral arch hemangioma producing spinal cord compression in pregnancy. *Spine* 1989;14:888–890.

67. Liu CL, Yang DJ. Paraplegia due to vertebral hemangioma during pregnancy. *Spine* 1988;13:107–108.

68. AbiFadel W, Afif N, Farah S, et al. Vertebral hemangioma symptomatic during pregnancy: a case report and review of the literature. *J Gynecol Obstet Biol Reprod* 1997;26:90–94.

69. Cioffi F, Buric J, Carnesecchi S, et al. Spinal meningiomas in pregnancy: report of two cases and review of the literature. *Eur J Gynaecol Oncol* 1996;17:384–388.

70. Castel E, Lazennec JY, Chiaras J, et al. Acute spinal cord compression due to intraspinal bleeding from a vertebral hemangioma: two case-reports. *Eur Spine J* 1999;8:244–248.

71. Glantz MJ, Cole BF, Forsyth PA, et al. Practice parameter: anticonvulsant prophylaxis in patients with newly diagnosed brain tumors. *Neurology* 2000;54:1886–1893.

72. Posner JB. *Neurologic complications of cancer*. FA Davis Co, Philadelphia, 1985.

73. Hall EJ (Ed). Effects of radiation on the embryo and fetus. In: *Radiology for the radiologist*. 3rd ed. JB Lippincott Co, Philadelphia, 1988.

74. Hopkins EL, Hendricks CH, Cibils LA. Cerebrospinal fluid pressure in labor. *Am J Obstet Gynecol* 1965;93: 907–916.

75. Marx GF, Zemaitis MT, Orkin LR. Cerebrospinal fluid pressures during labor and obstetrical anesthesia. *Anesthesiology* 1961;22:348–354.

76. Kempers RD, Miller RH. Management of pregnancy associated with brain tumors. *Am J Obstet Gynecol* 1963; 87:858–864.

77. Finfer SR. Management of labour and delivery in patients with intracranial neoplasms. *Br J Anaesth* 1991; 67:784–787.

78. Crawford JS. Extradural blockage and intracranial pressure. *Br J Anaesth* 1986;58:579.

79. Gast MJ, Grubb RL Jr, Strickler RC. Maternal hydrocephalus and pregnancy. *Obstet Gynecol* 1983;62:29S.

80. Wisoff JH, Kratzert KJ, Handwerker SM, et al. Pregnancy in patients with cerebrospinal fluid shunts: report of a series and review of the literature. *Neurosurgery* 1991;29:827–831.

81. Liakos AM, Bradley NK, Magram G, et al. Hydrocephalus and the reproductive health of women: the medical implications of maternal shunt dependency in 70 women and 138 pregnancies. *Neurol Res* 2000;22:69–88.

82. Sylvestre G, Harrison EA, Chazotte C. Outcomes of pregnancies complicated by the presence of maternal cerebrospinal fluid shunts. *Obstet Gynecol* 2000;95:S67.

Neurological Complications of Pregnancy, Second Edition, edited by Brian Hainline and Orrin Devinsky. Lippincott Williams & Wilkins, Philadelphia, © 2002.

13

Endocrine Aspects of Epilepsy

Steven C. Schachter

Department of Neurology, Harvard Medical School and Beth Israel Deaconess Medical Center, Boston, Massachusetts, U.S.A.

Endocrinologic changes during pregnancy contribute to the neurologic complications encountered by some pregnant women with epilepsy (WWE). To introduce the endocrine aspects of epilepsy in women, this chapter focuses on the relationships between cerebral function and hormones in nonpregnant WWE. A brief review of the anatomic connections between the brain and the hypothalamus is followed by an outline of the neuroendocrine aspects of single seizures. The reproductive endocrine disorders described in nonpregnant epileptic women then are presented, together with discussions of contraception and catamenial epilepsy.

The anatomic connections between the hypothalamus and the brain, especially limbic structures, are reciprocal. Neural outputs from limbic structures (mesial and inferior portions of the temporal and frontal lobes) regulate the hypothalamo-pituitary-adrenal (HPA) axis via the fornix and gonadotropin synthesis (and therefore reproductive behavior) via the stria terminalis under the control of estrogen. Another bundle, the ventral amygdalofugal pathway, counters the effect of the stria terminalis on gonadotropin synthesis and influences the HPA axis as well as secretion of prolactin (PRL) and growth hormone (GH). Another pathway, the median forebrain bundle, also affects the HPA axis.

The hypothalamus, in turn, influences limbic structures by the mamillothalamic tract as well as via control of glandular hormone secretion. Most systemically produced hormones bind to specific limbic sites and exert neurophysiologic effects (1–6). Estrogen concentrates in limbic regions critical for gonadotropin regulation and reproductive behavior (7,8), and progesterone concentrates in the hippocampus, among other sites (9).

ANTIEPILEPTIC DRUGS AND GONADAL HORMONES

The pharmacokinetics of gonadal hormones are altered in the presence of antiepileptic drugs (AEDs). Estradiol-17-OH binds to sex-hormone binding globulin (SHBG; 30%) and albumin (68%), leaving 2% free; progesterone is bound to albumin (53%) and transcortin (45%), leaving 2% free (10). In women, 66% of testosterone binds to SHBG, and changing SHBG concentrations affect serum free testosterone. With a fixed amount of total testosterone, higher levels of SHBG result in lower free testosterone levels (11). Enzyme-inducing seizure medications such as phenytoin (PHT), carbamazepine (CBZ), and phenobarbital increase SHBG (12–17) and, therefore, may lower free testosterone. CBZ also may lower luteinizing hormone (LH) levels (13) and promote heightened LH responses to luteinizing hormone releasing hormone (LHRH) (18).

SEIZURE-INDUCED HORMONE CHANGES

The reciprocal anatomic and physiologic connections between the brain and the endocrine system may become pathologic in the context of epilepsy arising from limbic structures. Further, transient hormonal elevations occur after seizures. For more than 20 years, postictal hormonal changes have been studied in association with several different seizure types—partial seizures, generalized seizures, induced (electroconvulsive) seizures, and nonepileptic (psychogenic) seizures. These hormonal effects, which are superimposed on normal circadian variations and the effects of AEDs (19), have been more fully reviewed elsewhere (20–24).

Partial seizures originate from a discrete region (or regions) of the brain. Simple partial seizures (SPS) do not impair consciousness and are usually unilateral, whereas complex partial seizures (CPS) impair consciousness and are usually bilateral, affecting temporal or frontal lobes. Limbic structures, including hippocampus, amygdala, cingulate cortex, and orbitofrontal cortex, are common sites of origin for CPS, particularly in patients with seizures refractory to AEDs. Trimble (25) first reported increased serum PRL levels in association with partial seizures, especially within 20 minutes after the seizure. In their studies, Dana-Haeri and colleagues (26), along with others (27–31), correlated PRL elevations with CPS rather than SPS, principally CPS of temporal lobe origin (32). Sperling and associates (33) recorded CPS in patients using depth electrodes and found those seizures that involved bilateral mesial temporal structures resulted in serum PRL levels nearly doubling, whereas SPS associated with unilateral mesial temporal involvement were not followed by elevations of PRL. Depth electrodes can stimulate brain tissue as well as record brain electrical activity. Stimulation of amygdala and hippocampus for 10 to 15 minutes by depth electrodes elevated PRL (34,35) and adrenocorticotropic hormone (ACTH), peaking 15 to 20 minutes after the stimulation and remaining elevated up to an hour (35). In contrast, eliciting epileptiform spike discharges in similar patients with transcranial magnetic stimulation did not elevate PRL (36).

A smaller number of studies have evaluated other hormonal changes after partial seizures. Levels of LH and GH, but not of follicle-stimulating hormone (FSH) or thyroid-stimulating hormone (TSH), may increase significantly compared to baseline (26,28). Two series (28,37) documented postictal cortisol elevations compared to expected values, whereas two other studies (38,39) of nocturnal CPS could not confirm these findings.

In contrast to partial seizures, generalized seizures affect the entire cortex, including limbic structures. The best-known subtype is the tonic-clonic seizure. Generalized seizures also are associated with hormonal changes, most notably PRL. Many studies (25,27,40–43) have demonstrated greater increases in PRL after generalized seizures than after partial seizures, including alcohol-withdrawal seizures (44). Similar findings may be seen in children (45,46). GH and ACTH increase immediately after generalized seizures (44), and significant elevations of LH and FSH may occur in females (26).

Among the hormonal changes associated with electroconvulsive seizures (ECT), the most consistent is PRL elevation 15 to 20 minutes after ECT (25,47–50). Longer seizures result in greater PRL elevations than shorter seizures (41). Acute changes in LH and FSH levels following ECT may be seen in reproductive-age women compared to postmenopausal women (50,51) and GH may (50) or may not (49,51,52) increase. ACTH levels may increase after ECT (52,53).

Patients with psychogenic seizures—behaviors mimicking seizures but lacking simultaneous electroencephalographic (EEG) confirmation (54,55)—are a challenging group to evaluate and treat. Because appropriate therapy requires accurate diagnosis, many investigators have attempted to determine whether postictal hormonal changes reliably discriminate between psychogenic and epileptic seizures. PRL levels do not increase after simulated tonic-clonic seizures (42), either in patients with normal EEGs while demonstrating episodic stereotyped behaviors (29) or in patients with induced motor or behavioral attacks without simultaneous EEG changes (37). However, the diagnostic usefulness of postictal hormonal assays is limited. PRL concentrations may not rise after a series of seizures (56), and lack of PRL elevation after an apparent generalized or partial seizure does not exclude epileptic seizures (26,30,33,44,57). In addition, cortisol measurements are unhelpful because fluctuations can occur after simulated seizures (42), and cortisol may be elevated after nonepileptic psychogenic events (46). Further, postictal elevations may take more than an hour to be recordable (44). Similarly, changes in LH, FSH, growth hormone, and TSH are too inconsistent to be useful clinically. However, an elevation of PRL following an apparent par-

tial seizure is useful diagnostically and suggests a seizure involving limbic structures (33).

REPRODUCTIVE ENDOCRINE DISORDERS

The above data suggest some women with frequent seizures are subjected to repeated surges of PRL, gonadotropins, or both, perhaps beginning as early as childhood (45,46). It is interesting that a variety of reproductive endocrine disorders occur in female (as well as male) patients with epilepsy (14,58–62), especially those with temporal lobe epilepsy (63). In general, these disorders are associated with abnormalities in the usual cycling of LH, FSH, progesterone, and estrogen (E2), shown in Figs. 13.1 and 13.2.

Abnormal menstrual function in WWE was described as early as 1853 (64). Jensen and Vaernet (65) found abnormal menstrual pat-

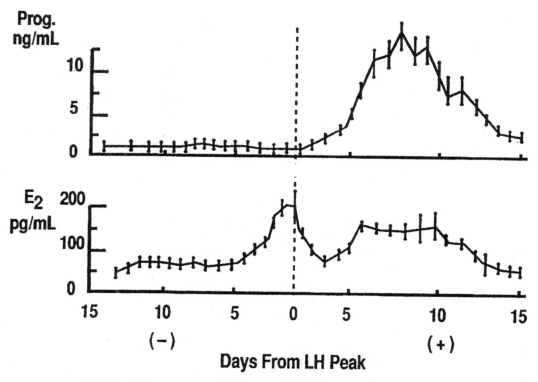

FIG. 13.1. Fluctuations in hormone levels during the menstrual cycle.

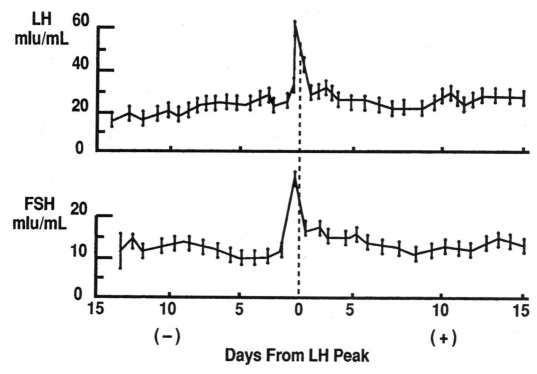

FIG. 13.2. Fluctuations in hormone levels during the menstrual cycle.

terns in more than 50% of WWE undergoing temporal lobectomies. More recently, the associated endocrinologic profile of these patients has been studied. Herzog and associates (66) found that five of 20 consecutive women with temporal lobe epilepsy (TLE) had oligomenorrhea and hirsutism; two had ovarian cysts, and another two had significantly elevated testosterone levels. LH was increased in two of three patients. In a subsequent, larger series, Herzog and colleagues (67) showed that 28 of 50 consecutive women with TLE had menstrual dysfunction, and 19 of these 28 had abnormal neuroendocrine testing: ten had elevated LH and total or free testosterone with relatively low FSH (suggestive of polycystic ovarian syndrome), two had low estradiol and elevated LH and FSH (gonadal insufficiency or premature menopause), one had elevated PRL, and six amenorrheic women had low LH levels (hypogonadotropic hypogonadism). Bilo and associates (68)

studied women with primary generalized epilepsy and found that five of 20 had reproductive endocrine disorders: three had polycystic ovarian syndrome and two had hypogonadotropic hypogonadism

Several authors (67,69,70) have observed a high frequency of anovulatory cycles or inadequate luteal phases in WWE. This finding is of interest given Backstrom's (71) assertion that seizures increase during periods of high ratios of estrogen to progesterone, the same hormonal ratio seen during anovulatory cycles caused by inadequate luteal phase progesterone levels.

Do seizures cause anovulation, or does anovulation cause seizures? Although these two mechanisms are not mutually exclusive and could both be operative in any given patient, the cause-and-effect relationship in women has not been proved. It is known, however, that stimulation of rat amygdala blocks ovulation (72), and bilateral ablation of the amygdaloid basolateral nucleus in female deer mice produces anovulatory cycles and polycystic ovarian changes (73).

Two other pathologic neurophysiologic processes possibly are related to the development of reproductive endocrine disorders. First, brief subclinical electrical cortical discharges might adversely affect hormonal function. In 85 presumably nonepileptic women with anovulation and infertility, Sharf and colleagues (74) found that more than half had abnormal EEGs. Treatment with the antiestrogen clomiphene normalized many of the EEGs, and those patients with normal EEGs after clomiphene therapy had higher rates of ovulation and pregnancy than EEG nonresponders. Second, WWE may have abnormal baseline hormone levels or cyclical hormonal function unrelated to overt seizures. Herzog (75) found abnormal LH responses to LHRH in two of three women with temporal lobe epilepsy. Bilo and associates (76) studied normally cycling, drug-free epileptic women and found abnormally high LH pulse frequencies during the midfollicular phase compared to controls. Nocturnal PRL levels were lower than controls among WWE in one study (77), whereas in another study (68), women with primary generalized epilepsy and normal menstrual cycles had elevated basal FSH and PRL levels as well as decreased LH responses to LHRH. Whether women with any or all of these abnormalities are at increased risk for developing reproductive endocrine disorders compared to women with seizures and no baseline or cyclical hormonal alterations remains to be proved. Herzog (78) has further proposed that patients with right temporal lobe dysfunction may develop different reproductive endocrine disorders than those with left temporal lobe dysfunction.

ORAL CONTRACEPTIVES AND ANTIEPILEPTIC DRUGS

WWE often ask their doctors about the advisability of taking birth control pills (BCP). There are two separate issues: (i) Do BCPs make seizures worse? and (ii) Are BCPs an effective form of contraception for this group of women? With respect to the first question, oral contraceptives usually do not exacerbate seizures (79), especially progesterone-only pills such as norethindrone (80). Concerning the second question, there is an increased incidence of oral-contraceptive failure among women taking AEDs (79,81), which is probably a result of the effect of enzyme-inducing medications, such as PHT, CBZ, oxcarbazepine, phenobarbital, and primidone, on increasing the metabolism of estrogen. Therefore, effective contraception in WWE, especially those taking enzyme-inducing medications, may require use of barrier or other methods. One indication of enhanced estrogen metabolism in this setting may be breakthrough bleeding (79). Another hormonal contraceptive, levonorgestrel, currently is used in a subdermal form. Simultaneous use of PHT enhances the metabolism of levonorgestrel (82), perhaps accounting for low levonorgestrel levels in women taking PHT who become pregnant despite use of this form of contraception (83).

CATAMENIAL EPILEPSY

Catamenial epilepsy indicates a significant relationship between gonadal hormones and epilepsy. Animal studies suggest that estrogen lowers and progesterone raises seizure threshold, but a model for cyclical seizures associated with menstrual fluctuations is lacking (84,88).

The clinical relevance of the menstrual cycle in WWE was written about in the 19th century (64) and has been carefully studied over the past 40 years. In an exhaustive study, Laidlaw (89) found that seizures were reduced during the luteal phase and increased perimenstrually. Two other series (90,91) found an increase in seizures perimenstrually. Three patterns of catamenial epilepsy were described by Herzog and associates (92). Seizure exacerbations tended to cluster in the perimenstrual or preovulatory phase in women with ovulatory cycles and throughout the second half of the cycle in women with anovulatory cycles.

Laidlaw (89) suspected that progesterone had an anticonvulsant effect in women. Mattson and colleagues (70) found support for this in a group of 14 women who had maximal seizure frequency at menstruation, when progesterone levels were lowest.

High ratios of estrogen to progesterone, in addition to low progesterone levels, may be associated with catamenial epilepsy. Backstrom (93) found a direct relationship between secondarily generalized seizures and ratios of estrogen to progesterone in seven women with partial seizures—increased seizures with high ratios and decreased seizures during periods of high progesterone levels. However, Rosciszewska and associates (91) could not confirm this mechanism.

Some women with catamenial exacerbation of seizures have perimenstrual fluctuations of AED levels, which may predispose to increased seizures when AED levels are low (91,94,95). For example, Rosciszewska and associates (91) studied women with catamenial seizures and found PHT levels on day 28 to be more than 30% lower than at midcycle in more than half of the women, whereas phenobarbital levels were more stable. This effect probably is related to menstrual-related fluctuations in AED clearance and may have some relevance to gestational epilepsy.

The diagnosis of women with catamenial seizures starts with awareness of the temporal association of seizures with the menses. This may be difficult in patients with irregular periods or in patients who have other triggers besides menses. It may be useful for women to keep track of their seizures on a calendar, noting onset of menses and basal body temperature, which may help to determine the luteal phase.

Treatment in women with clear catamenial exacerbation often consists of supplementing AEDs during the premenstrual period if levels are consistently low and if the patient's menstrual onset is predictable. Specific hormonal therapy may be efficacious by lowering the ratio of estrogen to progesterone or by replacing progesterone for women with pathologically low luteal-phase progesterone levels.

Several uncontrolled series of hormonal treatment for catamenial epilepsy have been published. Mattson and associates (96) treated 14 women with oral medroxyprogesterone for an average of 12 months. Of 11 women who developed amenorrhea, seven had an average of 52% fewer seizures. Because none of the patients without amenorrhea had any reduction in seizure frequency, the use of medroxyprogesterone for catamenial epilepsy appears limited. Herzog (69) treated eight women with CPS and anovulatory cycles or an inadequate luteal phase with progesterone suppositories. Six women had fewer seizures and overall monthly seizure frequency dropped 68% during 3 months of treatment compared with pretreatment. Other studies found favorable effects of clomiphene (97) and clobazam (98).

POLYCYSTIC OVARIAN SYNDROME: POSSIBLE PATHOPHYSIOLOGIC MECHANISMS

Polycystic ovarian syndrome (PCOS) usually is diagnosed based on the presence of hyperandrogenism with menstrual, ultrasound, or endocrine evidence of anovulatory cycles. The prevalence of PCOS in the general female population ranges from 3% to 19%, depending on the definition used and population studied. Hyperandrogenism is characterized by elevated serum concentrations of testosterone, androstenedione, or dehydroepiandrosterone in its free or conjugated sulfated form. Hirsutism usually is present but varies considerably in relation to ethnic origin even in the presence of hyperandrogenemia. Chronic anovulation is represented by (i) menstrual disorder, namely amenorrhea, oligomenorrhea, abnormal menstrual cycle intervals, or menometrorrhagia, and often by (ii) ultrasound evidence of enlarged ovaries with multiple follicular cysts and increased stroma, and (iii) abnormally low serum progesterone levels during the midluteal phase. Affected women, however, commonly revert spontaneously to having fertile ovulatory cycles.

Epilepsy and seizure therapy (in particular, valproate) have been implicated in the pathogenesis of PCOS in women with seizures. As noted above, the possible association of PCOS and epilepsy was first suggested by Herzog and colleagues (66,67) who more recently reported that eight of 36 (22.2%) consecutive women with unilateral temporolimbic epilepsy had PCOS as compared with 5% of control women (*p*=.001) (99).

The laterality and focality of temporolimbic discharges may be related to the development of PCOS; in particular, it may be significantly more common in women with left (rather than right) temporolimbic epileptiform discharges and possibly with right-sided nontemporolimbic discharges (100). Drislane and associates (101) and Herzog and colleagues (99) demonstrated higher gonadotropin releasing hormone pulse frequencies with left-sided temporal foci than with right-sided temporal foci. Kiely and colleagues found increased LH pulse amplitude in WWE (102). Increased LH pulse frequency, amplitude, or both may promote LH secretion over that of FSH and thereby promote gonadal steroid secretion without maturation of the follicle (103,104). This results in hyperandrogenism because the immature follicle is deficient in aromatase, which converts androgens to estrogens. Incomplete follicular maturation also results in anovulation and the collection of follicular cysts in the ovary. These features and the resulting menstrual disorder and hirsutism form the cardinal features of PCOS.

In 1993, Isojärvi and associates found evidence of polycystic ovaries in more than 60% of WWE who used valproate alone or in combination (105). The frequency was significantly greater than among WWE who took CBZ alone (33%) or other drugs (14%) and was particularly high among women who started treatment before 20 years of age. Among 23 women who took valproate and had ultrasound and endocrine investigations, four (17%) had hyperandrogenism (i.e., elevated serum testosterone levels) with three (13%) of these women having the combination of hyperandrogenism and menstrual disorder suggestive of PCOS. Of note, none of the 67 women taking other AEDs or controls had hyperandrogenism. Moreover, none of the 15 untreated WWE were found to have menstrual disorders in comparison to eight of 51 (16%) normal controls. In a subsequent controlled study, Murialdo and colleagues compared 65 women who had epilepsy, 21 on valproate monotherapy, with 20 normal controls and found that valproate use was associated with substantially and statistically significant higher body mass index, androgen levels, and more ovulatory dysfunction (low luteal phase progesterone levels in 64%) than with CBZ or phenobarbital use or for normal controls (106).

Based on their work, Isojärvi and colleagues have suggested that the overrepresentation of PCOS among valproate-treated WWE may be attributable to valproate-induced weight gain and the resultant endocrine concomitants of insulin resistance, namely hyperinsulinemia, increased insulinlike growth factor, and decreased insulinlike growth factor binding protein and SHBG (107). These endocrine changes increase gonadal steroidogenesis and permit a greater proportion of the released serum testosterone to be bioactive. Increased bioactive androgen may act locally in the ovary to block ovulation or may accomplish this through aromatization to estrogen and negative feedback on FSH secretion. An interactional effect between AEDs and epilepsy in the pathogenesis of PCOS also has been proposed (108).

CONCLUSION

This chapter has reviewed the interactions between seizures, AEDs, and the endocrine system in nonpregnant WWE. Specific postictal hormonal alterations and epilepsy-related neuroendocrine disorders have been identified, and pathophysiologic mechanisms have been suggested, which remain under study. Future work may use computer-automated detection of interictal epileptiform discharges to correlate their frequency and location with neuroendocrine dysfunction. Such techniques, in conjunction with neuroendocrine assays, eventually may be used prospectively to identify women at risk for catamenial seizures and neuroendocrine disorders.

Until then, neurologists and gynecologists must suspect the possibility of catamenial epilepsy and reproductive endocrine disorders when evaluating WWE, especially focal epilepsy of temporal lobe origin. In addition, the finding of weight gain, reproductive dysfunction, or a reproductive endocrine disorder should be recognized, evaluated, and treated appropriately. The contribution of AED use should be considered, and decisions regarding AED selection should weigh the importance of a particular selection for seizure control against its consequences on reproductive endocrine function. Finally, future double-blinded studies evaluating hormonal treatment of seizures and longitudinal evaluations of AEDs on hormonal function will further our understanding of epilepsy-related neuroendocrine disorders and the treatment of affected women.

REFERENCES

1. Rey M, Carlier E, Soumireu-Mourat B. Effects of corticosterone on hippocampal slice electrophysiology in normal and adrenalectomized BALB/c mice. *Neuroendocrinology* 1987;46:424–429.
2. Nabekura J, Oomura Y, Minami T, et al. Mechanism of the rapid effect of 17 beta-estradiol on medial amygdala neurons. *Science* 1986;233:226–228.
3. Majewska MD, Harrison NL, Schwartz RD, et al. Steroid hormone metabolites are barbiturate-like modulators of the GABA receptor. *Science* 1986;232:1004–1007.
4. McEwen BS, Wallach G. Corticosterone binding to hippocampus: nuclear and cytosol binding in vitro. *Brain Res* 1973;57:373–386.
5. McEwen BS, Weiss JM, Schwartz LS. Selective retention of corticosterone by limbic structures in rat brain. *Nature* 1968;220:911–912.
6. Joels M, de Kloet ER. Effects of glucocorticoids and norepinephrine on the excitability in the hippocampus. *Science* 1989;245:1502–1505.
7. Pfaff DW. Autoradiographic localization of radioactivity in rat brain after injection of tritiated sex hormones. *Science* 1968;161:1355–1356.
8. Pfaff D, Keiner M. Atlas of estradiol-concentrating cells in the central nervous system of the female rat. *J Comp Neurol* 1973;151:121–158.
9. Wade GN, Harding CF, Feder HH. Neural uptake of (1,2-3H)progesterone in ovariectomized rats, guinea pigs and hamsters: correlation with species differences in behavioral responsiveness. *Brain Res* 1973;61:357–367.
10. Mattson RH, Cramer JA. Epilepsy, sex hormones, and antiepileptic drugs. *Epilepsia* 1985; 26:S40–51.
11. Rosenfield RL. Plasma testosterone binding globulin and indexes of the concentration of unbound plasma androgens in normal and hirsute subjects. *J Clin Endocrinol Metab* 1971;32:717–728.
12. Backstrom CT, Sodergard R. Testosterone-estradiol-binding globulin, unbound and total estradiol and testosterone, and total progesterone during the menstrual cycle in women with epilepsy taking antiepileptic drugs. *J Endocrinol Invest* 1979;2:359–366.
13. Isojärvi JIT. Serum steroid hormones and pituitary function in female epileptic patients during carbamazepine therapy. *Epilepsia* 1990;31:438–445.
14. Toone BK, Wheeler M, Fenwick PBC. Sex hormone changes in male epileptics. *Clin Endocrinol (Oxf)* 1980;12:391–395.
15. Barragry JM, Makin HLJ, Trafford DJH, et al. Effect of anticonvulsants on plasma testosterone and sex hormone binding globulin levels. *J Neurol Neurosurg Psychiatry* 1978;41:913–914.
16. Isojärvi JIT, Pakarinen AJ, Ylipalosaari PJ, et al. Serum hormones in male epileptic patients receiving anticonvulsant medication. *Arch Neurol* 1990;47:670–676.
17. Victor A, Lundberg PO, Johansson EDB. Induction of sex hormone binding globulin by phenytoin. *BMJ* 1977;2:934–935.
18. Dana-Haeri J, Oxley J, Richens A. Pituitary responsiveness to gonadotrophin-releasing and thyrotrophin-releasing hormones in epileptic patients receiving carbamazepine or phenytoin. *Clin Endocrinol (Oxf)* 1984; 20:163–168.
19. Invitti C, Danesi L, Dubini A, et al. Neuroendocrine effects of chronic administration of sodium valproate in epileptic patients. *Acta Endocrinol(Copenh)* 1988; 118:381–388.
20. Kling MA, Kellner CH, Post RM, et al. Neuroendocrine effects of limbic activation by electrical, spontaneous, and pharmacological modes: relevance to the pathophysiology of affective dysregulation in psychiatric disorders. *Prog Neuropsychopharmacol Biol Psychiatry* 1987;11:459–481.
21. Schachter SC. Neuroendocrine aspects of epilepsy. In: Devinsky O, Theodore WH, eds. *Epilepsy and behavior.* New York: Alan R Liss, 1991;303–333.
22. Zimmerman AW. Hormones and epilepsy. *Neurol Clin* 1986;4:853–861.
23. Pritchard PB. The effect of seizures on hormones. *Epilepsia* 1991;32:546–550.
24. Stuenkel CA. Neural regulation of pituitary function. *Epilepsia* 1991;32:S2–S10.
25. Trimble MR. Serum prolactin in epilepsy and hysteria. *BMJ* 1978;2:1682.
26. Dana-Haeri J, Trimble MR, Oxley J. Prolactin and gonadotropin changes following generalised and partial seizures. *J Neurol Neurosurg Psychiatry* 1983;46: 331–335.
27. Collins WCJ, Lanigan O, Callaghan N. Plasma prolactin concentrations following epileptic and pseudoseizures. *J Neurol Neurosurg Psychiatry* 1983;46: 505–508.
28. Pritchard PB, Wannamaker BB, Sagel J, et al. Endocrine function following complex partial seizures. *Ann Neurol* 1983;14:27–32.
29. Laxer KD, Mullooly JP, Howell B. Prolactin changes

after seizures classified by EEG monitoring. *Neurology* 1985;35:31–35.

30. Wyllie E, Luders H, MacMillan JP, et al. Serum prolactin levels after epileptic seizures. *Neurology* 1984; 34:1601–1604.

31. Mattson RH, Cramer JA, Toftness BR, et al. Postictal changes in prolactin and luteinizing hormone. *Neurology* 1986;36:444.

32. Meierkord H, Shorvon S, Lightman S, et al. Comparison of the effects of frontal and temporal lobe partial seizures on prolactin levels. *Arch Neurol* 1992;49: 225–230.

33. Sperling MR, Pritchard PB, Engel J, et al. Prolactin in partial epilepsy: an indicator of limbic seizures. *Ann Neurol* 1986;20:716–722.

34. Parra A, Velasco M, Cervantes C, et al. Plasma prolactin increase following electric stimulation of the amygdala in humans. *Neuroendocrinology* 1980;31: 60–65.

35. Gallagher BB, Flanigin HF, King DW, et al. The effect of electrical stimulation of medial temporal lobe structures in epileptic patients upon ACTH, prolactin, and growth hormone. *Neurology* 1987;37:299–303.

36. Hufnagel A, Eiger CE, Klingmuller D, et al. Activation of epileptic foci by transcranial magnetic stimulation: effects on secretion of prolactin and luteinizing hormone. *J Neurol* 1990;237:242–246.

37. Pritchard PB, Wannamaker BB, Sagel J, et al. Serum prolactin and cortisol levels in evaluation of pseudoepileptic seizures. *Ann Neurol* 1985;18:87–89.

38. Molaie M, Culebras A, Miller M. Nocturnal plasma prolactin rise in patients with complex partial seizures. *Ann Neurol* 1985;18:719–722.

39. Molaie M, Culebras A, Miller M. Nocturnal plasma prolactin and cortisol levels in epileptics with complex partial seizures and primary generalized seizures. *Arch Neurol* 1987;44:699–702.

40. Mishra V, Gahlaut DS, Kumar S, et al. Value of serum prolactin in differentiating epilepsy from pseudoseizure. *J Assoc Physicians India* 1990;38:846–847.

41. Johansson F, Knorring LV. Changes in serum prolactin after electroconvulsive and epileptic seizures. *Eur Arch Psychiatry Neurol Sci* 1987;236:312–318.

42. Abbott RJ, Browning MCK, Davidson DLW. Serum prolactin and cortisol concentrations after grand mal seizures. *J Neurol Neurosurg Psychiatry* 1980;43: 163–167.

43. Takeshita H, Kawahara R, Nagabuchi T, et al. Serum prolactin, cortisol and growth hormone concentrations after various epileptic seizures. *Jpn J Psychiatry Neurol* 1986;40:617–623.

44. Aminoff MJ, Simon RP, Wiedemann E. The hormonal responses to generalized tonic-clonic seizures. *Brain* 1984;107:569–578.

45. Bye AME, Nunn KP, Wilson J. Prolactin and seizure activity. *Arch Dis Child* 1985;60:848–851.

46. Zelnik N, Kahana L, Rafael A, et al. Prolactin and cortisol levels in various paroxysmal disorders in childhood. *Pediatrics* 1991;88:486–489.

47. Ohman R, Walinder J, Balldin J, et al. Prolactin response to electroconvulsive therapy. *Lancet* 1976;2: 936–937.

48. O'Dea JPK, Gould D, Hallberg M, et al. Prolactin changes during electroconvulsive therapy. *Am J Psychiatry* 1978;135:609–611.

49. Arato M, Erdos A, Kurcz M, et al. Studies on the prolactin response induced by electroconvulsive therapy in schizophrenics. *Acta Psychiatr Scand* 1980;61: 239–244.

50. Skrabanek P, Balfe A, Webb M, et al. Electroconvulsive therapy (ECT) increases plasma growth hormone, prolactin, luteinising hormone and follicle-stimulating hormone but not thyrotropin or substance P. *Psychoneuroendocrinology* 1981;6:261–267.

51. Ryan RJ, Swanson DW, Faiman C, et al. Effects of convulsive electroshock on serum concentrations of follicle stimulating hormone, luteinizing hormone, thyroid stimulating hormone and growth hormone in man. *J Clin Endocrinol Metab* 1970:30:51–58.

52. Allen JP, Denny D, Kendall JW, et al. Corticotropin release during ECT in man. *Am J Psychiatry* 1974;131: 1225–1228.

53. Ylikorkala O, Kauppila A, Haapalahti J, et al. The effect of electric convulsion therapy on the circulating concentrations of pituitary hormones, cortisol and cyclic adenosine monophosphate. *Clin Endocrinol (Oxf)* 1976;5:571–574.

54. Fenton GW. Epilepsy and hysteria. *Br J Psychiatry* 1986;149:28–37.

55. Trimble MR. Pseudoseizures. *Neurol Clin* 1986;4: 531–548.

56. Jackel RA, Malkowicz D, Trivedi R, et al. Reduction of prolactin response with repetitive seizures. *Epilepsia* 1987;28:588.

57. Yerby MS, van Belle G, Friel PN, et al. Serum prolactins in the diagnosis of epilepsy: sensitivity, specificity, and predictive value. *Neurology* 1987;37: 1224–1226.

58. Morrell MJ. Sexual dysfunction in epilepsy. *Epilepsia* 1991;32:S38–45.

59. Cramer JA, Jones EE. Reproductive function in epilepsy. *Epilepsia* 1991;32:519–526.

60. Fenwick PBC, Toone BK, Wheeler MJ, et al. Sexual behaviour in a centre for epilepsy. *Acta Neurol Scand* 1985;71:428–435.

61. Toone BK, Edeh J, Nanjee MN, et al. Hyposexuality and epilepsy: a community survey of hormonal and behavioural changes in male epileptics. *Psychol Med* 1989;19:937–943.

62. Hierons R, Saunders M. Impotence in patients with temporal-lobe lesions. *Lancet* 1966;2:761–763.

63. Shukla GD, Srivastava ON, Katiyar BC. Sexual disturbances in temporal lobe epilepsy: a controlled study. *Br J Psychiatry* 1979;134:288–292.

64. Romberg MH. *A manual of the nervous diseases of man.* London: New Sydenham Society; 1853:2.

65. Jensen I, Vaernet K. Temporal lobe epilepsy: follow-up investigation of 74 temporal lobe resected patients. *Acta Neurochir (Wien)* 1977;37:173–200.

66. Herzog AG, Seibel MM, Schomer D, et al. Temporal lobe epilepsy: an extrahypothalamic pathogenesis for polycystic ovarian syndrome? *Neurology* 1984;34: 1389–1393.

67. Herzog AG, Seibel MM, Schomer DL, et al. Reproductive endocrine disorders in women with partial seizures of temporal lobe origin. *Arch Neurol* 1986;43: 341–346.

68. Bilo L, Meo R, Nappi C, et al. Reproductive endocrine disorders in women with primary generalized epilepsy. *Epilepsia* 1988;29:612–619.

69. Herzog AG. Intermittent progesterone therapy and frequency of complex partial seizures in women with menstrual disorders. *Neurology* 1986;36:1607–1610.

70. Mattson RH, Kramer JM, Cramer JA, et al. Seizure frequency and the menstrual cycle: a clinical study. *Epilepsia* 1981;22:242.

71. Backstrom T, Carstensen H, Sodergard R. Concentration of estradiol, testosterone and progesterone in cerebrospinal fluid compared to plasma unbound and total concentrations. *J Steroid Biochem* 1976;7:469–472.

72. Beltramino C, Taleisnik S. Facilitatory and inhibitory effects of electrochemical stimulation of the amygdala on the release of luteinizing hormone. *Brain Res* 1978; 144:95–107.

73. Herzog AG. A hypothesis to integrate partial seizures of temporal lobe origin and reproductive endocrine disorders. *Epilepsy Res* 1989;3:151–159.

74. Sharf M, Sharf B, Bental E, et al. The electroencephalogram in the investigation of anovulation and its treatment by clomiphene. *Lancet* 1969;1:750–753.

75. Herzog AG, Russell V, Vaitukaitis JL, et al. Neuroendocrine dysfunction in temporal lobe epilepsy. *Arch Neurol* 1982;39:133–135.

76. Bilo L, Meo R, Valentino R, et al. Abnormal pattern of luteinizing hormone pulsatility in women with epilepsy. *Fertil Steril* 1991;55:705–711.

77. Rao ML, Stefan H, Bauer J. Epileptic but not psychogenic seizures are accompanied by simultaneous elevation of serum pituitary hormones and cortisol levels. *Neuroendocrinology* 1989;49:33–39.

78. Herzog AG. Lateralized asymmetry of the cerebral control of endocrine secretion in women with epilepsy. *Neurology* 1991;41[Suppl 1]:366.

79. Mattson RH, Cramer JA, Darney PD, et al. Use of oral contraceptives by women with epilepsy. *JAMA* 1986; 256:238–240.

80. Dana-Haeri J, Richens A. Effect of norethisterone on seizures associated with menstruation. *Epilepsia* 1983; 24:377–381.

81. Coulam CB, Annegers JF. Do anticonvulsants reduce the efficacy of oral contraceptives? *Epilepsia* 1979;20: 519–525.

82. Odlind V, Olsson SE. Enhanced metabolism of levonorgestrel during phenytoin treatment in a woman with Norplant implants. *Contraception* 1986;33: 257–261.

83. Haukkamaa M. Contraception by Norplant subdermal capsules is not reliable in epileptic patients on anticonvulsant treatment. *Contraception* 1986;33:559–565.

84. Nicoletti F, Speciale C, Sortino MA, et al. Comparative effects of estradiol benzoate, the antiestrogen clomiphene citrate, and the progestin medroxyprogesterone acetate on kainic acid-induced seizures in male and female rats. *Epilepsia* 1985;26:252–257.

85. Terasawa E, Timiras PS. Electrical activity during the estrous cycle of the rat: cyclic changes in limbic structures. *Endocrinology* 1968;83:207–216.

86. Julien RM, Fowler GW, Danielson MG. The effects of antiepileptic drugs on estrogen-induced electrographic spike-wave discharge. *J Pharmacol Exp Ther* 1975; 193:647–656.

87. Marcus EM, Watson CW, Goldman PL. Effects of steroids on cerebral electrical activity: epileptogenic effects of conjugated estrogens and related compounds in the cat and rabbit. *Arch Neurol* 1966;15:521–532.

88. Landgren S, Backstrom T, Kalistratov G. The effect of progesterone on the spontaneous interictal spike evoked by the application of penicillin to the cat's cerebral cortex. *J Neurol Sci* 1978;36:119–133.

89. Laidlaw J. Catamenial epilepsy. *Lancet* 1956;2: 1235–1237.

90. Ansell B, Clarke E. Epilepsy and menstruation. *Lancet* 1956;271:1232–1235.

91. Rosciszewska D, Buntner B, Guz I, et al. Ovarian hormones, anticonvulsant drugs, and seizures during the menstrual cycle in women with epilepsy. *J Neurol Neurosurg Psychiatry* 1986;49:47–51.

92. Herzog AG, Klein P, Ransil BJ. Three patterns of catamenial epilepsy. *Epilepsia* 1997;38:1082–1088.

93. Backstrom T. Epileptic seizures in women related to plasma estrogen and progesterone during the menstrual cycle. *Acta Neurol Scand* 1976;54:321–347.

94. Shavit G, Lerman P, Korczyn AD, et al. Phenytoin pharmacokinetics in catamenial epilepsy. *Neurology* 1984;34:959–961.

95. Kumar N, Behari M, Ahuja GK, et al. Phenytoin levels in catamenial epilepsy. *Epilepsia* 1988;29:155–158.

96. Mattson RH, Cramer JA, Caldwell BV, et al. Treatment of seizures with medroxyprogesterone acetate: preliminary report. *Neurology* 1984;34:1255–1258.

97. Herzog AG. Clomiphene therapy in epileptic women with menstrual disorders. *Neurology* 1988;38:432–434.

98. Feely M, Calvert R, Gibson J. Clobazam in catamenial epilepsy: a model for evaluating anticonvulsants. *Lancet* 1982;2:71–73.

99. Herzog AG, Coleman AE, Jacobs AR, et al. Menstrual disorders, reproductive endocrine dysfunction and interictal discharge frequency in women with temporolimbic epilepsy. *Neurology* 1999;52:24–25.

100. Herzog AG. A relationship between particular reproductive endocrine disorders and the laterality of epileptiform discharges in women with epilepsy. *Neurology* 1993;43:1907–1910.

101. Drislane FW, Coleman AE, Schomer DL, et al. Altered pulsatile secretion in women with epilepsy. *Neurology* 1994;44:306–310.

102. Kiely J, Bertram EH, Quigg MS, et al. Effect of epilepsy on pulsatile secretion of luteinizing hormone. *Epilepsia* 2000;54:353.

103. Spratt DI, Finkelstein JS, Butler JP, et al. Effects of increasing the frequency of low doses of gonadotropin releasing hormone (GnRH) on gonadotropin secretion in GnRH-deficient men. *J Clin Endocrinol Metab* 1987;64:1179.

104. Knobil E. The neuroendocrine control of the menstrual cycle. *Recent Prog Horm Res* 1980;36:53–80.

105. Isojärvi JIT, Laatikainen TJ, Pakarinen AJ, et al. Polycystic ovaries and hyperandrogenism in women taking valproate for epilepsy. *N Engl J Med* 1993;329: 1383–1388.

106. Murialdo G, Galimberti CA, Gianelli MV, et al. Effects of valproate, phenobarbital and carbamazepine on sex steroid setup in women with epilepsy. *Clin Neuropharmacol* 1998;21:52–58.

107. Isojärvi JIT, Laatikainen TJ, Knip M, et al. Obesity and endocrine disorders in women taking valproate for epilepsy. *Ann Neurol* 1996;39:579–584.

108. Herzog AG. Polycystic ovarian syndrome in women with epilepsy: epileptogenic or iatrogenic? *Ann Neurol* 1996; 39:559–560.

Neurological Complications of Pregnancy, Second
Edition, edited by Brian Hainline and Orrin Devinsky.
Lippincott Williams & Wilkins, Philadelphia, © 2002.

14

Epilepsy

Vicky Bassi, *Mark S. Yerby, and †Orrin Devinsky

*University of Florida College of Medicine, Gainesville, Florida; *Oregon Comprehensive Epilepsy
Program, Portland Oregon; and †Departments of Neurology, Neurosurgery, and Psychiatry, New York
University School of Medicine, New York, New York, U.S.A.*

Epilepsy affects 1% of the population (1). Approximately 2.8 million people in the United States have epilepsy; 1.1 million of these individuals are women of childbearing age. Prejudice and discrimination against people with epilepsy have significantly diminished in our society over the past decades, but the stigma persists. The basic rights of marriage and parenthood usually are taken for granted, but for women with epilepsy (WWE) marriage and childbearing have not always been acceptable or legal. Social stigmas, popular mores, taboos, and misinformation concerning seizures have forced people living with epilepsy to shy away from conventional lifestyles. Furthermore, ideation that epilepsy is a psychiatric condition associated with progressive mental decline or aggression, and that epilepsy results from defective genes that must be eliminated (i.e., eugenics), has led some authorities to conclude that people with epilepsy are unfit to conceive (2).

In the past, almost every state in the United States developed legislation discriminating against people with epilepsy. As late as 1982, Missouri repealed legislation making it illegal for people with epilepsy to marry. Up until 1986, involuntary sterilization was legal in South Carolina for WWE. Until recently, some WWE still were encouraged by physicians not to consider pregnancy and, rarely, to undergo sterilization solely because they have epilepsy. Fortunately, public education and

new research have reduced discrimination against WWE who desire pregnancy (3). However, old habits and outlooks are difficult to relinquish, and although rare, even today some physicians "forbid" WWE from conceiving simply because they have epilepsy or take an antiepileptic drug (AED). In some cases, such recommendations lead women to discontinue their AEDs if they desire to become pregnant, regardless of their seizure history. Despite many forward strides in education regarding epilepsy, prejudice against people with epilepsy continues to exist with regards to issues such as child custody and adoption.

Even with advances in knowledge of epilepsy and pregnancy as a result of newer AEDs, utilization of vitamin supplements (especially folate) and improved prenatal diagnosis, pregnancies in WWE still are considered to be high risk. WWE have higher incidences of complications of pregnancy and labor and delivery, and their children display higher rates of adverse outcomes as a consequence of the pregnancy. Also, during pregnancy 20% to 35% of WWE will have an increase in seizure frequency—a result of changes in AED metabolism, noncompliance, stress, and/or sleep deprivation—making epilepsy management more difficult. This chapter provides an overview of epilepsy and pregnancy and addresses issues such as potential complications, effects of AEDs, management of WWE in the childbearing years, and other related topics.

EPILEPSY, PREGNANCY, AND POSSIBLE COMPLICATIONS

The vast majority (80% to 95%) of WWE have normal vaginal deliveries (4–7). However, WWE have an increased risk of certain obstetric complications (8–12). Over the past four decades the rate of complications has declined (8,12–13). Table 14.1 summarizes the most commonly reported obstetric complications and interventions in WWE. Most complications occur 1.5 to 4 times more commonly in WWE. Recent studies show complication rates of less than 2.5 times that of control groups.

Vaginal bleeding is more frequent among WWE, (3,9,11), especially during the first and third trimesters (12). Approximately 7% to 10% of WWE experience vaginal bleeding during pregnancy. Anemia is more common in pregnant WWE (3,15). Hyperemesis gravidarum may be more common in WWE (3,9,12), especially those on high doses of AEDs, and this can impair administration and absorption of oral medications. Yerby and associates (8) found a six-fold increase in maternal herpes among WWE.

Preeclampsia is also more common in WWE, with the increased risk ranging from 50% to 250% (8,9,12,16–18). Other studies, however, have found no difference between the frequency of preeclampsia in epilepsy and control groups (7,19,20). A recent Italian study also failed to establish a difference in frequency of preeclampsia between WWE and controls (13).

Slightly increased rates of placental complications may occur in WWE. Several studies find a slight but statistically significant increase in the rate of placenta previa and abruption in WWE (8,12,13).

The labor and delivery processes can offer more difficulty for WWE. Numerous studies found premature labor to occur more frequently in WWE than in controls. Also, uterine contractions are weaker in women taking AEDs such as carbamazepine and phenytoin (3,21–23), possibly contributing to the more frequent need for medical and surgical interventions in WWE. Induced labor, the use of forceps or vacuum assistance, mechanical rupture of membranes, and cesarean sections are all more common in these pregnancies (24–26). Additionally, one study found an elevated rate of breech presentation among WWE (27).

INCIDENCE OF SEIZURES DURING PREGNANCY

Pregnancy often alters seizure frequency. More than 30 studies report on seizure frequency during pregnancy (13,28,29). In the past, studies established trends in which seizure frequency increased in 37% to 45% of patients, decreased in 5% to 23% of patients, and remained unchanged in 42% to 53% of patients during pregnancy relative to their nonpregnant state (30–35). More recent trends indicate that 20% to 35% of WWE will experience increased seizure frequency, 3% to 22% experience decreased seizure frequency, and 60% to 85% experience no change in seizure frequency during pregnancy relative to their nonpregnant state (3,7,13,17,23,26, 30,32–42). The seizure frequency appears to be unrelated to seizure type, duration of

TABLE 14.1. *Obstetric complications and interventions in women with epilepsy*

Vaginal bleeding
Anemia
Hyperemesis gravidarum
Preeclampsia
Placental complications
    Placenta previa
    Placental abruption
Intrauterine growth restriction
Amniocentesis (2nd and 3rd trimester)
Induced labor
Cesarean section (primary and repeat)
Birthweight <2,500g
1-minute Apgar <5
5-minute Apgar <7
Toxemia
Premature rupture of membranes

more serious problems of alcohol abuse persist among a small group of pregnant women. Although the rates of alcoholism are lower among people with epilepsy than the general population, (115) there are pregnant WWE who abuse alcohol. These women are at increased risk of having seizures. Chronic alcohol use can induce the hepatic enzymes and lower plasma levels of AEDs such as carbamazepine, phenytoin, and phenobarbital. In people with epilepsy, moderate to heavy alcohol consumption (greater than 3 to 4 drinks per occasion) is associated with an increase in seizure frequency during the next several days (116,117). Also, intoxication predisposes to medication noncompliance and alteration of sleep–wake cycles, either of which can lead to an increase in seizure frequency.

Obstetric Interventions, Labor, and Delivery

Obstetric interventions are more common in WWE. Yerby and colleagues (8) found that amniocentesis during the second and third trimesters are 2.5 to 4.5 times more commonly performed on WWE than controls. Labor was induced two to four times as often among WWE in most (8,13,118), but not all (7), studies. Epilepsy alone is not an indication to induce labor because most WWE can have normal spontaneous labor and deliveries. However, in selected situations, it may be prudent to induce labor in WWE. This must be weighed against the risks of an induced labor, including prolonged labor and uterine and physical exhaustion, which can lead to the need for cesarean section (4,119).

Cesarean section is performed approximately twice as often in WWE in the United States (8). However, epilepsy is uncommonly a reason to perform an elective cesarean section. Tonic-clonic seizures occurring during labor or delivery occur in less than 1% to 4% of WWE, and another 1% to 2% will have seizures within 24 hours after delivery (33,89–91). Hiilesmaa (4) recommended criteria for elective and emergency cesarean sections, which are summarized in Table 14.4.

TABLE 14.4. *Epilepsy as an indication for cesarean section*

Elective cesarean section
  Substantial neurologic or mental defect
  Reduced cooperation of the patient in labor
  Very poor seizure control in late pregnancy
  Daily complex partial seizures
  Weekly tonic-clonic seizures
  Prior severe seizures
  Heavy physical or mental stress while taking
    medications
Emergency cesarean section
  Tonic-clonic seizure during labor
  Threat of fetal asphyxia
  Lack of maternal active contribution

Modified from Hiilesmaa VK. Pregnancy and birth in women with epilepsy. *Neurology* 1992;42 (Suppl 5):8–11, with permission.

EFFECTS OF MATERNAL SEIZURES ON OFFSPRING

Adverse Pregnancy Outcomes

Children of mothers, and less so with fathers, with epilepsy have an increased risk for developing epilepsy. Maternal age of epilepsy onset may be a contributing factor. Women whose epilepsy started before age 18 were twice as likely to have a child with epilepsy as women whose seizures began in adulthood. Having seizures during pregnancy also increases the risk of epilepsy in the offspring by a factor of two (3,109,120,121).

Population-based studies (8,9,12,14–16, 24–26,38,46,65,86,87,89,104,118,122–133), most of which were retrospective, showed that infants of mothers with epilepsy (IME) were approximately twice as likely to have adverse pregnancy outcomes. These complications include reduced viability and growth parameters, preterm delivery, neonatal complications, and maldevelopment. Possible mechanisms include the effect of seizures or AED therapy, the increased rate of pregnancy complications or labor interventions, and the higher incidence of congenital malformations. However, more recent large prospective studies (45,79,134–139) have shown no difference between IME and the general population with regards to poor pregnancy outcomes, with the exception of maldevelopment.

Decreased Viability

Older reports found Apgar scores were lower in IME in comparison to control children (8,9,11). Stillbirths as well as neonatal and perinatal death rates were approximately twice as common as in the general population (3,5,6,12,65,86,118,122–124,136,140). Studies suggest that stillbirth rates in infants of WWE range from 1.3% to 14.0% compared to 1.2% to 7.8% in infants of mothers without epilepsy (3,36,123,125). During the first year of life the mortality rate of IME remains higher than in infants whose mothers do not have epilepsy (65,138,139). Previous studies reported perinatal mortalities of 2.7% to 4.7% (6,132,133). Perinatal mortality has diminished from 4.7% during 1977 to 1981 to 2.1% during 1987 to 1991. However, the perinatal mortality was two to three times that of controls in both periods (43,66,78,141). More recent studies suggest that perinatal death rates range from 1.3% to 7.8%, compared to 1.0 % to 3.9% for controls (3)

Newborn Complications

Most newborn infants have low vitamin K-dependent coagulation activity. Although only a minority develops hemorrhagic disease of the newborn (HDN), it can cause death and handicap (142–145). It differs from other hemorrhagic disorders in that there is an increased risk of bleeding in IME within the first 24 hours of life. Prevalence figures average 10% in older studies, but more recent studies have found HDN in IME is very rare (7,108,146–151). These children usually bleed into internal body cavities; neonatal hemorrhage in this setting has a high morbidity and mortality because the disorder goes unnoticed until the child is in shock (3). This finding initially was reported in children exposed to barbiturates (phenobarbital or primidone) in utero and subsequently to children exposed to other AEDs including phenytoin, carbamazepine, diazepam, mephobarbital, amobarbital, and ethosuximide (109,122,152–156).

Hemorrhage results when newborn infants have decreased plasma levels of vitamin K-dependent clotting factors II, VII, IX, and X (157). The infant, but not the mother, has prolonged prothrombin and partial thromboplastin times. AEDs competitively inhibit vitamin K transport across the placenta, such that concentrations are predominantly below the detection limit. PIVKA-II (protein induced by vitamin K absence for factor II), which is a biochemical marker for vitamin K deficiency, is significantly more frequently detectable in newborns exposed to AEDs, and thus newborns exposed in utero to AEDs are at most risk for vitamin K deficiency (158).

The competitive inhibition imposed by AEDs can be overcome by administration of large doses of vitamin K. Maternal administration of oral vitamin K during the last week of pregnancy prevents this neonatal hemorrhage. However, because WWE have a higher rate of premature delivery, vitamin K (10 mg/day) should be administered during the last 2 to 4 weeks of pregnancy (143,158–163). Intramuscular injection of vitamin K to the infant at birth does not prevent hemorrhage if any two clotting factors have levels below 5% of normal (164). If these neonates bleed, they require treatment with fresh frozen plasma.

Drug withdrawal can occur in infants exposed to barbiturates in utero. When drug withdrawal occurs, symptoms begin approximately 7 days after delivery. Affected children become irritable, restless, tremulous, and hyperexcitable; have a voracious appetite; and frequently vomit after eating. Symptoms gradually increase in intensity, peaking in 2 to 6 weeks. Despite the increased appetite, these children often gain weight poorly (165).

Decreased Growth Parameters

The birthweight of IME was reported to be lower than control children, and IME are more likely to be small for various gestational periods when compared to controls. This difference occurs in IME exposed to AEDs and for IME not exposed. Approximately 8.5% of IME have low birthweight (less than 2,500 grams). Of these babies, 4% to 11% are premature (8,9,12,43,77,122,124,166). Several more recent prospective studies (7,39,83,134, 135,159) have failed to show these differences, however.

Maldevelopments

Children of WWE have a higher risk for congenital malformations than do children in the general population. Congenital malformations remain the most commonly reported adverse outcome in the pregnancies of WWE. Malformation rates in the general population range from 2% to 3% (3,109,146,167–170). Reports of malformation rates in various populations of IME range from 1.1% to 18.6% (3,7,108,125,126,146–151,171). These combined estimates yield a risk of malformations in an individual pregnancy of a WWE of 4% to 8% (109). These studies used diverse methodologies, but a consistent trend emerges (172). IME have approximately two to three times the number of malformations when compared with the general population. Several factors can contribute to the increased rates of malformations in IME, but AEDs appear most important. Other factors include maternal seizures during pregnancy, the genetics of maternal epilepsy, falls and injuries secondary to the seizures, lower socioeconomic status, and limited access to prenatal care. Several observations support the thesis that AEDs are the major cause of increased malformation among IME (109). Comparisons of the malformation rates of children of WWE treated with AEDs as opposed to those with no AED treatment consistently reveal higher rates of malformation in children of WWE receiving AED therapy (63,108,110, 148,173). Additionally, mean plasma AED concentrations are higher in WWE with malformed infants than in mothers with healthy children (174). And, infants of mothers on polytherapy have higher malformation rates than those exposed to monotherapy (109,175, 176).

Several studies found that idiopathic generalized epilepsy syndromes have a common genetic origin. Linkage studies have localized relevant gene defects on chromosomes 6p, 15q (67,177), and 1p (178). Also, a link between the genetics of idiopathic epilepsy and birth defects has been suggested. Recent genetic studies in families of patients with neural tube defects (NTDs) and cleft lip (with and without cleft palate), as well as genetic studies in families with a history of epilepsy, show evidence for the possible existence of genes on the short arm of chromosome 6. The suspected genes for cleft lip and cleft palate are linked to factor XIIIa and are neither identical with nor linked to a gene for idiopathic generalized epilepsy, which is located near the HLA region. The short arm of chromosome 6 also contains a human homologue of the mouse t-complex. Alterations of the mouse t-complex are involved in the defects of neural-crest development in mice. Relationships between a human homologue of the mouse t-complex, epilepsy, and malformations have yet to be proven (172).

Congenital Malformations

A variety of congenital malformations are more common in IME (174,179). Major congenital malformations are the most widely reported and extensively studied adverse outcomes. These include cleft lip, cleft palate, cardiac defects, NTDs, and urogenital defects. Minor congenital malformations include nail and phalangeal hypoplasia, high forehead, flat nasal bridge, and brachycephaly (180–182).

Orofacial clefts are the most commonly reported malformations in IME (approximately 30% of all major congenital malformations), followed by midline heart defects and NTDs (127,201,206,207). Table 14.5 summarizes the major and minor congenital malformations in IME.

Overall, the risk of malformations in any individual pregnancy in a WWE treated with a single AED is 4% to 8% (109), although modern care with the use of the most effective AED dose, multivitamins, and folate may reduce this substantially (7,183). Among WWE, the congenital malformation

TABLE 14.5. *Major and minor congenital abnormalities in epilepsy*

Major
  Congenital heart defects
  Transposition of great vessels
  Ventricular septal defect
  Pulmonalis stenosis
  Wolff-Parkinson-White syndrome
  Tetralogy of Fallot
  Neural tube defects
  Spina bifida aperta
  Anencephaly
  Spina bifida cystica
  Spina bifida occulta
  Hypospadias
  Polydactyly
  Cleft lip
  Cleft palate
  Congenital megacolon
  Urogenital malformations
  Esophageal stenosis
  Nonrotation
  Craniosynostosis
Minor
  Epicanthus
  Hypertelorism
  Ptosis
  Prominent metopic ridge
  Short, low-bridged nose
  Long, shallow philtrum
  Wide mouth with full lips
  Low-set/abnormal ears
  Distal digit hypoplasia
  Webbed neck
  Hirsutism/low hairline
  Anteverted nares

rates are higher in children of those who were treated with an AED than in children of untreated mothers with epilepsy (44,81,97, 125,127,128,141,184–197). Serum AED levels tend to be higher (and serum folate levels lower) in women with malformed infants when compared with mothers of healthy infants (191,198,199). Higher rates of congenital malformation are observed in IME when mothers received AED polytherapy rather than monotherapy (44,123,189–191,200, 201). Shakir and colleagues found that mothers with the highest risk of conceiving offspring with major congenital malformations were those with a longstanding history of epilepsy. Additionally, this group found that patients on polytherapy regimens had a significantly higher risk of major congenital

malformations (20.2%) compared to those receiving monotherapy (1.3%) (141). It also has been established that seizures during pregnancy do not increase the malformation rates in IME (3,43,44,97,109,125,127). However, another group found increased rates of malformations and central nervous system injuries in IME exposed to maternal seizures in utero (202).

All AEDs cross the placenta. The transport of maternal AED through the placenta cannot be detected in the early stages of pregnancy, but it is well documented at delivery with simultaneous collection of maternal and umbilical blood specimens. The unbound drug levels in the maternal and umbilical blood are almost equal or, as in the case of phenytoin, phenobarbital, and carbamazepine, the umbilical level is slightly lower than the maternal level (203,204). In cases treated with valproic acid, higher valproic acid levels in umbilical blood than maternal blood have been observed (201,204–206). AEDs also are excreted into breast milk, thus exposing breastfed infants to varying concentration of AEDs. Also, with the exception of ethosuximide and carbamazepine, the elimination half-life of AEDs tends to be prolonged in neonates in comparison to adults (3).

All of the AEDs marketed in the United States prior to 1990 have been associated with an increased risk of congenital malformations. Unfortunately, there are currently insufficient human data regarding AEDs marketed after 1990. No congenital malformations are associated unequivocally with specific AEDs, with the exception of NTDs with valproate and carbamazepine.

AED monotherapy is preferred over combination therapies (7,44,97,121,175,176,206, 208–210), although not all AEDs in monotherapy can be considered equally safe (72,211,212). An association between AED dose and increased risk of teratogenicity was shown for valproate (186,209,213–215) and possibly for phenobarbital (216). The teratogenic risk also may be different between specific polytherapy regimens and also may depend on specific pharmacokinetic and pharmacodynamic interactions and on genetic variation in drug metabolism (153,186,209).

Some specific combination therapies may be especially teratogenic, such as carbamazepine + valproate and phenytoin + primidone + phenobarbital (175,209,217–220). A potentiating effect of benzodiazepines on the expression of valproate-induced teratogenicity recently was suggested (221). Samren and colleagues reported a significantly increased risk of major congenital abnormalities for carbamazepine and valproate monotherapy, with evidence of a significant dose-response relationship for valproate. The group also reported that the risk of major congenital abnormalities was nonsignificantly increased for phenobarbital monotherapy when caffeine comedication was excluded, but was increased significantly when caffeine was included. Increased risks were found for several AED combinations, but clonazepam in combination with other AEDs showed a significantly increased relative risk. Additionally, there was a significantly increased malformation rate among IME combination of carbamazepine and valproate and the combination of phenobarbital and caffeine and other AEDs. Valproate ± other AEDs and valproate + carbamazepine were significantly associated with spina bifida (222). This finding is supported by earlier studies, which found that NTDs are more frequent in IME exposed to valproic acid (97,203,214,223,224) and carbamazepine in utero (225). The specific NTD associated with valproic acid and carbamazepine exposure is spina bifida aperta (97,138,140,226,227). Methodologic problems make frequency estimates imprecise (225), but spina bifida occurs in approximately 1% to 2% of IME exposed to valproate (228) and 0.5% exposed to carbamazepine (225). However, a prospective study in Holland discerned that IME exposed to valproate had a 5.4% prevalence rate of spina bifida. This high rate of spina bifida was associated with higher average daily valproate levels in IME with spina bifida (1,640±136 mg/day) compared to unaffected IME (941±48 mg/day). In light of this evidence, the authors

recommend lowering the valproate whenever valproate must be used in pregnancy (229). Kaneko and colleagues found that total daily valproate dosages of 1,000 mg or less and serum levels of 70 µg/ml or less are associated with significantly lower rates of congenital malformations (209).

AED Syndromes

Various syndromes of minor congenital malformations are associated with AED exposure. These anomalies are infrequent (<4%) in the general population and are structural deviations from the norm that do not constitute a threat to health (181). Clinical syndromes of minor anomalies have been reported for six AEDs. However, the evidence supporting the occurrence of specific minor anomalies with certain drugs and the actual existence of specific drug-induced syndromes varies for different AEDs.

The fetal trimethadione syndrome, first reported by Zackai and colleagues (230), describes infants with short stature, microcephaly, V-shaped eyebrows, epicanthal folds, low-set ears, anteriorly folded helices, irregular teeth, inguinal hernias, and simian creases. A retrospective study of trimethadione exposure revealed that 87% of 53 pregnancies displayed fetal loss or major malformations (231). Follow-up studies have reported significant rates of mental retardation (232). Currently, trimethadione rarely is used in treatment of epilepsy and should be avoided in women of childbearing years.

The fetal hydantoin syndrome (FHS), first described by Loughnan and colleagues (233), initially was characterized by hypoplasia and irregular ossification of the distal phalanges (219). Hanson and Smith (234) named the syndrome in 1975, but only one of the five children they reported was exposed to phenytoin monotherapy. Four of these IME also were exposed to barbiturate in utero. These infants displayed facial dysmorphism (epicanthal folds, hypertelorism, broad flat nasal bridges, an upturned nasal tip, and wide prominent lips), distal digital hypoplasia

(DDH), mental retardation, and intrauterine growth restriction. Hanson and colleagues (235) subsequently reported the FHS in 11% of exposed children, with an additional 30% expressing some syndromic features. These findings were refuted by later prospective studies. Gaily found no association between infants exposed to phenytoin and FHS; hypertelorism and DDH were the only dysmorphic features associated with phenytoin exposure in utero (236).

Benzodiazepine exposure in utero was associated with dysmorphism, convulsions, severe mental retardation, distortion of neuronal migration, cerebral pachygyria, polycystic kidneys, voiding difficulties, submucosal cleft hard palate, and perceptive disorders (237). Subsequent studies have not consistently found significantly elevated frequencies of malformations in IME exposed to benzodiazepines in utero (238). However, additional data are needed to resolve whether benzodiazepines are safe during pregnancy.

The primidone syndrome includes hirsute forehead, thick nasal roots, anteverted nostrils, long philtrums, straight thin upper lips, and DDH. Also, these children tend to have low birthweight for gestational age and have an increased risk for developmental delay and heart defects (195,239,240). In a recent multicenter study of 983 IME, primidone monotherapy had the highest percentage (14.3%) of malformations (209).

Phenobarbital exposure in utero has been associated with minor anomalies, including facial dysmorphism and other physical changes, pre- and postnatal growth deficiency, and developmental delay (41,97,192,197). The clinical features resemble those seen with fetal phenytoin and alcohol exposure, and investigators felt that these changes did not represent a specific syndrome (97,197,241). Investigators also observed that phenobarbital, phenytoin, and alcohol can cause folate deficiency, and this deficiency may contribute to the pathogenesis for the dysmorphism seen with such exposures in utero.

A valproate syndrome with dysmorphic features in children exposed in utero was first described by DiLiberti and colleagues (242). These children had inferior epicanthal folds, flat nasal bridges, upturned nasal tips, a shallow philtrum, thin vermilion borders, and inferior-turned mouths (243). Long thin overlapping fingers and toes and hyperconvex nails can occur. Isolated cases of fetal valproate exposure and radial ray aplasia have been observed (244). Also, children exposed to valproate in utero may have an increased rate of perinatal distress, low Apgar scores, postnatal growth deficiency, and microcephaly (245,246). Other possible clinical features of fetal valproate syndrome include stridor, genital anomalies, hand anomalies, hypotonia, abnormal external ears, midfacial hypoplasia (72,97,194,215,224), NTDs, congenital heart disease, cleft lip and palate, genitourinary malformations, tracheomalacia, and abdominal wall defects (196,203,211, 227). In a recent multicenter study of 983 IME, valproate monotherapy was associated with malformations in 11.1% (209).

A carbamazepine syndrome, reported by a single group of investigators (247), is characterized by dysmorphic features, including epicanthal folds, upslanting palpebral fissures, short nose, long philtrum, DDH, and microcephaly (18,248). Developmental delay also was found in 20% of exposed children, although the authors used one standard deviation from the mean as the cut off for abnormality, rather than the customary two standard deviations in defining developmental delay. Using conventional definitions, their data revealed no increased risk of developmental delay following in utero carbamazepine exposure. Recently, children exposed in utero to carbamazepine had increased rates of developmental delay or intelligence quotient (IQ) scores below 90— ten points lower than the control group (70,193,249). Thus, in utero exposure to carbamazepine may reduce intelligence, although the methodology of these studies has been questioned and findings await replication in a controlled study.

Cognition, Intelligence, and Psychomotor Development

IME have higher rates of mental retardation relative to control children (12,68–71,122, 250–254). Several factors, including intrauterine growth restriction, major and minor malformations, maternal seizures, in utero AED exposure, increased dose and numbers of AEDs, decreased parental education and socioeconomic status, and poor maternal–child relation may impair brain development during gestation and after birth (68–71, 251–255). A prenatal developmental disorder can present globally as subnormal intelligence (252) or as specific cognitive deficits with normal general intelligence (68,253). The type of dysfunction may depend on the nature of the agent, the stage at which the effect occurs, and other modifying intrinsic and extrinsic factors.

Beck-Mannagetta and colleagues found that 35% of AED exposed IME required special education because of mental deficiencies compared to 8% of controls (256). Unfortunately, most of these types of studies did not control for socioeconomic status, parental intelligence, or the number of seizures during pregnancy. Prospective controlled studies have documented only minor differences in cognitive function between IME and controls (257). Holmes and colleagues investigated the contribution of the mother's predisposition to epilepsy on her child's intelligence and physical features. They studied cognitive dysfunction in children whose mothers had epilepsy but did not take AEDs during pregnancy and control children of nonepileptic mothers. The results showed no significant differences in the full-scale IQ and several additional subsets of intelligence between a sample of children whose mothers had epilepsy and a comparison group of control children. The study also did not support the suggestion that the seizure history of the child and his or her mother was associated with an increased frequency of the AED syndrome (258).

Learning disabilities are more common among IME than control children. Psychometric testing revealed a learning disability in 48% of 23 IME followed to age 4 years (259). A prospective Finnish study (260) found that IME had lower scores on tests of block design (<5th percentile on the Weschler Preschool & Primary Scale of Intelligence) and auditory closure (<5th percentile on the Illinois Test of Psycholinguistic Ability) than control subjects. Cognitive dysfunction was diagnosed in 23% of IME and 7% of controls and was associated with maternal partial seizures, seizures during pregnancy, and low levels of parental education, but not with exposure to AED. Leavitt and colleagues found that IME have impaired language development at 2 years of age, with about half the vocabulary as controls despite equivalent IQ scores (261). In another study, 23 infants previously exposed to AEDs in utero were followed until the age of 4 years, and 48% of these infants were diagnosed as having a learning disability based on standardized psychometric testing (262). Other studies found that 35% of children who were exposed to AEDs in utero required special education compared to 8% of children who were not exposed (263); the studies also found that 23% of children of mothers with epilepsy had cognitive dysfunction compared with 7% of the control subjects (264). Katz and colleagues found that 6.2% of children exposed to AEDs in utero had pervasive developmental delay (7).

Long-term neuropsychologic consequences of maternal epilepsy and AED treatment during pregnancy also were studied for older children and adolescents. Across all measures of neurophysiologic function, controls displayed the best performance and the risk groups had the worst performance. In this study the group of at-risk children displayed lower cognitive functioning compared with a control group, which was recognizable at age 5 years. Although AED teratogenicity was postulated as the mechanism for developmental delay, with increasing age the family socioeconomic status appeared to play a pivotal role. At age 5 years, family social background was a better predictor of the child's intellectual functioning than the type of AED taken by the mother (255). In conclusion, this study showed that maternal epilepsy and AED therapy during pregnancy appear to have longterm effects on the offspring well into adolescence, as evinced by electroencephalogram patterns, minor neurologic dysfunction, and intellectual performance. Severity of effects increased from control group to epilepsy/no-drug group to monotherapy group and was most marked in the polytherapy group. These differences are thought to reflect differences in neural vulnerability to social and family factors (249).

NEW AEDS

New AEDs include clobazam, felbamate, gabapentin, lamotrigine, oxcarbazepine, tiagabine, topiramate, and zonisamide. Clobazam is a benzodiazepine chemically related to diazepam. It is mainly an add-on drug in partial epilepsy, but also has been helpful for some patients with generalized epilepsies. Felbamate is effective in treating partial and secondary generalized tonic-clonic seizures and for Lennox-Gastaut syndrome. Felbamate use commonly is associated with anorexia, nausea, vomiting, headaches, dizziness, insomnia, and behavioral disturbances. Major adverse effects of felbamate include aplastic anemia and hepatoxicity (265). Gabapentin is an amino acid that is chemically related to gamma-aminobutyric acid and is effective for partial and generalized seizures. Common side effects of gabapentin use include dizziness, fatigue, somnolence, ataxia, tremor, and weight gain. Both felbamate and gabapentin do not decrease concentration of contraceptive steroids (265). Lamotrigine is a phenyltriazine AED structurally unrelated to other conventional AEDs. There are no known active metabolites of lamotrigine in humans, and the major metabolite is an inactive 2–N-glucoronide conjugate (266). Common side effects of lamotrigine use include dizziness, headache, diplopia, ataxia, somnolence, vomiting, and rash. Major adverse effects include severe rash and acute kidney failure (267). Lamotrigine does not interfere with hormonal contraception (265). Oxcarbazepine is closely related to carbamazepine. It is used to treat complex partial seizures and secondary generalized tonic-clonic seizures, and it may be better tolerated than carbamazepine (51). Common side effects of oxcarbazepine include fatigue, headaches, dizziness, ataxia, and hyponatraemia. Other adverse effects of this AED include skin rashes (265). Tiagabine is indicated for people ages 12 or older with partial seizures. Common side effects include tremor, nervousness, and emotional changes (267). Tiagabine does not interfere with hormonal contraception (265). Topiramate is a sulfamate-substituted monosaccharide. It exerts its antiseizure effects by preventing abnormal activity in the cellular sodium pump, blocking the effects of excitatory neurotransmitters, and increasing the effects of inhibitory neurotransmitters in the brain. Topiramate is approved as adjunctive therapy for the treatment of adults with partial onset seizures, and recent data indicate that it may be effective in treating partial onset seizures in children, as well as Lennox-Gastaut syndrome and primary generalized tonic-clonic seizures in adults and children. It also has been shown to reduce the contraceptive concentration by approximately 30% (268). Topiramate commonly causes fatigue, dizziness, somnolence, impaired concentration, ataxia, and weight loss. The main adverse effect, which can result from topiramate use, is nephrolithiasis (265). Zonisamide is used to treat simple and complex partial seizures, primary and secondary generalized tonic-clonic seizures, tonic seizures, atypical absence seizures, and certain types of progressive myoclonic epilepsy. Zonisamide use commonly causes anorexia, ataxia, dizziness, fatigue, somnolence, impaired concentration, and confusion (265).

A number of these new AEDs may increase seizure frequency or severity or change seizure type. It is difficult to be certain that an AED exacerbates or worsens a seizure type, but accurate counts of seizures preceding the introduction of a new AED have helped clinicians in identifying this adverse effect.

Gabapentin and lamotrigine have been shown to increase the frequency of myoclonic seizures. Gabapentin also has been shown to increase the frequency of absence seizures (267).

Overall, these new AEDs have good safety and similar efficacy in men and women. It is not known whether the new AEDs affect bone health, fertility, the menstrual cycle, and sexuality. Whether these new AEDs are good choices for pregnant women and whether they have any major teratogenic properties await further experience in human pregnancy. However, animal reproductive toxicology studies appear promising. In prospective reports on lamotrigine, there were no birth defects in 34 pregnancies associated with the first-trimester exposure to lamotrigine monotherapy. In another study, however, 5.6% of 107 pregnancies consisting of patients treated with lamotrigine alone or lamotrigine and other AEDs evinced birth defects. However, no consistent pattern of malformations was reported (40,41).

BALANCING RISKS OF SEIZURES AND AEDS

Clinicians and their patients of childbearing age with epilepsy face difficult decisions. Antiepileptic drug therapy is associated with an increased risk of complicated pregnancies, major malformations, minor anomalies, neonatal hemorrhage, and delayed fetal growth and development. Maternal seizures also are associated with risks to the mother (loss of job or driver's license, declining neuropsychologic performance, and prolonged tonic-clonic seizures) and fetus (increased risks of miscarriage, premature labor, intracranial hemorrhage, and possibly developmental or learning disabilities). Therefore, either AEDs or seizures can cause difficulties. For most women, however, cessation of medication is not a viable option.

The current tendency for some practitioners, especially obstetricians and gynecologists, to use phenobarbital instead of nonsedating AEDs is not supported by experience, observation, or animal studies. Phenobarbital monotherapy can cause dysmorphic features (241). Cleft lip and palate are more frequent (0.6% to 3.9%) in mice exposed to phenobarbital in utero than controls (0.3%) (269). Phenobarbital inhibits hippocampal dendrite formation in the fetus (270). Phenobarbital treatment produces greater cognitive impairment compared to other AEDs, and its effects may be greater in the immature brain. Two recent studies found that in utero phenobarbital exposure may produce a lifelong reduction in IQ (254). Phenobarbital is the AED most strongly associated with neonatal hemorrhagic disorder (153) and neonatal withdrawal symptoms following intrauterine exposure. These withdrawal symptoms include irritability, restlessness, altered sleep and feeding patterns, increased startle and hyperreflexia and are similar to those witnessed in infants exposed to opiates during pregnancy. Withdrawal symptoms to barbiturates tend to develop later than those to opiates, with a median onset of 7 days after delivery and duration of up to 3 months (271).

During pregnancy there is a decline in serum AED levels. However, this decline in total plasma AED levels should not prompt an immediate and automatic increase in AED dosage. Most AEDs are bound to plasma proteins, but it is the "free" or unbound portion of the drug that is biologically active. Therefore, one must recognize the difference in the relative decline of total versus free AED levels. Free AED levels correlate best with both seizure control and central nervous system toxicity because only this portion traverses the blood–brain barrier. As total AED levels are most commonly available, the relationship between total and free levels must be considered in the management of pregnant WWE. We recommend that baseline total and free AED levels be obtained prior to conception. Preferentially free (or total) levels then should be obtained regularly once every 4 to 8 weeks during the duration of the pregnancy. However, dosage adjustments should be based primarily on the patient's clinical status (82). Also, during follow-up of a pregnant WWE, the principles of sound AED therapy should be applied. That is, use the first-choice drug for seizure type and use epileptic AED as monotherapy at the lowest effective dose. Avoid polytherapy and avoid valproate and carbamazepine if there is a history of NTDs. In cases of valproate administration, ensure that doses are divided over three to four administrations per day to avoid plasma toxicity. Try to maintain total daily dose under 1,000 mg and serum levels less than 70 µg/ml, especially during the first trimester (209). Also, continue daily folate supplements to ensure normal plasma levels, especially during the period of organogenesis in the first trimester (272).

Breastfeeding is generally considered safe for infants of WWE because it confers immunologic and nutritional advantages to the baby. However, all AEDs are present in breast milk. The percentage of the major AEDs found in breast milk is indicated in Table 14.6. The relative concentration of AED present is in proportion to the plasma-binding affinity of the drug (82,272,273). Thus, the AEDs that are highly protein bound are present in lower concentrations in breast milk, whereas AEDs that are largely present in the unbound form are present in higher concentrations in breast milk. As previously mentioned, the AEDs that are most often implicated in toxicity resulting from breastfeeding are primidone and phenobarbital because they have sedative properties and can cause lethargy, irritability, poor suck-

ling, sedation in the child, and cessation of feeding before satiation (82,272). This causes the child to awaken, hungry and irritable, and repeat the process (3).

PHARMACOKINETIC CHANGES IN AEDS DURING PREGNANCY

Plasma concentrations of AEDs decrease during the course of pregnancy despite constant, and, in some cases, increasing doses (274–278). Plasma levels of AEDs tend to rise during the first few postpartum weeks and may require a reduction of AED dosage. Although total plasma AED levels decline in all pregnant women, seizure frequency usually remains unchanged. However, almost all women with increased seizures during pregnancy have subtherapeutic AED levels (37,38, 88,279,280).

Several mechanisms may contribute to the decline in AED levels during pregnancy (Table 14.2). One woman who had normal phenytoin metabolism when not pregnant failed to absorb the drug during pregnancy (281). This resulted in a marked decline in plasma levels and status epilepticus. Impaired absorption is uncommon, and this appears to be an isolated case. Late pregnancy is associated with decreased gastrointestinal motility, which may delay gastric emptying and alter the time to peak levels in some women (282). However, slower passage through the gas-

TABLE 14.6. *Neonatal pharmacokinetics of antiepileptic drugs*

AED	Breast milk/plasma concentration (%)	Elimination half-life (hours)	
		Adult	Neonate
Carbamazepine	50	8–25	8–28
Ethosuximide	90	40–60	40
Phenobarbital	50	75–126	45–500
Phenytoin	30	12–50	15–105
Primidone	80	4–12	7–60
Valproate	10	6–18	30–60
Lamotrigine	61	6–30	6–11
Topiramate	100	20–30	—
Zonisamide	90	50–62	—
Gabapentin	—	5–9	—
Vigabartin	—	5–7	—

From Yerby MS. Pregnancy and epilepsy. *Epilepsia* 1991;3, with permission.

trointestinal tract can increase absorption of some drugs, especially those that are poorly soluble.

The volume of distribution increases throughout the course of pregnancy and may in part account for the reduction of AED levels when dosage is held constant. However, if the volume of distribution was a major factor in changing AED concentration, then one would predict a similar decline in both total and free levels, which is not the case (see below). Decreased plasma protein binding (78,85,203,278,283,284), reduced concentrations of albumin, and increased drug clearance (82,87,274,276–278,280,281,285) may be the most important mechanisms of lowering AED levels during pregnancy. The rate of clearance is maximal during the last trimester (276).

The decline in serum albumin levels and changes in plasma protein binding lead to an increase in the percentage of unbound (free) AEDs. The reduction in plasma protein binding of phenytoin and phenobarbital correlate positively with gestational age and negatively with serum albumin level (82,286). Because the free drug is available for metabolic degradation, an increased proportion of the drug is metabolized. The increased clearance of AEDs during pregnancy may result from induction of hepatic microsomal enzymes by elevated levels of steroid hormones such as estrogen and progesterone (42,78,287). Toward the end of the third trimester, as the fetal liver becomes functional, fetal hepatic metabolism may make a small contribution to the breakdown of AEDs. If this were a major factor, one would expect that AED levels would return to baseline within several days after delivery, particularly for AEDs with short half-lives such as carbamazepine. Such changes, however, often take several weeks (18,203, 288,289).

AED DOSAGES, PLASMA LEVELS, AND CLINICAL MANAGEMENT

The decline in plasma AED levels during the course of pregnancy presents a clinical challenge. During pregnancy, AED levels decline in almost all women, even in the face of constant doses and good compliance. However, the majority of these women do not experience an increase in seizure frequency (13,29). Therefore, a decline in the total plasma AED level should not reflexively trigger an increase in dosage. This is especially important because there is a difference in the amount of decline in total versus free AED levels. Adjustment in AED dosage should be based primarily on the clinical status of the patient.

Tables 14.7–14.9 summarize the pharmacokinetic data for AEDs during pregnancy. These and other summaries present group means; significant interindividual differences can occur. There is a decline in total levels for all major AEDs. However, the decline in the free level is less than that for the total level for all AEDs except phenobarbital. The percentage of free (unbound) drug therefore increases for most AEDs. However, although the ratio of unbound:bound drug increases, the amount of AED in the free form actually declines for all AEDs except valproate. For valproate, although the total level declines, the free level actually increases, particularly during the last trimester of pregnancy. In managing individual patients, understanding patterns of changes in AED can be helpful, but in difficult cases, there is no substitute for obtaining free levels, which will provide the most accurate information.

Three representative examples of typical clinical management problems are presented:

TABLE 14.7. *Proportionate decline in levels of antiepileptic drugs during pregnancy*

AED	Total (%)	Free (%)
Carbamazepine	42*	28
Phenytoin	56*	31
Phenobarbital	55*	50*
Valproic acid	39*	+25

*Significantly different from baseline *p* < 0.005.
From Yerby MS, Freil PN, McCormick K. Antiepileptic drug disposition during pregnancy. *Neurology* 1992;42:12–16, with permission.

TABLE 14.8. *Period of pregnancy with greatest decline in antiepileptic drug levels*

AED	Trimester	Total decline (%)
Carbamazepine		
Total	3	52
Free	3	83
Phenytoin		
Total	1	66
Free	1	102
Phenobarbital		
Total	1	80
Free	1	98
Valproic acid		
Total		Consistent decline throughout
Free		Consistent decline throughout
Lamotrigine		
Total	1	Consistent decline throughout
Free	1	Consistent decline throughout

From Yerby MS, Freil PN, McCormick K. Antiepileptic drug disposition during pregnancy. *Neurology* 1992;42:12–16, with permission.

1. A 30-year-old woman with tonic-clonic seizures controlled on phenytoin becomes pregnant. Her nonpregnant baseline trough total and free phenytoin levels are 14 μg/ml and 1.4 μg/ml, respectively (10% is unbound). During the course of pregnancy, she remains seizure-free, but during the beginning of the third trimester, the neurologist obtains a trough total phenytoin level of 7.5 μg/ml. However, the trough free phenytoin level is 1.1 μg/ml. Therefore, the free level remains in the low "therapeutic" range (1 to 2 μg/ml). Because seizures are well controlled, it is reasonable to monitor phenytoin levels and continue the same dosage of medication.

2. A woman with recurrent tonic-clonic seizures during the first trimester is taking carbamazepine monotherapy. Baseline nonpregnant trough carbamazepine levels were 9.0 (total) and 6.5 (free). After her second tonic-clonic seizure during pregnancy, carbamazepine levels were 7.0 (total) and 5.5 (free). In this case, there has been both an increase in seizures and a decline in the free carbamazepine level. Therefore, carbamazepine should be increased.

TABLE 14.9. *Percent free fraction of antiepileptic drug or metabolite during pregnancy*

	Carbamazepine	Carbamazepine epoxide (n = 22)	Dihydrodiol (n = 22)	Phenytoin (n = 18)	Phenobarbital (n = 11)	Valproic acid (n = 9)	Lamotrigine
Baseline trimester	21.4	42	63.7	7.7	52	11	9
1	23.9[a]	47.1	65.1	9.1	51.2	8	5
2	25[c]	50.5[c]	73.5[c]	9.3[c]	57.4[a]	10	7
3	25.5[c]	52.3[c]	75.6[c]	10.1[c]	59.3[c]	13	5
Delivery	27.6[c]	57.1[c]	74.5[c]	13[c]	61.8[c]	11	3
Postpartum	21.4	43	64.4	8[c]	52.6[b]	25	22
Decreased binding	29	36	17	69	19	—	—

[a]Significant at $p < 0.05$.
[b]Significant at $p < 0.025$.
[c]Significant at $p < 0.005$.
From Yerby MS, Freil PN, McCormick K. Antiepileptic drug disposition during pregnancy. *Neurology* 1992;42 (Suppl 5):12–16, with permission.

3. A woman with juvenile myoclonic epilepsy is seizure-free on valproate monotherapy, with baseline nonpregnant levels of 80 µg/ml (total) and 8 µg/ml (free). During the second trimester of pregnancy the woman reports no seizures but states that she is tremulous and excessively tired; valproate levels are 70 µg/ml (total) and 11 µg/ml (free). The rise in the free level—despite a decline in total level—accounts for her side effects and justifies a judicious reduction in valproate dose. Thus, in some women, an increase in the ratio of unbound:bound drug causes toxicity despite total levels which remain constant or even decline.

The frequency with which AED total or free levels should be obtained, and the criteria for adjusting AED dosage during pregnancy, cannot be precisely specified. In part, these decisions are influenced by the availability and cost of certain studies such as free AED levels and, in the case of changing AED dosage, the patient's input regarding the costs and benefits associated with balancing seizure control and adverse drug effects. We suggest the following general principles for management, which may require modification for individual patients.

Frequency of AED Levels

1. Baseline total and free levels should be obtained in all women before pregnancy. Trough levels should be obtained in women on stable doses for at least 4 to 5 half-lives.
2. Obtain monthly free levels (or total levels if free levels are not readily available) when patients have
   a. Uncontrolled tonic-clonic seizures during the year prior to conception
   b. Uncontrolled complex partial seizures or other seizure types that significantly interfere with activities of daily life during the year prior to conception
   c. Previously controlled seizures, but tonic-clonic seizures begin during pregnancy

d. Controlled seizures but total AED levels decline by more than 50% on routine screens
3. Obtain total levels every other month when patients have
   a. Complex partial, absence, myoclonic, or other seizure types that do not interfere with activities of daily life
   b. Well-controlled forms of epilepsy

Changing AED Dosage

The goal of therapy is to avoid changes in the AED regimen after patients become pregnant unless there are drug side effects or seizures that can be dangerous for the mother, the fetus, or both.

1. Reasons not to change AED dosage:
   a. Decline in total AED level in a woman with well-controlled seizures (unless there has been a greater than 30% decline in the free levels *and* the woman has a history of poorly controlled seizures prior to pregnancy)
   b. A woman taking two or more AEDs discovers she is pregnant (the time to change to monotherapy is before she becomes pregnant). In many cases, the critical developmental period of organogenesis has passed. For example, clefting defects in the lip and palate develop prior to day 49 of gestation. A woman who learns she is pregnant in the 6th to 7th week of pregnancy and is taking carbamazepine and phenobarbital should not have one medication suddenly discontinued (unless the dose is very small and the serum level is clinically insignificant) because this increases the risk of having a seizure, but does little to lower the risk of major congenital defects in the baby. This is especially true for phenobarbital and primidone (which is metabolized to phenobarbital) in which sudden discontinuation is likely to cause seizures; and the drug will persist in

the maternal and fetal circulations for weeks because of the long half life of phenobarbital.

2. Reasons to change AED dosage:
    a. Tonic-clonic seizures increase
    b. Complex partial or other seizure types interfere with activities of daily life and the patient wants seizures controlled with additional medication
    c. A greater than 50% decline in total level (60% for valproate) or a greater than 30% decline in free level in a woman who is free of tonic-clonic or other disabling seizure types during pregnancy but has had such seizures during the year prior to becoming pregnant
    d. Troublesome or disabling side effects (consider lowering AED dosage if seizure control permits)

PRINCIPLES OF MANAGEMENT

All women of childbearing age with epilepsy should be educated about risks associated with pregnancy and ways to minimize those risks. Nonepileptic seizures, syncope, and other syndromes mimic epilepsy; therefore, the diagnosis of epilepsy in WWE should be firm. The need for continued AED therapy should be reevaluated. Because many women of childbearing age have unplanned pregnancies, changing AEDs to monotherapy should be attempted.

The AED Pregnancy Registry was created in an effort to provide information and resources to pregnant WWE. Ninety-five percent of enrollments are WWE, and prospective enrollments constitute 59% of all cases. The registry seeks to enroll women who are taking AEDs before conception to avoid selection bias. This registry was designed to identify what risks are associated with different therapies. It responds to inquiries regarding fetal risk from AED use during pregnancy and provides information about the potential risk of each AED as monotherapy. Women who are pregnant and are taking AEDs can enroll by calling toll free (1-888-233-2334).

Each participant is provided a general guideline sheet concerning planning and perinatal care. Additionally, postpartum interviews are conducted. Information collected is analyzed to assess fetal risk from all AEDs during pregnancy. To date, there have not been sufficient data collected by the registry to provide WWE and their doctors with teratogenic risks associated with new AEDs.

Approximately 20% to 35% of WWE will have an increased seizure frequency during pregnancy. This risk can be minimized by compliance with medications and avoidance of seizure precipitants such as sleep deprivation. Compliance is often a problem during pregnancy, and women should be educated about risks of seizures to both the mother and fetus. There is a 1.5- to 2-fold increased risk of vaginal hemorrhage, eclampsia, premature labor, cesarean section, miscarriage, and stillbirth. Their children are at increased risk for prematurity, developmental delay, hemorrhage (7%), dysmorphism (10%), and major malformations (4% to 6%).

Seizures should be controlled without clinical toxicity. Monotherapy and use of the lowest effective dose reduces the risk of adverse outcomes. Growing evidence suggests that the preconceptual use of multivitamins with folate can reduce the risk of major malformations. We encourage all women of childbearing age to take multivitamins with folate.

Folate supplementation before and during pregnancy is being more commonly prescribed. There is evidence that folate can reduce plasma levels of phenobarbital and phenytoin (290–293). Periconceptual supplementation with folic acid at the pharmacologic dose of 4mg/day reduces the risk of recurrence of NTDs after one child has been born with a NTD from 3.5% to 0.7% without resulting in signs of adverse fetal effects (191). However, no study has examined the relationships between the amount of folate supplementation (e.g., 0.4 mg vs.1 mg vs. 4 mg), plasma folate levels, AED dosage and plasma levels, and seizure frequency in pregnant women. Additionally, it is not known whether AEDs are teratogenic by interfering with folic acid-related pathways. Pregnancy is associated with a physiologic decrease in folic acid levels—a response that can be aggravated by AED treatment. However, the AEDs that induce the most profound changes in folic acid status, phenytoin and barbiturates, paradoxically have a lower risk for fetal NTDs than valproate and carbamazepine (191). Thus, additional investigation is needed to define the relationship between folic acid and AED teratogenesis.

After conception, changing or stopping AEDs in a woman whose seizures are controlled does not clearly reduce the risk of malformations, but it does increase the risk of increased seizures. If changes are made, they should be gradual. Women with a family history of NTDs should probably avoid valproic acid and carbamazepine and should probably take high doses of folic acid (2 to 4 mg/day), regardless of whether they are taking an AED. When an AED is taken during pregnancy, ultrasonographic evaluation at 16 to 18 weeks should be performed to rule out spina bifida aperta, cardiac anomalies, or limb defects. If ultrasound is inconclusive, amniocentesis should be performed, and alpha fetoprotein and acetylcholinesterase levels should be obtained. In the detection of NTDs, high-resolution ultrasound and amniocentesis have approximate resolutions of 90% and 95%, respectively. Vitamin K1 should be administered (10 mg/day) beginning 2 to 4 weeks before expected delivery until birth to prevent neonatal hemorrhage.

AED levels should be monitored, and dosage should be adjusted as necessary. We prefer patients to enter their last month of gestation with therapeutic free AED levels to reduce the risk of seizures during labor and delivery. The patient's neurologist and obstetrician need to work together to establish a plan for treating acute seizures, particularly during labor. Short-acting benzodiazepines control acute seizures best in this setting. AED levels should be followed through the eighth postpartum week because they can increase and cause toxicity.

Pediatricians following IME need to be alert for the possibility of hemorrhage and drug withdrawal, especially in children exposed to phenobarbital. Children of WWE also need to be carefully and regularly evaluated for any developmental delay.

After the child is born, parents with epilepsy should consider how their condition might affect their child's care. In parents with well-controlled seizures, restrictions rarely are needed. However, parents with poorly controlled seizures that impair consciousness or motor control need to take special precautions. For example, changing and feeding the baby are safer on the floor and bathing should be supervised.

Fortunately, more than 90% of WWE have normal, healthy babies. New AEDs are now available, and although they hold great promise for improving seizure control, we know little about their teratogenic effects in humans. Doctors must continue to monitor their patients carefully. There is no substitute for sound clinical judgment. In this litigious era we must refrain from practicing to protect ourselves but must attempt to find a balanced approach that offers the best chance of a successful outcome for all of our patients. Effective communication remains essential to providing good patient care while minimizing the risk of malpractice suits.

REFERENCES

1. Hauser WA, Hesdorffer DC. *Epilepsy: frequency, causes, and consequences.* Landover, MD: Epilepsy Foundation of America, 1990:1–53.
2. Betts TA. Neuropsychiatry. In: Laidlaw J, Richens A, Oxley J, eds. *A textbook of epilepsy.* Edinburgh: Churchill Livingstone, 1988:350–385.
3. Yerby MS. Pregnancy and epilepsy. *Epilepsia* 1991;32:51–59.
4. Hiilesmaa VK. Pregnancy and birth in women with epilepsy. *Neurology* 1992;42:8–11.
5. Delgado-Escueta AV, Janz D. Consensus guidelines: preconception counseling, management, and care of the pregnant woman with epilepsy. *Neurology* 1992;42:149–160.
6. Kallen B. A register study of maternal epilepsy and delivery outcome with special reference to drug use. *Acta Neurol Scand* 1986;73:253–259.
7. Katz JM, Devinsky O. Current management of epilepsy and pregnancy: fetal outcome, congenital malformations, and developmental delay. Submitted.

8. Yerby M, Koepsell T, Daling J. Pregnancy complications and outcomes in a cohort of women with epilepsy. *Epilepsia* 1985;26:631–635.

9. Bjerkdal T, Bahna SL. The course and outcome of pregnancy in women with epilepsy. *Acta Obstet Gynecol Scand* 1973;52:245–248.

10. Monson RR, Rosenberg L, Hartz SC. Diphenylhydantoin and selected congenital malformations. *New Engl J Med* 1973;289:1049–1052.

11. Montouris GD, Fenichel GM, McLain LW Jr. The pregnant epileptic. *Arch Neurol* 1979;36:601–603.

12. Nelson KB, Ellenberg JH. Maternal seizure disorder, outcome of pregnancy and neurologic abnormalities in the children. *Neurology* 1982;32:1247–1254.

13. Tanganelli P, Regesta G. Epilepsy, pregnancy, and major birth anomalies: an Italian prospective, controlled study. *Neurology* 1992;42:89–93.

14. Sabin M, Oxorn H. Epilepsy and pregnancy. *Obstet Gynecol* 1956;7:175–199.

15. Svigos JM. Epilepsy and pregnancy. *Aust NZ J Obstet Gynaecol* 1984;24:182–185.

16. Vert AP, Deblay MF. Infants of epileptic mothers. In: Stern L, ed. *Intensive care in the newborn II.* New York: Masson, 1979:347–360.

17. Wilhelm J, Morris D, Hotham N. Epilepsy and pregnancy: a review of 98 pregnancies. *Aust NZ J Obstet Gynaecol* 1990;4:290.

18. Eller DP, Patterson A, Webb G. Maternal and fetal implications of anticonvulsive therapy during pregnancy. *Obstet Gynecol Clin NA* 1997;24:523–534.

19. Hiilesmaa VK, Bardy A, Teramo K. Obstetric outcome in women with epilepsy. *Am J Obstet Gynecol* 1985;152:499–504.

20. Kallen B. A register study of maternal epilepsy and delivery outcome with special reference to drug use. *Acta Neurol Scand* 1986;73:253–259.

21. Woolley DE, Timiras PS. Estrous and circadian periodicity and electroshock convulsions in rats. *Am J Physiol* 1962;202:379–382.

22. Medeiros YS, Calixto JB. Inhibitory effect of diphenylhydantoin on myometrium from pregnant women in vitro. A comparative study with nicardipine and trifluoperazine. *Pharmacol Res* 1990;22:597–603.

23. Sabin M, Oxorn H. Epilepsy and pregnancy. *Obstet Gynecol* 1956;7:175–179.

24. Bjerkdal T, Bahna SL. The course and outcome of pregnancy in women and epilepsy. *Acta Obstet Gynecol Scand* 1973;52:245–248.

25. Yerby MS, Koepsell T, Daling J. Pregnancy complications and outcomes in a cohort of women with epilepsy. *Epilepsia* 1985;26:631–635.

26. Egenaes J. Outcome of pregnancy in women with epilepsy—Norway 1967 to 1978: complications during pregnancy and delivery. In: Janz D, Dam M, Richens A, et al, eds. *Epilepsy, pregnancy, and the child.* New York: Raven Press, 1982:81–85.

27. Robertson IG. Breech presentation associated with anticonvulsant drugs. *J Obstet Gynaecol* 1984;4:174–177.

28. Schmidt D. The effect of pregnancy on the natural history of epilepsy: a review of the literature. In: Janz D, Dam M, Richens A, et al, eds. *Epilepsy, pregnancy, and the child.* New York: Raven Press, 1982:3–14.

29. Yerby MS. Pregnancy and epilepsy. *Epilepsia* 1991:32:51–59.

30. Swartjes JM, van Geijn HP. Pregnancy and epilepsy. *Eur J Obstet Gynecol Reprod Biol* 1998;79:3–11.

31. Knight AH, Rhind EG. Epilepsy and pregnancy: a study of 153 pregnancies in 59 patients. *Epilepsia* 1975;16:99–110.

32. Schmidt D, Canger R, Avanzini G. Change in seizure frequency in pregnant epileptic women. *J Neurol Neurosurg Psychiatry* 1983;46:751–755.

33. Katz JM, Devinsky O. Primary generalized epilepsy: a risk factor for seizures in labor and delivery. Submitted.

34. Yerby MS, Devinsky O. Epilepsy and pregnancy. *Adv Neurol* 1994;64:45.

35. Yerby MS. Treatment of epilepsy during pregnancy. In: Wyllie E, ed. *The treatment of epilepsy: principles and practice.* Philadelphia: Lea & Febiger, 1993:844–857.

36. Svigos JM. Epilepsy and pregnancy. *Aust NZ J Obstet Gynaecol* 1984;24:182–185.

37. Otani K. Risk factors for the increased seizure frequency during pregnancy and the puerperium. *Folia Psychiatr Neurol Jpn* 1985;39:33–42.

38. Gjerde IO, Strandjord RE, Ulstein M. The course of epilepsy during pregnancy: a study of 78 cases. *Acta Neurol Scand* 1988;78:198–205.

39. Mastroiacovo P, Bertollini R, Licata D. Fetal growth in the offspring of epileptic women: results of an Italian multicentric cohort study. *Acta Neurol Scand* 1988;78:110–114.

40. Morrell JM. Maximizing the health of women with epilepsy: science and ethics in new drug development. *Epilepsia* 1997;38:32–41.

41. Nulman I, Laslo D, Koren G. Treatment of epilepsy in pregnancy. *Drugs* 1999;4:535–544.

42. Morrell M. Hormones and epilepsy through the lifetime. *Epilepsia* 1992;33:49–61.

43. Sabers A, a'Rogvi-Hansen B, Dam M, et al. Pregnancy and epilepsy: a retrospective study of 151 pregnancies. *Acta Neurol Scand* 1998;97:164–170.

44. Dravet C, Julian C, Legras C, et al. Epilepsy, antiepileptic drugs, and malformations in children of women with epilepsy: a French prospective cohort study. *Neurology* 1992;42:72–82.

45. Tanganelli P, Regesta G. Epilepsy, pregnancy, and major birth anomalies. *Neurology* 1992;42:89–93.

46. Schmidt D. The effect of pregnancy on the natural history of epilepsy: review of the literature. In: Janz D, Dam M, Richens A, et al, eds. *Epilepsy, pregnancy, and the child.* New York: Raven Press, 1982:3–14.

47. Schmidt D. The effect of pregnancy on the natural history of epilepsy: Review of the literature. In Janz D, Dam M, Richens A, et al, eds. *Epilepsy, pregnancy, and the child.* New York: Raven Press, 1982:21–32.

48. Schmidt D. The effect of pregnancy on the course of epilepsy: a prospective study. In: Janz D, Dam M, Richens A, et al, eds. *Epilepsy, pregnancy, and the child.* New York: Raven Press, 1982:39–49.

49. Brady AH. Seizure frequency in epileptic women during pregnancy and puerperium: results of the prospective Helsinki study. In: Janz D, Dam M, Richens A, et al, eds. *Epilepsy, pregnancy, and the child.* New York: Raven Press, 1982:27–31.

50. Canger R, Avanzini G, Battino D, et al. Modifications of the seizure frequency in pregnant patients with epilepsy: a prospective study. In: Janz D, Dam M, Richens A, et al, eds. *Epilepsy, pregnancy, and the child.* New York: Raven Press, 1982:33–38.

51. Devinsky O. *A guide to understanding and living with epilepsy.* Philadelphia: FA Davis Co, 1994:18–29.

52. Bardy AH. Incidence of seizures during pregnancy, labor and puerperium in epileptic women: a prospective study. *Acta Neurol Scand* 1987;75:356–360.

53. Leavitt AM, Yerby MS, Robinson N, et al. Epilepsy in pregnancy: developmental outcome of offspring at 12 months. *Neurology* 1992;42:141–143.

54. Gjerde IO, Strandjord RE, Ulstein M. The course of epilepsy during pregnancy: a study of 78 cases. *Acta Neurol Scand* 1988;78:198–205.

55. Earnest MP, Thomas GE, Eden RA, et al. The sudden unexplained death syndrome in epilepsy: demographic, clinical and postmortem features. *Epilepsia* 1992;33:310–316.

56. Farmer DL, Adzick S, Crombleholme WR, et al. Fetal trauma: relation to maternal injury. *J Ped Surg* 1990; 25:711–714.

57. Rogers FB, Roxycki GS, Osler TM, et al. A multi-institutional study of factors associated with fetal death in injured pregnant patients. *Arch Surg* 1999;134: 1274–1277.

58. Corsi PR, Rasslan S, de Oliveira LB, et al. Trauma in pregnant women: analysis of maternal and fetal mortality. *Epilepsy Res* 1999;30:239–243.

59. Drost TF, Rosemurgy AS, Sherman HF, et al. Major trauma in pregnant women: maternal/fetal outcome. *J Trauma* 1990;30:574–578.

60. McDuffie RS, Bader T. Fetal meconium peritonitis after maternal hepatitis A. *Am J Obstet Gynecol* 1999; 180:1031–1032.

61. Pak LL, Reece EA, Chan L. Is adverse pregnancy outcome predictable after blunt abdominal trauma? *Am J Obstet Gynecol* 1998;179:1140–1144.

62. Pearlman MD, Tintinalli JE, Lorenz RP. Blunt trauma during pregnancy. *N Engl J Med* 1990;323: 1609–1613.

63. Speidel BD, Meadow SR. Maternal epilepsy and abnormalities of the fetus and newborn. *Lancet* 1972;2:839–843.

64. Higgins TA, Commerford JB. Epilepsy and pregnancy. *J Irish Med Assoc* 1974;67:317–320.

65. Beaussart-Defaye J, Basten N, Demarca C, et al. *Epilepsies and reproduction. II.* Grine Lille, France: Nord Epilepsy Research and Information Group, 1986.

66. Shuster EA. Epilepsy in women. *Mayo Clin Proc* 1996;71:991–999.

67. Janz D, Beck-Mannagetta G, Sander T. Do idiopathic epilepsies share a common susceptibility gene? *Neurology* 1992;42:48–55.

68. Cohen M, Campbell R, Yaghmai F. Neuropathological abnormalities in developmental dysphasia. *Ann Neurol* 1989;25:567–570.

69. Laegreid L, Olegard R, Walstrom J, et al. Teratogenic effects of benzodiazepine use during pregnancy. *J Pediatr* 1989;114:126–131.

70. Jones KL, Lacro RV, Johnson KA, et al. Pattern of malformation in the children of women treated with carbamazepine during pregnancy. *N Engl J Med* 1989; 320:1661–1666.

71. Granstrom ML, Gaily E. Psychomotor development in children of mothers with epilepsy. *Neurology* 1992;42: 144–148.

72. Kaneko S, Battino D, Andermann E, et al. Congenital malformations due to antiepileptic drugs. *Epilepsy Res* 1999;33:145–158.

73. Teramo K, Hiilesmaa V, Bardy A. Fetal heart rate during a maternal grand mal epileptic seizure. *J Perinat Med* 1979;7:3–6.

74. Nei M, Daly S, Liporace J. A maternal complex partial seizure in labor can affect fetal heart rate. *Neurology* 1998;51:904–906.

75. Katz J, Devinsky O. Primary generalized epilepsy: a risk factor for seizures in labor and delivery. Submitted.

76. Minkoff H, Schaffer RM, Delke I, et al. Diagnosis of intracranial hemorrhage in utero after a maternal seizure. *Obstet Gynecol* 1985;64:22–24.

77. Battino D, Granata T, Binelli S, et al. Intrauterine growth in the offspring of epileptic mothers. *Acta Neurol Scand* 1992;86:555–557.

78. Morrell M. The new antiepileptic drugs and women: efficacy, reproductive health, pregnancy and fetal outcome. *Epilepsia* 1996;37:34–44.

79. Steegers-Theunissen PMR, Renier WO, Borm FG, et al. Factors influencing the risk of abnormal pregnancy outcome in epileptic women: a multi-centre prospective study. *Epilepsy Res* 1994;18:261–269.

80. Nei M, Daly S, Liporace J. A maternal complex partial seizure in labor can affect fetal heart rate. *Neurology* 1998;51:904–906.

81. Remillard G, Dansky L, Andermann E, et al. Seizure frequency during pregnancy and the puerperium. In: Janz D, Dam M, Richens A, et al, eds. *Epilepsy, pregnancy, and the child.* New York: Raven Press, 1982: 15–26.

82. Devinsky O, Yerby MS. Women with epilepsy—reproduction and effects of pregnancy on epilepsy. *Neurol Clin* 1994;12:479–495.

83. Gaily E, Granstrom ML. A transient retardation of early postnatal growth in drug-exposed children of epileptic mothers. *Epilepsy Res* 1989;4:147–155.

84. Bruni J. Women's issues in the treatment of epilepsy. *Can J Neurol Sci* 1998;25:19–23.

85. Yerby MS. Problems and management of the pregnant woman with epilepsy. *Epilepsia* 1987;28:29–36.

86. Knight AH, Rhind EG. Epilepsy and pregnancy: a study of 153 pregnancies in 59 patients. *Epilepsia* 1975;16:99–110.

87. Philbert A, Dam M. The epileptic mother and her child. *Epilepsia* 1982;23:85–99.

88. Schmidt D, Conyen R, Avanzini G, et al. Change of seizure frequency in pregnant epileptic women. *J Neurol Neurosurg Psychiatry* 1983;46:751–755.

89. Bardy AH. Seizure frequency in epileptic women during pregnancy and the puerperium: results of the prospective Helsinki Study. In: Janz D, Bossi L, Dam M, et al, eds. *Epilepsy, pregnancy, and the child.* New York: Raven Press, 1982:27–31.

90. Bardy AH. Seizure frequency in epileptic women during pregnancy and the puerperium: results of the prospective Helsinki study. In: Janz D, Bossi L, Dam M, et al, eds. *Epilepsy, pregnancy, and the child.* New York: Raven Press, 1982:27–37.

91. Sabers A, a'Rogvi-Hansen B, Dam M, et al. Pregnancy and epilepsy: a retrospective study of 151 pregnancies. *Acta Neurol Scand* 1998;97:164–170.

92. Woolley DE, Timiras PS. The gonad-brain relationship: effects of female sex hormones on electroshock

convulsions in the rat. *Endocrinology* 1962;70: 196–209.

93. Stitt SL, Kinnard WJ. The effect of certain progestins and estrogens on the threshold of electrically induced seizure patterns. *Neurology* 1968;18:213–216.

94. Logothetis J, Harner R, Morrell F, et al. The role of estrogens in catamenial exacerbation of epilepsy. *Neurology* 1959;9:352–360.

95. Landgren S, Backstrom T, Kalistratov G. The effect of progesterone on the spontaneous interictal spike evoked by topical application of penicillin to the cat's cerebral cortex. *Acta Physiologica Scand* 1978;102:81–83.

96. Backstrom T, Zetterlund B, Blom S, et al. Effects of intravenous progesterone infusions on the epileptic discharge frequency in women with partial epilepsy. *Acta Neurolgica Scand* 1984;69:240–248.

97. Koch S, Losche G, Jager-Roman E, et al. Major and minor birth malformations and antiepileptic drugs. *Neurology* 1992;42:83–88.

98. Cramer J, Jones E. Reproductive function in epilepsy. *Epilepsia* 1991;32:19–26.

99. Herzog AG, Klein P, Ransil BJ. Three patterns of catamenial epilepsy. *Epilepsia* 1997;38:1082–1088.

100. Backstrom T. Epileptic seizures in women related to plasma estrogen and progesterone during the menstrual cycle. *Acta Neurol Scand* 1976;54:321–347.

101. Backstrom T. Premenstrual tension syndrome, catamenial epilepsy and their relation to plasma estrogen and progesterone. *Senologia* 1978;3:15–26.

102. Loiseau P, Legroux M, Henry PO. Epilepsies et grossesses. *Bordeaux Med* 1974;7:1157–1164.

103. Maroni E, Markoff R. Epilepsie and schwangerschaft. *Gynaecologia* 1969;168:418–421.

104. Canger R, Avanzini G, Battino D, et al. Modifications of seizure frequency in pregnant patients with epilepsy: a prospective study. In: Janz D, Bossi L, Dam M, et al, eds. *Epilepsy, pregnancy, and the child.* New York: Raven Press, 1982:33–38.

105. McClure JH. Idiopathic epilepsy in pregnancy. *Am J Obstet Gynecol* 1955;70:296–301.

106. Suter C, Klingman WO. Seizure states and pregnancy. *Neurology* 1957;7:105–118.

107. Ansell B, Clarke E. Epilepsy and menstruation. *Lancet* 1956;2:1232–1235.

108. Nakane Y, Oltuma T, Takahashi R. Multi-institutional study on the teratogenicity and fetal toxicity of anticonvulsants: a report of a collaborative study group in Japan. *Epilepsia* 1980;21:663–680.

109. Yerby MS. Pregnancy, teratogenesis, and epilepsy. *Neurol Clin* 1994;12:749–771.

110. South J. Teratogenic effects of anticonvulsants. *Lancet* 1972;2:1154.

111. Temkin NR, Davis GR. Stress as a risk factor for seizures among adults with epilepsy. *Epilepsia* 1984; 25:450–456.

112. Fenwick P. The influence of mind on seizure activity. In: Devinsky O, Theodore WH, eds. *Epilepsy and behavior.* New York: Wiley-Liss, 1991:405–419.

113. Mattson RH. Emotional effects on seizure occurrence. In: Smith D, Treiman D, Trimble M, eds. *Neurobehavioral problems in epilepsy.* New York: Raven Press, 1991:453–460.

114. Luciano D, Perrine K, Clayton B, et al. Stress as a seizure precipitant and its relationship to ictal focus. *Epilepsia* 1992;33:130.

115. Hauser WA. Epidemiology of alcohol use and epilepsy: The magnitude of the problem. In: Porter RJ, Mattson RH, Cramer JA, Diamond I, eds. *Alcohol and seizures.* Philadelphia: FA Davis Co, 1990:12–21.

116. Hoppener RJ, Kuyer A, van der Lugt PJ. Epilepsy and alcohol: the influence of social alcohol intake on seizures and treatment in epilepsy. *Epilepsia* 1983;24:459–467.

117. Mattson RH, Fay ML, Sturman JK, et al. The effect of various patterns of alcohol use on seizures in patients with epilepsy. In: Porter RJ, Mattson RH, Cramer JA, Diamond I, eds. *Alcohol and seizures.* Philadelphia: FA Davis Co, 1990:233–240.

118. Egenaes J. Outcome of pregnancy in women with epilepsy—Norway 1967–1978: complications during pregnancy and delivery. In: Janz D, Dam M, Richens A, et al, eds. *Epilepsy, pregnancy, and the child.* New York: Raven Press, 1982:81–85.

119. Hiilesmaa VK, Bardy AH, Teramo K. Obstetrical outcome in women with epilepsy. *Am J Obstet Gynecol* 1985;152:499–504.

120. Ottman R, Annegers JF, Hauser WA, et al. Higher risk of seizures in offspring of mothers than fathers with epilepsy. *Am J Hum Genet* 1988;43:357–364.

121. Seale SG, Morrell MJ, Nelson L, et al. Analysis of prenatal and gestational care given to women with epilepsy. *Neurology* 1998;51:1039–1045.

122. Speidel BD, Meadow SR. Maternal epilepsy and abnormalities of the fetus and the newborn. *Lancet* 1972; 2:839–843.

123. Nakane Y. Congenital malformations among infants of epileptic mothers treated during pregnancy. *Folia Psychiatr Neurol Jpn* 1979;33:363–369.

124. Fedrick J. Epilepsy and pregnancy: a report from the Oxford Record Linkage Study. *BMJ* 1973;2:442–448.

125. Nakane Y, Okuma T, Takahashi R. Multi-institutional study on the teratogenicity and fetal toxicity of anticonvulsants: a report of a collaborative study group in Japan. *Epilepsia* 1980;21:663–680.

126. Philbert A, Dam M. The epileptic mother and her child. *Epilepsia* 1982;23:85–99.

127. Annegers JF, Hauser WA, Elveback LR, et al. Congenital malformations and seizure disorders in the offspring of parents with epilepsy. *Int J Epidemiol* 1978; 7:241–247.

128. Lowe CR. Congenital malformations among infants born to epileptic women. *Lancet* 1973;1:9–10.

129. Egenaes J. Outcome of pregnancy in women with epilepsy—Norway, 1967–1978: complications during pregnancy and delivery. In: Janz D, Bossi L, Dam M, et al, eds. *Epilepsy, pregnancy, and the child.* New York: Raven Press, 1982:75–80.

130. Hill RM, Tennyson L. Premature delivery, gestational age, complications of delivery, vital data at birth on newborn infants of epileptic mothers: a review of the literature. In: Janz D, Bossi L, Dam M, et al, eds. *Epilepsy, pregnancy, and the child.* New York: Raven Press, 1982:167–173.

131. Kalter H, Warkany J. Congenital malformations. *N Engl J Med* 1983;308:491–497.

132. Knight AH, Rhind EG. Epilepsy and pregnancy: a study of 153 pregnancies in 59 patients. *Epilepsia* 1975;16:99–110.

133. Akhtar N, Millac P. Epilepsy and pregnancy: a study of 188 pregnancies in 92 patients. *Br J Clin Pract* 1987; 41:862–864.

134. Canger R, Battino D, Canevini MP, et al. Malformations in offspring of women with epilepsy: a prospective study. *Epilepsia* 1999;40:1231–1236.
135. Olafsson E, Hallgrimsson JT, Hauser WA, et al. Pregnancies of women with epilepsy: a population-based study in Iceland. *Epilepsia* 1998;39:887–892.
136. Sabers A, a'Rogvi-Hansen B, Dam M, et al. Pregnancy and epilepsy: a retrospective study of 151 pregnancies. *Acta Neurol Scand* 1998;97:164–170.
137. Olafsson E, Hallgrimsson TJ, Hauser AW, et al. Pregnancies of women with epilepsy: a population-based study in Iceland. *Epilepsia* 1998;39:887–892.
138. Canger R, Battino D, Canevini PM, et al. Malformations in offspring of women with epilepsy: a prospective study. *Epilepsia* 1999;40:1231–1236.
139. Battino D, Binelli S, Caccamo ML, et al. Malformations in offspring of 305 epileptic women: a prospective study. *Acta Neurol Scand.* 1992;85:204–207.
140. Waters CH, Belai Y, Gott PS, et al. Outcomes of pregnancy associated with antiepileptic drugs. *Arch Neurol* 1994;51:250–253.
141. Shakir RA, Abdulwahab B. Congenital malformations before and after onset of maternal epilepsy. *Acta Neurol Scand* 1991;84:153–156.
142. Najmaldin A, Francis J, Postle A, et al. Vitamin K coagulation status in surgical newborns and the risk of bleeding. *J Pediatr Surg* 1993;28:138–143.
143. Lane PA, Hathaway WE. Vitamin K in infancy. *J Pediatr* 1985;106:351–359.
144. Verity CM, Carswell F, Scott GL. Vitamin K deficiency causing infantile intracranial hemorrhage after the neonatal period. *Lancet* 1983;1:1439.
145. Shapiro DA, Jacobson JL, Armon EM, et al. Vitamin K deficiency in the newborn infant: prevalence and perinatal risk factors. *J Pediatr* 1968;109:675–680.
146. Kalter H, Warkany. J. Congenital malformations. *N Engl J Med* 1983;308:491–497.
147. Philbert A, Dam M. The epileptic mother and her child. *Epilepsia* 1982;23:85–99.
148. Dansky LV, Finnel RH. Parental epilepsy, anticonvulsant drugs and reproductive outcome: epidemiological and experimental findings spanning three decades. II Human studies. *Reprod Toxicol* 1991;5:281–299.
149. Janz D, Fuchs U. Are antiepileptic drugs harmful when given during pregnancy? *German Medicine Monthly* 1964;9:20–22.
150. Meadow SR. Anticonvulsant drugs and congenital abnormalities. *Lancet* 1968;2:1296.
151. Meyer JG. The teratological effects of anticonvulsants and the effects of pregnancy and birth. *Eur Neurol* 1973;10:179–180.
152. Mountain KR, Hirsh J, Gallus AS. Maternal coagulation defect due to anticonvulsant treatment in pregnancy. *Lancet* 1970;1:265–268.
153. Monnet P, Rossenberg D, Bovier-Lapierre M. Therapeutique anticomitiere pendant la grossesse et maladie hemorragique du nouveau ne. *Rev Fr Gynecol Obstet* 1968;63:695–702.
154. Traggis DG, Maunz DL, Baroudy R. Hemorrhage in a neonate of a mother on anticonvulsant therapy. *J Pediatr Surg* 1984;19:598–599.
155. Van Creveld S. Nouveaux aspects de la maladie hemorragique du nouveau ne. *Ned Tijdschr Geneeskd* 1957;101:2109–2112.
156. Vert P, Deblay MF. Hemorrhagic disorders in infants of epileptic mothers. In: Janz D, Dam M, Richens A, et al., eds. *Epilepsy, pregnancy, and the child.* New York: Raven Press, 1982:53–60.
157. Hathaway WE, Bonnar J. *Perinatal coagulation.* New York: Grune & Stratton, 1978:27–43.
158. Cornelissen M, Steegers-Theunissen R, Kolleée L, et al. Supplementation of vitamin K in pregnant women receiving anticonvulsant therapy prevents neonatal vitamin K deficiency. *Am J Obstet Gynecol* 1993;168:884–888.
159. Leavitt MA, Yerby SM, Robinson N, et al. Epilepsy in pregnancy: developmental outcome of offspring at 12 months. *Neurology* 1992;42:141–143.
160. Motohara K, Takagi S, Endo F, et al. Oral supplementation of vitamin K for pregnant women and effects on levels of plasma vitamin K and PIVKA-II in the neonate. *J Pediatr Gastroenterol Nutr* 1990;11:32–36.
161. Deblay MF, Vert P, Andre M, et al. Transplacental vitamin K prevents haemorrhagic disease of infant of epileptic mother. *Lancet* 1982;1:1247.
162. Davies VA, Argent AC, Staub H, et al. Precursor prothrombin status in patients receiving anticonvulsant drugs. *Lancet* 1985;1:126–128.
163. Hey E. Effect of maternal anticonvulsant treatment on neonatal blood coagulation. *Arch Dis Child Fetal Neonatal Ed* 1999;81:208–210.
164. Srinivasan G, Seeler RA, Tiruvury A, et al. Maternal anticonvulsant therapy and hemorrhagic disease of the newborn. *Obstet Gynecol* 1982;59:250–252.
165. Desmond MM, Schwanecke RP, Wilson GS, et al. Maternal barbiturate utilization and neonatal withdrawal symptomatology. *J Pediatr* 1972;80:190–197.
166. Hiilesmaa VK, Teramo K, Granstrom ML, et al. Fetal head growth retardation associated with maternal antiepileptic drugs. *Lancet* 1981;2:165–167.
167. Kalter H, Warkany J. Congenital malformations. *N Engl J Med* 1983;308:491–497.
168. Weber M. Medicaments antiepileptiques et teratogenese. *Rev Neurol (Paris)* 1987;143:413–419.
169. Fris ML. Malformations in children of epileptic patients. In: Dam M, Gram L, eds. *Comprehensive epileptologie.* New York: Raven Press, 1990:309–319.
170. Kelly TE. Teratogenicity of anticonvulsant drugs I: review of the literature. *Am J Med Genet* 1984;19:413–434.
171. Meadow SR. Anticonvulsant drugs and congenital anomalies. *Lancet* 1968;2:1269.
172. Druner M, Greenburg DA, Delgado-Escueta A. Is there a genetic relationship between epilepsy and birth defects? *Neurology* 1992;42:63–67.
173. Monson RR, Rosenberg, Hartz SC. Diphenyhydantoin and selected congenital malformations. *N Engl J Med* 1973;289:1049–1052.
174. Dansky LV, Andermann E, Sherwin AL. Maternal epilepsy and congenital malformations: a prospective study with monitoring of plasma anticonvulsant levels during pregnancy. *Neurology* 1980;3:15.
175. Lindhout D, Hoppener RJ, Meinardi H. Teratogenicity of antiepileptic drug combinations with special emphasis on epoxidation (of carbamazepine). *Epilepsia* 1984;25:77–83.
176. Nakane Y. Congenital malformation among infants of epileptic mothers treated during pregnancy. *Folia Psychiatric Neurol Jpn* 1979;33:363–369.
177. Greenberg DA, Durner M, Delgado-Escueta AV. Evi-

dence for multiple gene loci in the expression of the common generalized epilepsies. *Neurology* 1992;42: 56–62.

178. Delgado-Escueta AV, Gee MN, Medina MT, et al. *Genetics of common idiopathic generalized epilepsies.* (Abstract)

179. Lindhout D, Meinardi H, Meijer WA, et al. Antiepileptic drugs and teratogenesis in two consecutive cohorts: Changes in prescription policy paralleled by changes in pattern of malformations. *Neurology* 1992;42: 94–110.

180. Squier W, Hope PL, Lindenbaum RH. Neocerebellar hypoplasia in a neonate following intrauterine exposure to anticonvulsants. *Dev Med Child Neurol* 1990; 32:725–742.

181. Marden PM, Smith DW, McDonald MJ. Congenital anomalies in the newborn infant, including minor variations. *J Pediatr* 1964;64:357.

182. Koch S, Losche G, Jager-Roman E, et al. Major and minor birth malformations and antiepileptic drugs. *Neurology* 1992;42:83–88.

183. McGarth C, Buist A, Norman TR. Treatment of anxiety during pregnancy: effects of psychiatric drug treatment on the developing fetus. *Drug Saf* 1999;20: 171–186.

184. Monson RR, Rosenberg L, Hartz SC. Diphenylhydantoin and selected congenital malformations. *N Engl J Med* 1973;289:1049–1052.

185. South J. Teratogenic effects of anticonvulsants. *Lancet* 1972;2:1154.

186. Kaneko S, Otani K, Kondo T, et al. Malformation in infants of mothers with epilepsy receiving antiepileptic drugs. *Neurology* 1992;42:68–74.

187. Yerby MS, Leavitt A, Erickson DM, et al. Antiepileptics and the development of congenital anomalies. *Neurology* 1992;42:132–140.

188. Eskazan E, Aslan S. Antiepileptic therapy and teratogenicity in Turkey. *Int J Clin Pharmacol Ther Toxicol* 1992;30:261–264.

189. Kaneko S, Otani K, Fukushima, et al. Teratogenicity of antiepileptic drugs: analysis of possible risk factors. *Epilepsia* 1988;29:459–467.

190. Holmes LB, Harvey EA, Brown KS, et al. Anticonvulsant teratogenesis: I. A study design for newborn infants. *Teratology* 1994;49:202–207.

191. Lindhout D, Omtzigt JG. Pregnancy and the risk of teratogenicity. *Epilepsia* 1992;33:41–48.

192. Kaneko S, Otani K, Kondo T, et al. Malformations in infants of mothers with epilepsy receiving antiepileptic drugs. *Neurology* 1992;42:68–74.

193. Ornoy A. Outcome of children born to epileptic mothers treated with carbamazepine during epilepsy. *Arch Dis Child* 1996;75:517–520.

194. Lu MCK, Sammel MD, Cleveland R, et al. Digit effects produced by prenatal exposure to antiepileptic drugs. *Teratology.* 2000;61:277–283.

195. Gaily E, Granstrom MJ. Minor anomalies in children of mothers with epilepsy. *Neurology* 1992;42: 128–131.

196. Omtzigt JGC, Los FJ, Grobbee DE, et al. The risk of spina bifida aperta after first-trimester exposure to valproate in a prenatal cohort. *Neurology* 1992;42: 119–125.

197. Nulman I, Dionne L, Gideon K. Treatment of epilepsy in pregnancy. *Drugs* 1999;57:535–544.

198. Bossi L, Assael BM, Avanzini G, et al. Plasma levels and clinical effects of antiepileptic drugs in pregnant epileptic patients and their newborns. In: Johannessen SI, Morselli PL, Pippenger CE, et al, eds. *Antiepileptic therapy: advances in drug monitoring.* New York: Raven Press, 1980:9–18.

199. Dansky LV, Andermann E, Sherwin AL, et al. Maternal epilepsy and congenital malformations: a prospective study with monitoring of plasma anticonvulsant levels during pregnancy. *Neurology* 1980;3:15–18.

200. Lindhout D, Rene JE, Hoppener A, et al. Teratogenicity of antiepileptic drug combinations with special emphasis on epoxidation of carbamazepine. *Epilepsia* 1984;25:77–83.

201. Dickinson RG, Harland RC, Lynn RK, et al. Transmission of valproic acid (Depakene) across the placenta: half-life of the drug in the mother and baby. *J Pediatr* 1979;94:832–835.

202. Majewski F, Raft W, Fischer P, et al. Teratogenicity of anticonvulsant drugs (author's trans). *Dtsch Med Wochenschr* 1980;105:719–723.

203. Lindhout D, Omtzigt J, Cornel M. Spectrum of neural-tube defects in 34 infants prenatally exposed to antiepileptic drugs. *Neurology* 1992;42:111–118.

204. Takeda A, Okada H, Izumi M, et al. Protein binding of four antiepileptic drugs in maternal and umbilical cord serum. *Epilepsy Res* 1992;13:147–151.

205. Dravet C, Julian C, Legras C, et al. Epilepsy, antiepileptic drugs, and malformations in children with epilepsy: A French prospective cohort study. *Neurology* 1992;42:75–82.

206. Froescher W, Gugler R, Niesen M, et al. Protein binding of valproic acid in maternal and umbilical cord serum. *Epilepsia* 1984;25:244–249.

207. Anderson RC. Cardiac defects in children of mothers receiving anticonvulsant therapy during pregnancy. *J Pediatr* 1976;89:318–319.

208. Fris ML, Broeng-Nielsen B, Hein Sindrup EH, et al. Facial clefts among epileptic patients. *Arch Neurol* 1981;38:227–229.

209. Kaneko S, Battino D, Andermann E, et al. Congenital malformations due to antiepileptic drugs. *Epilepsy Res* 1999;33:145–158.

210. Samren EB, van Duijn CM, Christiaens GC, et al. Antiepileptic drug regimens and major congenital abnormalities in the offspring. *Ann Neurol* 1999;46: 739–746.

211. Samren EB, van Duijn C, Christiaens GCM, et al. Antiepileptic drug regimens and major congenital abnormalities in the offspring. *Ann Neurol* 1999;46: 739–746.

212. Delgado-Escueta AV, Janz D. Consensus guidelines: preconception counseling, management, and care of the pregnant woman with epilepsy. *Neurology* 1992; 42:211–222.

213. Janz D. Are antiepileptic drugs harmful when taken during pregnancy? *J Perinat Med* 1994;22:267–277.

214. Lindhout D, Meinardi H. Spina bifida and in utero exposure to valproate. *Lancet* 1984;2:396.

215. Robert E, Rosa F. Valproate and birth defects. *Lancet* 1983;2:1142.

216. Roas FW. Spina bifida in infants of women treated with carbamazepine during pregnancy. *N Engl J Med* 1991;324:674–677.

217. Dansky LV, Andermann E, Rosenblatt D. Anticonvulsants, folate levels, and pregnancy outcome: a prospective study. *Ann Neurol* 1987;21:176–182.

218. Omtzigt JG, Los FJ, Meijer JW, et al. The 10,11–epoxide-10,11–idol pathway of carbamazepine in early pregnancy in maternal serum, urine, and amniotic fluid: the effect of dose, comedication, and relation to outcome of pregnancy. *Ther Drug Monit* 1993;15: 1–10.

219. Strickler SM, Dansky LV, Miller MA. Genetic predisposition to phenytoin-induced birth defects. *Lancet* 1985;2:746–749.

220. Lindhout D, Meinardi JW, Nau H. Antiepileptic drugs and teratogenesis in ten consecutive cohorts: changes in prescription policy paralleled by changes in pattern of malformations. *Neurology* 1992;42:94–110.

221. Laegreid L, Kellerman M, Hedner T. Benzodiazepine amplification of valproate teratogenic effects in children of mothers with absence epilepsy. *Neuropediatrics* 1993;24:88–92.

222. Samren EB, van Duijn CM, Koch S. Maternal use of antiepileptic drugs and the risk of major congenital malformations: a joint European prospective study of human teratogenesis associated with maternal epilepsy. *Epilepsia* 1997;38:981–990.

223. Robert E, Guibaud P. Maternal valproic acid and congenital neural-tube defects. *Lancet* 1982;2:937.

224. Omtzigt JG, Nau H, Los FJ. The disposition of valproate and its metabolites in the late first trimester and early second trimester of pregnancy in maternal serum, urine, and amniotic fluid: effect of dose, comedication, and the presence of spina bifida. *Eur J Clin Pharmacol* 1992;43:381–388.

225. Rosa F. Spina bifida in infants of women treated with carbamazepine during pregnancy. *N Engl J Med* 1991;324:674–677.

226. Lindhout D, Omzigt JGC, Cornel MC. Spectrum of neural-tube defects in 34 infants prenatally exposed to antiepileptic drugs. *Neurology* 1992;42:111–118.

227. Clayton Smith J, Donnai D. Fetal valproate syndrome. *J Med Genet* 1995; 32: 724–727.

228. Lindhout D, Schmidt D. In-utero exposure to valproate and neural-tube defects. *Lancet* 1986;2:1392–1393.

229. Omtzigt JCG, Los FJ, Grobbee DE. et al. The risk of spins bifida aperta after first-trimester exposure to valproate in a prenatal cohort. *Neurology* 1992;42: 119–125.

230. Zackai EH, Mellman WJ, Neiderer B, et al. The fetal trimethadione syndrome. *J Pediatr* 1975;87:280–284.

231. Feldman GL, Weaver DD, Lovrien EW. The fetal trimethadione syndrome: report of an additional family and further delineation of this syndrome. *Am J Dis Child* 1977;131:89–92.

232. Goldman AS, VanDyke DC, Gupta C, Katsumata M. Elevated glucocorticoid receptor levels in lymphocytes of children with the fetal hydantoin syndrome. *Am J Med Genet* 1987;28:607–618.

233. Loughnan PM, Gold H, Vance JC. Phenytoin teratogenicity in man. *Lancet* 1973;1:70–72.

234. Hanson JW, Smith DW. The fetal hydantoin syndrome. *J Pediatr* 1975;87:285–290.

235. Hanson JW, Myrianthopoulos NC, Sedgwich MA, et al. Risks to the offspring of women treated with hydantoin anticonvulsants with emphasis on the fetal hydantoin syndrome. *J Pediatr* 1976;89:662–668.

236. Gaily E, Granstrom ML, Hiilesmaa V, et al. Minor anomalies in offspring of epileptic mothers. *J Pediatr* 1988;112:520–529.

237. Laegreid L, Olegard R, Whalstrom J, et al. Abnormalities in children exposed to benzodiazepines in utero. *Lancet* 1987;1:108–109.

238. Oguni M, Dansky L, Andermann E, Sherwin A, Andermann F. Improved pregnancy outcome in epileptic women in the last decade: relationship to maternal anticonvulsant therapy. *Brain Dev* 1992;14:371–380.

239. Rudd NL, Freedom RM. A possible primidone embryopathy. *J Pediatr* 1979;94:835–837.

240. Gustavson EE, Chen H. Goldenhar syndrome. Enteroencephalocele and aqueductal stenosis following fetal primidone exposure. *Teratology* 1985;32:13–17.

241. Seip M. Growth retardation, dysmorphic facies and minor malformations following massive exposure to phenobarbital in utero. *Acta Paediatr Scand* 1976;65: 617–621.

242. DiLiberti JH, Farndon PA, Dennis NR, et al. The fetal valproate syndrome. *Am J Med Genet* 1984;19: 473–481.

243. Christianson A, Chester N, Kromberg J. Fetal valproate syndrome: clinical and neuro-developmental features in two sibling pairs. *Dev Med Chil Neurol* 1994;36:357–369.

244. Bron JTJ, Van DerHarten HJ, Van Geiin HP. Prenatal ultrasonographic diagnosis of radial-ray reduction malformations. *Prenat Diagn* 1990;10:279–288.

245. Jager-Roman E, Deichi A, Jakob S, et al. Fetal growth major malformations and minor anomalies in infants born to women receiving valproic acid. *J Pediatr* 1986; 108:997–1004.

246. Ardinger HH, Atkin JF, Blacston RD, et al. Verification of the fetal valproate syndrome phenotype. *Am J Med Genetics* 1988;29:171–185.

247. Jones KL, Lacro RV, Johnson KA, et al. Pattern of malformations in the children of women treated with carbamazepine during pregnancy. *N Engl J Med* 1989;320:1661–1666.

248. Tomson T, Lindbom U, Ekquist D, et al. Disposition of carbamazepine and phenytoin in pregnancy. *Epilepsia* 1994;35:131–135.

249. Koch S, Titze K, Zimmermann RB, et al. Long-term neuropsychological consequences of maternal epilepsy and anticonvulsant treatment during pregnancy for school-age children and adolescents. *Epilepsia* 1999;40:1237–1243.

250. Hill RM, Berniam WM, Morning MG, et al. Infants exposed in utero to antiepileptic drugs. *Am J Dis Child* 1974;127:645–652.

251. Barth PG. Disorders of neuronal migration. *Can J Neurol Sci* 1987;14:1–16.

252. Volpe JJ. Neuronal proliferation, migration, organization and myelinization. In: Volpe JJ, ed. *Neurology of the newborn.* Philadelphia: WB Saunders, 1981: 28–51.

253. Galaburda AM, Sherman GF, Rosen GD, et al. Developmental dyslexia: four consecutive patients with cortical anomalies. *Ann Neurol* 1985;18:222–223.

254. GRANT.

255. Losche G, Steinhausen HC, Koch S, et al. The psychological development of children of epileptic parents: II differential impact of intrauterine exposure to anticonvulsant drugs and further influential factors. *Acta Paediatr* 1994; 83:961–966.

256. Beck-Mannagetta G, Dress B, Janz D. Malformations and minor anomalies in the children of epileptic mothers: Preliminary results of the prospective Helsinki study. In Janz D, Dam M, Richens A, et al., eds.

Epilepsy, pregnancy and the child. New York, Raven Press. 1982:317–323.

257. Gaily E, Kantula-Sorsa E, Granstrom ML. Intelligence of children of epileptic mothers. *J Pediatr* 1988;113:677–684.

258. Holmes LB, Rosenberger PB, Harvey EA, et al. Intelligence and physical features of children of women with epilepsy. *Teratology* 2000;61:196–202.

259. Hill RM, Verniaud WM, Retting GM, et al. Relationship of antiepileptic drug exposure of the infant and developmental potential. In Janz D, Dam M, Richens A, et al, eds. *Epilepsy, pregnancy, and the child.* New York: Raven Press, 1982:IQ10.

260. Gaily E, Kantola-Sorsa E, Granstrom ML. Specific cognitive dysfunction in children with epileptic mothers. Developmental and child *Neurology* 1990;32:403–414.

261. Leavitt AM, Yerby MS, Robinson N, et al. Epilepsy and pregnancy: Developmental outcomes at 12 months. *Neurology* 1992;42:141–143.

262. Gaily E, Kantola-Sorsa E, Granstrom ML. Specific cognitive dysfunction in children with epileptic mothers. *Dev Child Neurol* 1990; 32:403–414.

263. Beck-Managetta. Malformations and minor anomalies in children of epileptic mothers: preliminary results of the prospective Helinsky study. In: Janz D, Dam M, Richens A, eds. *Epilepsy, pregnancy and the child.* New York: Raven Press, 1982:317–323.

264. Hill RM, Vernaiud WM, Retting GM. Relationship of antiepileptic drug exposure of the infant and developmental potential. In Janz D, Dam M, Richens A, eds. *Epilepsy, pregnancy and the child.* New York: Raven Press, 1982:325–332.

265. Percucca E. The new generation of antiepileptic drugs: advantages and disadvantages. *Br J Clin Pharmacol* 1996;42:531–543.

266. Ohman I, Vitols S, Tomson T. Lamotrigine in pregnancy: pharmacokinetics during delivery, in the neonate, and during delivery. *Epilepsia* 2000;41:709–713.

267. Greenwood RS. Adverse effects of antiepileptic drugs. *Epilepsia* 2000;41:42–52.

268. Data on File. Ortho-McNeil Pharmaceuticals. Raritan, NJ, 1996.

269. Sullivan FM, McElhatton PR. Teratogenic activity of the antiepileptic drugs, phenobarbital, phenytoin, and primidone in mice. *Toxicol Appl Pharmacol* 1975;34:271–282.

270. Jacobson CD, Autolick CL, Scholey R, et al. The influence of prenatal phenobarbital exposure on the growth of dendrites in the rat hippocampus. *Dev Brain Res* 1988;44:233–239.

271. Desmond MM, Schwanecke RP, Wilson GS, et al. Maternal barbiturate utilization and medical withdrawal symptomatology. *J Pediatr* 1972;80:190–197.

272. Delgado-Escueta A, Janz D. Consensus guidelines: preconception, counseling, management, and care of the pregnant woman with epilepsy. *Neurology* 1992; 42:149–160.

273. Rochester JA, Kirchner JT. Epilepsy in pregnancy. *Am Fam Physician* 1997;56:1631–1636.

274. Eadie MJ, Lander CM, Tyrer JH. Plasma drug level monitoring in pregnancy. *Clin Pharmacokinet* 1977; 2:427–436.

275. Lander CM, Edwards VE, Eadie MJ, et al. Plasma an-

ticonvulsant concentrations during pregnancy. *Neurology* 1977;27:71–78.

276. Dam M, Christiansen J, Munck O, et al. Antiepileptic drugs: metabolism in pregnancy. *Clin Pharmacokinet* 1979;4:53–62.

277. Nau H, Kuhnz W, Egger HJ, et al. Anticonvulsants during pregnancy and lactation. Transplacental, maternal and neonatal pharmacokinetics. *Clin Pharmacokinet* 1982;7:508–543.

278. Yerby MS, Friel PN, McCormick K. Antiepileptic drug disposition during pregnancy. *Neurology* 1992;42:12–16.

279. Dansky L, Andermann E, Sherwin AL, et al. Plasma levels of phenytoin during pregnancy and the puerperium. In: Janz D, Bossi L, Dam M, et al, eds. *Epilepsy, pregnancy, and the child.* New York: Raven Press, 1982,155–162.

280. Janz D. Antiepileptic drugs and pregnancy: altered utilization patterns and teratogenesis. *Epilepsia* 1982;23:53–62.

281. Ramsay RE, Strauss RG, Wilder BJ, et al. Status epilepticus in pregnancy: effect of phenytoin malabsorption on seizure control. *Neurology* 1978;28:85–89.

282. Parry E, Shields R, Turnbull AC. Transit time in the small intestine in pregnancy. *J Obst Gynaecol Brit Comm* 1970;77:900–901.

283. Perucca E, Crema A. Plasma protein binding of drugs in pregnancy. *Clin Pharmacokinet* 1982;7:336–352.

284. Yerby MS, Friel PN, McCormick KB, et al. Pharmacokinetics of anticonvulsants in pregnancy: alterations in plasma protein binding. *Epilepsy Res* 1990;5:223–238.

285. Dam M, Christiansen J, Munck O. Antiepileptic drugs: metabolism in pregnancy. *Clin Pharmacokinet* 1979; 4:53–62.

286. Chen SS, Perucca E, Lee JN, et al. Serum protein binding and free concentration of phenytoin and phenobarbitone in pregnancy. *Brit J Clin Pharmacol* 1982;13:547–552.

287. Krauer B, Krauer F. Drug kinetics in pregnancy. *Clin Pharmacokinet* 1977;2:167–181.

288. Lindhout D, Meinardi H, Meijer J, et al. Antiepileptic drugs and teratogenesis in two consecutive cohorts: changes in prescription policy paralleled by changes in pattern of malformations. *Neurology* 1992;42:94–110.

289. Ohman I, Vitols S, Tomson T. Lamotrigine in pregnancy: pharmacokinetics during delivery, in the neonate and during lactation. *Epilepsia* 2000;41:709–713.

290. Jensen ON, Olsen OV. Subnormal serum folate due to anticonvulsant therapy: a double-blind study of the effect of folic acid treatment in patients with drug-induced subnormal serum folate. *Arch Neurol* 1970;22:181–182.

291. Olsen OV, Jensen DN. The influence of folic acid on phenytoin (DPH) metabolism and the 24-hours fluctuation in urinary output of 5-(p-hydroxyphenyl)-5 phenyl-hydantoin (HPPH). *Acta Pharmacol Toxicol* 1970;28:265–269.

292. Baylis EM, Crowley JM, Preece JM, et al. Influence of folic acid on blood-phenytoin levels. *BMJ* 1971;1:62–64.

293. Strauss RG, Bernstein R. Folic acid and Dilantin antagonism in pregnancy. *Obstet Gynecol* 1974;44:345–348.

Neurological Complications of Pregnancy, Second Edition, edited by Brian Hainline and Orrin Devinsky. Lippincott Williams & Wilkins, Philadelphia, © 2002.

15

Movement Disorders

Alireza Minagar, Alejandro Rabinstein, Lisa M. Shulman, and William J. Weiner

Department of Neurology, University of Maryland School of Medicine, Baltimore, Maryland, U.S.A.

The occurrence of movement disorders during pregnancy represents an unusual clinical problem. The effect of pregnancy on individual movement disorders and the effect of treatment of the movement disorder on the outcome of the pregnancy are poorly studied. Some movement disorders (Parkinson's disease and parkinsonism) occur for the most part in postmenopausal women; other movement disorders (Wilson's disease and Huntington's disease) if manifest and untreated often have decreased fertility rates associated with them; and some movement disorders (chorea gravidarum) are associated with underlying disorders. This chapter provides an overview of movement disorders pertinent to women of childbearing ages, and addresses management issues relevant to pregnancy and the developing fetus.

PREGNANCY AND PARKINSON'S DISEASE

Parkinson's disease (PD) is a common progressive neurologic disease first described in 1817 by James Parkinson, an English physician. The exact incidence and prevalence of PD is unknown. Estimates of the prevalence in the United States vary from 300,000 to 1 million individuals. The incidence ratio ranges from 4.5 to 21.0 per 100,000 population, reflecting in part a variation of study designs, case ascertainment, and definition of disease. PD is uncommon before age 50, and both the prevalence and incidence rise sharply

thereafter. Most cases of PD start between 50 and 70 years of age (1,2).

Clinically, PD is characterized by resting tremor, bradykinesia, rigidity, and loss of postural reflexes. Resting tremor is the most easily recognized sign of PD and is often asymmetric. Bradykinesia is among the most disabling symptoms of PD and manifests with difficulties in activities of daily living such as writing, shaving, and buttoning buttons. Muscle tone is increased in both flexor and extensor muscles of parkinsonian patients, providing constant resistance to passive movements of the joints. When rigidity is superimposed on tremor, a ratchet-like phenomenon, known as cogwheeling, may be detected. Loss of postural reflexes in more advanced PD causes imbalance and falls. Dystonia can occur in PD. Dystonia in PD patients may be an initial manifestation of the disease process or a side effect of drug treatment. Nonmotor symptoms of PD include cognitive decline, sleep disturbances, sensory alterations, akathesia and restless legs syndrome, decreased olfactory ability, diminished visual contrast sensitivity, and autonomic dysfunction.

The major histopathologic finding in PD consists of degeneration of pigmented neurons of the pars compacta of the substantia nigra. The changes in the substantia nigra correlate with motor symptomatology. Another prominent histopathologic feature of PD is the Lewy body. Lewy bodies are a distinctive intraneuronal inclusion of complex biochemical composition found in neurons of the sub-stantia nigra and regarded as a diagnostic hallmark that helps distinguish idiopathic PD from other parkinsonian syndromes. Histo-pathologic diagnosis of PD requires both neu-rodegenerative alterations and the presence of Lewy bodies.

The etiology of PD is unknown. The pres-ence of genetic susceptibility factors are strongly suspected. In recent years, well-doc-umented pedigrees with dominant inheritance have been reported, but this pattern is clearly exceptional. One large pedigree of familial parkinsonism has been linked to a mutation of alpha-synuclein. Two genes—alpha-synuclein and ubiquitin carboxy-terminal hydrolase L1 (3)—and two gene loci on chromosomes 2p13 and 4p14–16.3 have been implicated in the pathogenesis of autosomal dominant PD (4,5). Recently, mutations in another gene designated as Parkin have been identified in several families with autosomal recessive early-onset PD (6).

Pregnancy in women with PD is uncom-mon, and our knowledge of the effects of pregnancy on PD is limited. The majority of PD patients are beyond childbearing age, and only 2% of patients with PD are diagnosed before age 50 (7). There are many unanswered questions about the interaction of pregnancy and PD, including the possible teratogenicity of levodopa/carbidopa and dopamine agonists and the effect of the pregnancy on the pa-tient's clinical course. Information about pregnancy in the context of PD is important for counseling of patients and to better under-stand the physiologic changes of pregnancy on parkinsonism. Levodopa crosses the pla-centa and is metabolized by the fetus, whereas carbidopa does not (8). Another factor is the influence(s) of rising female sex hormones on dopaminergic transmission and sensitivity of basal ganglia (9–12).

A review of the literature reveals a total of 36 pregnancies among 27 women with PD (7,13–20). In eight of these pregnancies, the patients did not receive any antiparkinsonian medications (7,13,15). In 17 (47%) of the pregnancies, worsening of PD symptoms or

occurrence of new symptoms during or shortly after pregnancy were reported (Table 15.1). Reported complications of pregnancy in women with PD who were treated with an-tiparkinsonian agents include (i) first trimester spotting (7,13); (ii) nausea and vomiting (7); (iii) spontaneous miscarriage (7,16); and (iv) preeclampsia, breech presen-tation, and an infant with inguinal hernia (7). In one patient, levodopa dosage rose pro-gressively through pregnancy, reaching a peak does of nearly twice the pre-pregnancy dose at 2 months postpartum (20). The dete-rioration or onset of PD symptoms during pregnancy might imply that there is a risk of worsening PD during pregnancy. The tempo-ral relationship reported in some patients be-tween deterioration of PD with advancing pregnancy further supports the impression that pregnancy may not only worsen symp-toms of PD, but may do so for periods ex-ceeding the normally defined postpartum pe-riod.

The mechanism responsible for progres-sion of PD symptoms in some women both during pregnancy and in the early postpartum period remains unknown. There exist various reports of both dopaminergic and anti-dopaminergic effects of estrogen (21,22). However, more recent reports have suggested that estrogen replacement therapy may have a beneficial effect on PD (23). Estrogen may have dopamine-sparing properties that result

TABLE 15.1. *Reported changes in parkinsonian symptoms during pregnancy*

Changes (reference number)	Number of pregnancies
Worsening/onset of symptoms (14,17,21)	10
Transient worsening/onset of symptoms (14,15,17)	5
Worsening/onset of symptoms postpartum (14,18)	2
Transient worsening of L-dopa-induced chorea (14)	1
Transient improvement of dexterity (14)	1
Prolonged L-dopa effect (19)	1
None (13,14,20)	16

from inhibition of catechol-O-methyltransferase (COMT) gene expression (24) as well as the interaction of the estrogen metabolite, catecholestrogen, with COMT (25). This observation may explain the prominent increase of levodopa dosage sometimes observed in the early postpartum period when estrogen levels are declining rapidly.

The majority of reports lend support to the idea that levodopa/carbidopa does not have an adverse effect on the growing fetus. Cook and Klawans reported two PD patients with four pregnancies in which levodopa/carbidopa had no teratogenic effects (13). There are also four additional reports of healthy infants born to mothers receiving levodopa/benserazide (14,17,19,26).

There are reports of ten pregnancies in women without PD who were treated with levodopa during pregnancies for other reasons (26–29). Only one patient with dopa-responsive dystonia who was treated with levodopa-carbidopa developed toxemia; however, she delivered a normally developed child after 34 weeks of gestation (27). All other patients had full-term pregnancies and delivered normal children.

Administration of the D2 receptor agonists bromocriptine and lisuride to nonparkinsonian pregnant women was not associated with increased risk of complications of pregnancy, teratogenicity, or withdrawal symptoms in the newborn (30–33). One woman, who was treated with only bromocriptine during pregnancy, had no change in her parkinsonian motor status, had no complications of pregnancy, and delivered a normal infant (34). In preliminary studies of pergolide for endocrine disorders, two major and three minor congenital abnormalities among 38 pregnancies were found; however, a causal relationship was never established (35).

Other Antiparkinsonian Medications in Pregnancy and Lactation

Amantadine may be associated with first-trimester obstetric complications. There are four anecdotal reports of complications associated with amantadine use. These include a miscarriage, hydatiform mole, preeclampsia, and first-trimester hemorrhage (7). Nora and associates (36) reported an infant with single cardiac ventricle and pulmonary atresia whose mother had received amantadine during the first trimester. In one surveillance study, five major birth defects occurred among 51 infants exposed to amantadine during the first trimester (37).

Dopamine agonists potentially can inhibit physiologic lactation and are contraindicated in breastfeeding mothers. However, there exists one report of a patient who was able to breastfeed her infant while she was taking bromocriptine 5 mg daily for a pituitary tumor (38). Amantadine enters the breast milk in small quantities, but there have not been any reports of adverse effects on breastfed children (39). It is unknown whether levodopa or selegiline are excreted in milk.

Drug-Induced Parkinsonism

Clinicians caring for pregnant women should be alert to the possibility that drug-induced parkinsonism (DIP) can occur in this setting. DIP can present with bradykinesia, rigidity, tremor, and gait disturbance. This, of course, is an unusual group of signs to present in this age group, but parkinsonism can be induced by antiemetics used to treat nausea and vomiting associated with pregnancy. DIP usually can be distinguished from idiopathic PD because its onset is subacute (over weeks), the motor signs are bilateral and usually symmetric, and there is a history of starting a new drug with potential dopamine receptor blocking activity. Treatment of DIP in this setting should be withdrawal of the offending agent.

PREGNANCY AND WILSON'S DISEASE

Wilson's disease (WD) is an autosomal recessive inherited disease of copper metabolism (40–41). It is a rare but widespread disease, believed to occur in 1 out of 40,000 individuals in most populations (40). Copper is an essential trace element, and most modern diets contain 1.0 mg/day (40). This amount is 25% more than the amount required, and almost 0.25 mg/day must be excreted (40). In contrast to most other cations whose balance is regulated by the intestine, the kidney, or both, copper balance exclusively involves the liver. The normal mechanism for elimination of excess copper is hepatic excretion into the bile for removal in the stool (42). Patients with WD have a defect in this excretory pathway (43–44). As a result of the defect in the excretory pathway, patients with WD accumulate minute amounts of copper everyday of their lives. The excess copper is stored in the liver. Eventually, the storage capacity of the liver is exceeded, resulting in hepatic damage and spillover of copper into widespread organs in the body.

WD is caused by a homozygous state for a mutation or mutations in the WD locus on the long arm of the chromosome 13q14.3. The gene recently has been cloned and is a copper-binding, membrane-associated, ATPase protein (45–48). The full-length DNA sequence reveals a predicted 1411 amino acid protein. It contains a WD protein and has a high degree of homology to the Menkes' disease product. Both are members of a cation-transporting P-type ATPase subfamily. The overall homology is 56%, but it is even greater in the phosphatased domain (78%) and the transduction-phosphorylation domains. Menkes' disease is an x-linked recessive disorder in which copper absorption is impaired, with consequent copper deficiency in body tissues, including the liver and brain. Ceruloplasmin also is reduced in Menkes' disease.

WD typically presents between the ages of 10 and 40 years, although presentations in early childhood and late in life also occur (40,41). Patients may present with hepatic, neurologic, or psychiatric disease, or a combination of these.

Prior to the introduction of penicillamine, successful pregnancy was almost unknown in patients with untreated symptomatic WD, although an occasional patient, with late onset, may have earlier carried a pregnancy to term successfully. However, most untreated patients even prior to the clinical manifestation of WD, and almost invariably after development of clinical signs of WD, will miscarry (49). This rarity of successful pregnancies in women with WD before treatment of WD has been attributed to menstrual irregularities and amenorrhea, the progressive course of hepatic disease, and neurologic and psychiatric abnormalities, which reduced the fertility rate and probability of conception among these patients (50–52). However, with early diagnosis of WD and proper treatment with anticopper medications, the prognosis and fertility rate have improved (49,53). Only patients with advanced hepatic disease, esophageal varices, or both are advised to avoid pregnancy because risks of bleeding are increased during pregnancy due to increased blood volume and intraabdominal pressure from an enlarging uterus. Apart from patients with severe hepatic disease, patients with WD can tolerate pregnancy. Restrictions on patients with severe hepatic disease due to WD are no different than restrictions on patients with other kinds of hepatic diseases.

The available anticopper medications include chelator-type drugs (such as penicillamine and trientine), zinc acetate (which blocks copper absorption), and tetrathiomolybdate (54). The initial treatment of patients presenting with neurologic or psychiatric disease is a source of current controversy. Tetrathiomolybdate, zinc, or both often are recommended because penicillamine carries the risk of severe neurologic worsening when used in this setting. Some patients deteriorate with penicillamine treatment and may never recover to their prepenicillamine baseline. Because trientine shares the mechanism of action of penicillamine, there is concern that it may share this deleterious effect. Tetrathiomolybdate blocks copper absorption and is absorbed in the blood, rendering copper into a nontoxic form. Tetrathiomolybdate is available as an experimental agent. In the majority of patients, treatment leads to a remarkable reduction or to a complete remission of symptoms so that the probability of a successful pregnancy increases. There are several reports of women discontinuing treatment during pregnancy to reduce the risk of teratogenicity; unfortunately, the patients suffered severe relapses, including death. (40,55). D-penicillamine also has been used in the chronic management of cystinuria. There is more experience with D-penicillamine in pregnancy as compared to other anticopper medications. D-penicillamine is a known teratogen in humans (56,57) and animals (58), and trientine is teratogenic in animals (58). Zinc has been found not to be teratogenic, and it is the treatment of choice for pregnant patients (54).

Successful pregnancies in patients with WD have been observed under treatment with D-penicillamine, zinc, and trientine. Drug therapy for WD should be continued during pregnancy because the advantages of continuation far outweigh the dangers of interruption. Pregnancies of patients with WD should be monitored carefully and closely.

CHOREA GRAVIDARUM

Chorea, derived from the Latin term chorus (to dance), consists of irregular, rapid, unpredictable, involuntary, and usually distal movements, which move randomly from one part of the body to another. This hyperkinetic movement may affect small muscle groups around the face and mouth.

Pregnancy rarely may present with chorea, known as chorea gravidarum (CG). Patients typically present with the abrupt onset of chorea during an otherwise uneventful pregnancy. CG is the symptom of underlying central nervous system dysfunction rather than a separate disease (Table 15.2). CG more frequently manifests in women with a prior history of Sydenham's chorea (SC), or the chorea may herald systemic lupus erythematosus (SLE) (59) or even Huntington's disease (HD) (60). Symptoms, which are often unilateral, include choreiform movements of the face, arm, and leg. Psychiatric symptoms such as emotional lability, subtle mental status changes, and psychosis may precede the movement disorder. Patients may appear restless and assume postures with crossed legs and clasped hands to suppress the chorea. The chorea may progress to hemiballismus, and in severe cases rhabdomyolysis, hyperthermia, and self-injury can occur. The chorea subsides with sleep. Prognosis depends on the underlying etiology, with an overall mortality rate of less than 1% (61).

The majority of cases are associated with autoimmune and rheumatic diseases. The patients with rheumatic CG have a history of rheumatic heart disease, recurrent tonsillitis, or Sydenham's chorea (62–64). The clinical syndrome manifests during the first trimester and often subsides in the mid to late second trimester. Neuroimaging studies usually are unremarkable. Serum antistreptolysin–O antibodies titers are elevated and may continue to rise during pregnancy. Patients frequently have overt cardiac involvement.

Autoimmune causes of CG include SLE, anticardiolipin antibody, and lupus anticoagulant (65–69). In this group, CG manifests during the second or third trimester with mental status changes such as agitation and confusion. These patients may develop strokes, transient ischemic attacks, rhabdomyolysis, seizures, hemiplegia, migraines, recurrent spontaneous abortion, venous thrombosis, cardiac valvular dysfunction, thrombocytopenia, and coma. Presence of hyperthermia is a poor prognostic factor. There is no history of autoimmunity. Patients with antiphospholipid antibodies and lupus anti-coagulant are predisposed to strokes; therefore, a complete workup is mandatory, especially in patients with a history of previous spontaneous abortion. In these patients no specific marker of disease activity, such as sedimentation rate, ANA titer, or complement

TABLE 15.2. *Etiologies of chorea gravidarum*

Rheumatic disease
Systemic lupus erythmatosus
Lupus anticoagulant
Anticardiolipin antibody
Wilson's disease
Huntington's disease
Thyrotoxicosis
Neuroacanthocytosis
Cerebrovascular accidents

level, is a reliable indicator of central nervous system involvement.

Neuroimaging may be normal or reveal focal abnormalities of the basal ganglia and caudate nucleus. Cerebrospinal fluid may be normal or reveal elevated protein or pleocytosis. Postmortem examinations have disclosed diffuse foci of hemorrhage throughout the brain, most evident in the basal ganglia and caudate nucleus. The main treatment modalities include immunosuppression with corticosteroids, but neuroleptics also may be effective. In patients with lupus anticoagulant, aspirin treatment may be indicated (70). Recurrence of CG with subsequent pregnancies, with occasional fatal outcome, has been reported.

Etiology

Chorea in the context of pregnancy has various etiologies with different treatment approaches and prognoses (Table 15.2). The concurrent widespread use of oral contraceptives and an increase in reports of chorea in young women points to estrogen as a possible cause. It is hypothesized that high estrogen states modify postsynaptic dopamine receptors and cause dopamine hypersensitivity (71). In the majority of cases, detailed history and neurologic examination as well as pertinent investigations reveal the diagnosis. Laboratory evaluation for diagnosis of CG includes complete blood count, serum electrolytes, hepatic function tests, toxicology screen, coagulation profile, lupus anticoagulant and anticardiolipin antibody, blood culture, antinuclear antibody, antistreptolysin–O antibody, echocardiography, peripheral blood smear for acanthocytes, and slit light examination of the eyes. Neuroimaging studies are of limited value in diagnosis and should be performed only in obscure cases when stroke, hemorrhage, or mass lesions are suspected.

Treatment

Treatment of CG is not usually necessary because chorea resolves postpartum or following correction of the underlying endocrine or metabolic disorder. However, in CG (that is clinically significant) due to rheumatic diseases the neuroleptics are useful. Tetrabenazine and sodium valproate also have been used as antichoreic agents. However, during the first trimester and especially during the limb-genesis period, neuroleptics, including haloperidol, should be avoided. For patients with CG in which treatment during the second and third trimesters is required, haloperidol is preferred because of a relative lack of embryotoxicity (72,73). Fetal limb deformity has been reported with the use of haloperidol during the limb-genesis period of the first trimester, although sufficient evidence to prove cause and effect is lacking (74,75). Tetrabenazine remains an investigational drug in the United States, and sodium valproate is not used for treatment of CG because of its potential embryotocxicity. The relapse rate during subsequent pregnancies is 25% (62).

PREGNANCY AND RESTLESS LEGS SYNDROME

Restless legs syndrome (RLS) is probably the most frequent movement disorder during pregnancy, occurring in 10% to 20% of pregnancies (76–77). RLS is described as an unpleasant crawling and burning sensation in the legs and sometimes in the arms associated with an irresistible desire to move the legs. It occurs most frequently at night while the patient is relaxed. RLS symptoms commence during the second or third trimester of pregnancy and improve after delivery (78). The pathophysiology of RLS remains an enigma, and neurologic examination is always normal. Recommended treatments include diazepam, clonazepam, and levodopa/carbidopa (79).

PREGNANCY AND DYSTONIA

Dystonia is characterized by sustained muscle contractions, frequently causing repetitive movements and abnormal postures or gestures. Dystonic movements can vary from slow to rapid and can be worse with exercise. Dystonia can present as focal, segmental, or generalized movements causing variable degrees of disability (80).

There is a higher prevalence of idiopathic focal dystonia in women than in men in all categories of focal dystonia (81), and it has been suggested that these differences could be related to the effect of the female reproductive hormones on the central nervous system (82). Menstruation- and pregnancy-related fluctuations in symptoms also have been described in patients with Parkinson's disease and Tourette syndrome (TS) (83–85). In a recent study, Gwinn-Hardy and colleagues (86) surveyed 204 women with dystonia in an attempt to determine if any relationship existed between the severity of their symptoms and female reproductive hormonal variations. The authors found that although there was no consistent hormonal effect on the patients' assessments of their dystonia symptom severity, 42% of premenstrual patients noted some change of their symptoms just before or during their menses. The majority of these women (38.7% of the total group) reported perimenstrual worsening of the dystonia. However, those women also reported symptoms of premenstrual syndrome more frequently. A definite relationship between menses and dystonia severity could not be firmly established. No significant influence on the severity of the symptoms of dystonia was associated with pregnancy, menopause, or the use of oral contraceptives or hormone replacement therapy. The authors concluded that the biologic basis of dystonia may be influenced by female reproductive hormones, and some patients might have a greater susceptibility to those influences. In addition, Robinson and associates (87) reported a young woman with monthly exacerbations of her dystonia in relationship to reductions in her serum estradiol level who improved after treatment with estradiol. However, no effect of estrogen treatment in eight patients with dystonia (although six of these patients were male) was found (88).

In pregnant women the most common cause of acute generalized dystonia is secondary to the use of dopamine blocking agents, frequently used during pregnancy as antiemetics. Pregnancy does not appear to significantly alter the course of dystonia either during gestation or after delivery in patients with dystonia. Rogers and Fahn (89) reported their experience with ten pregnant patients with dystonia (nine with focal forms). Three patients suffered onset or exacerbation of the dystonia during pregnancy, and in another the dystonia appeared in the postpartum period. Four patients enjoyed a partial or complete remission during pregnancy, and two others had no changes. All attempts to taper medications during pregnancy were hampered by worsening of the symptoms.

In a review by Nygaard and colleagues (27) on patients with dopa-responsive dystonia (DRD), the authors report 12 pregnant women with untreated DRD of whom three experienced symptomatic worsening during the first two trimesters. Two of these women with initial worsening and two of the women with no initial change reported improvement of symptoms during the third trimester. None of the patients felt that the dystonia symptoms were significantly different when asked to compare their severity before and after pregnancy. Four patients with DRD became pregnant while taking levodopa (two patients) or levodopa/carbidopa (two patients). Three of these women had uncomplicated pregnancies, whereas another had premature delivery secondary to toxemia (a 38-year-old woman treated with a combination of levodopa and carbidopa). There were no symptomatic complaints related to the dystonia during these pregnancies, and all children were born normal. Ten women in this series reported premenstrual exacerbation of symptoms prior to initiation of treatment. These premenstrual fluctuations disappeared in all cases once patients were receiving optimal doses of levodopa.

Idiopathic torsion dystonia and idiopathic dystonias of early adulthood commonly are treated with anticholinergic agents (trihexyphenidyl, benztropine, diphenhydramine), baclofen, tetrabenazine, diazepam, clonazepam, and reserpine. In most cases, insufficient data on the safety of these drugs during pregnancy are available. However, it is well known that diazepam can produce neonatal depression, clonazepam can be teratogenic when used during the first trimester, and reserpine is also teratogenic and is excreted in human milk (89). In view of the lack of information regarding their safety during pregnancy, it appears prudent to taper and discontinue these oral medications prior to contemplated conception (90).

Botulinum toxin A is a very useful alternative for the symptomatic treatment of patients with focal dystonias. It has not been tested properly for safety during pregnancy (91). Scott (92) reported nine patients with blepharospasm treated with injections of botulinum toxin during pregnancy and found no abnormalities on pregnancy, delivery, or neonatal health, except for one premature delivery most likely unrelated to the drug.

Levodopa has been shown to be teratogenic in rats (bone dysplasias, visceral abnormalities, abortions) at doses of 200 mg/kg. However, there are no clinical reports of teratogenicity related to the use of levodopa or levodopa/carbidopa during human pregnancy (26,93). In view of the available data, there is no reason to withhold levodopa during pregnancy (20,26,93), particularly considering that cessation of levodopa increases the disability of patients and can cause harmful effects on the later stages of pregnancy and labor. A single report has suggested that combination therapy with carbidopa potentially could be associated with unsuccessful pregnancy, suggesting that levodopa alone could be a better option for patients with recurrent miscarriages (93).

Genetic Counseling

Idiopathic dystonia may be familial or sporadic. There is a higher prevalence of dystonia in the Ashkenazi Jewish population. In both Jewish (94) and non-Jewish patients, dystonia may be inherited as an autosomal dominant disorder (9q32–q34) (95). Dopa-responsive dystonia also can be inherited as an autosomal dominant disorder (27). Therefore, the genetic risk of dystonia in the child should be discussed in advance with a genetic counselor.

PREGNANCY AND NEUROLEPTIC MALIGNANT SYNDROME

Neuroleptic drugs frequently are used in the treatment of psychotic disorders during pregnancy. These agents are considered relatively safe to the mother and fetus when their use is weighed against the potential danger imposed by untreated psychosis (96–97). However, neuroleptic use is associated with the risk of significant adverse effects, including the threat of neuroleptic malignant syndrome (NMS). NMS typically presents with altered consciousness and a variable combination of extrapyramidal and autonomic dysfunction, including muscle rigidity, fever, tachycardia, labile blood pressure, and diaphoresis. Levels of creatine phosphokinase are characteristically elevated. NMS severity can be variable, and mild forms with insidious presentation have been reported (98). However, the diagnosis of NMS can place the pregnancy at a high risk and may constitute an obstetric emergency requiring aggressive in-hospital management.

Reports of NMS in pregnancy or postpartum are very scarce (99–100). This is somewhat surprising because estimates of NMS incidence as high as 3% have been reported in psychiatric inpatients receiving neuroleptic drugs (101). Therefore, the possibility of underdiagnosis or underreporting cannot be excluded.

The treatment of NMS should include immediate discontinuation of the neuroleptic drug and vigorous hydration. Several medications are used to treat this condition, including bromocriptine, dantrolene, and, less commonly, amantidine and benzodiazepines. Bromocriptine exposure in human pregnancy has resulted in no significant elevations in the rate of spontaneous abortions, premature deliveries, intrauterine growth restriction, or congenital malformations (102–103). Dantrolene is capable of producing fetal abnormalities when given in high doses to laboratory animals, but no adverse consequences were observed in neonates exposed to this drug in utero (104). Maternal exposure to amantadine has been associated, at least once, with cardiovascular malformations (36).

Maternal use of antipsychotics has been associated with extrapyramidal and dysautonomic symptoms in the infant. These may include poor arousal and responsiveness, bradykinesia, fine tremor, and changes in the color of the extremities. Symptoms may last for weeks or even several months, but they eventually resolve (96,99).

TOURETTE SYNDROME AND PREGNANCY

Tourette Syndrome (TS) is defined as a neurobehavioral disorder involving motor and vocal tics, with onset before 21 years of age and duration of symptoms for more than a year. Tics may range from simple, brief, involuntary movements most commonly involving the head or face (e.g., grimacing, eye blinking, or head shaking) to more complex and coordinated patterns of motor activity that may spread to the limbs. Vocal or phonic tics are usually sounds (e.g., grunting, sniffing, or barking) but can be words (coprolalia being typical but actually quite infrequent). Tics are often voluntarily suppressible for brief periods and may be preceded by an unpleasant sensation that builds up until relieved by the occurrence of the tic. These patients often have associated behavioral disturbances in the form of obsessive-compulsive or attention-deficit disorders (105). The inherited nature of TS generally is accepted, but the pattern of transmission remains elusive and no genetic site has been linked to the disease (106). The dopaminergic system has been implicated in the pathogenesis of TS for a long time; how-

ever, available data have failed to confirm any consistent abnormality of dopaminergic transmission in these patients (106).

Although generally thought of as a chronic and potentially lifelong condition, the course of TS may be variable. Symptoms characteristically are waxing and waning, and some patients show spontaneous remission or marked improvement over time (106). Maximum tic severity tends to occur between 8 and 12 years of age, followed frequently by a progressive decline in the symptoms (107).

Very limited information is available in the literature concerning the effects of pregnancy on TS. From a survey of 63 women with TS, it was found that 12 of those patients (26%) experienced exacerbation of tic severity during the premenstrual phase of the menstrual cycle and eight of them during menstruation. An increase in tics at the time of menarche was predictive of premenstrual tic exacerbation. However, most patients showed no change in their tics related to the phases of the menstrual period. In this same study, nine of ten women had no change in tic frequency or severity during pregnancy or postpartum. Oral contraceptives or the presence of premenstrual syndrome did not appear to have any significant effect on TS symptoms (108). Overall, these results seem to support the concept of an estrogen-related increase in tic severity in a subgroup of TS patients. In addition, conjugated estrogen has been reported to be useful as adjunctive treatment in TS, probably by preventing the cyclic rise in the level of endogenous estrogen (109).

There are no collected data on the effects of TS on pregnancy outcome. However, anecdotal experience appears to indicate that no detrimental effects occur.

A variety of pharmacotherapeutic options are available for the treatment of tics, including alpha-adrenergic agonists (such as clonidine and guanfacine) and dopamine receptor blockers (such as haloperidol, pimozide, fluphenazine, olanzepine, and risperidone). All of these agents should be restricted during pregnancy. Clonazepam may be useful and is probably safer in pregnant women. Newer treatment alternatives such as baclofen and botulinum toxin should be tested further before they can be formally recommended (110).

PREGNANCY AND TREMOR

Essential tremor (ET) consists of rhythmic and involuntary oscillations of a body part, usually an extremity, while held in a sustained position or during movement. Tremor results from simultaneous or alternating contraction of agonist and antagonist muscle groups. Four types of tremors may be observed during pregnancy: physiologic tremor, drug-induced tremor, essential tremor, and tremor associated with multiple sclerosis.

Physiologic tremor is frequent and may be accentuated by anxiety, fatigue, exercise, and caffeine intake. The frequency of physiologic tremor is 10 to 12 Hz with small amplitude.

A host of medications used during pregnancy, labor, or delivery may induce physiologic tremor, including sympathomimetic agents such as epinephrine and oxytocin. Occasionally, general anesthetic agents have induced rhythmic myoclonus that may simulate tremor.

Essential tremor has a tendency to run in families, and family history positivity varies from 17% to 70%. Larsson and Sjögren (111) conducted a comprehensive genetic population study in a region of northern Sweden. In this study, 210 cases of ET were traced to nine ancestral families in this geographically and ethnically restricted area. The pattern of occurrence of ET was consistent with autosomal dominant inheritance. Onset of tremor is usually during adolescence or early adulthood, and tremor amplitude increases with age. ET has as its sole manifestation tremor. The diagnosis is raised either incidentally or when the patient presents because of the mechanical or social disability resulting from the tremor. Other neurologic signs and symptoms typically are absent. Mild abnormalities of tone or gait occasionally are reported. In one study, 50% of ET patients exhibited tandem gait abnormalities, as compared to 28% of age-matched controls (112). Tremor, indistinguishable in appearance from ET, can be seen in association with other neurologic disorders. Usually, conditions that exacerbate physiologic tremor also will accentuate the ET. In many patients, ingestion of a small amount of an alcoholic beverage lessens the tremor for short periods. ET remits during sleep, and the appearance of tremor in a given patient may vary, not only with passage of years, but even over the course of a single day. Although tremor has minimal impact on pregnancy, the condition may deteriorate during pregnancy.

Multiple sclerosis occurs with greatest frequency in women of childbearing age. The demyelinating plaques in the subcortical, brainstem, and cerebellar white matter occasionally cause a coarse intention tremor known as a rubral or cerebellar outflow tremor.

Many patients with ET require no specific treatment except education and reassurance that their illness has a benign nature and that some more ominous disease is not present. Current medications that are effective in suppressing ET include propranolol (and other beta-adrenergic blockers) and primidone (113). It is unclear which should be the drug of first choice. As many as 20% of patients will suffer adverse effects for several days after the first dose of primidone. If the patient is informed of these potential adverse reactions and encouraged to continue to take the drug, only a minority will discontinue the primidone. Side effects with chronic therapy are uncommon with primidone but are much more of a concern with propranolol. Many elderly patients cannot take beta-adrenergic blockers. It appears that marked tremor reduction is more often achieved with primidone than with propranolol. Some patients may require both propranolol and primidone therapy. In cases of propranolol and primidone failure, alprazolam may be tried. Botulinum toxin type A is effective for a variety of movement disorders such as dystonia and hemifacial spasms. The drug appears to possess some efficacy for ET of the head, voice, and hand. Surgical approaches for treatment of tremors include thalamotomy and deep brain stimulation.

The available information on treatment of tremor during pregnancy is limited. Pregnancy may intensify tremor. Antitremor medications should be used with caution because they may have adverse effects on the fetus.

PREGNANCY AND HUNTINGTON'S DISEASE

Huntington's disease (HD) is an autosomal dominant progressive neurodegenerative disorder that is characterized by extrapyramidal movement disorder (chorea and dystonia), subcortical dementia, and varying degrees of psychiatric and behavioral dysfunction. HD was originally described by George Huntington in 1872 under the title of "hereditary chorea" (114). HD typically begins in middle adult life (although about 10% of patients have onset of illness before age 20 and about another 10% after age 55). Approximately 30,000 individuals in North America are affected by HD, and a further 150,000 unaffected individuals are considered at immediate 50:50 risk for developing the disease because of having an affected parent (115).The polymorphic DNA marker linked to HD was identified in 1983 (116), and later the mutation was characterized as an excessive number of trinucleotide CAG repeats that code for a polyglutamine (Huntington) on chromosome 4 (117). The size of the CAG expansion in the mutant gene has significant implications for age at onset, penetrance, and the stability of the gene between generations. Neuropathologically, HD is characterized by atrophy of the neostriatum (caudate and putamen) and cerebral cortex and microscopically by neuronal loss and gliosis.

Treatment of HD demands a coordinated effort on the part of the medical, social service, and physical therapy teams. Most patients are managed symptomatically. Depression usually responds to standard antidepressants, and carbamazepine and valproate may improve patients with manic disorder. Neuroleptics often lessen chorea and should be used cautiously because neuroleptics may impair motor function, swallowing, and cognitive capacities. Maintaining adequate nutrition is significant in HD patients because their metabolic demands may be remarkably increased.

There are no specific concerns about pregnancy or delivery in patients with HD. Individuals at risk for HD or carriers of the HD gene should be offered genetic counseling prior to pregnancy. Prenatal diagnostic testing for HD is available at many centers.

REFERENCES

1. Kessler II. Parkinson's disease in epidemiologic perspective. *Adv Neurol* 1978;19:355–384.
2. Kuopio AM, Marttila RJ, Helenius H, et al. Changing epidemiology of Parkinson's disease in southwestern Finland. *Neurology* 1999;52:302–308.
3. Leroy E, Boyer R, Auburger G, et al. The ubiquitin pathway in Parkinson's disease. *Nature* 1998;395: 451–452.
4. Gasser T, Muller-Myhsok B, Wszolek ZK, et al. A susceptibility focus for Parkinson's disease maps to chromosome 2p13. *Nat Genet* 1998;18:262–265.
5. Farrer M, Gwinn-Hardy K, Muenter M, et al. A chromosome 4p haplotype segregating with Parkinson's disease and postural tremor. *Hum Mol Genet* 1999;8: 81–85.
6. Lucking CB, Durr A, Bonifati V, et al. Association between early-onset Parkinson's disease and mutations in the parkin gene. French Parkinson's Disease Genetics Study Group. *N Engl J Med* 2000;342:1560–1567.
7. Golbe LI. Parkinson's disease and pregnancy. *Neurology* 1987;37:1245–1249.
8. Merchant CA, Cohen G, Mytilineou C, et al. Human transplancental transfer of carbidopa/levodopa. *J Neural Transm Park Dis Dement Sect* 1995;9:239–242.
9. Nausieda PA, Koller WC, Weiner WJ, et al. Modification of postsynaptic dopaminergic sensitivity by female sex hormones. *Life Sci* 1979;25:521–526.
10. Nausieda PA, Koller WC, Weiner WJ, et al. Chorea induced by oral contraceptives. *Neurology* 1979;29: 1605–1609.
11. Koller WC, Barr A, Biary N. Estrogen treatment of dyskinetic disorders. *Neurology* 1982;32:547–549.
12. Caviness JN, Muenter MD. An unusual case of recurrent chorea. *Mov Disord* 1991;4:355–357.
13. Cook DG, Klawans HL. Levodopa during pregnancy. *Clin Neuropharmacol* 1985;8:93–95.
14. Allain H, Bentue-Ferrer D, Milon D, et al. Pregnancy and parkinsonism. A case report without problem. *Clin Neuropharmacol* 1989;12:217–219.
15. Tobiassen D, Brasso K, Kohler OM. [Pregnancy and Parkinson's disease]. *Ugeskr Laeger* 1991;153: 1210–1211.
16. Gershanik OS, Leist A. Juvenile onset Parkinson's disease. *Adv Neurol* 1986;45:213–216.
17. Bauherz G. Pregnancy and Parkinson's disease: a case report. *New Trends in Clin Neuropharmacol* 1994;8:142.
18. Kupsch A, Oertel WH. Selegiline, pregnancy and Parkinson's disease. *Mov Disord* 1998;13:175–176.

19. Hagell P, Odin P, Vinge E. Pregnancy in Parkinson's disease: a review of the literature and a case report. *Mov Disord* 1998;13:34–38.

20. Shulman LM, Minagar A, Weiner WJ. The effect of pregnancy in Parkinson's disease. *Mov Disord* 2000; 15:132–135.

21. Bedard PJ, Langelier P, Dankova J, et al. Estrogens, progesterone and the extrapyramidal system. In: Poirier LJ, Sourkes TL, Bedard PJ, eds. *Advances in neurology.* New York: Raven Press, 1979.

22. Koller WC, Barr A, Biary N. Estrogen treatment of dyskinetic disorders. *Neurology* 1982;32:547–549.

23. Saunders-Pullman R, Gordon-Elliot J, Paredes M, et al. The effect of estrogen replacement on early Parkinson's disease. *Neurology* 1999;52:1417–1421.

24. Tao X, Shu-Leong H, Ramsden D. Estrogen can down-regulate the human catechol-o-methyltransferase gene expression: its implication in Parkinson's disease [Abstract]. *Mov Disord* 1998;13:114.

25. Fishman J. Biological action of catecholestrogens. *J Endocrinol* 1981;89:59–65.

26. Ball MC, Sagar HJ. Levodopa in pregnancy. *Mov Disord* 1995;10:115.

27. Nygaard TG, Marsden CD, Fahn S. Dopa-responsive dystonia: long-term treatment response and prognosis. *Neurology* 1991;41:174–181.

28. Chajek T, Berry EM, Friedman G, et al. Treatment of acute hepatic encephalopathy with L-Dopa. *Postgrad Med J* 1997;53:262–265.

29. Pujol-Amat P, Gamissans O, Calaf J, et al. Influence of L-Dopa on serum prolactin, human chorionic somaomammotrophin (HCS) and human chorionic gonadotrophin (HCG) during the last trimester of pregnancy. In: Pasteels JL, Robyn C, eds. *Human prolactin.* New York: Elsevier, 1973:316–320.

30. Weil C. The safety of bromocriptine in long-term use: a review of the literature. *Curr Med Res Opin* 1986; 10:25–51.

31. Raymond JP, Goldstein E, Konopka P, et al. Follow-up of children born of bromocriptine-treated mothers. *Horm Res* 1985;22:239–246.

32. Rojanasakul A, Sirimongkolkasem R, Chailurkit LO. The efficacy of lisuride in the treatment of hyperprolactinemic amenorrhea. *J Med Assoc Thai* 1990;73: 42–46.

33. Scialli AR. The reproductive toxicity of ovulation induction. *Fertil Steril* 1986;45:315–323.

34. Benito-Leon J, Bermejo F, Porta-Etessam J. Pregnancy in Parkinson's disease: a review of the literature and a case report. *Mov Disord* 1999;14:194.

35. Product information. Permax (pergolide). San Francisco: Athena Neurosciences, 1995.

36. Nora JJ, Nora AH, Way CL. Cardiovascular maldevelopment associated with maternal exposure to amantadine. *Lancet* 1975;2:607.

37. Briggs GG, Freeman RK, Yaffe SJ. *Drugs in pregnancy and lactation.* 4th ed. Baltimore: Williams & Wilkins, 1994.

38. Canales ES, Garcia IC, Ruiz JE, et al. Bromocriptine as prophylactic therapy in prolactinoma during pregnancy. *Fertil Steril* 1981;36:524–526.

39. Kacew S. Adverse effects of drug and chemicals in breast milk on the nursing infant. *J Clin Pharmacol* 1993;33:213–221.

40. Brewer GJ, Yuzbasiyan-Gurkan, V. Wilson disease. *Medicine (Baltimore)* 1992;71;139–164.

41. Schilsky ML. Wilson disease: genetic basis of copper toxicity and natural history. *Semin Liver Dis* 1996;16: 83–95.

42. Cartwright GE, Wintrobe MM. Copper metabolism in normal subjects. *Am J Clin Nutr* 1964;14:224–232.

43. Frommer DJ. Defective biliary excretion of copper in Wilson's disease. *Gut* 1974;15:125–129.

44. Gibbs K, Walshe JM. Biliary excretion of copper in Wilson's disease. *Lancet* 1980;2:538–539.

45. Bull PC, Thomas GR, Rommens JM, et al. The Wilson disease gene is a putative copper transporting P-type ATPase similar to the Menkes gene. *Nat Genet* 1993;5: 327–337.

46. Tanzi RE, Petrukhin K, Chernov I. The Wilson's disease gene is a copper transporting ATPase with homology to the Menke's disease gene. *Nat Genet* 1993; 5:344–350.

47. Yamaguchi Y, Heiny ME, Gitlin JD. Isolation and characterization of a human liver cDNA as a candidate gene for Wilson disease. *Biochem Biophys Res Commun* 1993;197:271–277.

48. Dupont P, Irion O, Beguin F. Pregnancy in a patient with treated Wilson's disease: a case report. *Am J Obstet Gynecol* 1990;23:1527–1528.

49. Sherwin A. The course of Wilson's disease during pregnancy and after delivery. *Can Med Assoc J* 1960; 83:160.

50. Walshe JM. Pregnancy in Wilson's disease. *Q J Med* 1977;181:73–83.

51. Klee JG. Undiagnosed Wilson's disease as a cause of unexplained miscarriage (Letter). *Lancet* 1979;2:423.

52. Mason AL, Marsh W, Alpers DH. Intractable neurological Wilson's disease treated with orthotopic liver transplantation. *Dig Dis Sci* 1993;38:1764–1750.

53. Hatard C, Kunze K. Pregnancy in a patient with Wilson's disease treated with D-penicillamine and zinc sulfate. *Eur Neurol* 1994;34:337–340.

54. Brewer GJ, Fink JK, Hedera P. Diagnosis and treatment of Wilson's disease. *Sem Neurol* 1999;3: 261–270.

55. Scheinberg IH, Sternlieb I. Pregnancy in penicillamine-treated patients with Wilson's disease. *N Eng J Med* 1975;293:1300–1302.

56. Mjolnerod OK, Dommerud SA, Rasmussen K, et al. Congenital connective tissue defect probably due to D-penicillamine treatment in pregnancy. *Lancet* 1971;1: 673–675.

57. Solomon L, Abrams G, Dinner M, et al. Neonatal abnormalities associated with D-penicillamine treatment during pregnancy. *N Eng J Med* 1977;296:54–55.

58. Keen CL, Lonnerdal B, Hurley LS. Teratogenic effect of copper deficiency and excess. In: Sorenson JR, ed. *Inflammatory diseases and copper.* Clifton, NJ: Humana Press, 1982:109–121.

59. Donaldson IM, Espiner EA. Disseminated lupus erythematosus presenting as chorea gravidarum. *Arch Neurol* 1971;25:240–244.

60. Bolt JM. Abortion and Huntington's chorea. *BMJ* 1968;1:840.

61. Lewis BV, Parsons M. Chorea gravidarum. *Lancet* 1966;1:284–286.

62. Wilson P, Preece AA. Chorea gravidarum. *Arch Int Med* 1932;471:671–697.

63. Zegart KN, Schwartz RH. Chorea gravidarum. *Obstet Gynecol* 1968;32:24–27.

64. Winkelbauer RG, Kimsly LR. Chorea gravidarum

treated with chlorpromazine. *Am J Obstet Gyn* 1956; 1353–1354.

65. Donaldson IM, Espiner EA. Disseminated lupus erythematosus presenting as chorea gravidarum. *Arch Neurol* 1971;25:240–244.

66. Ichikawa K, Kim RC, Givelber H, et al. Chorea gravidarum—report of a fatal case with neuropathological observations. *Arch Neurol* 1980;37:429–432.

67. Lubbe WF, Butler WS, Palmer SJ, et al. Lupus anticoagulant in pregnancy. *Br J Obstet Gynaecol* 1984;91:357–363.

68. Lubbe WF, Walker EB. Chorea gravidarum associated with circulatory lupus anticoagulant-successful outcome of pregnancy with prednisone and aspirin therapy. Case report. *Br J Obstet Gynaecol* 1983;90:487–490.

69. Beresford OD, Graham AM. Chorea gravidarum. *J Obstet Gyn* 1950;57:616–625.

70. Lubbe WE, Walker EB. Chorea gravidarum associated with circulatory lupus anticoagulant—successful outcome of pregnancy with prednisone and aspirin therapy. Case report. *Br J Obstet Gynaecol* 1983;90:487–490.

71. Nausieda PA, Koller WC, Weiner WJ, et al. Modification of postsynaptic dopaminergic sensitivity by female sex hormones. *Life Sci* 1979;25:521–526.

72. Donaldson JO. Control of chorea gravidarum with haloperidol. *Obstet Gynecol* 1982;59:381–382.

73. Patterson JF. Treatment of chorea gravidarum with haloperidol. *South Med J* 1979;72:1220–1221.

74. Hanson J. Haloperidol and limb deformity. *JAMA* 1975;231:26.

75. Kopelman A, McCullar F, Heggeness L. Limb malformations following maternal use of haloperidol. *JAMA* 1975;231:62–64.

76. Ekbom KA. Restless legs syndrome. *Neurology* 1960; 10:868–873.

77. Lang AE. Akathisia and the restless legs syndrome. In: Jankovic J, Tolosa E, eds. *Parkinson's disease and movement disorders.* Baltimore: Williams & Wilkins, 1993:399–418.

78. Earley CJ. Sleep disorders. In: Johnson RT, Griffen JW, eds. *Current therapy in neurologic disease.* 4th ed. St Louis: Mosby-Year Book, 1993.

79. Walters AS, Hening WA, Chokroverty S. Review and videotape recognition of idiopathic restless legs syndrome. *Mov Disord* 1988;6:105–110.

80. Weiner WJ, Lang AE. *Movement disorders: a comprehensive survey.* Mount Kisco, NY: Futura Publishing Co, 1989.

81. Soland VL, Bhatia KP, Marsden CD. Sex prevalence of focal dystonias. *J Neurol Neurosurg Psychiatry* 1996; 60:204–205.

82. Duane DD. Spasmodic torticollis: clinical and biologic features and their implications for focal dystonia. *Adv Neurol* 1988;50:473–492.

83. Quinn NP, Marsden CD. Menstrual-related fluctuations in Parkinson's disease. *Mov Disord* 1986;1:85–87.

84. Schwabe MJ, Konkol RJ. Menstrual cycle-related fluctuations of tics in Tourette syndrome. *Pediatr Neurol* 1992;8:43–46.

85. Weiner WJ, Shulman LM, Singer C, et al. Menopause and estrogen replacement therapy in Parkinson's disease. *Neurology* 1996;46:376–377.

86. Gwinn-Hardy KA, Adler CH, Weaver AL, et al. Effect of hormone variations and other factors on symptom severity in women with dystonia. *Mayo Clin Proc* 2000;75:235–240.

87. Robinson RO, Stutchfield P, Hicks B, et al. Estrogens and dyskinesia. *Neurology* 1984;34:404–405.

88. Koller WC, Barr A, Biary N. Estrogen replacement of dyskinetic disorders. *Neurology* 1982;32:547–549.

89. Rogers JD, Fahn S. Movement disorders and pregnancy. In: Devinsky O, Feldmann E, Hainline B, eds. *Neurological complications of pregnancy. (Advances in neurology,* vol 64). New York: Raven Press, 1994: 163–178.

90. Golbe LI. Pregnancy and movement disorders. *Neurol Clin* 1994;12:497–508.

91. Tsui JK. Botulinum toxin as a therapeutic agent. *Pharmacol Ther* 1996;72:13–24.

92. Scott AB. Clostridial toxins as therapeutic agents. In: Simpson LL, ed. *Botulinum neurotoxin and tetanus toxin.* New York: Academic Press, 1989:399–412.

93. Nomoto M, Kaseda S, Iwata S, et al. Levodopa in pregnancy. *Mov Disord* 1997;12:261.

94. Bressman SB, de Leon D, Brin MF, et al. Idiopathic torsion dystonia among Ashkenazi Jews: evidence for autosomal dominant inheritance. *Ann Neurol* 1989;26: 612–620.

95. Ozelius L, Kramer PL, Moskowitz CB, et al. Human genome for torsion dystonia located on chromosome 9q32–q34. *Neuron* 1989;2:1427–1434.

96. Goldberg HL, DiMascio A. Psychotropic drugs in pregnancy and lactation. In: Lipton MA, Di Mascio A, Killam KF, eds. *Psychopharmacology: a generation of progress.* New York: Raven Press, 1978:1047–1055.

97. Lewis PJ: The effect of psychotropic drugs in the fetus. In: Sandler M, ed. *Mental illness in pregnancy and the puerperium.* New York: Oxford University Press, 1978:99–111.

98. Addonizio G, Susman VL, Roth SD. Symptoms of neuroleptic malignant syndrome in 82 consecutive inpatients. *Am J Psychiatry* 1986;143:1587–1589.

99. James ME. Neuroleptic malignant syndrome in pregnancy. *Psychosomatics* 1988;29:119–122.

100. Price DK, Turnbull GJ, Gregory RP, et al. Neuroleptic malignant syndrome in a case of post-partum psychosis. *Br J Psychiatry* 1989;155:849–852.

101. Pelonero AL, Levenson JL, Pandurangi AK. Neuroleptic malignant syndrome: a review. *Psychiatr Serv* 1998;49:1163–1172.

102. Turkalj I, Braun P, Krupp P. Surveillance of bromocriptine in pregnancy. *JAMA* 1982;247: 1589–1591.

103. Weil C. The safety of bromocriptine in long-term use: a literature review. *Curr Med Res Opin* 1986;10: 25–51.

104. Cupryn JP, Kennedy A, Byrick RJ. Malignant hyperthermia in pregnancy. *Am J Obstet Gynecol* 1984;150: 327–328.

105. Kurlan R. Tourette's syndrome: current concepts. *Neurology* 1989;39:1625–1630.

106. Singer HS. Current issues in Tourette Syndrome. *Mov Disord* 2000;15:1051–1063.

107. Goetz CG, Tanner CM, Stebbins GT, et al. Adult tics in Gilles de la Tourette syndrome. *Neurology* 1992;42: 784–788.

108. Schwabe MJ, Konkol RJ. Menstrual cycle-related fluctuations of tics in Tourette syndrome. *Pediatr Neurol* 1992;8:43–46.

109. Sandyk R, Bamford CR. Estrogen as adjuvant treatment of Tourette syndrome. *Pediatr Neurol* 1987;3:122.

110. Kurlan R. New treatments for tics? *Neurology* 2001; 56:580–581.

111. Larsson T, Sjögren T. Essential tremor. A clinical and genetic population study. *Acta Psychiatry Neurol Scand* 1960;36:1–176.

112. Singer C, Sanchez-Ramos J, Weiner WJ. Gait abnormalities in essential tremor. *Mov Disord* 1994;9:193–196.

113. Larsen TA, Calne DB. Essential tremor. *Clin Neuropharmacol* 1983;6:185–206.

114. Huntington G. On chorea. *Med Surg Rep* 1872;26: 320.

115. Conneally PM. Huntington disease: genetics and epidemiology. *Am J Hum Genet* 1984;36:506–526.

116. Gusella JF, Wexler NS, Conneally PM, et al. A polymorphic DNA marker genetically linked to Huntington's disease. *Nature* 1983;306:234–237.

117. Huntington's Disease Collaborative Research Group. A novel gene containing a trinucleotide repeat that is expanded and unstable on Huntington's disease chromosomes. *Cell* 1993;72:971–983.

Neurological Complications of Pregnancy, Second Edition, edited by Brian Hainline and Orrin Devinsky. Lippincott Williams & Wilkins, Philadelphia, © 2002.

16

Peripheral Nerve Disorders

Aleksandar Berić

Department of Neurology, New York University School of Medicine, Hospital for Joint Diseases, New York, New York, U.S.A.

Peripheral nerve disorders have diverse etiologies but are usually divided into hereditary and acquired forms. During pregnancy, delivery, and puerperium several peripheral nerve disorders may occur but are unaffected by this different physiologic state and may not pose any threat to or complicate the pregnancy. Most of the hereditary disorders fall into this low-impact or nonimpact category. However, some disorders, such as compression neuropathies, have a higher incidence during pregnancy or result from delivery, and they are discussed in this chapter. Also covered are disorders, such as diabetic neuropathy, that may not be influenced by pregnancy but require special precautions during pregnancy and delivery.

Acquired peripheral nerve disorders can be broadly divided into traumatic and compressive; inflammatory and immune; associated with systemic diseases; and metabolic (including malnutrition) and toxic (1). The incidence and clinical relevance of these disorders to pregnancy depends on socioeconomic factors, especially availability and quality of prenatal and general medical care. Malnutrition is not a significant cause of neuropathy in pregnancy in developed countries (2), where, because of more specialized medical care, women with serious preexisting conditions may carry their pregnancies to term, bringing new challenges to medical care.

Traumatic nerve lesions can cause scattered damage to the axons, called axonot-

mesis, (3,4) with distal axonal degeneration (i.e., anterograde Wallerian degeneration). This type of lesion requires regeneration of axons from the lesion site to the target before full recovery can be expected. However, if the lesion is only partial, collateral intramuscular reinnervation may occur and may provide a full functional recovery in a shorter time, as in the case of muscle reinnervation after proximal nerve damage in radicular lesions. The degree of recovery depends on the degree of the initial damage. Minor damage may be clinically unrecognizable at the time of initial trauma. However, repetitive mild trauma such as a pudendal nerve lesion resulting from repeated mild traumatic compression during multiple pregnancies ultimately may become manifest clinically (5). However, more than 50% of fiber loss or complete lesions cause immediate functional loss and protracted recovery.

With *neurotmesis* (3,4), the entire nerve, including its sheaths, is lesioned. Neurotmesis (3,4) usually carries a poor prognosis and may require nerve grafting, which at best will result in only partial recovery. *Neurapraxia* refers to nerve injury that may show no histologic changes and has an excellent prognosis because there is no loss of continuity of either nerve or axons. Neurapraxia is recognized electrophysiologically by the presence of a conduction block across the lesion, which may reverse within minutes, hours, or days, but definitely earlier than regeneration. Compression of the nerve may cause demyelination with consequent conduction slowing due to loss of saltatory conduction from one node of Ranvier to the next. Neurapraxia is accompanied by a functional deficit, in part also due to conduction block. These lesions also have a good outcome unless there is repeated or prolonged compression, which ultimately can result in axonal damage.

Nontraumatic lesions can be exclusively or predominantly *axonal* or *demyelinating* (6). Most inflammatory neuropathies are demyelinating, whereas most toxic neuropathies are axonal. Neuropathies can be of different types in time domain (acute, chronic, relapsing-remitting), as well as in regard to their distribution within the body. Dying-back or distal neuropathies are usually symmetric and can be either acute or chronic. Diabetic neuropathy is an example of a metabolic type, usually with combined demyelinating-axonal pathology. Another frequent distal neuropathy is caused by alcohol, which is a toxic type and exclusively axonal. *Mononeuropathies* involve only one peripheral nerve, such as Bell's palsy of the facial nerve or meralgia paresthetica with involvement of the lateral cutaneous femoral nerve. *Mononeuropathy multiplex* involves any combination and number of peripheral nerves in diseases such as lupus erythematosus, other connective tissue disorders, paraneoplastic syndromes and as a form of diabetic neuropathy.

Axons in peripheral nerves can be categorized on the basis of their diameter and presence or absence of a myelin sheath. They are most commonly classified as A, B, and C groups. The A group represents myelinated somatic fibers and is further divided into alpha, beta, gamma, and delta, from largest to smallest, respectively. The B group represents preganglionic autonomic fibers, and C fibers are unmyelinated. Clinically relevant classification divides all fibers into two groups: large and small fibers. *Large fibers* include all afferent and efferent myelinated fibers except those of the smallest diameter, mostly A delta. A delta fibers, together with unmyelinated fibers, represent a *small fiber* group. This dis-

tinction is important; most painful neuropathies and most of the autonomic neuropathies present as small-fiber dysfunction.

In addition to clinical evaluation, the diagnosis of neuropathy includes extensive metabolic testing. Sometimes the diagnosis can be confirmed only by nerve biopsy, which is usually not entertained during pregnancy. Noninvasive techniques such as neurophysiologic tests are preferable. *Nerve conduction velocity (NCV) study* and *electromyography* (EMG) are usually sufficient to document the extent and type of lesion (e.g., axonal vs. demyelinating) (6). These tests are not appropriate for evaluation of a small-fiber neuropathy because they assess only the function of large myelinated fibers. *Quantitative sensory testing* (7) can reveal a small-fiber dysfunction through testing of temperature perception and, if necessary, thermal pain perception. Additionally, autonomic fiber function is tested by analyzing the variability of electroencephalography frequency, changes in blood pressure on standing up, and more sophisticated tests of sweating function such as QSART (quantitative sudomotor axon reflex test) (8).

Management of nontraumatic neuropathies primarily involves removing the offending agent and treating the underlying metabolic or inflammatory abnormality. There are no drugs to treat neuropathy, and vitamins are useful only if the neuropathy is caused by a specific vitamin deficiency.

Treatment of traumatic lesions depends on the cause. In pregnancy the cause is usually compression due to swelling and, because this condition is temporary, surgical intervention is not warranted. Nerve lesions during delivery are almost always incomplete and therefore have a good prognosis without surgical intervention. Physical therapy or, if necessary, orthosis is usually sufficient. Surgical intervention may be contraindicated because nerve exposure and neurolysis also might impair microvascular nerve supply and inadvertently compress further the fragile axons and sheaths. A reversible conduction block can be easily converted to the axonal damage that would require axonal regeneration and protracted recovery and probably result in a less complete functional outcome.

PERIPHERAL NERVE DISORDERS WITH HIGHER INCIDENCE IN PREGNANCY

Carpal Tunnel Syndrome

The most frequent neuropathy during pregnancy is carpal tunnel syndrome (CTS). It is reported (9,10) in 1% to as many as 50% of pregnancies. In a few prospective studies (9,10,11,12), the incidence varied from 2.3% to 25%, which is still too wide a range to know the real occurrence. In the most recent study using very strict inclusion criteria, only 0.34% of 14,579 pregnancies were identified as having *de novo* CTS (13). Another factor is how sensitive the variables are. In one of the studies (14) 35% of pregnant women complained of hand symptoms, and a surprising 30% of the age-matched control group also had hand pain, although none of the control group required any treatment. This suggests a milder intensity of pain in the control group. This study exemplifies the difficulty in rating sensory symptoms and consequent comparisons between different studies.

CTS typically begins in the third trimester and usually involves the thumb and index and middle fingers with symptoms of numbness, tingling, and pins and needles. Patients shake their hands in an attempt to alleviate symptoms, which are usually worse during the night or morning and frequently awaken patients. Pain is less frequently present and may involve the wrist and sometimes even more proximal areas such as the deltoid region. Symptoms are often bilateral, although rarely symmetric. The intensity is usually mild and does not require specific treatment. However, there is no reason not to treat a patient who loses sleep or is annoyed with symptoms. Because CTS in pregnancy is reversible within 2 weeks after delivery, surgery is not indicated. In most clinical series (9,14) surgical release was not performed. Wrist splints are most ef-

fective (15,16,17); other treatments include local corticosteroid injection or a low-dose tricyclic antidepressant as a neurogenic analgesic, but medication should be avoided, if possible, during pregnancy. However, if symptoms persist after puerperium and do not respond to conservative treatment, surgery might be indicated (13,18,19).

The cause of CTS is compression of the median nerve in the carpal tunnel (Fig. 16.1). The cause of compression is multifactorial; however, a correlation between the presence of CTS and generalized edema during pregnancy has been found, making it the most likely underlying mechanism (11,20,21). Its disappearance immediately after delivery as edema resolves supports this mechanism. However, a subpopulation of patients may demonstrate axonal damage, (22) and these patients may benefit from CTS surgery.

In approximately 10% of patients with hand symptoms, the distribution of paresthesias develops primarily in the ulnar nerve and rarely involves the entire hand (14). Focal neuropathies such as CTS may be a sign of more severe and widespread abnormality, such as diabetic neuropathy; therefore, some workup might be necessary. Because the incidence of most neuropathies is not increased in pregnancy and CTS usually is self-limited, a balanced use of ancillary techniques is recommended.

CTS can be confirmed by neurophysiologic testing (23), which should include transcarpal nerve conduction study. The palmar interdigital nerve branches are stimulated, and nerve action potential is recorded proximally over the median nerve at the wrist for the I, II, and III branch and over the ulnar nerve for the IV branch (Fig 16.2). As the conduction is over the same distance, the latencies are compared, and absolute values over 2 ms and a difference between the ulnar and median nerve innervated branches over 0.3 ms confirm compression of the sensory portion of the median nerve. If the compression is severe, the routine digital median nerve conduction study is also abnormal. At this point the distal motor latency to the abductor pollicis brevis muscle

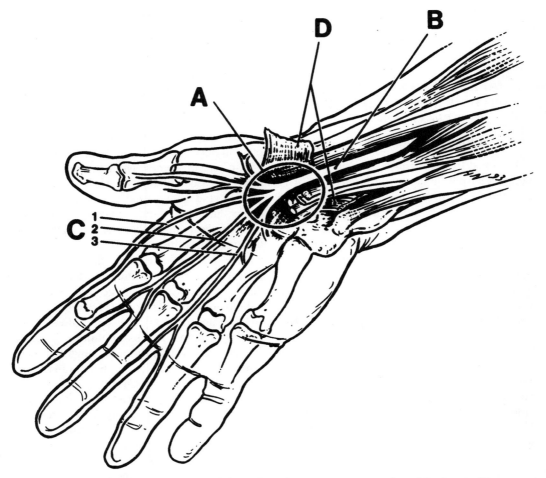

FIG. 16.1. Median nerve in the hand. **(A)** Site of median nerve compression at the level of the carpal tunnel, **(B)** median nerve, **(C)** palmar interdigital nerves, and **(D)** transverse carpal ligament cut to show the relationship of median nerve to long flexor tendons.

also becomes abnormally prolonged. Needle EMG is not necessary to confirm the diagnosis of CTS and should not be performed except to exclude some other suspected neuromuscular abnormality.

Facial Mononeuropathy: Bell's Palsy

The idiopathic form of facial palsy (Bell's palsy) appears with slightly higher incidence in pregnancy than in the general population. It involves all three peripheral motor branches—frontal, ocular, and oral—and ap-

pears as a sudden onset of asymmetric facial expression and an inability to close the eye (2). Most cases of Bell's palsy have a good prognosis, with early and complete or almost complete recovery. A small number of patients require a long recovery as a result of severe axonal damage, usually hypothesized as the result of prolonged swelling within the facial canal (6). True reinnervation is required for recovery to occur with regeneration of axons from the site of lesion to the corresponding muscle. Even this is followed by excellent recovery because the facial muscles, even

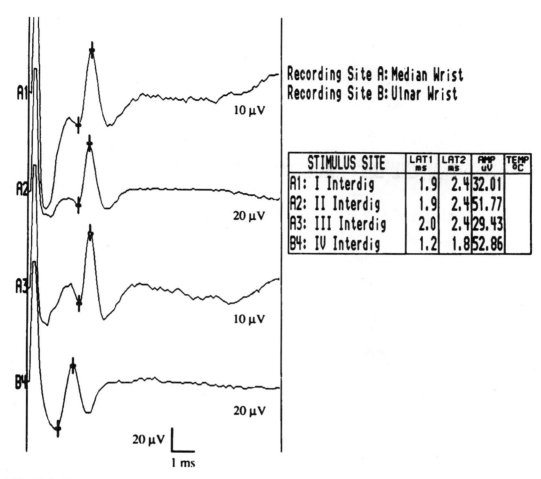

Recording Site A: Median Wrist
Recording Site B: Ulnar Wrist

STIMULUS SITE	LAT1 ms	LAT2 ms	AMP uV	TEMP °C
A1: I Interdig	1.9	2.4	32.01	
A2: II Interdig	1.9	2.4	51.77	
A3: III Interdig	2.0	2.4	29.43	
B4: IV Interdig	1.2	1.8	52.86	

FIG. 16.2. Transcarpal orthodromic nerve conduction study. **(A1)** I interdigital nerve stimulation; **(A2)** II interdigital nerve stimulation; **(A3)** III interdigital nerve stimulation; **(B4)** IV interdigital nerve stimulation—ulnar nerve branch. Note the 0.6-msec difference in peaks of median nerve contributing branches compared to short, normal latency of ulnar nerve contributing branch (LAT2 column).

when denervated, do not atrophy. Treatment is usually symptomatic and oculoprotective. Careful neurologic examination always is indicated to exclude a symptomatic cause of the facial nerve lesion, which may require otoneurosurgical care.

Lateral Femoral Cutaneous Nerve Neuropathy: Meralgia Paresthetica

Meralgia paresthetica is a purely sensory neuropathy believed to be the result of nerve compression under the lateral part of the in-guinal ligament (Fig. 16.3). Swelling during pregnancy has been postulated as a cause of compression. Also, a major change in the patient's weight leads to a change in the local amount of protective fat padding tissue. Patients complain of dysesthetic pain: unpleasant sensations, pins and needles, and burning pain. There is no weakness. The sensory deficit usually localizes to the upper and middle part of the lateral thigh above the tensor fasciae latae and vastus lateralis muscles.

Treatment is difficult if local anesthetic blocks with or without corticosteroids at the fractory deafferentation syndrome. A similar approach is taken for pregnancy-induced intercostal and abdominal wall neuralgias (24,25)

Chronic Inflammatory Demyelinating Polyneuropathy

Chronic inflammatory demyelinating polyneuropathy is a relatively rare, autoimmune peripheral nerve myelin disorder characterized by diffuse asymmetric nerve involvement (26). Sometimes upper extremities are more involved, and paresthesias may overshadow the weakness. Incidence is slightly higher in pregnancy, raising speculations about changes in the immune system during pregnancy (27).

Metabolic Neuropathies

Malnutrition and vitamin deficiency may cause severe neuropathies; however, the clinical picture usually is dominated by central nervous system dysfunction. With available prenatal care and easy access to vitamins, these disorders rarely occur during pregnancy (2). Vitamin B_{12} and folate deficiency cause an axonal neuropathy that is prevented during pregnancy with standard vitamin supplements.

Porphyria, especially the acute intermittent form, may by chance appear for the first time during pregnancy and therefore represents a diagnostic challenge and a major emergency. In some women with porphyria, exacerbations can appear in pregnancy, most frequently in early pregnancy (2). The less frequent late pregnancy crises are, however, more serious and are accompanied by increased fetal and maternal morbidity and mortality. Neuropathy results from porphyria but is neither a medical emergency nor a frequent problem. Similarly, thyroid neuropathy, usually seen with hypothyroidism, might occur during pregnancy; however, other clinical manifestations are of more importance than the mild neuropathy.

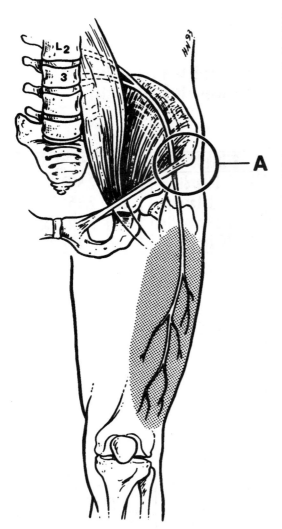

FIG. 16.3. Lateral femoral cutaneous nerve. **(A)** Site of lateral cutaneous nerve compression at the level of the inguinal ligament. Shaded area represents skin distribution of nerve.

inguinal ligament level fail to alleviate discomfort. Sometimes antidepressants in low dosages are useful. Carbamazepine and phenytoin are usually not necessary and are relatively contraindicated for this disorder in pregnancy. Neurectomy is never indicated in pregnancy and generally should not be done because it may result in a treatment re-

PERIPHERAL NERVE DISORDERS IN PREGNANCY WITH THE SAME INCIDENCE AS IN THE GENERAL POPULATION BUT REQUIRING SPECIAL PRECAUTIONS

Acute Inflammatory Demyelinating Neuropathy: Guillaine-Barré Syndrome

Acute inflammatory demyelinating neuropathy (AIDP) is an acute autoimmune antimyelin disorder that usually has a favorable recovery after a few weeks of progressive paralysis (28). In such cases it does not interfere with pregnancy, and weakness is not as severe or relevant for delivery because it does not involve small-caliber fibers of the uterine plexus. However, more severe forms, which often include respiratory paralysis, do require artificial respiration and as a general medical problem may interfere with pregnancy. It appears that, if anything, risk of AIDP is lower during pregnancy (29). In patients who suffer from AIDP during pregnancy, some deliveries are by cesarean section (30), although there is a concern that induction of labor and cesarean section in the acute phase of AIDP may delay and affect recovery (31). So-called hyperacute forms, which may represent axonal forms of Guillaine-Barré syndrome (GBS), or alternatively, severe distal conduction blocks leading to early axonal degeneration, are followed by severe paralysis and even death (33,33). Fortunately, they represent only 3% to 5% of all cases of GBS and do not occur more frequently during pregnancy.

Treatment of GBS in pregnancy is no different than in any other clinical situation, including early and, if necessary, repeated plasmapheresis, repeated administration of gammaglobulin, or both (34,35,36). Steroids have been phased out completely as an initial treatment option. Because an early aggressive treatment must be instituted, early diagnosis is extremely important and should be made on the basis of observation of characteristic albuminocytologic dissociation in the spinal fluid and early absence of F-waves in the nerve conduction study followed by, or concomitant with, focal slowing of motor conduction velocities seen diffusely. This is one of the rare instances when a nerve conduction study may be needed urgently and should be widely available.

Brachial Plexopathy: Parsonage-Turner Syndrome

Brachial plexopathy is an idiopathic, usually painful condition followed by atrophy of the shoulder girdle muscle and medium to protracted recovery times (37,38). A similar abnormality in the lower extremities represents lumbar plexopathy with most severe involvement of femoral nerve innervated muscles. The recurrent form of brachial plexopathy is often hereditary with focal nerve enlargements in a form of tomaculous neuropathy, also called hereditary neuropathy with tendency for pressure palsies (39). It recurs frequently during pregnancy or in early puerperium (40,41). Nonhereditary forms also have been described (42).

Diabetic Neuropathy

Diabetic neuropathy, seen in juvenile-onset diabetes mellitus, can take many different forms. It may be asymptomatic with mild fiber loss across the entire range of fibers, or it can be in the form of painful diabetic neuropathy with dysfunction restricted to small-caliber fibers (A delta and unmyelinated) (43). There are also several forms of large-fiber, combined axonal and demyelinating neuropathies that may in time contribute to the development of diabetic foot or Charcot's joint. Pregnancy has not been shown to trigger or aggravate diabetic neuropathy, and in the absence of specific treatment, glucose control is the regimen of choice. Even when nerve function was followed prospectively by repeated nerve conduction studies (44) in asymptomatic pregnant women with diabetes, no changes in this sensitive subclinical measure of nerve function were found (45). In comparison to diabetic retinopathy and nephropathy, neuropathy is less troublesome and less clinically significant during pregnancy (46). Pregnancy may accelerate neuropathy in the short term, but it does not lead to long-term diabetes complications (47). Treatment is symptomatic (i.e., foot orthosis for a footdrop or pain-control measures for neuropathic pain, including low-dose tricyclic antidepressants for severe pain).

Diabetic neuropathy can have an adverse effect on pregnancy. The most dangerous form is diabetic autonomic neuropathy, which may lead to blood pressure fluctuations and visceral organ dysfunction (48). Gastroparesis with severe and intractable vomiting may be a contraindication for continuing pregnancy because there is risk to both mother and fetus (49). In a few reported cases (50) it appears that gastroparesis worsens, although the effect on orthostatic hypotension has been reported to even improve in one case. Autonomic function should be assessed in pregnant women with diabetes because of the potential complications. Further study of the effects of diabetic autonomic neuropathy on pregnancy would assist in developing diagnostic and therapeutic guidelines.

POSTPARTUM PERIPHERAL NERVE DISORDERS

Different focal neuropathies result from different delivery techniques. They all have in common compression as the underlying

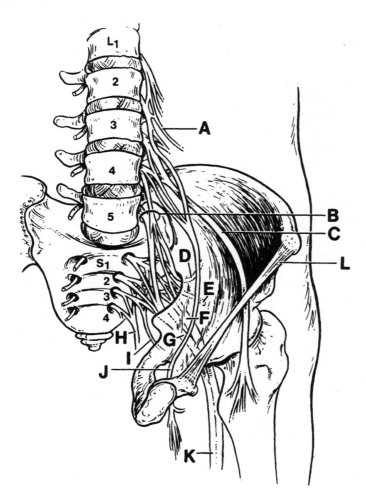

FIG. 16.4. The lumbar, lumbosacral, and sacral plexus and branches. **(A)** Lateral femoral cutaneous nerve, **(B)** lumbosacral trunk, **(C)** femoral nerve, **(D)** superior gluteal nerve, **(E)** inferior gluteal nerve, **(F)** common peroneal nerve, **(G)** tibial nerve, **(H)** pudendal nerve, **(I)** posterior femoral cutaneous nerve, **(J)** obturator nerve, **(K)** sciatic nerve, and **(L)** inguinal ligament.

cause. Forceps delivery is especially prone to cause compression mononeuropathy. Speed of delivery and disproportion of the fetal head to the pelvis are the major determinants in compression neuropathy development. Also, prolonged or obstructed labor can lead to tissue compressions, including fistulas, that have concomitant, usually bilateral, lumbosacral plexus lesions. Cesarean section, however, has a small incidence of nerve injuries (16). A schematic representation of the lumbar, lumbosacral, and sacral plexus is shown in Fig. 16.4.

Obturator Nerve Lesions

The obturator nerve is formed from branches of the L2–L4 roots, runs under the psoas muscle, and reaches the true pelvis after crossing the sacroiliac joint. The fetal head can compress it as it travels along the lateral pelvic wall before entering the obturator canal (Fig. 16.5). Its anterior branch supplies the motor innervation to the obturator muscles, pectineus, adductor longus and brevis, and gracilis muscles. The anterior branch terminates with a cutaneous branch that has a variable distribution. Most frequently, it innervates part of the inner thigh. The posterior branch innervates the adductor magnus and frequently has an articular branch to supply the posterior knee joint.

Acute obturator nerve compression is followed by sharp pain in the upper thigh and groin accompanied by a variable degree of adductor weakness because the femoral and sciatic nerves also contribute to adductor longus and magnus innervation (51,52). The paresis may be prominent only during gait, when preserved abductors predominate, resulting in leg circumduction. The lesion is usually incomplete, and functional recovery is typically good due to reinnervation as well as compensation through the femoral and sciatic nerves. However, severe lesions can be accompanied by femoral nerve paralysis resulting in major, although usually temporary, deficit. However, obturator nerve lesions may result in a chronic pain syndrome with inner thigh pain, local-

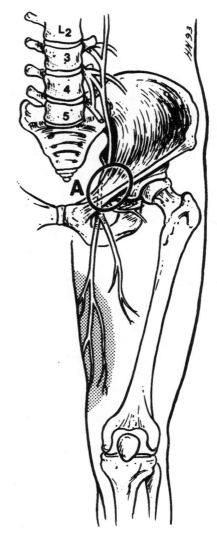

FIG. 16.5. Obturator nerve. **(A)** Site of obturator nerve compression on the lateral wall of the true pelvis. Shaded area represents skin distribution of nerve.

ized hyperesthesia, and occasional posterior knee pain. Clinical exam is sufficient for early diagnosis. In the case of chronic pain, obturator nerve block is indicated for both diagnosis and treatment (53).

Femoral Nerve Lesions

The femoral nerve is formed from the L2–L4 roots, descends through the psoas muscle, reaches the groove between the psoas and iliac muscles, and exits to the thigh under the inguinal ligament (Fig. 16.6). It provides motor innervation to the iliopsoas muscle, although a major supply appears from direct plexus branches. In the thigh the femoral nerve innervates the quadriceps femoris and sartorius muscles. Its anterior cutaneous branches innervate the anterior and medial thigh, whereas the major terminal branch represents the saphenous nerve innervating the medial knee and inner foreleg distal to the medial foot.

Postpartum femoral neuropathy can be either unilateral or bilateral (54). Its incidence has decreased significantly during the past five decades; it was reported in up to 4.7% of postpartum cases in the early 1900s (55). It is usually a painless condition that becomes obvious when the patient walks for the first time after delivery. Anterior thigh paresthesia is common. There is some hip flexion weakness and more profound knee extension weakness. Walking up stairs is very difficult. The cause of the injury is unclear (56,57,58), although prolonged labor and cephalopelvic disproportion certainly contribute (59). Another possible cause is ischemia of the vasa nervorum, which are considered branches of the intrapelvic internal iliac artery (60). Lithotomy position possibly may provoke femoral neuropathy (61). Primiparas may be more prone to develop femoral nerve injury (59). According to Donaldson and colleagues (59), consequent deliveries should be managed by cesarean section unless the baby's head is small.

Diagnosis is clinical, and because most lesions have a good prognosis, no specific therapy is necessary. Even complete femoral nerve compressions have excellent prognosis. If the timing of recovery is to be assessed, an EMG study is indicated to show the extent of axonal damage. Usually it takes 2 to 3 weeks for full denervation to develop; hence early EMG is not indicated. If necessary, EMG can follow the extent and the speed of nerve recovery.

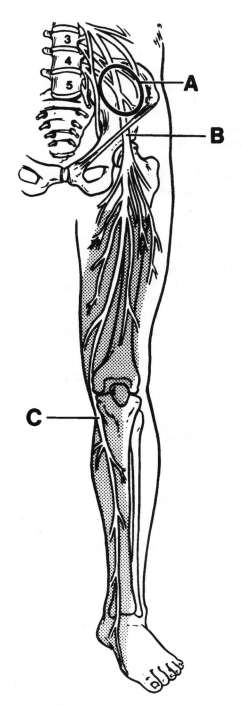

FIG. 16.6. Femoral nerve. **(A)** Site of femoral nerve compression inside pelvis, **(B)** femoral nerve, **(C)** saphenous nerve. Shaded area represents skin distribution of nerve.

Lumbosacral Plexus Lesions

The most frequent postpartum dysfunction is of the peroneal nerve (62,63,64). It appears unilaterally or bilaterally and usually results from pelvic compression, not from lumbosacral disc herniation and compression (65). In addition, common peroneal nerve lesions at the knee level can occur, although they are uncommon (66).

The lumbosacral plexus is formed from the L4–S2 roots (Fig. 16.7). The L4 and L5 roots form the lumbosacral trunk that enters the true pelvis to join the sacral roots. This is the point where it can be compressed easily, resulting in footdrop without major tibial nerve dysfunction. Frequently peroneal and tibial nerves already are separated at the level of the piriform muscle before entering the posterior thigh. Branches of the plexus innervate the piriform muscle and gemelli. The superior gluteal nerve passes through the suprapiriform foramen supplying the gluteus medius and minimus muscles to distally innervate the tensor fasciae latae muscle. The inferior gluteal nerve leaves the pelvis through the infrapiriform foramen together with the sciatic nerve and innervates the gluteus maximus muscle. The tibial portion innervates the semimembranosus and

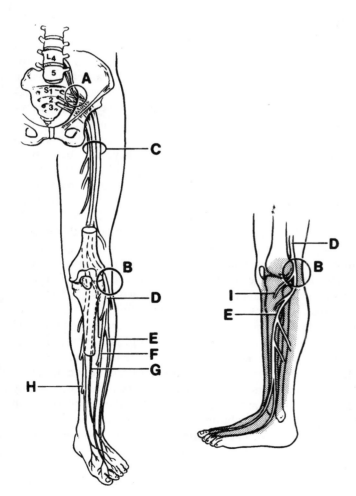

FIG. 16.7. Lumbosacral plexus and its branches. **(Left)** Sciatic nerve and its branches. **(Right)** Common peroneal nerve and superficial peroneal nerve. **(A)** Site of sciatic nerve—lumbosacral trunk compression in the pelvis, **(B)** site of common peroneal nerve compression at the knee, **(C)** sciatic nerve, **(D)** common peroneal nerve, **(E)** superficial peroneal nerve, **(F)** deep peroneal nerve, **(G)** sural nerve, **(H)** tibial nerve, **(I)** lateral cutaneous nerve of the calf. The shaded area represents skin distribution of the common peroneal nerve.

semitendinosus muscles and the long head of the biceps femoris muscle, further distally innervating the entire posterior foreleg compartment and intrinsic foot muscles. The short head of the biceps femoris muscle is innervated by the most proximal branch of the peroneal nerve. At the fibular head, this nerve divides into the deep peroneal branch, which innervates the foot and toe dorsiflexors including the intrinsic foot toe extensor (extensor digitorum brevis). The superficial peroneal branch innervates the peroneal muscles, which evert the foot. Sensory innervation of the posterior thigh comes from the posterior thigh nerve as a branch of the sciatic nerve. The anterior and lateral foreleg skin innervation comes from the common peroneal and superficial peroneal nerves, with the latter innervating most of the foot dorsum. The calf skin is innervated by the tibial nerve, which covers the sole of the foot and together with a variable peroneal nerve contribution forms a sural nerve that innervates the lateral foot.

Postpartum footdrop, the first sign of the lesion, often is accompanied by a variable sensory deficit in the peroneal nerve distribution. The lesion may be preceded by intermittent pain in the buttocks during the last trimester (52). If possible compression is anticipated, cesarean section is the method of choice. The reason is that footdrop might be severe, and because the lesion is very proximal, recovery is incomplete. Short primigravidas are at risk especially if the baby is large. Forceps delivery is another risk, as are a narrow pelvis and occipitoposterior rotation (2). Similar clinical presentation can result from improper position of legs and leg holders during delivery or excessive hand pressure over the lateral knee and fibular head by the patient during later stages of delivery (2,66,67). Prolonged squatting prior to delivery also may lead to common peroneal neuropathy (68). Nerve conduction study can distinguish between these two situations, which may have different outcomes. If footdrop persists, EMG is recommended to assess the extent and amount of axonal damage. Paresis

with minimal axonal damage has a good prognosis, whereas complete footdrop with severe axonal loss, especially with a pelvic lesion, has a poor prognosis. Physical therapy and foot orthosis may be necessary. In milder cases boots are sufficient support for functional gait.

Pudendal Nerve Lesions

The pudendal plexus is formed from the S2–S4 roots. Its short branches innervate the levator ani and coccygeus muscles. The pudendal nerve exits the pelvis through the infrapiriform foramen to innervate the perineal skin, labia majora, clitoris, external anal and urethral sphincters, transversal perineal muscles, and superficial pelvic floor-bulbocavernosus muscle.

The acute lesions are not well characterized, although it is well known that prolonged fetal head pressure can cause tissue necrosis and vesicovaginal fistulas that result in nerve damage. Large episiotomies result in local nerve damage and sensory loss as well as possible anal sphincter disturbances. These lesions have not been fully characterized neurologically. Most of the urogenital prolapses as well as urinary stress and other incontinences are considered the result of anatomic changes. These disorders are more common in women with multiple pregnancies. Symptoms do not appear immediately postpartum and may develop years later as a result of repeated pudendal plexus trauma. Snooks and coworkers (5) first suggested this mechanism with long-term neurophysiologic follow-up studies that revealed a high incidence of mild pudendal nerve lesions that may contribute to urogenital problems. The magnitude of female incontinence and odd pelvic pain syndromes certainly warrant more detailed studies of nerve lesion contributions to these situations. Although available techniques are not completely noninvasive and involve assessment, recordings, and stimulations within a sensitive area, they nevertheless should be judiciously used in diagnosing this important clinical problem.

PERIPHERAL NERVE DISORDERS IN PUERPERIUM

Most of the peripheral nerve disorders in puerperium represent progression of lesions that occurred during pregnancy or delivery. Most improve spontaneously and do not require special treatment. CTS may, however, develop during puerperium.

CTS can appear for the first time in puerperium and usually is seen in primiparae who are breastfeeding their infants (69,70). It also appears in older primiparae. There are no clear explanations for the cause because edema is not a feature in these women as it is in women with CTS during pregnancy (21). A combination of hormonal changes, local swelling, and possible aggravation of compression by handling of infants is most likely (70). CTS in the puerperium has a good prognosis and does not require surgical release. It subsides after discontinuation of breastfeeding and normalization of prolactin levels.

In one woman, incomplete breast emptying and consequent breast engorgement leading to fluctuating asymmetric bilateral brachial plexus compression was postulated (71). She developed hand and arm numbness and Tinel's sign on plexus compression in axilla.

There is some recent evidence that GBS might have a higher incidence in puerperium, especially during the first 2 weeks (72). There also are reported cases of more severe GBS, including axonal variant, in early puerperium (73), suggesting that health professionals should stay vigilant for possible disabling peripheral nerve disorders following delivery.

REFERENCES

1. Dyck PJ, Thomas PK, Griffin JW, et al, eds. *Peripheral neuropathy.* 3rd ed. Philadelphia: WB Saunders, 1993.
2. Donaldson JO. Neuropathy. In: Donaldson JO, ed. *Neurology of pregnancy.* Philadelphia: WB Saunders, 1978: 23–55.
3. Seddon HJ. Classification of nerve injuries. *BMJ* 1942; 11:237–239.
4. Seddon HJ. Three types of nerve injury. *Brain* 1943;66: 237–288.
5. Snooks SJ, Swash M, Mathers SE, et al. Effect of vaginal delivery on the pelvic floor: a 5-year follow-up. *Br J Surg* 1990;77:1358–1360.
6. Kimura J. *Electrodiagnosis in diseases of nerve and muscle: principles and practice.* 2nd ed. Philadelphia: FA Davis Co, 1989.
7. Lindblom U. Quantitative testing of sensibility including pain. In: Stalberg E, Young RR, eds. *Clinical neurophysiology.* London: Butterworths, 1981:168–190.
8. Low PA. Laboratory evaluation of autonomic failure. In: Low PA, ed. *Clinical autonomic disorders: evaluation and management.* Rochester, NY: Little, Brown, 1993.
9. Gould JS, Wissinger HA. Carpal tunnel syndrome in pregnancy. *South Med J* 1978;71:144–146.
10. Voitk AJ, Mueller JC, Farlinger DE, et al. Carpal tunnel syndrome in pregnancy. *Can Med Assoc J* 1983;128: 277–281.
11. Ekman-Ordeberg G, Sälgeback S, Ordeberg S. Carpal tunnel syndrome in pregnancy. *Acta Obstet Gynecol Scand* 1987;66:233–235.
12. Nicholas GG, Noone RB, Graham WP III. Carpal tunnel syndrome in pregnancy. *Hand* 1971;3:80–83.
13. Stolp-Smith KA, Pascoe MK, Ogburn PL Jr. Carpal tunnel syndrome in pregnancy: frequency, severity, and prognosis. *Arch Phys Med Rehabil* 1998;79:1285–1287.
14. McLennan HG, Oats JN, Walstab JE. Survey of hand symptoms in pregnancy. *Med J Aust* 1987;147:542–544.
15. Massey EW. Carpal tunnel syndrome in pregnancy. *Obstet Gynecol Surv* 1978;33:145–147.
16. Graham JG. Neurological complications of pregnancy and anaesthesia. *Clin Obstet Gynaecol* 1982;9:333–350.
17. Nygaard IE, Saltsman CL, Whitehouse MB, et al. Hand problems in pregnancy. *Am Fam Physician* 1989;39: 123–126.
18. al Qattan MM, Manktelow RT, Bowen CV. Pregnancy-induced carpal tunnel syndrome requiring surgical release longer than 2 years after delivery. *Obstet Gynecol* 1994;84:249–251.
19. Stahl S, Blumenfeld Z, Yarnitsky D. Carpal tunnel syndrome in pregnancy: indications for early surgery. *J Neurol Sci* 1996;136:182–184.
20. Tobin SM. Carpal tunnel syndrome in pregnancy. *Am J Obstet Gynecol* 1967;97:493–498.
21. Wand JS. Carpal tunnel syndrome in pregnancy and lactation. *J Hand Surg* 1990;15:93–95.
22. Seror P. Pregnancy-related carpal tunnel syndrome. *J Hand Surg [Br]* 1998;23:98–101.
23. Melvin JL, Burnett CN, Johnson EW. Median nerve conduction in pregnancy. *Arch Phys Med Rehabil* 1969; 50:75–80.
24. Samlaska S, Dews TE. Long-term epidural analgesia for pregnancy-induced intercostal neuralgia. *Pain* 1995; 62:245–248.
25. Peleg R, Gohar J, Koretz M, et al. Abdominal wall pain in pregnant women caused by thoracic lateral cutaneous nerve entrapment. *Eur J Obstet Gynecol Reprod Biol* 1997;74:169–171.
26. Dyck PJ, Prineas J, Pollard J. Chronic inflammatory demyelinating polyradiculoneuropathy. In: Dyck PJ, Thomas PK, Griffin JW, et al, eds. *Peripheral neuropathy.* 3rd ed. Philadelphia: WB Saunders, 1993:1498–1517.
27. McCombe PA, McManis PG, Frith JA, et al. Chronic inflammatory demyelinating polyradiculoneuropathy associated with pregnancy. *Ann Neurol* 1987;21:102–104.
28. Arnason BGW, Soliven B. Acute inflammatory demyelinating polyradiculoneuropathy. In: Dyck PJ, Thomas PK, Griffin JW, et al, eds. *Peripheral neuropathy.* 3rd ed. Philadelphia: WB Saunders, 1993:1437–1497.

29. Jiang GX, de Pedro-Cuesta J, Strigard K, et al. Pregnancy and Guillain-Barré syndrome: a nationwide register cohort study. *Neuroepidemiology* 1996;15:192–200.

30. Brooks H, Christian AS, May AE. Pregnancy, anaesthesia and Guillain-Barré syndrome. *Anaesthesia* 2000;55: 894–898.

31. Rockel A, Wissel J, Rolfs A. Guillain-Barré syndrome in pregnancy—an indication for caesarian section? *J Perinat Med* 1994;22:393–398.

32. Feasby TE, Gilbert JJ, Brown WF, et al. An acute axonal form of Guillain-Barré syndrome. *Brain* 1986;109: 1115–1126.

33. Triggs WJ, Cros D, Gominak SC, et al. Motor nerve inexcitability in Guillain-Barré syndrome. *Brain* 1992; 115:1291–1302.

34. Yaginuma Y, Kawamura M, Ishikawa M. Landry-Guillain-Barré-Strohl syndrome in pregnancy. *J Obstet Gynaecol Res* 1996;22:47–49.

35. Breuer GS, Morali G, Finkelstein Y, et al. A pregnant woman with hepatitis A and Guillain-Barré. *J Clin Gastroenterol* 2001;32:179–180.

36. Yamada H, Noro N, Kato EH, et al. Massive intravenous immunoglobulin treatment in pregnancy complicated by Guillain-Barré Syndrome. *Eur J Obstet Gynecol Reprod Biol* 2001;97:101–104.

37. Parsonage MJ, Turner JWA. Neuralgic amyotrophy: the shoulder-girdle syndrome. *Lancet* 1948;1:973–978.

38. Turner JWA, Parsonage MJ. Neuralgic amyotrophy (paralytic brachial neuritis) with special reference to prognosis. *Lancet* 1957;2:209–212.

39. Windebank AL Inherited recurrent focal neuropathies. In: Dyck PJ, Thomas PK, Griffin JW, et al, eds. *Peripheral neuropathy.* 3rd ed. Philadelphia: WB Saunders, 1993:1137–1148.

40. Geiger LR, Mancall EL, Penn AS. Familial neuralgia amyotrophy. Report of three families with review of the literature. *Brain* 1974;97:87–102.

41. Simonetti S. Lesion of the anterior branch of axillary nerve in a patient with hereditary neuropathy with liability to pressure palsies. *Eur J Neurol* 2000;7:577–579.

42. Redmond JM, Cros D, Martin JB, et al. Relapsing bilateral brachial plexopathy during pregnancy. *Arch Neurol* 1989;46:462–464.

43. Thomas PK, Tomlinson DR. Diabetic and hypoglycemic neuropathy. In: Dyck PJ, Thomas PK, Griffin JW, et al, eds. *Peripheral neuropathy.* 3rd ed. Philadelphia: WB Saunders, 1993:1219–1250.

44. Nylund L, Brismar T, Lunell NO, et al. Nerve conduction in diabetic pregnancy: a prospective study. *Diabetes Res Clin Prac* 1985;1:121–123.

45. Lapolla A, Cardone C, Negrin P, et al. Pregnancy does not induce or worsen retinal and peripheral nerve dysfunction in insulin-dependent diabetic women. *J Diabetes Complications* 1998;12:74–80.

46. Berk MA, Miodovnik M, Mimouni F. Impact of pregnancy on complications of insulin-dependent diabetes mellitus. *Am J Perinatol* 1988; 5:359–367.

47. Hemachandra A, Ellis D, Lloyd CE, et al. The influence of pregnancy on IDDM complications. *Diabetes Care* 1995;18:950–954.

48. Steel JM. Autonomic neuropathy in pregnancy. *Diabetes Care* 1989;12:170–171.

49. Macleod AF, Smith SA, Sonksen PH, et al. The problem of autonomic neuropathy in diabetic pregnancy. *Diabet Med* 1990;7:80–82.

50. Scott AR, Tattersall RB, McPherson M. Improvement of postural hypotension and severe diabetic autonomic neuropathy during pregnancy. *Diabetes Care* 1988;11: 369–370.

51. Hopf HC. [Obturator nerve paralysis during parturition (author's transl)] *J Neurol* 1974;207:165–166.

52. Mumenthaler M, Schliack H, Mumenthaler M. *Peripheral nerve lesions: diagnosis and therapy.* New York: Thieme Medical Publishers, 1991.

53. Warfield CA. Obturator neuropathy after forceps delivery. *Obstet Gynecol* 1984;64:47-48.

54. Adelman JU, Goldberg GS, Puckett JD. Postpartum bilateral femoral neuropathy. *Obstet Gynecol* 1973;42: 845–850.

55. Vargo MM, Robinson LR, Nicholas JJ, et al. Postpartum femoral neuropathy: relic of an earlier era? *Arch Phys Med Rehabil* 1990;71:591–596.

56. O'Connell JE. Maternal obstetrical paralysis. *Surg Gynecol Obstet* 1944;79:374–382.

57. King AB. Neurologic conditions occurring as complications of pregnancy. *Arch Neurol Psychiatry* 1950;471: 611–644.

58. Montag TW, Mead PB. Postpartum femoral neuropathy. *J Reprod Med* 1981;26:563–566.

59. Donaldson JO, Wirz D, Mashman J. Bilateral postpartum femoral neuropathy. *Conn Med* 1985;49:496–498.

60. Allen LA. Maternal obstetric paralysis. *S Afr Med J* 1983;63:736–737.

61. al Hakim M, Katirji B. Femoral mononeuropathy induced by the lithotomy position: a report of 5 cases with a review of literature. *Muscle Nerve* 1993;16: 891–895.

62. Brunner C. Peroneaeusparese als seltene Indikaton zur Schnittentbindung. *Schweiz Med Wochenschr* 1941;71: 1243–1244.

63. Pommier M, Lecomte Cl. Die Peronaeuslähmung im Wochenbett. *Bull Féd Soc Gynéc Obstét Franç* 1959;11: 176–9.

64. Watson WJ, Beebe JE. Postpartum foot drop: a case report. *J Reprod Med* 1988;33:973–974.

65. Bademosi O, Osuntokun BO, Van de Werd HJ, et al. Obstetric neuropraxia in the Nigeria African. *Int J Gynaecol Obstet* 1980;17:611–614.

66. Adornato BT, Carlini WG. "Pushing palsy": a case of self-induced bilateral peroneal palsy during natural childbirth. *Neurology* 1992;42:936–938.

67. Colachis SC 3rd, Pease WS, Johnson EW. A preventable cause of foot drop during childbirth. *Am J Obstet Gynecol* 1994;171:270–272.

68. Babayev M, Bodack MP, Creatura C. Common peroneal neuropathy secondary to squatting during childbirth. *Obstet Gynecol* 1998;91:830–832.

69. Wand JS. The natural history of carpal tunnel syndrome in lactation. *J R Soc Med* 1989;82:349–350.

70. Snell NJ, Coysh HL, Snell BL. Carpal tunnel syndrome presenting in the puerperium. *Practitioner* 1980;224: 191–193.

71. Simkin P. Intermittent brachial plexus neuropathy secondary to breast engorgement. *Birth* 1988;15:102–103.

72. Cheng Q, Jiang GX, Fredrikson S, et al. Increased incidence of Guillain-Barré syndrome postpartum. *Epidemiology* 1998;9:601–604.

73. Vital A, Larriviere M, Lagueny A, et al. Severe axonal polyneuropathy with onset in the postpartum period. *Acta Neurol Scand* 1994;89:303–306.

Neurological Complications of Pregnancy, Second Edition, edited by Brian Hainline and Orrin Devinsky. Lippincott Williams & Wilkins, Philadelphia, © 2002.

17

Muscle Disease

James M. Gilchrist

Department of Neurosciences, Brown University School of Medicine;
Department of Neurology, Rhode Island Hospital, Providence, Rhode Island, U.S.A.

Muscle disease is a nonspecific term that for this chapter will include primary disorders of muscle, including the neuromuscular junction. This chapter addresses those muscle diseases for which a relationship to pregnancy is described in the literature and those muscle diseases not directly affecting the pregnant woman but for which prenatal genetic counseling and testing are important. Molecular genetics has made a significant impact on the field of neuromuscular disease, and advances continue. As such, specific mention of genetic localizations and counseling is limited to those diseases deemed of paramount importance. All patients with a presumption of genetic muscle disease should be seen by a physician or genetic counselor knowledgeable on the latest in genetic diagnosis and screening techniques. There is no unifying concept covering the affects of pregnancy on muscle disease, and vice versa, and this review will be largely phenomenological as a consequence. When cause and effect is known, it will be discussed.

MUSCULAR DYSTROPHY

There are several forms of muscular dystrophy, all being progressive, inherited muscular diseases. Most are inherited as autosomal dominant traits (myotonic dystrophy, proximal myotonic myopathy, facioscapulohumeral dystrophy, oculopharyngeal dystrophy), some as autosomal recessive (limb-girdle muscular dystrophy, congenital muscular dystrophy), and several as x-linked (Duchenne muscular dystrophy, Becker muscular dystrophy, Emery-Driefuss muscular dystrophy). All have had chromosomal localization, many have had genes localized, and some have had the affected genetic product elucidated. Discussion of genetic counseling will be limited to those dystrophies with a known gene product and accurate, easily available gene testing (i.e., Duchenne and Becker dystrophy, facioscapulo-humeral dystrophy, oculopharyngeal dystrophy, and myotonic dystrophy). In the near future such testing likely will be available for other dystrophies. Emery-Driefuss muscular dystrophy will not be discussed because there is no known effect of or on pregnancy.

Myotonic Dystrophy

Myotonic dystrophy (also known as dystrophica myotonica, myotonia atrophica, Steinert's disease) is a multisystem disorder characterized by variable expression of progressive, predominantly distal, skeletal muscle weakness; cataracts; frontal balding; cardiac conduction defects; clinical and electrical myotonia; smooth muscle weakness of esophagus, stomach, bowel, and uterus; and endocrine disturbances (1). Onset is usually in the second to third decade, but it can be much later (1) or as early as birth (2,3).

Myotonic dystrophy is inherited as an autosomal dominant trait. The abnormal gene has been localized to chromosome 19 (4–6). The disease is related to the presence of inserted triplet repeats in the gene, which increase in size in succeeding generations, explaining the clinical phenomenon of anticipation, in which subsequent generations manifest the disease more severely and at an earlier age (7). The gene encodes for myotonin, a member of the protein kinase family (4) whose function remains poorly understood.

The first issue to address regarding myotonic dystrophy and pregnancy is the matter of getting pregnant at all. Large sibships are not uncommon in families with myotonic dystrophy, and certainly fertility is not drastically reduced. However, amongst the abnormalities noted in myotonic dystrophy is testicular atrophy in approximately 80% of affected men (8). This atrophy is of primary gonadal origin, as shown by elevated FSH and LH levels (9–11), normal secondary sexual characteristics, and low testosterone levels (9), abnormalities that can be seen prepubertal (12). Seminiferous tubule destruction is seen histologically and comprises the bulk of the gonadal pathology; Leydig cells are normal until total tubular fibrosis is present (10,13). Despite this, men with testicular atrophy have been reported to father children (14). Women have few clinical or hormonal gonadal abnormalities (11,12), and in two studies of six women, there were no abnormalities of estrogen, gonadotropin, or testosterone (12,15). In a group of 33 women followed by Thomasen, menstrual irregularities correlated with severity of myotonic dystrophy (16), although others are not sure this is significant (11). Harper studied 44 affected females and compared them to 25 unaffected siblings and spouses. He found a tendency toward irregular and painful menses and an earlier onset of menopause (12). A case of amenorrhea from hypothalamic hypogonadism reported normal gonadal hormone levels (17). Fertility seems to be reduced to 75% of normal in both sexes. However, because this includes severely affected members who are unlikely to conceive, the fertility of less affected women may well be normal or even increased (18).

Pregnancy's Effect on Myotonic Dystrophy

Pregnancy uncommonly can have an ill effect on women with myotonic dystrophy (19). There is no evidence to suggest pregnancy has a beneficial effect on the disease. Several case reports indicate myotonia, muscle wasting, and weakness can first become symptomatic or dramatically worsen during pregnancy (20–24). This usually, but not exclusively, occurs during the third trimester (21,25), corresponding to the time of maximal progesterone levels, leading to speculation that progesterone is involved in the increased symptoms (21). The worsened clinical state is temporary with return to baseline after delivery. Fall and colleagues (26) report a unique case, of a pregnant myotonic woman who developed heart failure at 32 weeks gestation, with an endomyocardial biopsy consistent with myotonic dystrophy. She improved after delivery but died suddenly from cardiac arrhythmia 8 weeks later. Progressive loss of muscle function in the mother is expected regardless of pregnancy. Whether pregnancy accelerates permanent disability is unknown but if so, it occurs rarely (19).

Myotonic Dystrophy's Effect on Pregnancy

Myotonic dystrophy has a potentially devastating impact on the pregnant mother (Table 17.1) (19,20,23,25,27–32) and her fetus (19, 25,27,28,33,34). Postpartum hemorrhage related to failure of uterine contraction after delivery is particularly worrisome (28,31). Labor can be prolonged in both the first (21) and

TABLE 17.1. *Effects of myotonic dystrophy on the pregnant mother and her fetus*

Maternal effects	Fetal effects
Prolonged labor	Hydramnios
Premature labor	Increased neonatal
Uterine atony	mortality
Retained placenta	Reduced fetal
Placenta previa	movements
Spontaneous abortion	
Postpartum hemorrhage	
Variable response to oxytocin	

second stages, due to poor uterine contraction from myometrial involvement (20,25) and to inability to "bear down" because of voluntary muscle weakness (22,24). Despite this, labor is not prolonged for most women with myotonic dystrophy (19). Prolonged bed rest should be avoided because disuse of muscles will further weaken any patient with myotonic dystrophy.

Anesthesia and surgery carry special risks as well. Depolarizing neuromuscular blockers, such as succinylcholine, in patients with myotonic dystrophy have been reported to cause "myotonic spasm," (35,36) in which muscles diffusely contract and cannot be relaxed. This is temporary and without permanent sequelae. However, it may be impossible to ventilate the patient during the spasm. Nondepolarizing agents (e.g., curare) do not cause this reaction and can be used. Myotonic dystrophy does not place these patients at high risk for malignant hyperthermia (37). Thiopental has been noted to cause marked respiratory depression in patients with myotonic dystrophy (31). All things considered, local anesthesia is preferable to general anesthesia (31).

The major intraanesthetic and postoperative concerns are adequate ventilation and control of cardiac arrhythmias (37). Both problems arise from the multisystem nature of myotonic dystrophy (e.g., weakness of pharyngeal and other skeletal muscles) and cardiac conduction abnormalities. Preoperative clinical assessment of cardiac and respiratory function (including electrocardiogram, chest X-ray, and pulmonary function tests) and careful postoperative monitoring of ventilation and cardiac rhythm are the best ways to avoid trouble (37).

Congenital Myotonic Dystrophy

Myotonic dystrophy can present in utero, at birth, or in early childhood. For reasons still unexplained (38,39), this congenital myotonic dystrophy occurs almost exclusively when the mother is the affected parent (40). The risk of an affected woman having a congenitally affected child is 10%, but risk increases to near 40% if she already has had congenitally affected offspring (38). Women with multisystem disease at the time of pregnancy and delivery are at the highest risk for a child with congenital myotonic dystrophy (38), but even asymptomatic women have borne congenitally affected children (41). The mother's age at birth may have an effect on the severity of her offspring's disease, suggesting the older the woman the more severely affected are her children (42).

The disease can manifest in utero as polyhydramnios and reduced fetal movements, resulting in arthrogryposis multiplex congenita at birth (25,27,33,34,43). The first description of congenital myotonic dystrophy was in 1960 (44), and subsequently Dyken and Harper described congenital myotonic dystrophy in 38 patients from 24 families who had symptoms referable to myotonic dystrophy from birth (3). Symptoms varied from severe respiratory involvement at birth to clumsiness and mental retardation evident in early childhood. Neonatal onset of myotonic dystrophy is frequently fatal, due to respiratory failure (27,43). Survivors are impaired, with hypotonia, diffuse weakness, developmental delay, poor feeding, mental retardation (45), and arthrogryposis (43). Fetal muscle in these cases exhibits maturational arrest most severely involving limb, pharyngeal, and diaphragmatic muscles (46). Rutherford and associates found respiratory function at birth determined survival in congenital myotonic dystrophy, and duration of mechanical ventilation was the best guide to prognosis (47). Electrodiagnostic studies sometimes confirm the diagnosis (48) but often do not show myotonia and may be more informative when done on the mother than on the infant. A high index of suspicion for congenital myotonic dystrophy is important in the infant with respiratory failure and failure to feed because the mother commonly has not been previously diagnosed. Affected children without the fetal or neonatal presentation exhibit talipes, facial diplegia, mental retardation, developmental delay, weakness, clumsiness, strabismus, and dysarthria (2,3).

Genetic Counseling

In the absence of a foreseeable cure for myotonic dystrophy, genetic counseling offers an opportunity to improve a patient's understanding of the disease, establish individual risk for symptoms, determine the risk for myotonic dystrophy, and offer advice for dealing with these risks. Carrier and prenatal detection now can be done with near 100% accuracy by measuring trinucleotide repeat length (7), thereby allowing better genetic counseling and the option of elective abortion of affected fetuses. For prenatal detection, chorionic villus sampling circa 10 weeks, or amniocentesis circa 16 weeks, is required to establish fetal genotype. Trophoblast cells from endocervical canal flushing between 7 and 9 weeks gestation also can provide fetal DNA (49). Expansion of the trinucleotide repeat in fetal compared to maternal tissue does not reliably predict congenital myotonic dystrophy (50).

Proximal Myotonic Myopathy

Accurate genetic testing for myotonic dystrophy has revealed families without either a triplet repeat expansion or linkage to DNA markers on chromosome 19. These patients are clinically similar to those with myotonic dystrophy except for proximal rather than distal weakness, thus the newly coined diagnosis of proximal myotonic myopathy (PROMM) (51). PROMM has been linked to a locus on chromosome 3q, as have two other myotonic entities—proximal myotonic dystrophy and myotonic dystrophy 2 (52). Whether the three diseases are allelic or represent phenotypic variation of a single genetic mutation is unknown (52). A new classification proposes calling myotonic dystrophy linked to chromosome 19q "myotonic dystrophy type 1" and the entities linked to chromosome 3q "myotonic dystrophy type 2" (52). Newman and associates report three sisters with PROMM who had myotonia present during pregnancy but the disease disappeared after delivery (53). PROMM affects genetic counseling because asymptomatic patients with a family history of myotonic dystrophy and normal cytosine-thymidine-guanine (CTG) triplet repeat numbers cannot be definitely excluded as carriers until an affected family member has been shown to have an expanded triplet repeat region.

Duchenne and Becker Muscular Dystrophy

Duchenne and Becker muscular dystrophy are allelic x-linked recessive disorders arising from defects in a gene coding for a large structural protein called dystrophin (54,55). Boys become symptomatic for Duchenne dystrophy around 5 years of age, become wheelchair-bound around 10 to 12 years of age, and die by their early 20s. Becker dystrophy is milder and the symptoms, although similar, reach the same milestones a decade or so later (56). Females, by nature of the chromosomal location, are at risk for being carriers but not for the dystrophy (infrequently, carrier females can manifest a milder form of the disease) (57,58). Female carriers have an increased incidence of breech deliveries, regardless of the genetic status of the neonate, indicating a maternal factor, such as subtle uterine or pelvic floor muscle weakness (59).

Prenatal Diagnosis and Counseling

Because of the devastating impact of an affected boy and the lack of a cure, pre-pregnancy genetic counseling for women with affected offspring, siblings, or other relatives regarding risk is important. Unfortunately, the dystrophin gene region is quite large, and up to one-third of cases of Duchenne and Becker dystrophy are new mutations (56). In families with known dystrophinopathies, however, carrier detection and prenatal diagnosis of affected fetuses is available (60). The risk of being a carrier is dependent on the pedigree (i.e., the number of affected males and their relationship to the woman in question). Baysian analysis is usually the basis for calculating the genetic risk for carrier status (56). For a known carrier, each of her offspring, male or female, carry a 50% chance of inheriting the abnormal gene. The situation is often not so straightforward (56) and the risk calculation may be improved by DNA analysis (60).

Abnormal dystrophin quantity and quality are the *sine qua non* of Duchenne and Becker muscular dystrophy, and this can be determined by muscle assay (61). Female carriers are not diagnosed reliably by dystrophin quantitation, however (58). Immunostaining of muscle for dystrophin may be useful in that regard, but a normal examination does not exclude being a carrier (58). Thus, DNA analysis must be used to establish carrier status. Approximately 60% of Duchenne cases arise from a deletion of the dystrophin gene, and another 7% arise from duplications (62). If either is present in the affected male(s) of a family, the presence or absence of the deletion or duplication can be determined in at-risk females by a blood test for DNA analysis. Absence of the DNA abnormality can exclude the risk, although germline or placental mosaicism (63) also must be considered. Presence of the DNA defect indicates the female is a carrier. If a deletion or duplication is not found in the affected male, then DNA linkage analysis is indicated (60). This necessitates obtaining blood from members of the family and, most especially, from affected males, if alive. Prenatal testing can be used to significantly lower the risk of affected boys in families known to be at risk. If the fetus is male, DNA linkage using polymerase chain reaction (PCR) techniques can be done to determine if the fetus carries the defective gene. This can be accomplished by chorionic villus sampling or amniocentesis. Other approaches include fetal muscle biopsy for dystrophin analysis (64), cleavage cell embryo biopsy (65), and dystrophin deletion analysis of nucleated maternal erythrocytes (66). These tests are only helpful if therapeutic abortion is being considered.

Limb-Girdle Muscular Dystrophy

A diagnosis of limb-girdle muscular dystrophy (LGMD) in the past often was given to patients with muscle disease not otherwise explained. In the past several years, the molecular genetics of LGMD have been much clarified, with localization of eight autosomal recessive forms and three autosomal dominant forms (67,68). Several of the genes code for proteins of the dystrophin-associated glycoprotein complex, which, with dystrophin, comprise the major underlying structural support of the muscle fiber membrane (69). This has enabled a genetic classification of the LGMD syndromes (67,69).

Typically, LGMD appears in the second and third decade of life, with proximal legs then arms affected over a prolonged course. Ambulation may be lost, but not until 20 years or so after onset. LGMD is sporadic or inherited as an autosomal recessive trait in 95% of patients, with the remaining cases inherited in an autosomal dominant pattern (70). Less commonly, a severe childhood form of the disease is seen, looking very much like Duchenne dystrophy but distinguishable from it by an autosomal recessive pattern of inheritance (severe childhood autosomal recessive muscular dystrophy, or SCARMD).

LGMD and Pregnancy

Delivery can be very difficult when a patient with LGMD is severely affected and wheelchair bound (71). In an unpublished study, Lauren Donald and Gilchrist did a retrospective survey of 38 women with autosomal recessive LGMD from 31 families. There were 59 pregnancies in 22 women with 38 children and a known spontaneous abortion rate of 31%, with one perinatal death. Difficulty with labor and delivery was reported in 29% of births without other complications. Seven women suffered significant and permanent decline in function while pregnant, most frequently in the more severely affected women and usually in the first two trimesters.

Similar findings were reported from a retrospective review of nine LGMD women with 15 pregnancies (72). Therapeutic abortion occurred in three (20%), with no miscarriages noted. Operative delivery was necessary in five of the remaining 12 pregnancies, of which two were emergencies. Five of the nine women experienced worsening weakness during pregnancy, one of whom improved after delivery. Five of the women required assistance in child care after delivery because of physical limitations. Women with LGMD therefore should be counseled that pregnancy may increase spontaneous abortion and may significantly and permanently increase weakness, the risk being greater with increasing disease severity.

Genetic Counseling

The majority of LGMD patients have an autosomal recessively inherited trait. Therefore, the risk of their offspring inheriting the disease is increased only marginally over the general population, as long as the mating is not consanguineous. The real question arises in families wishing another child who already have one child with SCARMD. The risk of any further children having the disease is 25% if there is no consanguinity. Prenatal screening is possible but requires linkage analysis, mutation analysis, or fetal muscle biopsy at a center able to do the testing, which is not widely available (73–75).

Facioscapulohumeral Dystrophy

Facioscapulohumeral muscular dystrophy (FSHD) is inherited as an autosomal dominant trait. Approximately 95% of families have been linked to chromosome 4q35, near the telomere (76). FSHD is a muscular dystrophy of characteristic and defining weakness involving the face and scapular muscles. The age of onset is variable, from childhood (these patients are frequently more severely affected) to the early third decade. The weakness is slowly progressive and may arrest for several years or more. However, the disease also may progress in sudden accelerations.

Despite the relative frequency of FSHD, there is only one report of 26 pregnancies in 11 patients (72). There were three miscarriages (12%), two preterm births, and six operative deliveries. Three women had symptomatic worsening during gestation, but all recovered after delivery and there were no long-term sequelae.

Genetic Counseling

As with any autosomal dominant inherited trait, the risk of intergenerational transmission is 50% for each child. The gene for FSHD has not been found nor is the gene product known. However, more than 90% of FSHD patients have a deletion on chromosome 4q35 resulting in a small EcoRI restriction fragment, which can be used to confirm the disease and for prenatal diagnosis (77).

Congenital Muscular Dystrophy

Congenital muscular dystrophy (CMD) comprises a group of inherited disorders with progressive muscular weakness and variable amounts of central nervous system (CNS) involvement. CMD has been classified into the classical form without CNS involvement and Fukuyama muscular dystrophy. The classical form has been further divided by the presence or absence of merosin, a protein that connects the dystrophin-associated glycoprotein complex to the extracellular matrix. Merosin-deficient CMD has been linked to the locus of the laminin alpha-2 chain of merosin on chromosome 6q2 (78). Merosin-deficient and merosin-positive CMD share similar characteristics of hypotonia, muscle weakness, and developmental delay with onset in early infancy (79). Imaging studies of the brain reveal white-matter changes but no malformations. Mental retardation occurs in a minority of patients with classical CMD. The progressive weakness and the mental retardation may be milder in the merosin-positive patients (79). Fukuyama CMD has early infantile onset of severe weakness, brain malformation, severe mental retardation, and early death. It has been linked to a locus on chromosome 9q31(80).

The finding of a genetic locus for merosin-negative CMD and for Fukuyama CMD has made prenatal genetic determination possible in families at risk. Trophoblast tissue immunocytochemistry and DNA linkage analysis have been used to determine affected and unaffected merosin-negative CMD fetuses (81,82). Linkage analysis using PCR markers has been used in Fukuyama CMD for the same purpose (83,84).

CHANNELOPATHIES

Channelopathy (myotonia congenita, periodic paralysis, malignant hyperthermia) refers to a group of inherited muscle disorders caused by genetic defects of muscle membrane channels. These include the SCN4A gene on chromosome 17q23 coding for the adult sodium channel α-subunit (85), the CLCN1 gene on chromosome 7q35 encoding the chloride channel (85), the CACNL1A3 gene on 1q31–32 coding for the dihydropyridine receptor of the calcium channel (85), and the RYR1 gene on 19q coding for the ryanodine receptor of the calcium release channel (86). Mutations of the SCN4A gene result in several autosomal dominant phenotypes, including hyperkalemic periodic paralysis, normokalemic periodic paralysis, and paramyotonia congenita (85). These diseases cause transient paralysis of muscles, beginning in the legs and progressing to involve arm and even facial muscles, and rarely, muscles of respiration. Each attack lasts hours to days and onset is in childhood. All have electrical, and to a lesser extent, clinical myotonia. Mutations of the CLCN1 gene cause either autosomal dominant (Thomsen disease) or autosomal recessive (Becker-type myotonia) myotonia congenita (85). The former is the more common. Both are characterized by electrical and clinical myotonia of skeletal muscles, with normal muscle strength. Patients complain of stiffness, which abates with continued use of the muscle (i.e., after "warming up"). Sudden movement, however, may result in falls. Mutations of the calcium channel gene result in hypokalemic periodic paralysis in which patients suffer transient weakness of limbs, as in the hyperkalemic form, but have no myotonia.

They are associated with low serum potassium. Mutations of the RYR1 gene result in malignant hyperthermia.

The effect of pregnancy on myotonia congenita in two women was temporary worsening in the second half of the pregnancy (87, 88). As with myotonic dystrophy, increased symptoms in the pregnant woman occur but are probably uncommon. Obstetric problems have not been described. Exceptionally, patients with autosomal dominant myotonia congenita may develop weakness and fluctuating symptoms only during pregnancy (89).

Anesthetics pose some risks to the pregnant woman with myotonia congenita. "Myotonic spasms" may occur with depolarizing neuromuscular blockers such as succinylcholine (37). Malignant hyperthermia has been reported in two cases of myotonia congenita (90,91), although a connection between the two disorders remains doubtful (92).

There are no reports of pregnancy in periodic paralysis. In a multigeneration family with hyperkalemic periodic paralysis known to the author, affected women have had multiple uneventful pregnancies. It is uncertain whether certain anesthetics precipitate attacks of paralysis (92). Paralytic attacks with surgery may be related more to the stress of the operation, long periods of fasting, or overeating the night before surgery than to any anesthetic agent.

Malignant Hyperthermia

Malignant hyperthermia is a syndrome of hyperpyrexia, muscle rigidity, rhabdomyolysis, and death, triggered by certain anesthetic agents (e.g., depolarizing muscle relaxants, inhalation anesthetics), and, in malignant hyperthermia-susceptible patients, by stress and infection. The incidence in adults is 1:50,000 operative cases, and the question relating to pregnancy and malignant hyperthermia is why more cases are not encountered (93). Familial malignant hyperthermia has been linked to three different chromosomal loci so far (86). Only three cases of malignant hyperthermia during pregnancy have been reported, all during cesarean section (94–96) and all managed successfully with dantrolene. Malignant hyperthermia-susceptible patients can be managed uneventfully through labor and delivery, including cesarean section, by using agents not associated with malignant hyperthermia, careful monitoring (93), and prophylactic dantrolene if needed (97–99). Dantrolene crosses the placenta (99) and, although its effects on the newborn have not been well studied, one study of 20 exposed pregnancies found no adverse effect on the fetus or newborn (98).

MYASTHENIA GRAVIS

Myasthenia gravis is an autoimmune disorder in which polyclonal antibodies are directed against the nicotinic acetylcholine receptor of skeletal muscle (100). This results in degradation of the neuromuscular junction and failure of neuromuscular transmission (100). The clinical hallmark of the disease is fatigable weakness, causing intermittent symptoms, such as ptosis, diplopia, dysphagia, dysarthria, and facial and limb muscle weakness, usually following repetitive action. Respiratory compromise can occur in severe cases.

The disease has a bimodal peak incidence, affecting older men and young women of childbearing age. Although the clinical history and exam are often typical and highly suggestive, confirmation of the diagnosis rests on pharmacologic, immunologic, and electrodiagnostic grounds. Edrophonium (Tensilon) given intravenously will quickly but briefly reverse the signs of myasthenia gravis and serves as a good bedside test (101). Assay for the presence of serum acetylcholine receptor antibodies is very specific for myasthenia gravis and is abnormal in 70% to 90% of cases (102). Sensitivity is lower in patients with only ocular signs. Electrodiagnostic tests of neuromuscular transmission include repetitive nerve stimulation (abnormal in 50% to 75% of cases) (103) and single fiber electromyography (SFEMG); (abnormal in 98% of cases) (104).

Treatment may address symptoms only or may be curative. Anticholinesterases can be used to briefly abate or improve symptoms attributable to myasthenia gravis, but they will not affect the underlying immunologic dysfunction. These drugs work by inhibiting the breakdown of acetylcholine, the neurotransmitter released by terminal motor nerve fibers. Edrophonium, neostigmine, and pyridostigmine (Mestinon) are all anticholinesterases; the latter is used most commonly given its longer duration of action (2 to 4 hours) and lesser muscarinic side effects. A time-release form of pyridostigmine is also available, usually for overnight use. Pyridostigmine is commonly used by itself in mild cases and in conjunction with immune suppression in more severe cases. Side effects include diaphoresis, hypersalivation, diarrhea, nausea, abdominal cramping, bradycardia, and fasciculations. Pyridostigmine can enter the fetal circulation, at 85% to 90% of maternal levels (105). Despite this, only one case of presumed fetal teratogenicity has been reported in the 50 years it has been available, and that was in a woman taking four to eight times (1,500 to 3,000 mg daily) the recommended dose (106). At recommended doses (less than 600 mg per day) pyridostigmine is safe to use during pregnancy. Parenteral formulations of neostigmine and pyridostigmine are available when needed pre- or postsurgery, during labor, or early in pregnancy if emesis gravidarum is severe. Intravenous dosages are one-thirtieth the oral dose for both drugs.

Suppression of the immune system attack on the acetylcholine receptor is indicated when the disease is generalized, involves vital functions such as ventilation or swallowing, or is not amenable to symptomatic treatment alone. Various treatments can be used including corticosteroids, immune suppressants such as azathioprine and cyclosporine, plasmapheresis, intravenous human immuneglobulin, and thymectomy. In the pregnant patient, corticosteroids are preferred over the other immunosuppressants. Corticosteroids can cause worsening of symptoms at initiation of therapy and patients must be watched carefully early on, preferably as inpatients (107, 108). This worsening can be limited by starting patients on very low doses with a slow titration upwards in dose, although this delays clinical benefit (109). Plasmapheresis is indicated in the severely compromised patient, in the patient refractory to other treatment modalities, and in the patient in whom an immediate response is required. Plasmapheresis rapidly lowers acetylcholine antibody titers and may be indicated when high maternal titers threaten fetal development (110) or predict neonatal myasthenia. The technique has been used successfully to treat fulminant myasthenia gravis in a pregnant patient (111), and the low rate of complications is no different from nonpregnant patients (112).

Thymomas are present in 10% to 15% of patients with myasthenia gravis, and myasthenia gravis occurs in 30% of patients with thymomas (113). Thymic hyperplasia is present in another 70% of patients with myasthenia gravis (113). Malignant thymoma is uncommon in the pregnant patient but carries a poor prognosis when associated with pregnancy (114). The thymus gland is the likely site for initial sensitization to the acetylcholine receptor (115). Removal of thymic tissue increases the remission rate from 15% to 30% and results in significant clinical improvement in two-thirds of patients, although the improvement may take up to 5 years (116). Thymectomy favorably influences the incidence of neonatal myasthenia gravis (117). Thymectomy has been performed on pregnant women with refractory disease (118), and, if done before pregnancy, can decrease the incidence of disease exacerbation during pregnancy (119). If possible, it is advisable for a woman with generalized myasthenia gravis who is considering pregnancy to have thymectomy prior to becoming pregnant. Thymectomy should be considered in all patients between 18 and 55 years of age with generalized myasthenia gravis.

Drug Interactions

Many drugs can cause worsening of myasthenia gravis (Table 17.2) (120,121): Transient exacerbations may occur using several treatments for myasthenia, including anticholinesterases, steroids, and high-dose intravenous immuneglobulin. Iodinated contrast dye also has been noted to cause transient worsening of myasthenic symptoms (122).

Pregnancy's Effect on Myasthenia Gravis

Review of the literature reveals 31% of pregnancies in myasthenic women caused no change in the status of the myasthenia, 29% had improvement, and 41% had worsening of symptoms during the pregnancy or, most commonly, in the puerperium (123). Mortality of mothers was 10%, most commonly from myasthenic crisis, but also from cholinergic crisis and postpartum hemorrhage (123). These numbers reflect a reporting bias toward more severe disease but indicate pregnancy frequently has an adverse effect on the

TABLE 17.2. *Drugs potentially harmful in myasthenia gravis*

Antibiotics	Antiarrhythmics	Anticonvulsants	Antirheumatics	Psychotropics	Others
Aminoglycosides	Lidocaine	Dilantin	Chloroquine	Lithium	Neuromuscular blockers
Polymixin A & B	Quinidine	Trimethadione	D-penicillamine	Chlorpromazine	Magnesium
Colistin	Quinine			Phenelzine	Steroids
Lincomycin	Procainamide			Promazine	Thyroid replacement
Clindamycin	Beta blockers				Adrenocorticotropic hormone
Trimethoprim	Ca++ channel blockers				Intravenous immune globulin
Tetracyclines					Cholinesterase inhibitors

myasthenic patient. A study of 47 myasthenic women with 64 pregnancies from a single institution (124) showed that during pregnancy 39% improved, 42% remained unchanged, and 19% deteriorated or relapsed. However, after delivery 28% had worsening of symptoms. Exacerbations tend to be most sudden and dangerous in the postpartum period and are frequently accompanied by respiratory failure (123). Therapeutic abortion is of little benefit in the treatment of myasthenia gravis (125,126).

Alpha-fetoprotein (AFP) effectively inhibits binding of acetylcholine antibodies to the acetylcholine receptor (127). The presence of AFP in maternal serum during pregnancy may explain the symptomatic improvement often seen in the third trimester (117) and its absence may account for the frequent postpartum exacerbation of myasthenia gravis when AFP levels precipitously fall.

Effects of Myasthenia Gravis on Pregnancy

Myasthenia gravis increases the risk of premature delivery (123,128) slightly but does not effect the incidence of preeclampsia (128,129). Magnesium sulfate is contraindicated in the myasthenic patient because it interferes with neuromuscular transmission and muscle fiber excitability (130) and may lead to increased weakness.

Myasthenia gravis does not affect smooth muscle but may weaken voluntary muscles used during the second stage of labor; parenteral anticholinesterases (e.g., pyridostigmine intravenously 2 mg) may be useful at this point. Care must be taken to not push the myasthenic patient beyond her physical capabilities during labor, and criteria for cesarean section should be broadened (117). Myasthenia gravis does not appear to effect the overall length of labor (131). Women taking corticosteroids during pregnancy should have stress doses given during labor and delivery.

Regional anesthesia is preferred over other anesthetic methods. Myasthenic patients are particularly sensitive to even small doses of neuromuscular blocking agents, especially of the nondepolarizing type such as curare, and these drugs should be avoided. Lidocaine is the recommended local anesthetic because it is an aminoacyl amide and is not affected by the decreased cholinesterase activity seen in patients receiving anticholinesterase drugs (132,133). Combined spinal and epidural anesthesia using intrathecal opioids can provide analgesia without inhibiting muscular strength (134).

There is an increased perinatal death rate in myasthenia gravis (128) secondary to antenatal and neonatal myasthenia gravis. Both conditions are presumed secondary to transplacental transfer of maternal acetylcholine receptor antibodies (135), which affect fetal acetylcholine receptors much more so than adult receptors (136,137). Antenatal effects derive from inhibited skeletal muscle movement and development resulting in pulmonary hypoplasia, arthrogryposis multiplex, and polyhydramnios (110), consistent with the fetal akinesia deformation sequence (138). Mothers with previously affected infants or especially high titers of acetylcholine receptor antibodies are at higher risk of having such children, who have a very high perinatal mortality rate. Ultrasound monitoring of total fetal and diaphragmatic movement and assessment of acetylcholine receptor antibody titers, particularly determining the antifetal/antiadult receptor antibody titer ratio (139), may predict at-risk women in whom aggressive lowering of antibody load to the placenta, such as with plasmapheresis, could prevent congenital anomalies (110,140).

A less severe but more common occurrence is neonatal myasthenia gravis, characterized by transient weakness in the newborn infant (141). The disease affects up to 19% of children born to mothers with myasthenia gravis, manifests within the first 3 days of life, and can persist for weeks before improving (141). Symptoms include poor feeding, weak suck, feeble cry, floppiness, generalized weakness, and respiratory distress. Treatment is supportive but can be supplemented by cholinesterase inhibitors. Neostigmine 0.1 mg intramuscular (IM) or subcutaneous, or pyridostigmine 0.15 mg IM, will be effective but may increase oral secretions and should be used sparingly. Further therapeutic interventions (e.g., plasmapheresis) are rarely needed, and intravenous immunoglobulin has not been effective (142). The disease is self-limited and does not represent a risk to the infant of later myasthenia gravis. Subsequent infants are at higher risk for neonatal myasthenia gravis (141).

Nearly all infants born to mothers with myasthenia are exposed to maternal acetylcholine receptor antibodies in utero (143), yet only a minority develop symptoms. The acetylcholine receptor consists of five subunits, with the fetal and adult forms differing by an ε subunit instead of an alpha in the adult. An increased ratio of antibodies against the fetal form of the receptor predisposes to antenatal and neonatal myasthenia gravis and may explain why both conditions have occurred in infants born to mothers in remission (144). Because AFP binds acetylcholine receptor antibody (127), its decline after birth may result in the emergence of symptoms (123,128).

POLYMYOSITIS/DERMATOMYOSITIS

Polymyositis and dermatomyositis are inflammatory disorders affecting striated and cardiac muscle. Dermatomyositis differs clinically from polymyositis primarily by the presence of skin involvement, and it is thought to be a vasculopathy. The etiology of polymyositis and dermatomyositis is unknown. Both diseases can be seen in isolation or in conjunction with a variety of connective tissue diseases. Both are characterized by proximal weakness, elevated creatine phosphokinase (CPK) levels, myopathic EMG, and inflammatory myonecrosis on muscle biopsy.

Polymyositis and dermatomyositis are encountered uncommonly in the pregnant patient. Although females are affected twice as often as men, the bimodal age of onset largely spares the childbearing years and the average age of

onset of the inflammatory myopathies is 47 years (145). A review of the literature reveals 27 patients with 41 examined pregnancies, about evenly split between polymyositis and dermatomyositis antedating pregnancy or starting during pregnancy (146–165). Preexisting inflammatory myopathy generally does not result in gestational exacerbation, but when it does, it occurs in later pregnancy (146). This is in contrast with *de novo* disease, which usually occurs during the first trimester (146) but can appear postpartum (152). In preexisting polymyositis or dermatomyositis, the inflammatory myopathy is rarely fulminant or difficult to control. *De novo* inflammatory myopathy often is active throughout gestation, even on treatment, but with remission following close on the heels of delivery (146).

Several complications of pregnancy have been reported in patients with polymyositis or dermatomyositis, including postpartum microangiopathic hemolytic anemia (150), placental abruption, uterine atony, and postpartum maternal death (156, 165). More frequently encountered are intrauterine growth restriction, spontaneous abortion, and preterm labor, the latter being quite common (146).

Fetal wastage is increased in pregnancies complicated by inflammatory myopathies, with a rate of 50% and 60% found by Gutierrez and colleagues (152). The author's experience differs: in *de novo* disease 36% fetal deaths occurred, and in preexisting disease the rate was 21%.

Treatment of gestational polymyositis and dermatomyositis is determined by the clinical condition of the patient and the length of gestation. Mild disease may not need to be treated. For those patients who need treatment, corticosteroids are the drug of choice, in doses approximating 1 mg/kg per day. Although the effect of corticosteroids on fetal development is not clear, they are a much better choice than the antimetabolites, which in the first trimester almost invariably result in spontaneous abortion or fetal malformation (166). Unfortunately, even with corticosteroids, no controlled studies of efficacy are available.

In general, women with either mildly active inflammatory myopathy or women in remission should have a relatively uneventful pregnancy, using corticosteroids to manage exacerbations. Pregnancy should not be undertaken electively in severe disease or in any patient requiring antimetabolite therapy. In those patients with onset in pregnancy, attempts to manage the disease early with corticosteroids can be made, but unsuccessful attempts should lead to consideration of therapeutic abortion (167). Tapering of corticosteroids postpartum should be done conservatively to avoid exacerbations.

METABOLIC MYOPATHIES

Myophosphorylase Deficiency

Metabolic myopathies can be loosely defined as inborn errors of metabolism affecting muscle. Myophosphorylase deficiency, or McArdle's disease, is caused by lack of an enzyme in the muscle glycolytic pathway, manifesting as exercise-induced muscle contracture and myoglobinuria. There are several glycogen storage disorders, all of which are rare, and little is known of their effect on pregnancy. A single report documents an uneventful pregnancy and delivery in a woman with McArdle's disease (168). Dawson and associates (169) mention one multiparous woman with McArdle's disease who suffered leg "cramps" and myoglobinuria after her last delivery. Smooth muscle phosphorylase is normal in McArdle's patients (170), and uterine activity should be unimpaired. Neither deterioration nor exacerbation is expected during pregnancy.

Myoglobinuria

Myoglobinuria is a sign of rhabdomyolysis rather than a disease. Dramatically elevated levels of CPK in the serum and the presence of myoglobin in the urine are the biochemical hallmarks of the syndrome. Idiopathic and polymyositis-associated myoglobinuria have been reported during pregnancy (147,171). Increased estrogens decrease muscle enzyme efflux and are proposed to have some stabilizing effect on muscle (172), including lowering baseline CPK levels during pregnancy. Oral contraceptives have no effect on serum levels of CPK (173). Extreme unaccustomed exertion also can be associated with rhabdomyolysis, as illustrated by a woman with severe hyperemesis gravidarum (174).

Mitochondrial Myopathy

Mitochondrial encephalomyopathies are a heterogeneous group of diseases in which mitochondrial metabolism is defective. The disorders have been defined by both morphologic and biochemical means but at the present time are best grouped into four categories (175): defects of mitochondrial substrate transport, defects of the respiratory chain, defects of substrate utilization (including the pyruvate dehydrogenase complex and the Krebs cycle), and defects of energy transduction. Mitochondrial disorders also can be defined by mutations of the mitochondrial genome.

Intramitochondrial fatty acid oxidation is largely dependent on the transport of long-chain fatty acids across the mitochondrial membrane by attachment to carnitine. Deficiency of carnitine can be purely myopathic, in which case pregnancy is unlikely to be a factor, or systemic. Primary systemic carnitine deficiency is rare, with most deficiencies being secondary to other metabolic disorders (175). Weakness, predominantly of proximal muscles, is frequent, and muscle biopsy shows abnormal lipid storage. Rapid progression of weakness has been reported during pregnancy (176) and in the postpartum period (177,178) in three cases, two of which were fatal (176,178). The one patient treated with carnitine replacement, 2 gm daily, improved (177). A fourth patient with systemic carnitine deficiency and a defect in the respiratory chain had rapidly progressive worsening of weakness in the last trimester of her pregnancy. She improved following treatment with 6 gm carnitine daily (175). The dramatic worsening of disease probably is related to already low carnitine stores experienced normally by pregnant women (177), which are further depleted by lactation (177) and increased fetal demand. Carnitine is actively transported placentally to the fetus (179), which has relatively poor ability to produce carnitine (180). Untreated, systemic carnitine deficiency in pregnancy can be fatal; treated, patients do well.

A relatively common cause of myoglobinuria, but a rare disease nonetheless, is carnitine palmitoyltransferase deficiency (CPT). This enzyme attaches and detaches long-chain fatty acids to carnitine for transport across the mitochondrial membrane where they will undergo oxidation, providing a major source of muscle energy, especially during aerobic exercise (glycolysis is the main source of anaerobic energy production). The prolonged exertion required during labor would seem to make patients with CPT deficiency susceptible to rhabdomyolysis and myoglobinuria, but no reports of this exist. The author has experience of one woman with an uneventful pregnancy prior to her diagnosis, when she was mildly symptomatic, and there is one report of a woman with CPT who had cesarean section but an otherwise uncomplicated pregnancy (181). The disease is inherited as an autosomal recessive trait, but only 20% of documented cases are women (182), and some of those were diagnosed as siblings of affected males. A hormonal protective effect has been postulated (182).

There are many possible defects of the respiratory chain, and several syndromes have been described, some associated with particular mutations of the mitochondrial genome. As recognition of the syndromes and the ability to test the mitochondrial genome improve, more case reports of pregnancy in patients with defects of the respiratory chain appear. A frequent feature of mitochondrial syndromes is small stature, which by itself may explain an association with hypertension and preterm labor in several patients (183,184). Commonly, pregnancy proceeds normally or with mild exercise intolerance (185–188).

Two women had initial presentation of MELAS (mitochondrial myopathy, encephalopathy, lactic acidosis, and stroke-like episodes) during pregnancy. Both women had spontaneous improvement of symptoms as the pregnancy progressed and normal deliveries (189,190).

Deficiencies of numerous enzymes involved in mitochondrial substrate utilization have been reported, and a discussion of each is not relevant. At least one—long-chain 3–hydroxyacyl-CoA dehydrogenase deficiency—predisposes female carriers to preeclamptic complications of pregnancy. Carrier frequency has been reported in Finland to be 1:240 (191).

Mitochondrial Maternal Inheritance

Approximately 85% of the proteins comprising the mitochondrial respiratory chain are encoded by nuclear DNA, with 15% (in total, 13 proteins) encoded on DNA within the mitochondria itself (175). All human mitochondria arise from the ova because there are no mitochondria in spermatozoa. This results in maternal (nonmendelian) inheritance of many mitochondrial encephalomyopathies (192), although some follow mendelian inheritance patterns. Because mitochondria replicate autonomously, a range of mitochondrial genomes exist in any ovum. The presence and percentage of mutated mitochondria determine the expression of a particular mitochondrial defect, explaining the variable expression of mitochondrial encephalomyopathies (193). Only females pass the disease between generations, although all offspring of a carrier mother may carry the genetic defect and be affected. The higher the load of maternal mutant mitochondrial DNA, the higher the chance of affected offspring (193).

CONGENITAL MYOPATHY

There are a number of congenital myopathies, which usually require a muscle biopsy for diagnosis. These disorders reflect a developmental arrest of muscle, with the pathologic and clinical manifestations dependent on the timing of insult or the nature of the genetic defect. These diseases do not progress, although the patient may be severely affected or die. Myotubular myopathy frequently results in neonatal death of males and has been linked to the X-chromosome. Prenatal diagnosis is possible by mutation testing of the MTM1 gene (194) and linkage analysis of DNA markers in the Xq28 region (195).

Congenital nemaline myopathy is a static muscle disease of variable severity usually diagnosed in childhood. Antenatal onset may occur with consequences characteristic of the fetal akinesia sequence (138,196), including arthrogryposis, polyhydramnios, lung hypoplasia, and neonatal demise (196). Hypotonia, weakness, jaw and palatal abnormalities, and scoliosis are frequent findings in milder cases. Congenital nemaline myopathy is inherited as either an autosomal dominant or recessive trait. There are four cases of pregnant women with congenital nemaline myopathy: pregnancy was uneventful in all, and vaginal or cesarean deliveries were normal, except when micrognathia, prognathia, and high-arched palate made intubation difficult and scoliosis inhibited epidural anesthesia (197,198). All infants were unaffected.

A retrospective report (72) detailed the 12 pregnancies of five women with central core congenital myopathy and the two pregnancies of a woman with cytoplasmic body congenital myopathy. For the most part, the women had mild weakness, which was not progressive prior to pregnancy. Three of the patients with central core myopathy had worsening of weakness during pregnancy, with no improvement after delivery. There were no miscarriages, three preterm deliveries, and two assisted deliveries (prolonged labor in one and threatened fetal asphyxia in another), and no adverse fetal outcomes. Two of the children inherited central core myopathy. The chromosomal locus for central core myopathy is 19q13.1, and the gene product is the ryanodine receptor, the same as for one of the familial malignant hyperthermia types (199).

CRAMPS

Cramps are uncommonly a sign of muscle disease; rather they are a sign of nerve or metabolic disturbance. The word cramp often is misused to cover any type of muscle pain or myalgia. In fact, a muscle cramp is a specific clinical and electrophysiologic syndrome that must be differentiated from muscle contracture, myalgia, tetany, stiffness, spasticity, myotonia, neuromyotonia, and dystonia.

A cramp is a "sudden, forceful, painful, involuntary contraction of one muscle or part of a muscle, lasting anywhere from a few seconds to several minutes" (200). EMG during a cramp reveals a full interference pattern indistinguishable from a maximal voluntary contraction of the muscle. Cramps often begin and end with fasciculations, in contrast with muscle contractures, as in McArdle's disease, which are electrically silent.

Cramps can occur in normal individuals, at night or related to exercise. Several metabolic disorders also can cause cramps, including uremia, hypothyroidism, and hypoadrenalism. Acute extracellular volume depletion (perspiration, diarrhea, vomiting, diuresis, hemodialysis) also is associated with cramps (200). Pregnant women suffer an increased frequency of cramping, probably secondary to changes in metabolic and extracellular volume parameters. Cramps are seen most seriously in disorders of the motor neuron, (e.g., amyotrophic lateral sclerosis, radiculopathy, neuropathy, and old polio). Layzer (200) hypothesized the pathophysiology to be ectopic nerve excitation in the distal, intramuscular portion of the motor axon. Stretching the affected muscle is the best immediate treatment for cramping. If no correctable cause is present, recurrent cramps can be treated with quinine, oral magnesium (201), phenytoin, or carbamezepine for prophylaxis, although the latter two drugs carry some risk for teratogenesis. Demaerschalk and Strong (202) suggest Brewer's yeast and primrose oil as safe and possibly helpful but they offer no supportive literature.

REFERENCES

1. Harper PS. *Myotonic dystrophy,* 2nd ed. Philadelphia: WB Saunders, 1989:187–214.
2. Harper PS. *Myotonic dystrophy,* 2nd ed. Philadelphia: WB Saunders, 1989:187–214.
3. Dyken PR, Harper PS. Congenital dystrophica myotonica. *Neurology* 1973;23:465–473.
4. Brook JD, McCurrach ME, Harley HG, et al. Molecular basis of myotonic dystrophy: expansion of a trinucleotide (CTG) repeat at the 3' end of a transcript encoding a protein kinase family member. *Cell* 1992;68: 799–808.
5. Fu YH, Pizzuti A, Fenwick RG Jr, et al. An unstable triplet repeat in a gene related to myotonic muscular dystrophy. *Science* 1992;255:1256–1258.
6. Mahadevan M, Tsilfidis C, Sabourin L, et al. Myotonic dystrophy mutation: an unstable CTG repeat in the 3' untranslated region of the gene. *Science* 1992;255: 1253–1255.
7. Caskey CT, Pizzuti A, Fu YH, et al. Triplet repeat mutations in human disease. *Science* 1992;256:784–789.
8. Drucker WD, Rowland LP, Sterling K, et al. On the function of the endocrine glands in myotonic muscular dystrophy. *Am J Med* 1961;31:941–950.
9. Harper P, Penny R, Foley TP Jr, et al. Gonadal function in males with myotonic dystrophy. *J Clin Endocrinol Metab* 1972;35:852–856.
10. Febres F, Scaglia H, Lisker R, et al. Hypothalamic-pituitary-gonadal function in patients with myotonic dystrophy. *J Clin Endocrinol Metab* 1975;41:833–840.
11. Sagel J, Distiller LA, Morley JE, et al. Myotonia dystrophica: studies on gonadal function using luteinizing hormone-releasing hormone (LHRH). *J Clin Endocrinol Metab* 1975;40:1110–1113.
12. Harper PS. *Myotonic dystrophy,* 2nd ed. Philadelphia: WB Saunders, 1989:127–132.
13. Drucker WD, Blanc WA, Rowland LP, et al. *J Clin Endocrinol Metab* 1963;23:59.
14. Caughey JE, Myrianthopoulos NC. *Dystrophica myotonica and related disorders.* Springfield, Ill: Charles C. Thomas, 1963.
15. Marshall J. Observations on endocrine function in dystrophica myotonica. *Brain* 1959;82:221–231.
16. Thomasen E. *Myotonia: Thomsen's disease (myotonic congenita), paramyotonia, and dystrophica myotonica: a clinical and heredobiologic investigation.* London: MK Lewis, 1948.
17. Febres F, Scaglia H, Lisker R, et al. Hypothalamic-pituitary-gonadal function in patients with myotonic dystrophy. *J Clin Endocrinol Metab* 1975;41:833–840.
18. Harper PS. *Myotonic dystrophy,* 2nd ed. Philadelphia: W.B. Saunders, 1989:320.
19. O'Brien TA, Harper PS. Reproductive problems and neonatal loss in women with myotonic dystrophy. *J Obstet Gynecol* 1984;4:170–173.
20. Sciarra JJ, Steer CM. Uterine contractions during labor in myotonic muscular dystrophy. *Am J Obstet Gynecol* 1961;82:612–615.
21. Hopkins A, Wray S. The effect of pregnancy on dystrophica myotonica. *Neurology* 1967;17:166–168.
22. Gardy HH. Dystrophica myotonica in pregnancy. *Obstet Gynecol* 1963;21:441–445.
23. Jaffe R, Mock M, Abramowicz J, et al. Myotonic dystrophy and pregnancy: a review. *Obstet Gynecol Surv* 1986;41:272–278.
24. Davis HA. Pregnancy in myotonica dystrophica. *J Ob Gyn Brit Empire* 1958;65:479–480.
25. Shore RN, MacLachlan TB. Pregnancy with myotonic dystrophy: course, complications and management. *Obstet Gynecol* 1971;38:448–454.
26. Fall LH, Young WW, Power JA, et al. Severe congestive heart failure and cardiomyopathy as a complication of myotonic dystrophy in pregnancy. *Obstet Gynecol* 1990;76:481–485.
27. Broekhuizen FF, de Elejalde M, Elejalde R, et al. Neonatal myotonic dystrophy as a cause of hydramnios and neonatal death. A case report and literature review. *J Reprod Med* 1983;28:595–599.
28. Webb D, Muir I, Faulkner J, et al. Myotonia dystrophica: obstetric complications. *Am J Obstet Gynecol* 1978;132:265–270.
29. Maas O. Observations on dystrophica myotonica. *Brain* 1937;60:498–524.
30. Watters GV, Williams TV. Early onset myotonic dystrophy. Clinical and laboratory findings in five families and a review of the literature. *Arch Neurol* 1967; 17:137–152.
31. Hook R, Anderson EF, Noto P. Anesthetic management of a parturient with myotonia atrophia. *Anesthesiology* 1975;43:689–692.
32. Rudnik-Schoneborn S, Rohrig D, Zerres K. Increased risk for abnormal placentation in women affected by myotonic dystrophy. *J Perinat Med* 1998;26:192–195.
33. Sarnat HB, O'Connor T, Byrne PA. Clinical effects of myotonic dystrophy on pregnancy and the neonate. *Arch Neurol* 1976;33:459–465.
34. Esplin MS, Hallam S, Farrington PF, et al. Myotonic dystrophy is a significant cause of idiopathic polyhydramnios. *Am J Obstet Gynecol* 1998;179:974–977.
35. Thiel RE. The myotonic response to suxamethonium. *Brit J Anaesth* 1967;39:815–820.
36. Mitchell MM, Ali HH, Savarese JJ. Myotonia and neuromuscular blocking agents. *Anesthesiology* 1978;49: 44–48.
37. Harper PS. *Myotonic dystrophy,* 2nd ed. Philadelphia: WB Saunders, 1989:116.
38. Koch MC, Grimm T, Harley HG, et al. Genetic risks for children of women with myotonic dystrophy. *Am J Hum Genet* 1991;48:1084–1091.
39. Poulton J. Congenital myotonic dystrophy and mtDNA. *Am J Hum Genet* 1992;50:651–652.
40. Harper PS, Dyken PR. Early onset dystrophica myotonica: evidence supporting a maternal environmental factor. *Lancet* 1972;2:53–55.
41. Howeler CJ, Busch HF. An asymptomatic mother of children with congenital myotonic dystrophy. *J Neurol Sci* 1990;98:197.
42. Andrews PI, Wilson J. Relative disease severity in siblings with myotonic dystrophy. *J Child Neurol* 1992;7: 161–167.
43. Pearse RG, Howeler CJ. Neonatal form of dystrophica myotonica. Five cases in preterm babies and a review of earlier reports. *Arch Dis Child* 1979;54:331–338.
44. Vanier TM. Dystrophica myotonica in childhood. *BMJ* 1960;2:1284–1288.
45. Calderon R. Myotonic dystrophy: a neglected cause of mental retardation. *J Pediat* 1966;68:423–431.

46. Sarnat HB, Silbert SW. Maturational arrest of fetal muscle in neonatal myotonic dystrophy. *Arch Neurol* 1976;33:466–474.

47. Rutherford MA, Heckmatt JZ, Dubowitz V. Congenital myotonic dystrophy: respiratory function at birth determines survival. *Arch Dis Child* 1989;64:191–195.

48. Swift TR, Ignacio OJ, Dyken PR. Neonatal dystrophica myotonica: electrophysiological studies. *Am J Dis Child* 1975;29:734–737.

49. Massari A, Novelli G, Colosimo A, et al. Non-invasive early prenatal molecular diagnosis using retrieved transcervical trophoblast cells. *Hum Genet* 1996;97:150–155.

50. Geifman-Holtzman O, Fay K. Prenatal diagnosis of congenital myotonic dystrophy and counseling of the pregnant mother: case report and literature review. *Am J Med Genet* 1998;78:250–253.

51. Moxley RT. Proximal myotonic myopathy: mini-review of a recently delineated clinical disorder. *Neuromuscul Disord* 1996;6:87–93.

52. New nomenclature and DNA testing guidelines for myotonic dystrophy type 1 (DM1). The International Myotonic Dystrophy Consortium (IDMC). *Neurology* 2000;54:1218–1221.

53. Newman B, Meola G, O'Donovan DG, et al. Proximal myotonic myopathy (PROMM) presenting as myotonia during pregnancy. *Neuromuscul Disord* 1999;9:144–149.

54. Hoffman EP, Brown RH, Kunkel LM. Dystrophin: the protein product of the Duchenne muscular dystrophy locus. *Cell* 1987;51:919–928.

55. Diagnosis of Duchenne and Becker muscular dystrophies by polymerase chain reaction. A multicenter study. *JAMA* 1992;267:2609–2615.

56. Emery AEH. *Duchenne muscular dystrophy,* 2nd ed. New York: Oxford Press, 1993.

57. Barkhaus PB, Gilchrist JM. Duchenne muscular dystrophy manifesting carriers. *Arch Neurol* 1989;46:673–675.

58. Hoffman EP, Arahata K, Minetti C, et al. Dystrophinopathy in isolated cases of myopathy in females. *Neurology* 1992;42:967–975.

59. Geifman-Holtzman O, Bernstein IM, Capeless EL, et al. Increase in fetal breech presentation in female carriers of Duchenne muscular dystrophy. *Am J Med Genet* 1997;73:276–278.

60. Clemens PR, Fenwick RG, Chamberlain JS, et al. Carrier detection and prenatal diagnosis in Duchenne and Becker muscular dystrophy families, using dinucleotide repeat polymorphisms. *Am J Hum Genet* 1991;49:951–960.

61. Hoffman EP, Fischbeck KH, Brown RH, et al. Characterization of dystrophin in muscle-biopsy specimens from patients with Duchenne's or Becker's muscular dystrophy. *N Engl J Med* 1988;318:1363–1368.

62. Den Duneen JT, Grootscholten PM, Bakker E, et al. Topography of the Duchenne muscular dystrophy (DMD) gene: FIGE and cDNA analysis of 194 cases reveals 115 deletions and 13 duplications. *Am J Hum Genet* 1989;45:835–847.

63. Vondran S, Edelmann J, Holland H, et al. Pitfalls in prenatal diagnosis of DMD due to placental mosaicism of the X-chromosome: prenatal and postnatal findings in a fetus with a deletion of exons 67–71 of the dystrophin gene. *Prenat Diagn* 1999;19:64–67.

64. Heckel S, Favre R, Flori J, et al. In utero fetal muscle biopsy: a precious aid for the prenatal diagnosis of Duchenne muscular dystrophy. *Fetal Diagn Ther* 1999;14:127–132.

65. Liu J, Lissens W, Devroey P, et al. Cystic fibrosis, Duchenne muscular dystrophy and preimplantation genetic diagnosis. *Hum Reprod Update* 1996;2:531–539.

66. Sekizawa A, Kimura T, Sasaki M, et al. Prenatal diagnosis of Duchenne muscular dystrophy using a single fetal nucleated erythrocyte in maternal blood. *Neurology* 1996;46:1350–1353.

67. Bushby K. Towards the classification of the autosomal recessive limb-girdle muscular dystrophies. *Neuromuscul Disord* 1996;6:439–441.

68. Speer MC, Yamaoka LH, Gilchrist JM, et al. Confirmation of Genetic Heterogeneity in Limb-girdle Muscular Dystrophy: Linkage of an Autosomal Dominant Form to Chromosome 5q. *Am J Hum Genet* 1992;50:1211–1217.

69. Anderson LV. Optimized protein diagnosis in the autosomal recessive limb-girdle muscular dystrophies. *Neuromuscul Disord* 1996;6:443–446.

70. Morton NE, Chung CS. Discrimination of genetic entities in muscular dystrophy. *Am J Hum Genet* 1959;11:339.

71. Pash MP, Balaton J, Eagle C. Anesthetic management of a parturient with severe muscular dystrophy, lumbar lordosis and a difficult airway. *Can J Anaesth* 1996;43:959–963.

72. Rudnick-Schoneborn S, Glauner B, Rohrig D, et al. Obstetric aspects in women with facioscapulohumeral muscular dystrophy, limb-girdle muscular dystrophy, and congenital myopathies. *Arch Neurol* 1997;54:888–894.

73. Restagno G, Romero N, Richard I, et al. Prenatal diagnosis of limb-girdle muscular dystrophy type 2A. *Neuromuscul Disord* 1996;6:173–176.

74. Dincer P, Piccolo F, Leturcq F, et al. Prenatal diagnosis of limb-girdle muscular dystrophy type 2C. *Prenat Diagn* 1998;18:1300–1303.

75. Pegoraro E, Fanin M, Angelini C, et al. Prenatal diagnosis in a family affected with beta-sarcoglycan muscular dystrophy. *Neuromuscul Disord* 1999;9:323–325.

76. Fisher J, Upadhyaya M. Molecular genetics of facioscapulohumeral muscular dystrophy (FSH). *Neuromuscul Disord* 1997;7:55–62.

77. Galluzzi G, Deidda G, Cacurri S, et al. Molecular analysis of 4q35 rearrangements in facioscapulohumeral muscular dystrophy (FSHD): application to family studies for correct genetic advice and a reliable prenatal diagnosis of the disease. *Neuromuscul Disord* 1999;9:190–198.

78. Helbling-Leclerc A, Zhang X, Topaloglu H, et al. Mutation sin the laminin alpha 2–chain gene (LAMA 2) cause merosin-deficient congenital muscular dystrophy. *Nature Genet* 1995;11:216–218.

79. Kobayashi O, Hayashi Y, Arahata K, et al. Congenital muscular dystrophy: Clinical and pathologic study of 50 patients with classical (Occidental) merosin-positive form. *Neurology* 1996;46:815–818.

80. Toda T, Segawa M, Nomura Y, et al. Localization of a gene for Fukuyama type congenital muscular dystrophy to chromosome 9q31–33. *Nature Genet* 1993;5:283–286.

81. Naom I, Sewry C, D'Alessandro M, et al. Prenatal diagnosis of merosin-deficient congenital muscular dystrophy. *Neuromuscul Disord* 1997;7:176–179.

82. Nass D, Goldberg I, Sadeh M. Laminin alpha2 deficient congenital muscular dystrophy: prenatal diagnosis. *Early Hum Dev* 1999;55:19–24.

83. Kondo E, Saito K, Toda T, et al. Prenatal diagnosis of Fukuyama type congenital muscular dystrophy by polymorphism analysis. *Am J Med Genet* 1996;66:169–174.

84. Takai Y, Tsutsumi O, Harada I, et al. Prenatal diagnosis of Fukuyama-type congenital muscular dystrophy by microsatellite analysis. *Hum Reprod* 1998;13:320–323.

85. Lehmann-Horn F, Rudel R. Hereditary nondystrophic myotonias and periodic paralyses. *Curr Opin Neurol* 1995;8:402–410.

86. Kaplan J-C. Neuromuscular disorders: genetic location. *Neuromuscul Disord* 2000;10:I–VIII.

87. Gardiner CF. A case of myotonia congenita. *Arch Ped* 1901;18:925–928.

88. Hakim CA, Thomlinson J. Myotonia congenita in pregnancy. *J Obstet Gynaecol Br Commonw* 1969;76:561–562.

89. Lacomis D, Gonzales JT, Giuliani MJ. Fluctuating clinical myotonia and weakness from Thomsen's disease occurring only during pregnancies. *Clin Neurol Neurosurg* 1999;101:133–136.

90. Morley JB, Lambert TF, Kakulas BA. *Excerpta Medica International Congress Series* 1973;295:543.

91. Saidman LJ, Havard ES, Eger EI. Hyperthermia during anesthesia. *JAMA* 1964;190:1029–1032.

92. Miller JD, Lee C. Muscle diseases. In: Katz J, Benumof JL, Kadis LB, eds. *Anesthesia and uncommon diseases*. 3rd ed. Philadelphia: WB Saunders, 1990:622–626.

93. Kaplan RF, Kellner KR. More on malignant hyperthermia during delivery. *Am J Obstet Gynecol* 1985;152:608–609.

94. Liebenschutz F, Mai C, Pickerodt VW. Increased carbon dioxide production in two patients with malignant hyperthermia and its control by dantrolene. *Br J Anaesth* 1979;51:899–903.

95. Lips FJ, Newland M, Dutton G. Malignant hyperthermia triggered by cyclopropane during cesarean section. *Anesthesiology* 1982;56:144–146.

96. Cupryn JP, Kennedy A, Byrick RJ. Malignant hyperthermia in pregnancy. *Am J Obstet Gynecol* 1984;150:327–328.

97. Sorosky JI, Ingardia CJ, Botti JJ. Diagnosis and management of susceptibility to malignant hyperthermia in pregnancy. *Am J Perinatol* 1989;6:46–48.

98. Shime J, Gare D, Andrews J, et al. Dantrolene in pregnancy: lack of adverse effects on the fetus and newborn infant. *Am J Obstet Gynecol* 1988;159:831–834.

99. Morison DH. Placental transfer of dantrolene. *Anesthesiology* 1983;59:265.

100. Lindstrom JM. Acetylcholine receptors and myasthenia. *Muscle Nerve* 2000;23:453–477.

101. Daroff RB. The office Tensilon test for ocular myasthenia gravis. *Arch Neurol* 1986;43:843–844.

102. Lindstrom J, Shelton D, Fujii Y. Myasthenia gravis. *Adv Immunol* 1988;42:233–284.

103. Oh SJ, Eslami N, Nishihira T, et al. Electrophysiological and clinical correlation in myasthenia gravis. *Ann Neurol* 1982;12:348–354.

104. Sanders DB, Stalberg EV. Single fiber electromyography. *Muscle Nerve* 1996;19:1069–1083.

105. Lefvert AK, Osterman PO. Newborn infants to myasthenic mothers: a clinical study and an investigation of acetylcholine receptor antibodies in 17 children. *Neurology* 1983;33:133–138.

106. Niesen CE, Shah NS. Pyridostigmine-induced microcephaly. *Neurology* 2000;54:1873–1874.

107. Pascuzzi RM, Coslett HB, Johns TR. Long-term corticosteroid treatment of myasthenia gravis: report of 116 patients. *Ann Neurol* 1984;15:291–298.

108. Miller RG, Milner-Brown HS, Mirka A. Prednisone-induced worsening of neuromuscular function in myasthenia gravis. *Neurology* 1986;36:729–732.

109. Seybold ME, Drachman DB. Gradually increasing doses of prednisone in myasthenia gravis. *N Engl J Med* 1974;290:81–84.

110. Carr SC, Gilchrist JM, Abuelo D, et al. Antenatal treatment of myasthenia gravis. *Obstet Gynecol* 1991;78:485–489.

111. Levine SE, Keesey JC. Successful plasmapheresis for fulminant Myasthenia gravis during pregnancy. *Arch Neurol* 1986;43:197–198.

112. Watson WJ, Katz VL, Bowes WA. Plasmapheresis during pregnancy. *Obstet Gynecol* 1990;76:451–457.

113. Castleman B. The pathology of the thymus gland in myasthenia gravis. *Ann N Y Acad Sci* 1966;135:496–503.

114. Goldman KP. Malignant thymomas in pregnancy. *Brit J Dis Chest* 1974;68:279–283.

115. Hohlfeld R, Wekerle H. The immunopathogenesis of myasthenia gravis. In: Engel AG, ed. *Myasthenia gravis and myasthenic disorders*. New York: Oxford University Press, 1999:87–110.

116. Perlo VP, Arnason B, Poskanzer D, et al. The role of thymectomy in treatment of myasthenia gravis. *Ann N Y Acad Sci* 1971;183:308–315.

117. Genkins G, Kornfeld P, Papatestas AE, et al. Clinical experience in more than 2000 patients with myasthenia gravis. *Ann N Y Acad Sci* 1987;505:500–513.

118. Ip MS, So SY, Lam WK, et al. Thymectomy in myasthenia gravis during pregnancy. *Postgrad Med J* 1986;62:473–474.

119. Eden RD, Gall SA. Myasthenia gravis and pregnancy: a reappraisal of thymectomy. *Obstet Gynecol* 1983;62:328.

120. Kaeser HE. Drug-induced myasthenic syndromes. *Acta Neurol Scand Suppl* 1984;100:39–47.

121. Argov Z, Mastaglia FL. Disorders of neuromuscular transmission caused by drugs. *N Engl J Med* 1979;301:409–413.

122. Chagnac Y, Hadani M, Goldhammer Y. Myasthenic crisis after intravenous administration of iodinated contrast agent. *Neurology* 1985;35:1219–1220.

123. Plauche WC. Myasthenia gravis in mothers and their newborn. *Clin Obstet Gynecol* 1991;34:82–99.

124. Batocchi AP, Majolini L, Evoli A, et al. Course and treatment of myasthenia gravis during pregnancy. *Neurology* 1999;52:447–452.

125. Hay DM. Myasthenia gravis and pregnancy. *J Obstet Gynaecol Br Commonw* 1969;76:323–329.

126. Viets HR, Schwab RS, Brazier MA. The effect of pregnancy on the course of Myasthenia gravis. *JAMA* 1942;119:236–242.

127. Brenner T, Beyth Y, Abramsky O. Inhibitory effect of

alpha fetoprotein on the binding of myasthenia gravis antibody to acetylcholine receptor. *Proc Natl Acad Sci USA* 1980;77:3635–3639.

128. Fennell DF, Ringel SP. Myasthenia gravis and pregnancy. *Obstet Gynecol Surv* 1987;42:414–421.

129. Duff GB. Preeclampsia and the patient with myasthenia gravis. *Obstet Gynecol* 1979;54:355–358.

130. delCastillo J, Engbaek L. The nature of neuromuscular block produced by magnesium. *J Physiol* 1954;124: 370.

131. Giwa-Osagie OF, Newton JR, Larcher V. Obstetric performance of patients with myasthenia gravis. *Int J Gynaecol Obstet* 1981;19:267.

132. Kalow W. Hydrolysis of local anesthetics by human serum cholinesterase. *J Pharm Exper Therap* 1952; 104:122–134.

133. Rolbin SH, Levinson G, Shnider SM, et al. Anesthetic consideration for myasthenia gravis and pregnancy. *Anesth Analg* 1978;57:441.

134. D'Angelo R, Gerancher JC. Combined spinal and epidural analgesics in a parturient with severe myasthenia gravis. *Reg Anesth Pain Med* 1998;23:201–203.

135. Keesey J, Lindstrom J, Cokely H. Anti-acetylcholine receptor antibody in neonatal myasthenia gravis. *N Engl J Med* 1977;296:55.

136. Vincent A, Newland C, Brueton L, et al. Arthrogryposis multiplex congenita with maternal autoantibodies specific for a fetal antigen. *Lancet* 1995;346:24–25.

137. Riemersma S, Vincent A, Beeson D, et al. Association of arthrogryposis multiplex congenita with maternal antibodies inhibiting fetal acetylcholine receptor function. *J Clin Invest* 1996;98:2358–2363.

138. Moessinger AC. Fetal akinesia deformation sequence: an animal model. *Pediatrics* 1983;72:857–863.

139. Gardnerova M, Eymard B, Morel F, et al. The fetal/adult acetylcholine receptor antibody ratio in mothers with myasthenia gravis as a marker for transfer of the disease to the newborn. *Neurology* 1997;48: 50–54.

140. Stoll C, Ehret-Mentre MC, Treisser A, et al. Prenatal diagnosis of congenital myasthenia with arthrogryposis in a myasthenic mother. *Prenat Diag* 1991;11: 17–22.

141. Namba T, Brown SB, Grob D. Neonatal myasthenia gravis: report of two cases and review of the literature. *Pediatrics* 1970;45:488–504.

142. Tagher RJ, Baumann R, Desai N. Failure of intravenously administered immunoglobulin in the treatment of neonatal myasthenia gravis. *J Pediatr* 1999; 134:233–235.

143. Eymard B, Morel E, Dulac O, et al. Myasthenia and pregnancy: a clinical and immunologic study of 42 cases (21 neonatal myasthenia gravis). *Rev Neurol (Paris)* 1989;145:696–701.

144. Elias SB, Butler I, Appel S. Neonatal myasthenia gravis in an infant of a myasthenic mother in remission. *Ann Neurol* 1979;6:72.

145. Bohan AJ, Peter JB, Pearson CM. A computer-assisted analysis of 150 patients with polymyositis and dermatomyositis. *Medicine* 1977;56:255.

146. Rosenzweig BA, Rotmensch S, Binette SP, et al. Primary idiopathic polymyositis and dermatomyositis complicating pregnancy: diagnosis and management. *Obstet Gynecol Surv* 1989;44:162–170.

147. Ditzian-Kadanoff R, Reinhard JD, Thomas C, et al.

148. Polymyositis with myoglobinuria in pregnancy: a report and review of the literature. *J Rheumatol* 1988; 15:513–514.

148. Ishii N, Ono H, Kawaguchi T, et al. Dermatomyositis and pregnancy. Case report and review of the literature. *Dermatologica* 1991;183:146–149.

149. Glickman FS. Dermatomyositis associated with pregnancy. *US Armed Forces Med J* 1958;9:417–425.

150. Tsai A, Lindheimer MD, Lamberg SI. Dermatomyositis complicating pregnancy. *Obstet Gynecol* 1973;41: 570–573.

151. Katz AL. Another case of polymyositis in pregnancy. *Arch Intern Med* 1980;140:1123.

152. Gutierrez G, Dagnino R, Mintz G. Polymyositis/dermatomyositis and pregnancy. *Arthritis Rheum* 1984; 27:291–294.

153. Barnes AB, Lisak DA. Childhood dermatomyositis and pregnancy. *Am J Obstet Gynecol* 1983;146:335–336.

154. Bauer KA, Siegler M, Lindheimer MA. Polymyositis complicating pregnancy. *Arch Intern Med* 1979;139: 449.

155. Houck W, Melnyk C, Gast MJ. Polymyositis in pregnancy. *J Reprod Med* 1987;32:208–210.

156. England MJ, Perlmann T, Veriava Y. Dermatomyositis in pregnancy. *J Reprod Med* 1986;31:633–636.

157. King CR, Chow S. Dermatomyositis and pregnancy. *Obstet Gynecol* 1985;66:589–592.

158. Emy PH, Lenormand V, Maitre F, et al. [Polymyositis, dermatomyositis and pregnancy: high-risk pregnancy. A further case report and review of the literature.] *J Gynecol Obstet Biol Reprod (Paris)* 1986;15:785.

159. Masse MR. Grossesses et dermatomyosite. *Bull Soc Franc Derm Syph* 1962;69:921.

160. Satoh M, Ajmani AK, Hirakata M, et al. Onset of polymyositis with autoantibodies to threonyl-tRNA synthetase during pregnancy. *J Rheumatol* 1994;21: 1564–1566.

161. Harris A, Webley M, Usherwood M, et al. Dermatomyositis presenting in pregnancy. *Br J Dermatol* 1995; 133:783–785.

162. Boggess KA, Easterling TR, Raghu G. Management and outcome of pregnant women with interstitial and restrictive lung disease. *Am J Obstet Gynecol* 1995; 173:1007–1014.

163. Kofteridis DP, Malliotakis PI, Sotsiou F, et al. Acute onset of dermatomyositis presenting in pregnancy with rhabdomyolysis and fetal loss. *Scand J Rheumatol* 1999;28:192–194.

164. Papapetropoulos T, Kanellakopoulou N, Tsibri E, et al. Polymyositis and pregnancy: report of a case with three pregnancies. *J Neurol Neurosurg Psychiatry* 1998;64:406.

165. Case records of the Massachusetts General Hospital. *N Engl J Med* 1999;340:455–464.

166. Nicholson HO. Cytotoxic drugs in pregnancy. *J Obstet Gynaecol Br Commonw* 1968;75:307–312.

167. Mintz G. Dermatomyositis. *Rheum Dis Clin North Am* 1989;15:375–382.

168. Cochrane P, Alderman B. Normal pregnancy and successful delivery in myophosphorylase deficiency (McArdle's disease). *J Neuro Neurosurg Psychiatry* 1973;36:225–227.

169. Dawson DM, Spong FL, Harrington JF. McArdle's disease: lack of muscle phosphorylase. *Ann Int Med* 1968;69:229–235.

170. Engel WK, Eyerman EL, Williams HE. Late-onset type of skeletal-muscle phosphorylase deficiency: a new familial variety with completely and partially affected members. *N Engl J Med* 1962;268:135–137.

171. Owens OJ, Macdonald R. Idiopathic myoglobinuria in the early puerperium. *Scott Med J* 1989;34:564–565.

172. Thomson WH, Smith I. Effects of oestrogens on erythrocyte enzyme efflux in normal men and women. *Clin Chim Acta* 1980;103:203–208.

173. Simpson J, Zellweger H, Burmeister LF, et al. Effect of oral contraceptive pills on the level of creatine phosphokinase with regard to carrier detection in Duchenne muscular dystrophy. *Clin Chim Acta* 1974;52:219–223.

174. Fukada Y, Ohta S, Mizuno K, et al. Rhabdomyolysis secondary to hyperemesis gravidarum. *Acta Obstet Gynecol Scand* 1999;78:71–73.

175. Morgan-Hughes JA. The mitochondrial myopathies. In: Engel AG, Franzini-Armstrong C, eds. *Myology*, 2nd ed. New York: McGraw-Hill, 1994:1610–1660.

176. Cornelio F, DiDonato S, Peluchetti D, et al. Fatal cases of lipid storage myopathy with carnitine deficiency. *J Neurol Neurosurg Psychiatry* 1977;40:170–178.

177. Angelini C, Govoni E, Bragaglia M, et al. Carnitine deficiency: acute postpartum crisis. *Ann Neurol* 1978; 4:558–561.

178. Boudin G, Mikol J, Guillard A, et al. Fatal systemic carnitine deficiency with lipid storage in skeletal muscle, heart, liver and kidney. *J Neurol Sci* 1976;30:313–325.

179. Hahn P, Skala JP, Secombe DW, et al. Carnitine content of blood and amniotic fluid. *Ped Res* 1977;11: 878–880.

180. Warshaw JB, Terry ML. Cellular energy metabolism during fetal development. II. Fatty acid oxidation by the developing heart. *J Cell Biol* 1970;44:354–360.

181. Dreval D, Bernstein D, Zakut H. Carnitine palmitoyl transferase deficiency in pregnancy—a case report. *Am J Obstet Gynecol* 1994;170:1390–1392.

182. Zierz S. Carnitine palmitoyltransferase deficiency. In: Engel AG, Franzini-Armstrong C, eds. *Myology*, 2nd ed. New York: McGraw Hill, 1994:1577–1586.

183. Ewart RM, Burrows RF. Pregnancy in chronic progressive external opthalmoplegia: a case report. *Am J Perinatol* 1997;14:293–295.

184. Torbergsen T, Oian P, Mathiesen E, et al. Pre-eclampsia—a mitochondrial disease? *Acta Obstet Gynecol Scand* 1989;68:145–148.

185. Berkowitz K, Monteagudo A, Marks F, et al. Mitochondrial myopathy and preeclampsia associated with pregnancy. *Am J Obstet Gynecol* 1990;162:146–147.

186. Rosaeg OP, Morrison S, MacLeod JP. Anaesthetic management of labour and delivery in the parturient with mitochondrial myopathy. *Can J Anaesth* 1996; 43:403–407.

187. Larsson N-G, Eiken HG, Boman H, et al. Lack of transmission of deleted mtDNA from a woman with Kearns-Sayre syndrome to her child. *Am J Hum Genet* 1992;50:360–363.

188. Blake LL, Shaw RW. Mitochondrial myopathy in a primigravid pregnancy. *Br J Obstet Gynaecol* 1999; 106:871–873.

189. Yanagawa T, Sakaguchi H, Nakao T, et al. Mitochondrial myopathy, encephalopathy, lactic acidosis, and stroke-like episodes with deterioration during pregnancy. *Intern Med* 1998;37:780–783.

190. Kokawa N, Ishii Y, Yamoto M, et al. Pregnancy and delivery complicated by mitochondrial myopathy, encephalopathy, lactic acidosis, and stroke-like episodes. *Obstet Gynecol* 1998;91:865.

191. Tyni T, Pihko H. Long-chain 3–hydroxyacyl-CoA dehydrogenase deficiency. *Acta Paediatr* 1999;88: 237–245.

192. Giles RE, Blanc H, Cann HM, et al. Maternal inheritance of human mitochondrial DNA. *Proc Natl Acad Sci USA* 1980;77:6715.

193. Chinnery PF, Howell N, Lightowlers RN, et al. MELAS and MERRF. The relationship between maternal mutation load and the frequency of clinically affected offspring. *Brain* 1998;121:1889–1894.

194. Tanner SM, Laporte J, Guiraud-Chaumeil C, et al. Confirmation of prenatal diagnosis results of X-linked recessive myotubular myopathy by mutational screening, and description of three new mutations in the MTM1 gene. *Hum Mutat* 1998;11:62–68.

195. Hu LJ, Laporte J, Kress W, et al. Prenatal diagnosis of X-linked myotubular myopathy: strategies using new and tightly linked DNA markers. *Prenat Diagn* 1996; 16:231–237.

196. Lammens M, Moerman P, Fryns JP, et al. Fetal akinesia sequence caused by nemaline myopathy. *Neuropediatrics* 1997;28:116–119.

197. Stackhouse R, Chelmow D, Dattel BJ. Anesthetic complications in a pregnant patient with nemaline myopathy. *Anesth Analg* 1994;79:1195–1197.

198. Wallgren-Pettersson C, Hiilesmaa VK, Paatero H. Pregnancy and delivery in congenital nemaline myopathy. *Acta Obstet Gynecol Scand* 1995;74:659–661.

199. Quane KA, Healey JM, Keating KE, et al. Mutations in the ryanodine receptor gene in central core disease and malignant hyperthermia. *Nat Genet* 1993;5:51–55.

200. Layzer RB. *Neuromuscular manifestations of systemic disease*. Philadelphia: FA Davis Co, 1985:19–22.

201. Dahle LO, Berg G, Hammar M, et al. The effect of oral magnesium substitution on pregnancy-induced leg cramps. *Am J Obstet Gynecol* 1995;173:175–180.

202. Demaerschalk BM, Strong MJ. Amyotrophic lateral sclerosis. *Curr Treat Options Neurol* 2000;2:13–22.

Neurological Complications of Pregnancy, Second
Edition, edited by Brian Hainline and Orrin Devinsky.
Lippincott Williams & Wilkins, Philadelphia, © 2002.

18

Developmental Disabilities

Debra Shabas and Danielle Chiaravalloti

*Department of Neurology, New York University Medical Center, and
The Women's Center at Premier HealthCare, New York, New York, U.S.A.*

There are 28 million women with disabilities in the United States, approximately half of whom are of childbearing age (1). Many women with disabilities are choosing to become pregnant. However, these women encounter various difficulties compared to nondisabled women. Unfortunately, we lack information about reproductive health issues in diverse disabling conditions. The belief that women with disabilities are asexual and the lack of focus on women's issues in disabling conditions contribute to this paucity of information.

Finding an appropriate physician is another challenge. Women with physical disabilities have difficulty finding a physician knowledgeable about their disability and able to care for them throughout their pregnancy (2). There is a lack of adequate counseling on sexuality, pregnancy, and childbirth from either obstetrician–gynecologists or rehabilitation professionals (3). Further, in one study, 31% of women with physical disabilities were turned away by physicians because of their disability (2). Architectural and transportation barriers also limit access to physicians able and willing to care for a pregnant, disabled woman.

Negative attitudes about pregnancy and women with disabilities are widespread. According to Barbra Waxman, "while a nondisabled woman's pregnancy is considered a miracle, a disabled woman's pregnancy is considered a crime against society" (4). Society believes that women with disabilities can-

not be good mothers (3). There is a pervasive and unwarranted fear that the children of women with disabilities also will have a disability and a belief that women with disabilities will harm, neglect, or be a burden to their children (3). This attitude compels many mothers with disabilities to stay in a bad marriage for fear of losing custody of their child (2).

Many barriers facing pregnant women with mental retardation and developmental disabilities (MR/DD) are similar to those facing women with physical disabilities. However, women with MR/DD have additional challenges. The past 30 years witnessed a movement toward community integration for people with MR/DD, which improved education and socialization, increased access to health care, emphasized dignity, and validated the expression of sexuality. However, the issue of pregnancy and parenting remains controversial. A deeply rooted bias pervades health care professionals and the general public: women with MR/DD should not have children (5). This belief was expressed in its extreme during the era of compulsory sterilization, fueled by the late 19th century popularity of eugenics. Mental retardation was attributed entirely to hereditary factors, and sterilization was routinely performed (6). In 1927 the United States Supreme Court ruling in *Buck v. Bell* supported the constitutionality of involuntary sterilization, a position reversed in 1942 (in *Skinner v. Oklahoma*) when the Court declared that reproduction is an "inalienable right" (7). Forced sterilization continued to be commonplace until the Department of Health, Education, and Welfare banned the use of federal funds for the procedure in 1974, following the highly publicized case of two young sisters (one with mental retardation) in Alabama who were sterilized involuntarily (6).

In addition to prejudicial attitudes, other barriers exist. There is a paucity of information specific to pregnancy in women with MR/DD. General information is most often not available in cognitively appropriate formats. Impaired comprehension coupled with communication and speech dysfunction make a dialogue with providers difficult for women with MR/DD. Significant fear of examination present in many women with MR/DD further limits their access to care. A wide range of cognitive ability, functional adaptation, and decisional capacity exists in women with MR/DD. Therefore, the ability to accomplish the necessary tasks of parenting varies and must be considered on a case-by-case basis.

Despite these issues and attitudes, many women with disabilities choose to have children. From an obstetric standpoint, women with disabilities do not have significant difficulty with pregnancy and delivery. There are potential complications in certain conditions that need close monitoring, although outcomes have been generally positive. Information on the subject of pregnancy and women with disabilities is very limited. This chapter reviews the available information on pregnancy and diverse disabilities including developmental disabilities, with and without MR (cerebral palsy, spina bifida, Down's syndrome).

GENERAL CONSIDERATIONS FOR WOMEN WITH PHYSICAL DISABILITIES PLANNING A PREGNANCY

Medications

Many of the medications that women with disabilities take chronically, including antispasticity medications, bladder medications, antiepileptic drugs, and antidepressants may be contraindicated in pregnancy. Safer alternative medications for these conditions must be evaluated prior to conception. The need for high dosage or multiple antiepileptic drugs should be reassessed. The lowest effective doses should be used, and drug levels need to be monitored closely.

Mobility Issues

For women with physical disabilities, pregnancy potentially can result in greater difficulties with balance and gait as a result of increases in weight and changes in the center of gravity. As with nondisabled pregnant women, the increase in weight also can result in low back pain, often a preexisting condition in women with diverse physical disabilities. Joint instability also can occur in pregnancy, adversely affecting mobility in some women with disabilities. For all these reasons, pregnant women with disabilities should be followed closely by their neurologists or rehabilitation professionals as well as by their obstetricians.

Urinary Dysfunction

Pregnancy is associated with changes in urinary function, which may exacerbate preexisting urinary dysfunction often present in several different disabling conditions (1). There is also an increased risk of urinary tract infections. Renal function and urine samples need to be screened regularly.

Pressure Sores

Pressure sores are issues for many women with disabilities. Increases in weight along with decreased mobility during pregnancy can increase the risk for decubiti. Close monitoring and prophylactic measures can help minimize these potential complications.

Genetic Counseling

Certain disabling conditions have a clear pattern of inheritance. In other conditions, such as spina bifida, there is an increased risk of having children with a neural tube defect as compared to the general population (8). Yet other conditions, like spinal cord injury, have no hereditary risks. To be properly prepared, all of these possibilities need to be discussed carefully and understood prior to conception.

CEREBRAL PALSY AND PREGNANCY

Information about pregnancy and cerebral palsy (CP) is sparse. One large retrospective study performed by Foley and colleagues included 132 pregnancies in women with CP. Although focused on the offspring of women with CP, information regarding pregnancy also was obtained (9). The largest study of obstetric issues in women with CP is a retrospective chart review of 22 women by Winch and associates (10). Much of the following information about pregnancy and delivery for women with CP is derived from these two studies.

Fertility

No information specifically relating to fertility was found in the literature.

Pregnancy

The general issues mentioned earlier (e.g., musculoskeletal pain and increased difficulty with balance and ambulation) during pregnancy can develop in women with CP (1). In some cases, increased spasticity can occur (1).

Early Pregnancy Failure

Of the 38 pregnancies in the Winch survey, two miscarried (5%) (10). In Foley's review of 132 pregnancies, there were 18 miscarriages (14%) (9).

Urinary Tract Dysfunction

Urinary tract infections were not a problem during pregnancy in this sample, although there were histories of urinary dysfunction and previous urinary tract infections (10).

Seizures

Seizures occur in 25% to 35% of people with CP (11). For these women, the medical issues related to pregnancy and epilepsy are important considerations. (See Chapter 14). Among other concerns, there may be an increase in seizure activity during pregnancy because of the changes in protein binding and metabolism of antiepileptic medications (12). Five women had seizure disorders in the Winch series (10). One of these women had two breakthrough seizures during her pregnancy.

Preeclampsia

Pregnancy was complicated by gestational hypertension in nine of 28 pregnancies; five of these (18%) had definite preeclampsia (10). This is greater than the 7% rate of preeclampsia in the general population (13). In the Foley series, however, only 5% of the women had preeclampsia (9).

Delivery

Uterine contractions, cervical dilatation, and the sensation of uterine contractions should not be affected by cerebral palsy (10).

Preterm Delivery

In the Winch study, there were two preterm deliveries out of 27 births (10). The rate of preterm births in the women with CP was not higher than that of the general population (14).

Vaginal vs. Cesarean Delivery

In Winch's series, there were nine cesarean sections out of 27 births (10). The indications for cesarean section included abnormal fetal position and cephalopelvic disproportion. Two vaginal deliveries required forceps or vacuum extraction. In Foley's series, 33 out of 132 births were by cesarean section (9). Of these, 28 were elective and may have been primarily a result of the anxiety on the part of the obstetrician in delivering a woman with a disability. The reasons for the five emergency cesarean sections included two fetal distress, difficult breech, spasms in the mother's legs, and one unspecified. The rate of cesarean sections in both series was identical, but it was higher than the 18% in the general population (14).

Anesthesia

Epidural anesthesia is presumed to be safe in women with CP (1). Spinal or epidural anesthesia can be difficult in some patients with CP with scoliosis or athetotic reactions. This often makes it necessary to use general anesthesia for cesarean sections. Some general anesthetics are associated with an increased risk of seizures (15). Barbiturates are safe in women with CP who are prone to seizures and remain the first choice for induction drugs for cesarean section (15). In one case, propofol was used in a woman with CP without complications (15).

Newborns

Neither series found an elevated risk for CP in the newborns of women with CP (9,10). Two infants in the Winch series had meconium passage into the amniotic fluid. This rate is comparable to the general population (16).

SPINA BIFIDA

There are many case reports in the literature regarding spina bifida and pregnancy. The larger series includes a study of 17 women with spina bifida (17) and one review article (8).

Genetic Counseling

Genetic counseling prior to pregnancy is necessary for women with spina bifida because of the increased risk of affected offspring (8). Folic acid supplementation is important. It is effective in the prevention of neural tube defects in women with prior affected children, but it is not definitely known whether this supplementation will decrease the risk of neural tube defects for the offspring of women with spina bifida (8).

Fertility

In the series of 17 women with spina bifida, two had infertility problems requiring ovulation induction with clomiphene. Their second pregnancies, however, occurred without intervention (17).

Pregnancy

Other than the previously mentioned general concerns that all pregnant women with physical disabilities share (e.g., back pain and mobility changes), the majority of health issues for pregnant women with spina bifida relate to spina bifida. The mild back pain (sciatica in nine out of 17 patients) in Arata's series was without any new neurologic dysfunction. Mobility issues (in two out of 17) were temporary and reverted to baseline after delivery (17). Early involvement of rehabilitation professionals is recommended.

Early Pregnancy Failure

In one study, there were three spontaneous first trimester abortions out of 29 pregnancies (17). Another study of obstetric issues for women who were cerebrospinal fluid (CSF) shunt dependent included four women with spina bifida. One woman had six pregnancies, four of which ended in miscarriage. Another had three pregnancies, all of which ended in miscarriage at 4 to 6 weeks (18).

Urinary Tract Dysfunction

Urinary tract dysfunction is common in women with spina bifida and potentially can be exacerbated by pregnancy. In Arata's series, seven women had a history of recurrent urinary tract infections prior to pregnancy (17). Many of these women had urinary diversion procedures performed to prevent upper urinary tract dysfunction or treat incontinence prior to the use of newer techniques including clean intermittent catheterization. Urinary tract infections were particularly frequent in nonpregnant women with ileal conduits.

Pregnancy, which predisposes to urinary stasis and ureteric dilatation, further increases the risk of infection and deterioration of renal function (8). In Arata's series, women with prior urinary tract infections developed urinary tract infections during pregnancy. All but one had an ileal conduit. Only one woman without a prior history of urinary tract infections developed a urinary tract infection during pregnancy (17). Potential complications during pregnancy related to previous urinary diversion procedures also include an increased risk for ureteric, ileal conduit, and mechanical bowel obstruction due to adhesions and the growing uterus (19,20,21). In Arata's series, only one out of 12 women with ileal conduits and a urinary undiversion had an ureteric obstruction requiring 1 month of an indwelling catheter (17).

Pressure Sores

Pressure sores occur in women with spina bifida and may be exacerbated by pregnancy (1). Prior to pregnancy, five out of 17 women had pressure sores in Arata's series. Two of these worsened during pregnancy and required hospitalization. However, only one new pressure sore during pregnancy was reported in the entire group (17).

Ventriculoperitoneal Shunts

Many women with spina bifida have ventricular shunts for hydrocephalus, which are another potential source of complications during pregnancy. Shunt malfunction may occur during pregnancy, most commonly in the third trimester (8). In a review of 19 pregnant women with spina bifida and shunts, nine women had symptoms of shunt malfunction (8). Symptoms of shunt malfunction include headaches, nausea, vomiting, gaze palsy, and,

occasionally, impaired consciousness. In most cases of malfunction, management was conservative and all patients improved postpartum (8). The etiologies of shunt malfunction may include the enlarging uterus impeding CSF flow as a result of increased intraabdominal pressure or compression of the peritoneal catheter between the enlarged uterus and other viscera (22). In Bradley's series of 56 live births (mothers with diverse causes of hydrocephalus), 83.9% of women had normal shunt function. Shunt malfunctions occurred before delivery in five women, and three of them required a shunt revision prior to delivery (18). In Arata's series, five women had ventriculoperitoneal shunts (17). None of these women had any problems with their shunts during their pregnancy. In another series of 25 pregnancies of mothers with shunts (for diverse conditions), none had shunt malfunction (23).

Preeclampsia

In Arata's series, six of 23 pregnancies had hypertension-related problems. Two women had preexisting hypertension, and one of these two developed superimposed severe preeclampsia necessitating premature delivery. In addition, three developed preeclampsia and one had pregnancy-induced hypertension (17)

Delivery

Uterine contractions are normal and unaffected by spina bifida (17). Failure to recognize the onset of labor occurred only in one woman in Arata's series (17).

Premature Labor

There has been a suspicion that women with spina bifida have an increased risk of premature labor due to congenital genital tract abnormalities (8). Rietberg reviewed 20 cases of pregnancy and spina bifida in the literature and found that seven women had nine spontaneous deliveries before 37 weeks (26 to 37 weeks) (8). In Arata's series, five pregnancies were complicated by threatened premature labor requiring admission and suppression with salbutamol. One delivered at 36 weeks, and the others delivered at term (17).

Vaginal vs. Cesarean Delivery

There is a significantly higher cesarean section rate in the spina bifida population compared to the general population. In one series, eight of 20 deliveries were by cesarean section (8). Four cesarean sections were performed because of pelvic disproportion (one due to breech, one due to recurrent renal infection and lack of the lower extremity abduction, and two for unclear reasons).

In Arata's series, 12 of 23 pregnancies were delivered by cesarean section (17). The reasons for emergency cesarean section included failure to progress, severe preeclampsia, and primigravida breech. The reasons for elective cesarean section included breech in primigravida, preeclampsia, marked pelvic contraction, high head at term, and maternal spina bifida.

Potential complications of cesarean section in this population include thromboembolic disease and abdominal adhesions from prior surgeries. Cesarean section was associated with significant complications in Arata's series. Ten of 12 cesarean sections were complicated by small bowel perforation, wound infections, chest infections, endometritis, sciatica, mastitis, urinary infection, and persistent hypertension associated with preeclampsia (17).

In view of the potential for significant complications, cesarean sections should be performed for specific obstetric reasons only. Spina bifida patients may have pelvic abnormalities that can complicate vaginal deliveries. Careful assessment of the pelvis is necessary. When this assessment reveals reduced measurements, a cesarean section should be planned (8).

In women with CSF shunts, vaginal delivery is preferable. Pushing during the second stage of labor is not contraindicated, and the stress of labor and bearing down does not appear to adversely affect the patient with a functioning shunt (8). Opening the peritoneal cavity at cesarean section carries the risk of septicemic infection of the CSF shunt. In addition, it has been suggested that shunt malfunction can occur with cesarean section due to fibrin deposition (24).

Antibiotic prophylaxis has been recommended for women with CSF shunts during vaginal delivery as a single administration immediately before delivery, which may be repeated once at 6 to 12 hours postpartum. The necessity and value of this prophylaxis is controversial (23).

Anesthesia

Regional anesthesia can be achieved, but often there are technical difficulties because of anatomic abnormalities including the identification of the proper space. Recommendations have been made that the puncture site be above the lesion (16,17). Inadequate anesthesia can occur (8,17,25). In Arata's series, 11 women with cesarean sections had general anesthesia, including one who had a failed epidural. Four women with vaginal deliveries had no anesthesia, two had nitrous oxide, four had pudendal anesthesia, and one had an epidural (17). Epidural anesthesia is not contraindicated in women with shunts (23).

Newborns

Meta-analysis of four studies found an overall risk of 4.1% that parents with spina bifida would have affected offspring (8). In one series of mothers with spina bifida, none of the 23 infants had spina bifida; however, three had other congenital malformations (17). This number of anomalies is higher than the general population risk of one in 30 (26).

MENTAL RETARDATION: DOWN'S SYNDROME

Mental retardation has multiple biologic and environmental etiologies. Biologic causes include perinatal insults, intrauterine alcohol exposure, and sex chromosomal abnormalities. Down syndrome (DS) is the most commonly identified genetic cause of mental retardation, affecting approximately 9.2 per 100,000 live births in the United States (27). The majority of cases of DS result from trisomy of chromosome 21 (90%), whereas the remainder occurs as a result of mosaicism or translocation. The risk of this chromosomal abnormality increases proportionally with increasing maternal age (28). As the majority of research available on MR/DD focuses on genetically identifiable causes, most of this discussion on pregnancy in MR/DD is limited to DS.

Most women do not receive adequate preconception counseling. Ideally, women with DS need genetic counseling and evaluation of disability-specific medical conditions, as well as general health optimization.

Preconception Medical Issues

DS is associated with a variety of medical complications that should be evaluated prior to conception because certain issues may have significant impact on future pregnancy. The most important consideration is congenital heart disease. Incidence estimates of cardiac disease in DS range from an average of 40% to as high as 70%, and females may have a higher incidence than males (28). Cardiac lesions associated with DS include (in descending order of frequency): atrioventricular canal, ventral septal defect, patent ductus arteriosus, atrial septal defect, tetralogy of Fallot, as well as a variety of other defects (28, 29). Pulmonary hypertension is a common companion of congenital cardiac anomalies, which potentially evolves into future pulmonary vascular obstructive disease. This evolution can occur earlier and more frequently in children with DS than in nonaffected children with similar cardiac lesions (28). Whereas dramatic cardiac anomalies would have received early and aggressive surgical intervention in childhood, less impressive defects may have been managed expectantly or even escaped detection. Goldhaber

and colleagues (30) examined 35 asymptomatic patients with DS considered clinically free of cardiac disease and found mitral valve prolapse in 57% (in combination with tricuspid valve prolapse in 25%) and aortic regurgitation in 11%.

Physiologic alterations during pregnancy may make a previously unnoticed cardiac defect apparent or destabilize already compromised cardiac reserves. All women with DS should be referred to a cardiologist for a precise anatomic and functional assessment prior to pregnancy.

Other medical issues common to women with DS include thyroid disease, obesity, joint laxity, and atlantoaxial subluxation. The incidence of thyroid disease in adult patients is approximately 40%, with the majority attributable to hypothyroidism. Women with DS may not exhibit clinical signs of hypothyroidism other than obesity, which is also quite common in DS. Therefore, routine screening should be performed prior to pregnancy.

Prenatal Counseling

Anticipatory guidance is key for pregnant women with DS. Prenatal and parent training curriculum may need adaptation for use with women with MR/DD. Choose simplified (but age-appropriate) teaching materials tailored to the woman's level of ability. Women with mild mental retardation are concrete thinkers who do not readily grasp concepts presented abstractly; internal body representation is more difficult for MR/DD patients to conceptualize than external body representation. The ability to generalize from experience may be greatly reduced or absent, necessitating patient explanation and repetition of ideas. Reinforcement of information via role-playing or interactive games in scenarios that approximate reality is most effective. Although women with MR/DD may have difficulty learning as easily as their nondisabled peers, opportunities to interact with perceived peers increase learning and retention. Levy and colleagues (31) describe a school-based prenatal program serving non-MR/DD pregnant elementary girls ages 11–15 and adolescents (ages 11–19) with mild to moderate mental retardation. The combination of groups proved effective as well as developmentally appropriate.

Genetic Counseling

Genetic counseling is a necessity for all women with chromosomal abnormalities. The theoretic risk of DS in the child of a woman with DS is 50% because of the genetic expectation that euploid 23,X and aneuploid 24,X, +21 will occur with equal frequency (32). Review of the 31 documented pregnancies in women with DS to date showed ten children with DS and 19 children without DS, resulting in an approximate risk of 30%. However, six of the 19 children without DS had other anomalies such as mental retardation and congenital malformations (32,33). Women with DS considering pregnancy need to consider the overall risk and to be aware that prenatal testing may not be sensitive to all potential malformations.

Fertility

Pregnancy in women with DS is uncommon. Women with DS develop secondary sexual characteristics, achieve menarche, and experience regular menstrual cycles in sequence and timing similar to women without chromosomal disorders (7,34). However, ovulatory function remains in question. Review of the literature reveals 31 pregnancies in 27 women with DS documented over the past 84 years, confirming the reproductive capacity of women with DS (32,33).

One study has investigated ovulatory patterns. Tricomi and associates (35) examined vaginal smears over a period of two theoretic menstrual cycles to attempt an indirect determination of ovulatory capacity in 13 women with DS. Two-thirds of the women exhibited signs of ovulation (38.5% definitely ovulated, whereas 15.4% probably and 15.4% possibly ovulated) (35). Elkins (7) found that irregular anovulatory cycles are a common problem in women with DS as a result of obesity or hy-

pothyroidism (7). Ovulatory disorders are among the most treatable causes of infertility.

Pregnancy

There is no literature available addressing intrapartum concerns specific to women with DS or MR/DD.

Delivery/Anesthesia

Consider early and adequate anesthesia for women who cannot cognitively cope with labor. The anesthesiologist should be made aware of any atlantoaxial subluxation in the event that intubation is necessary.

Newborns

See Genetic Counseling.

Postpartum Issues

As highlighted previously, meticulous anticipatory guidance and multiple psychosocial supports are crucial to ensure the parenting success of women with MR/DD. Newborns are completely dependent on their caregivers and communicate needs by nonverbal cues, which women with MR/DD may need assistance interpreting to respond appropriately. Stressors and demands normally associated with new motherhood can lead to frustration and erosion of self-confidence with catastrophic results if in-home training and assistance are not available. Finally, peer networks allow women with MR/DD to share common experiences and solve common problems while providing the opportunity to reinforce learning.

ACKNOWLEDGMENT

Special thanks to Diane McNally, research assistant.

REFERENCES

1. Welner S. Pregnancy in women with disabilities. In: Cohen WR, ed. *Cherry and Merkata's complications of*

pregnancy. 5th. Philadelphia: Lippincott Williams & Wilkins, 2000:829–838.

2. Nosek MA, Rintala DH, Young ME, et al. *National study of women with physical disabilities*. Houston: Center for Research on Women with Disabilities, 1997.

3. Fine M, Asch A, eds. *Women with disabilities*. Philadelphia: Temple University Press, 1988.

4. Waxman BF. The right to bear young. *The Disability Rag ReSource* 1993;3–11.

5. Lunsky Y, Reiss S. Health needs of women with mental retardation and developmental disabilities. *Am Psychol* 1998;53:319.

6. Kreutner AK. Sexuality, fertility, and the problems of menstruation in mentally retarded adolescents. *Pediatr Clin North Am* 1981;28:475–480.

7. Elkins TE. Gynecology. In: Pueschel SM, Pueschel JK, eds. *Biomedical concerns in persons with Down syndrome*. Baltimore: Paul Brookes, 1992:139–146.

8. Rietberg CC, Lindhout D. Adult patients with spina bifida cystica: genetic counselling, pregnancy and delivery. *Eur J Obstet Gynecol Reprod Biol* 1993;52:63–70.

9. Foley J. The offspring of people with cerebral palsy. *Dev Med Child Neurol* 1992;34:972–978.

10. Winch R, Bengtson L, McLaughlin J, et al. Women with cerebral palsy: obstetric experience and neonatal outcome. *Dev Med Child Neurol* 1993;35:974–982.

11. Taft LT. Cerebral palsy. *Pediatr Rev* 1995;16:411–418.

12. Morrell MJ. Hormones, reproductive health and epilepsy. In: Wyllie E, ed. *The treatment of epilepsy*. Baltimore: Williams & Wilkins, 1996:179–187.

13. Creasy RK, Resnick R. *Maternal-fetal medicine: principles and practice*. 2nd ed. Philadelphia: WB Saunders, 1989.

14. Notzon FC, Placek PJ, Taffel SM. Comparisons of national cesarean-section rates. *N Engl J Med* 1987;316: 386–389.

15. Kariya N, Toyoyama H, Furuichi, K, et al. Induction of general anesthesia using propofol for cesarean section of a woman with cerebral palsy. *J Clin Anesth* 1999;11: 672–674.

16. Brady JP, Goldman ST. Management of meconium aspiration syndrome. In: Thibeault DW, Gregory DA, eds. *Neonatal pulmonary care*. Norwalk, CT: Appleton-Century-Crofts, 1986:485.

17. Arata M, Grover S, Dunne K, et al. Pregnancy outcome and complications in women with spina bifida. *J Reprod Med* 2000;45:743–748.

18. Bradley NK, Liakos AM, McAllister JP, et al. Maternal shunt dependency: implications for obstetric care, neurosurgical management, and pregnancy outcomes and a review of selected literature. *Neurosurgery* 1998;43: 448–461.

19. Wynn JS, Mellor S, Morewood GA. Pregnancy in patients with spina bifida cystica. *Practitioner* 1979;222: 543–546.

20. Mann WJ, Jones DE. Pregnancy complicated by maternal neural tube defect and ileal conduit: a case report. *J Reprod Med* 1976;17:339–341.

21. Daw E. Pregnancy problems in a paraplegic patient with an ileal conduit bladder. *Practitioner* 1973;211: 781–784.

22. Hanakita J, Suzuki T, Yamamoto Y, et al. Ventriculoperitoneal shunt malfunction during pregnancy. *J Neurosurg* 1985;63:459–460.

23. Landwehr JB Jr, Isada NB, Pryde PG, et al. Maternal neurosurgical shunts and pregnancy. *Obstet Gynecol* 1994;83:134–137.

24. Cusimano MD, Meffe FM, Gentili F, et al. Ventriculoperitoneal shunt malfunction during pregnancy. *Neurosurgery* 1990;27:969–971.

25. Vaagenes P, Fjaerestad I. Epidural block during labour in a patient with spina bifida cystica. *Anaesthesia* 1981; 36:299–301.

26. Harper PS. *Practical genetic counseling*. 4th ed. Oxford: Butterworth Heinemann, 1993.

27. Centers for Disease Control. Down syndrome prevalence at birth—United States, 1983–1990. *MMWR Morb Mortal Wkly Rep* 1994;43:617–622.

28. Rogers PT, Coleman M. *Medical care in Down syndrome*. New York: Marcel Dekker, 1992.

29. Baciewicz FA Jr, Melvin WS, Basilius D, et al. Congenital heart disease in Down's syndrome patients: a decade of surgical experience. *Thorac Cardiovasc Surg* 1989;37:369–371.

30. Goldhaber SZ, Brown WD, Sutton MG. High frequency of mitral valve prolapse and aortic regurgitation among asymptomatic adults with Down's syndrome. *JAMA* 1987;258:1793–1795.

31. Levy SR, Perhats C, Nash-Johnson M, et al. Reducing the risks in pregnant teens who are very young and those with mild mental retardation. *Ment Retard* 1992; 30:195–203.

32. Bovicelli L, Orsini LF, Rizzo N, et al. Reproduction in Down syndrome. *Obstet Gynecol* 1982;59:13S–17S.

33. Shobda Rani A, Jyothi A, Reddy PP, et al. Reproduction in Down's syndrome. *Int J Gynaecol Obstet* 1990;31: 81–86.

34. Goldstein H. Menarche, menstruation, sexual relations and contraception of adolescent females with Down syndrome. *Eur J Obstet Gynecol Reprod Biol* 1988;27: 343–349.

35. Tricomi V, Valenti C, Hall JE. Ovulatory patterns in Down syndrome. *Am J Obstet Gynecol* 1964;89: 651–656.

Neurological Complications of Pregnancy, Second
Edition, edited by Brian Hainline and Orrin Devinsky.
Lippincott Williams & Wilkins, Philadelphia, © 2002.

19

Paraplegia

Bruce K. Young

*Department of Obstetrics and Gynecology, New York University School of Medicine,
New York, New York, U.S.A.*

Pregnancy and paraplegia do not coincide very often. When they do, most obstetricians and most neurologists are relatively unfamiliar with the problems caused by this combination. Advances in obstetrics, neurology, and rehabilitation medicine have improved the outcomes for patients with paraplegia.

Survival among women with spinal cord damage and paraplegia is common today. Rehabilitation techniques and equipment have improved the quality of life for them as well. Most of these patients sustained an injury to the spinal cord in an accident (Table 19.1), especially automobile or diving accidents, and were otherwise healthy. Compression of the spinal cord secondary to enlargement of hemangiomas during pregnancy also may produce spinal cord transection symptoms or paraplegia of rapid onset. Magnetic resonance imaging may help in diagnosis. Evaluation by spinal fluid examination suggests subarachnoid block. Hemangiomas typically will decrease in size postpartum. They are the most common spinal cord tumors in pregnancy, but other kinds of spinal cord tumors may produce similar symptoms in pregnant women (1,2). Von Hippel-Lindau disease has been associated with acute onset of paraplegia in pregnancy. It is an autosomal dominant disorder characterized by multiorgan hemangioblastomas and a predisposition to carcinoma. It has been reported as a cause of paraplegia with spinal hemorrhage as well as autonomic hyperreflexia in a pregnant woman (3). Other causes of paraplegia are transverse myelitis, tuberculosis, multiple sclerosis, Guillain-Barré syndrome, and poliomyelitis, although the latter is now rare (1–6).

Although amenorrhea often follows spinal cord injury, most premenopausal women resume menstruation within a few months. Their pregnancy rate and the risk of spontaneous abortion remain as they were before the spinal cord trauma (1,7). In fact, those who had dysmenorrhea may find that problem gone or much improved. Ovulation and fertility are the same as in other women once the transient amenorrhea of injury has abated. Pregnancy is not only possible but also quite likely when these women recuperate and try to achieve all of their potential despite paraplegia.

Thus, pregnancy in paraplegic women, while uncommon, is no longer a rarity, and physicians must be prepared to care for the paraplegic pregnancy. Preconception counseling for these women is essential. They must be advised of the potential complications that

TABLE 19.1. *Causes of paraplegia in young
women*

Spinal cord trauma
Spinal cord tumor
Spinal cord tuberculosis
Multiple sclerosis
Guillain-Barré syndrome
Transverse myelitis
Poliomyelitis

TABLE 19.2. *Complications of pregnancy in paraplegics*

Complication	Antepartum	Intrapartum	Postpartum
Urinary infection	✓	✓	✓
Urinary calculi	✓	✓	✓
Catheter obstruction	✓	✓	✓
Anemia	✓	✓	✓
Decubiti	✓	✓	✓
Muscle spasms	✓	✓	✓
Sepsis	✓	✓	✓
Autonomic hyperreflexia	✓	✓	✓
Uterine hyperactivity	✓	✓	
Preterm labor	✓	✓	
Precipitate labor		✓	
Painless cervical dilation	✓	✓	
Fetal stress	✓	✓	
Thrombophlebitis			✓
Exhaustion			✓

may arise antepartum, intrapartum, and postpartum (Table 19.2). Prenatal laboratory studies should be performed before pregnancy and should include urine cultures and sonography of the urinary tract as well as the usual prenatal tests. Patients need to plan for child care and devise practical means with regard to work or managing a home with a newborn as an added responsibility.

Specific problems should be addressed in counseling these patients. Those with long-standing paraplegia are usually very aware of the problems with which they must cope in daily living. However, pregnancy may increase and expand the problems of the paraplegic woman. The most common concerns are sexual activity, urinary infection and calculi, decubiti, sepsis, and autonomic hyperreflexia. All these concerns should be discussed fully with the patient before pregnancy.

Sexual activity in the pregnant paraplegic is not prohibited unless associated with the autonomic hyperreflexia response or a marked increase in uterine activity. Most women will have increased uterine contractions following sexual intercourse, and this is not usually accompanied by cervical dilation. However, the paraplegic woman is more susceptible to uterine hyperactivity and preterm labor and should be examined regularly for cervical changes. Spinal cord lesions at T10 are associated with painless labor, and the patient may not be aware of postcoital uterine contractions

(1–6). Cervical length measured sonographically may be helpful in evaluating for possible uterine hyperactivity.

Urinary infections are common and recurrent in paraplegics, and they are much more of a problem in those who require continuous urinary catheterization. Cystitis is almost ineradicable, with bladder and renal calculi and pyelonephritis the frequent consequence of urinary stasis and bacteriuria. Frequent urine cultures, antibiotics, and serial sonograms for calculi are important. A mild degree of hydroureter and hydronephrosis are normal in pregnancy and are more pronounced on the right than on the left because of uterine dextrorotation. This should not be overinterpreted. Long-term urinary antiseptic agents may be necessary but must be carefully selected, as with all drugs in pregnancy. Pyelonephritis is a very serious illness in the woman who is pregnant and paraplegic. Methylmandelic acid is a safe choice for prolonged use in pregnancy and may prevent pyelonephritis and a life-threatening gram-negative sepsis in these susceptible patients.

Decubiti often are exacerbated by pregnancy because of the increased weight, decreased mobility, and greater stasis and tissue edema. Decubitus ulcers must be prevented if possible and scrupulously cared for otherwise. They are a source of cellulitis, necrotizing infection, and sepsis if neglected. Pregnancy tends to detract from their care.

TABLE 19.3. *Autonomic hyperreflexia:*
symptoms and signs

Hypertension
Headache
Tachycardia
Bradycardia
Arrhythmias
Flushing
Diaphoresis
Dilated pupils
Piloerection
Nasal blockage
Muscle spasms
Unconsciousness
Seizures
Anxiety

Autonomic hyperreflexia (3–6) results from spinal cord transection. It develops when impulses from a distended viscus such as the bladder, intestine, or uterus enter the spinal cord but are not modulated by higher centers in the sensory cortex due to the transection. As a consequence, a relatively mild stimulus evokes a nonspecific massive autonomic reflex response. The syndrome of autonomic hyperreflexia usually is encountered in the patient with a spinal cord transection at the fifth to seventh thoracic vertebrae or higher, when there is acute distension of a hollow viscus, most often the bladder. However, it is very likely in such a patient during active labor because of the effects of uterine contractions. The mechanism is massive release of maternal catecholamines (8–11). This results in paroxysmal headache, flushing, anxiety, tachycardia, hypertension, bradycardia (8,9), diaphoresis, piloerection, pupillary dilation, cardiac arrhythmias, blocked nasal passages, muscle spasms, and, rarely, seizures and coma (Table 19.3). When severe and prolonged, autonomic hyperreflexia may cause cerebral hemorrhage or cardiac arrhythmia sufficient to be fatal (12,13).

ANTEPARTUM CARE

Anemia is common before pregnancy and should be treated vigorously when diagnosed. It often is exacerbated by pregnancy and predisposes to slow healing, decubiti, and de-creased resistance to infection. Therapy should aim for hemoglobin levels of at least 10 g/dL. Oral iron should be used along with stool softeners and bulking agents because of the adverse effects of both iron therapy and pregnancy on chronic constipation in paraplegics.

Frequent visits and careful assessment of these patients is wise. Evaluation for painless cervical dilation and decubiti should be performed at every visit. The urine should be cultured monthly, and treatment should be provided for bacteriuria. Serial sonography of the urinary tract as well as obstetric sonograms and cervical length measurements should be performed. Complete blood counts should be performed to monitor and treat anemia, and meticulous physiotherapy should be initiated and maintained throughout the pregnancy and puerperium. Monitoring uterine activity also is advisable to prevent preterm birth before 36 weeks, although its effectiveness is unproven. Beta blockade has been used to prevent recurrent symptoms in nonobstetric patients and may be considered in antepartum patients with recurrent episodes of preterm autonomic hyperreflexia. Metoprolol was successful in a nonpregnant patient (14). However, the onset of preterm labor may accompany the hyperreflexia in many cases. This poses a dilemma in pharmacologic management because the beta-blocker could augment uterine activity. Magnesium sulfate or indomethacin as usually used for preterm labor would seem to be appropriate agents, whereas the beta mimetics such as terbutaline and ritodrine are relatively contraindicated. The best single agent for treating both the symptoms of autonomic hyperreflexia and preterm labor is a calcium channel blocker, such as nicardipine or nifedipine (15).

INTRAPARTUM CARE

The onset of labor may be silent as a result of painless contractions, or it may be heralded by the syndrome of autonomic hyperreflexia as the first indication of labor (Table 19.4). When the lesion is at the tenth thoracic verte-

TABLE 19.4. *Autonomic hyperreflexia in labor*

Fetal heart rate decelerations
Fetal heart rate accelerations
Normal fetal pH
Uterine polysystole
Uterine hypertonicity
Perineal muscle spasms

bra or above, the contractions often are not recognized by the patient so that minor symptoms such as spotting; increased discharge; pelvic, back, or abdominal pressure; and leakage of fluid from the vagina must be investigated. In labor, mother and fetus should be closely monitored with a fetal monitor, and frequent maternal blood pressure readings should be performed. An indwelling Foley catheter should be placed if none is present. Analgesia is often unnecessary but may be used prophylactically.

Autonomic hyperreflexia in labor may be life-threatening for the mother but is usually well tolerated by the fetus as long as there is good maternal perfusion of the placenta (Fig. 19.1). Regional anesthesia is the most effec-

tive way to prevent or treat autonomic hyperreflexia (9,11,12,14,17). Other agents such as diphenhydramine, hydralazine, diazepam, trimethaphan camsylate, metoprolol, nicardipine, nifedipine, and guanethidine have been used successfully to treat the acute syndrome, but they require careful titration to prevent hypotension (14–17). Hypotension may be difficult to control with any of the therapeutic modalities. Both hypotension and hypertension can result in maternal and fetal stress (18). Nonpregnant patients also have responded to these therapeutic alternatives (13,16), as well as general anesthesia (17), but the laboring patient's symptoms are the most difficult to control.

The diagnosis of preeclampsia may be confused with the syndrome, but there is no increased incidence of toxemia of pregnancy in paraplegics. The fetus often is stressed (Table 19.4) and exhibits tachycardia and variable decelerations (11) during paroxysms of hyperreflexia. Despite the maternal catecholamine surge and the resultant hypertension, the fetal pH is usually normal and the

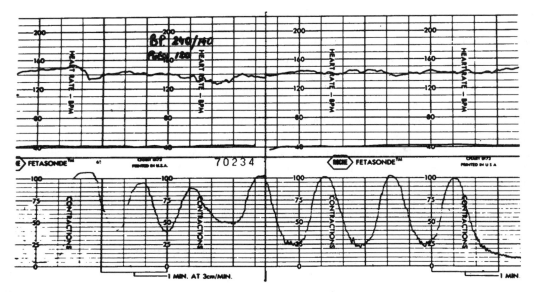

FIG. 19.1. This fetal monitoring record is from a patient in labor. The upper trace shows baseline fetal heart rate of 140 to 150 bpm with mild variable decelerations. The lower trace shows increased frequency and intensity of uterine contractions early in the first stage of labor. Maternal pulse is 120 bpm, blood pressure 245/140 mm Hg, due to autonomic hyperreflexia.

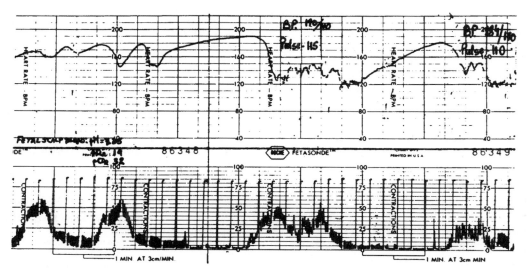

FIG. 19.2. Fetal monitoring record with continuous tissue pH, fetal heart rate, and uterine contractions. The upper trace shows baseline tachycardia of 160 to 180 bpm with accelerations and variable decelerations late in the second stage of labor. The lower trace shows both uterine contractions and tissue pH superimposed. The tissue pH is seen as a vertical bar every 15 seconds; pH 7.0 is at the zero line, and pH 7.40 is at the 100 line. Fetal scalp capillary blood sampling showed pH 7.35, pO_2 19 mm Hg, and pCO_2, 32 mm Hg, with tissue pH reading 7.33 to 7.35. Maternal pulse is 100 to 115 bpm, blood pressure 184 to 190/110 mm Hg, during a paroxysm of autonomic hyperreflexia.

stress usually is tolerated by the fetus without adverse outcome (Fig. 19.2). Complications of labor are not increased, except for rapid labor. The combination of preterm labor and uterine hyperactivity usually produces rapid labor and prompt delivery, often without pain or anesthesia. Low forceps may be used, especially to shorten the second stage in a woman with autonomic hyperreflexia. Cesarean delivery is performed only for specific obstetric indications, with regional anesthesia preferred where anesthesia is indicated. However, when autonomic hyperreflexia is recurrent in labor and delivery is not likely within a reasonable period of time, cesarean delivery may be considered because of difficulty in maintaining stability of the patient's condition. Under those circumstances, the patient must have adequate anesthesia and be symptomatically well controlled before undergoing cesarean delivery. An interval of good control may be an opportunity to achieve prompt delivery in an otherwise difficult labor. Nevertheless, the preferred management is vaginal

delivery with a closely monitored and well-controlled patient (19).

Placement of an epidural catheter 2 to 3 weeks before the expected date of delivery has been advocated to assure prompt control of autonomic hyperreflexia with the onset of labor. Because the incidence of autonomic hyperreflexia and the severity of symptoms are not predictable in most patients, but may be anticipated in many, routine prophylactic epidural placement has been suggested for paraplegic women (15).

POSTPARTUM CARE

Shortly after delivery, autonomic hyperreflexia usually will abate. Nevertheless, the maintenance of the epidural catheter for 24 to 48 hours postpartum is recommended to prevent autonomic hyperreflexia or treat it if it recurs. Postpartum uterine contractions, bladder distension, or constipation, all common occurrences, may trigger autonomic hyperreflexia (15,19). The risk of postpartum hemorrhage is not increased, but phlebitis and sepsis occur more commonly than in the usual obstetric patient. This period requires intensive physiotherapy to mobilize the exhausted gravida, prevent decubiti or treat them, and avoid phlebitis and embolism. Anemia and urinary infection must be treated. Postnatal therapy must be oriented to teaching both parents how to care for their infant as part of the patient's rehabilitation from childbirth. Occupational therapists and physiatrists should use programs designed for developing parenting techniques adapted to the mother with paraplegia. Spousal involvement is even more important in these patients than in the usual couple. Newborn and child care must be taught to these parents with special needs by a skilled and patient staff emphasizing the abilities of the mother rather than her disability, helping her to overcome her limitations with confidence. This will enable the new mother to cope with lactation and child care, which can proceed normally (20). The pregnant paraplegic is beset by exacerbations of the many conditions she has learned to tolerate. Of these, autonomic hyperreflexia, urinary infection and calculi, sepsis, and phlebitis pose serious risks. However, the prognosis is good for both mother and child when close attention is paid to their care. With careful monitoring and medical care, women with paraplegia may expect a healthy infant and a safe passage through pregnancy.

REFERENCES

1. Geller H, Paeslack V. Our experiences about pregnancy and delivery of the paraplegic woman. *Paraplegia* 1971; 8:161.
2. Divers S. A spinal cord neurolemmoma in pregnancy. *Obstet Gynecol* 1978;52:474–505.
3. Ogasawara KK, Ogasawara EM, Hirata G. Pregnancy complicated by von Hippel-Lindau disease. *Obstet Gynecol* 1995;85:829–831.
4. Berghella V, Spector T, Trauffer P, et al. Pregnancy in patients with pre-existing transverse myelitis. *Obstet Gynecol* 1996;87:809–812.
5. Vaidya MK, Shah GV, Bharucha KE. Pregnancy and its outcome in quadriplegia due to Pott's spine. *Int J Gynaecol Obstet* 1995;49:319–321.
6. Robertson DNS. Pregnancy and labour in the paraplegic. *Paraplegia* 1972;10:709–715.
7. Comarr AE. Observations on menstruation in pregnancy among female spinal cord injury patients. *Paraplegia* 1966;3:263–266.
8. Chiaou-Tan FY, Robertson CS, Chiou GL. Catecholamine assays in a rat model for autonomic dysreflexia. *Arch Phys Med Rehabil* 1998;79:402–404.
9. Stirt JA, Marco A, Conklin KA. Obstetric anesthesia for a quadriplegic patient with autonomic hyperreflexia. *Anesthesiology* 1979;51:560.
10. Naftchi NE, Wooten GF, Lowman EW, et al. Relationship between serum dopamine-β-hydroxylase activity, catecholamine metabolism, and hemodynamic changes during paroxysmal hypertension in quadriplegia. *Circ Res* 1974;35:850.
11. Young BK, Katz M, Klein SA. Pregnancy after spinal cord injury: altered maternal and fetal response to labor. *Obstet Gynecol* 1983;62:59–64.
12. Tabsh KMA, Brinkman CR III, Reff RA. Autonomic dysreflexia in pregnancy. *Obstet Gynecol* 1982;60:119.
13. McGregor JA, Meeuwsen J. Autonomic hyperreflexia: a mortal danger for spinal cord damaged women in labor. *Am J Obstet Gynecol* 1985;151:330–333.
14. Pasquina PF, Houston RM, Belandres PV. Beta blockade in the treatment of autonomic dysreflexia: a case report and review. *Arch Phys Med Rehabil* 1998;79:582–584.
15. Kobayashi A, Mizobe T, Tojo H, et al. Autonomic hyperreflexia during labour. *Can J Anaesth* 1995;42: 1134–1136.
16. Katz VL, Thorp JM, Cefalo RC. Epidural analgesia and autonomic hyperreflexia: a case report. *Am J Obstet Gynecol* 1990;162:471–472
17. Hambly PR, Martin B. Anaesthesia for chronic spinal cord lesions. *Anaesthesia* 1998;53:273–289
18. Antoine C, Young BK. Fetal lactic acidosis with epidural anesthesia. *Am J Obstet Gynecol* 1982;142: 55–58.
19. American College of Obstetricians and Gynecologists. *Obstetric management of patients with spinal cord injury.* ACOG Committee Opinion 121. Washington, DC: ACOG, 1993.
20. Verduyn WH. Pregnancy and delivery in tetraplegic women. *J Spinal Cord Med* 1997;20:371–374.

Neurological Complications of Pregnancy, Second Edition, edited by Brian Hainline and Orrin Devinsky. Lippincott Williams & Wilkins, Philadelphia, © 2002.

20

Psychiatric Disorders

Orrin Devinsky and Mary T. Miceli

Departments of Neurology, Neurosurgery, and Psychiatry, New York University School of Medicine, New York, New York, U.S.A.

Pregnancy and childbearing are complex psychosocial and biologic processes and raise issues of intense interest to both medical professionals and the public. The interplay between psychosocial and biologic factors is evident in the behavioral disorders complicating pregnancy and the postpartum period. Psychologic factors complicating pregnancy include a premorbid history of behavioral disorders and the unique psychodynamics of pregnancy and parenthood. Pregnancy and the immediate postpartum period are a time in a woman's life fraught with special psychologic meaning. Like other developmental stages, life changes in an irrevocable way (1). Psychosocial factors such as marital status, family support, and financial and employment status take on new meaning because of new responsibilities and expectations. Biologic factors that may influence behavioral changes during pregnancy and postpartum include hormonal, neurochemical, and physical changes, pain, sleep deprivation, and a genetic predisposition for behavioral disorders. The pathogenesis of peripartum psychiatric disorders is a tangled web. This chapter reviews some behavioral disorders unique to pregnancy and the postpartum period and discusses the use of psychotropic medications and electroconvulsive therapy (ECT) for these and other psychiatric problems encountered during pregnancy and postpartum.

COMPETENCY OF MOTHERS WITH CHRONIC PSYCHIATRIC DISORDERS

Most women with psychiatric disorders during pregnancy have preexisting psychiatric illness (2). Care of pregnant women with preexisting psychiatric disorders is complex because ethical and separate but overlapping health issues related to mother and fetus come into play. Family planning interventions to prevent pregnancy in women with chronic mental illness are controversial and need to be more fully addressed (3). Patients with serious, longstanding psychiatric disorders often have cognitive impairment, poor judgment, emotional instability, and impulsive behavior that places them at increased risk of contracting sexually transmitted diseases (4) and unwanted pregnancies (5,6). Poor prenatal care and exposure to psychotropic medication and illicit drugs are potential hazards to the fetus in these patients (7–11). Furthermore, children of chronic psychiatric patients are at increased risk of coexisting cognitive impairment (12,13). Existing guidelines for mentally retarded patients, however, cannot be applied to patients with psychiatric disorders. A simple dichotomy between patients capable and not capable of informed consent (14) does not adequately address the mentally ill population. New guidelines for dealing with these patients are needed.

PSYCHIATRIC PROBLEMS DURING PREGNANCY: AN OVERVIEW

Pregnancy confers no immunity against psychiatric disorders. Although not associated with an increased incidence of mental disorders (15), pregnancy imposes challenges in managing pregnant women with these disorders. All behavioral problems confronting women of childbearing age can occur in pregnancy. Emergent conditions such as acute psychosis, mania, depression with suicidal ideation, or homicidal ideation must be recognized and appropriately managed. Other psychiatric conditions such as eating disorders and substance abuse can present a danger to the fetus and mother. Psychiatric conditions such as anxiety, panic, and obsessive-compulsive disorders (OCDs) can continue into or become more refractory during pregnancy. Psychiatric conditions also can contribute to poor compliance with prenatal care (16).

Therapy of psychiatric disorders during pregnancy must balance the risks and benefits to the mother and fetus. Because there are so many interacting variables, cases must be approached individually. There have been several excellent reviews of therapy for these problems (16–20). In this chapter we will discuss psychiatric conditions unique to pregnancy and the postpartum period, the treatment of these conditions, as well as other psychiatric conditions that can complicate pregnancy and the postpartum period.

Hyperemesis Gravidarum

Emesis gravidarum refers to the mild to moderate degree of vomiting during the first trimester of pregnancy that affects approximately 40% to 70% of women. Hyperemesis gravidarum is a pathologic, self-limiting condition with severe vomiting that results in electrolyte imbalance, impaired nutrition, and weight loss. Pregnancy-related physiologic changes, particularly delayed gastric emptying secondary to high levels of cholecystokinin, influence both conditions (16–21). The incidence of hyperemesis gravidarum is three in 1,000 live births (22–24) with a recurrence rate of 26% to 50% (25–27), and it is more common in women with eating disorders (28). Prior to the availability of antiemetic drugs and intravenous fluid replacement, hyperemesis gravidarum occasionally resulted in pregnancy loss and maternal death (24).

Although no psychologic significance is attributed to normal morning sickness, psychologic factors are thought to play a role in up to four-fifths of patients with hyperemesis gravidarum (26–27). Earlier this century, psychoanalysts hypothesized that pernicious vomiting during pregnancy occurred in women who were pathologically close to their mothers (23,19) or was an unconscious attempt to abort the fetus (30,31). It is currently conceptualized as resulting from a combination of biologic, psychologic, and social factors (19). The condition has been linked to ambivalence about pregnancy, stress somatization disorder (32), and borderline and histrionic personality disorders (26). Other theories include thyroid dysfunction, adrenocortical or anterior pituitary insufficiency, and psychosomatic factors (29). Women who develop hyperemesis gravidarum are more likely to be unmarried, to have unplanned or unwanted pregnancies, and to find their significant others unsupportive (33). They are also more likely to have had a prior pregnancy loss (34) or to be carrying a multiple gestation (26). Hyperemesis gravidarum may result from a confluence of factors.

The treatment of hyperemesis gravidarum is supportive, ranging from hospitalization with nasogastric feeding, parenteral antiemetics, and intravenous fluid replacement; nutrition; vitamins; sedation; pharmacologic therapies; or simply placing the patient in a supportive, less stressful environment. Symptoms often cease shortly after the patient is hospitalized, without other interventions (32). Similarly, returning to the home of origin or having a close relative stay with the patient can help. Other useful treatments are supportive psychotherapy (35), behavior modification (36), placebo, and hypnosis (37,38). Benzodiazepines can reduce symptoms. Ditto and colleagues (29) showed a significantly shorter length of stay, lower readmission rate (4% compared to 27%, *n*=50, 25 treated with diazepam and 25 untreated), and less nausea in the diazepam treated group, but no teratogenic effects.

Dietary Changes, Cravings, and Eating Disorders

Proper nutrition during pregnancy is essential for healthy fetal development. Cravings and aversion for certain foods during pregnancy are normal and may actually benefit the pregnant woman and fetus by providing additional nutrients and protection from harmful substances (39,19). In some, cravings and compulsive eating may reflect the resurgence of old psychologic conflicts in pregnancy (19). Occasionally, pregnant women crave nonfood substances such as dirt and laundry starch ("pica") (39). Physicians should question pregnant women carefully about their dietary habits because women who develop bizarre cravings or dietary changes are unlikely to spontaneously report such symptoms.

There are limited data on pregnancy and eating disorders. Women with eating disorders often marry late in life if at all, may be unable to conceive because of amenorrhea, or may decide to have few or no children (40,16). Bulimia nervosa involves self-induced vomiting, extreme dieting, and compulsive diuretic or laxative use to prevent weight gain (41). Anorexia nervosa represents obsessive concerns about weight, eating, and dieting, despite an actual weight of less than 85% of the norm. Overall, women with a history of anorexia nervosa gain less weight during pregnancy, have significantly more low birthweight babies, and have higher rates of prematurity than controls (42,43).

Physicians should inquire about eating disorders in any woman who is underweight or who mentions concerns about dieting or weight (16). Best outcomes are obtained when the eating disorder is treated and remits prior to conception (44,45). Patients should be informed of the potential adverse consequences of failure to adequately gain weight, including prematurity, low birthweight infants, low Apgar scores, and small head circumference (46). Fetal growth and maternal weight gain should be monitored carefully during the last trimester in patients with an eating disorder.

Obsessive-Compulsive Disorder

Several studies document an association between pregnancy and onset or exacerbation of OCD (47–52); others have not confirmed this finding (53). Neziroglu and colleagues (52) surveyed 106 women with OCD and found that women with children have a later peak of onset than those without children (22 to 32 years compared to 13 to 15 years). Of 59 patients with at least one child, 23 (39%) experienced symptom onset during pregnancy (12 during their first pregnancy, eight in their second pregnancy, and three in their third pregnancy). Sichel's group (47) reported on 15 women with new-onset obsessive-compulsive symptoms during the puerperium. All patients reported intrusive obsessional thoughts to harm their babies and exercised some form of avoidance of their infants and modified their contact or behavior with them (e.g., not bathing their baby, avoiding knives, or staying physically away from them). Nine of the 15 women subsequently developed major depression with excellent response to selective serotonin reuptake inhibitors (SSRIs) (47). Obstetric complications may increase the risk of postpartum OCD (49).

Denial of Pregnancy

Patients who deny pregnancy have a strong unconscious motivation not to be pregnant and lack awareness of the obvious pregnant state. These patients exhibit less nausea, weight gain, and abdominal distention. True denial of pregnancy is different from the situation occasionally seen in massively obese women who present to the emergency room with sudden onset of abdominal pains from unsuspected labor. These latter patients do not dread the thought of having a baby and are usually pleased with the outcome.

Patients exhibiting true denial of pregnancy fall into three groups (54). First, patients with a history of schizophrenia or other psychoses use delusions to explain away the pregnancy. For example, "abdominal distention is due to overeating" (55,56). The patient usually resists the attempts of family and health care providers to convince her that she is pregnant.

The second group consists of women with borderline intelligence, borderline personality disorder, or both (54,55,57–59). These patients may give birth on the toilet and then, in a horrified state, kill the newborn by suffocation, drowning, or throwing the baby out the bathroom window. Amnesia of labor and the infanticide may result from a brief psychotic episode around delivery. Alternately, a denial or delusional syndrome also may contribute to the amnesia. Family members also commonly ignore the obvious symptoms and signs of pregnancy.

Finally, the third category includes young, relatively highly functioning women who, for various reasons, cannot bear the idea of being pregnant. These patients often come from religious families who stress sexual abstinence and dogmatic morality (54,58,60). Amnesia for sexual intercourse and subsequent labor and delivery are common. Treatment of denial of pregnancy must be individualized and ranges from psychotherapy and family counseling to hospitalization and use of psychotropic medications.

PSYCHOTROPIC MEDICATIONS IN PREGNANCY

Recognition and appropriate management of psychiatric conditions during pregnancy better ensures the physical and psychologic well being of the mother and infant. Although generally avoided during pregnancy, judicious use of medications is at times necessary for the health and safety of both the woman and unborn child. Risks associated with the use of psychotropic drugs include teratogenic effects, direct neonatal toxicity, and the potential for longer-term neurobehavioral sequelae, also called "behavioral teratogenesis" (61–63). As with epilepsy, dogmatic avoidance of medications for pregnant women can result in harm to both the mother and infant.

Metabolic changes during pregnancy can alter the pharmacokinetics of psychotropic medications. Volume of distribution increases and plasma albumin concentration decreases. Changes in plasma albumin concentrations increase the free (unbound) portion of psychotropic drugs such as benzodiazepines, tricyclic antidepressants, and antipsychotics. Induction of hepatic enzymes and increased glomerular filtration rate during pregnancy increase drug clearance (64,65), and gastrointestinal motility and transit time can alter absorption and time of peak serum drug levels (66). Cardiovascular changes during pregnancy, including increased heart rate and decreased mean arterial pressure (66), predispose women to the hypotensive effects of low-potency phenothiazines and tricyclic antidepressants.

All psychotropic drugs readily diffuse across the placenta to reach the fetus (20). In contrast to maternal pharmacokinetics, psychotropic drugs in the fetus have a higher unbound (free) fraction, easier penetration through the immature blood–brain barrier, and decreased hepatic and renal clearance. Together, these factors prolong serum half-life and increase the amount of drug reaching the fetal central nervous system.

Benzodiazepines

Benzodiazepines, which readily cross the placenta (67,68), are anxiolytics used to treat symptoms of anxiety and fear. Two studies demonstrated an increase in congenital malformations, including cleft lip or palate, among infants whose mothers took diazepam during the first trimester (69,70). However, subsequent larger prospective studies found no evidence that diazepam is teratogenic (71,72). Similarly, large series failed to demonstrate an increased rate of congenital malformations among offspring of mothers taking chlordiazepoxide (73–74). However, one series found a nonsignificant trend (11.4% vs. 2.6%) toward increased malformations in infants exposed to chlordiazepoxide in utero compared to controls (75). Other benzodiazepines such as oxazepam, alprazolam, and triazolam are associated with increased rates of major and minor congenital malformations and spontaneous abortions in small to moderate size series (76,77).

Occasional use of benzodiazepines in the second and early-mid portions of the third trimester has not been associated with any adverse fetal effects (78). However, chronic use during the latter two trimesters or small doses at parturition can cause neurobehavioral changes, including low Apgar scores, decreased tone, feeding difficulties with impaired suck reflex, and impaired temperature regulation (79–82).

Neonates and infants exposed to chronic benzodiazepines in utero can develop a withdrawal syndrome, including irritability, excessive crying, jitteriness, tremor, hyperactive suck reflex, diarrhea, and vomiting (83–87). These symptoms are most likely to develop in mothers who take the equivalent of 15 to 20 mg/day of diazepam for at least 12 weeks (87).

Benzodiazepines are excreted in breast milk and can cause sedation as well as impaired feeding and temperature regulation in neonates (88,89). Benzodiazepines are not conjugated with glucuronic acid during the first 3 to 5 days after delivery, thereby increasing the risk of neonatal jaundice (88,90).

Although a definite teratogenic effect of benzodiazepines has not been established, these drugs should not be used during the first trimester unless strongly indicated. If a woman taking moderate to high doses of benzodiazepines becomes pregnant, a gradual taper is recommended. Benzodiazepine use during the second and third trimesters should be restricted to occasional doses or low-dose regimens. Because benzodiazepines are excreted in breast milk and their effects on the newborn and infant are not known, women who regularly take these medications, especially at moderate to high doses, should not breastfeed.

Selective Serotonin Reuptake Inhibitors

The SSRIs are the newest class of antidepressant agents and are widely prescribed as firstline agents. They include fluoxetine, paroxetine, sertaline, fluvoxamine, and, most recently, citalopram. The SSRIs selectively inhibit the reuptake of serotonin. These drugs freely cross the placental barrier, exposing the fetus to the drug. SSRIs are used to treat depression and panic, obsessive-compulsive, and eating disorders. Adverse effects associated with the use of SSRIs include sedation, fatigue, nausea, diarrhea, weight loss, and sexual dysfunction. Citalopram may have a more favorable side-effect profile in some women. Combining SSRIs with monoamine oxidase inhibitors (MAOIs) should be avoided because of the potential for fatal serotonin syndrome (91).

Fluoxetine, the first SSRI to be marketed, has the most pregnancy outcome information available (>3,000 exposed cases). Currently, fluoxetine appears to be safe for use in all trimesters of pregnancy. Studies both retrospectively and prospectively suggest there is no evidence of increased risk over that of the general population of miscarriage, stillbirth, or major malformation to infants born from women exposed to SSRIs during pregnancy (92,61). Nulman and associates (93) prospectively studied preschool children exposed to the SSRI fluoxetine (*n*=55) or a tricyclic antidepressant (TCA) (*n*=80) in utero at a mean age of 33 months. They were compared to a nonexposed control group (*n*=84), and no significant differences in cognitive, language, and behavioral development in the groups exposed versus nonexposed were found. Because of the lower incidence of side effects and the safety data available during pregnancy, the use of fluoxetine as a first choice is encouraging.

SSRIs and their metabolites are excreted at low levels in breast milk, with paroxetine having the lowest milk-to-plasma ratio (94). Limited data collected thus far show no adverse effects in nursed infants (94,95). Fluoxetine and its metabolite, norfluoxetine, with serum levels within therapeutic range, were detected in one infant whose mother was taking fluoxetine while breastfeeding (96). This infant experienced vomiting, excessive crying, watery stools, and decreased sleep. Symptoms resolved when the mother began bottle-feeding (96). Because of their potential to affect neurobehavioral development, the American Academy of Pediatrics regards the SSRIs to be of special concern when given to breastfeeding mothers over a long period (97). Mothers should be informed that the risk of neonatal toxicity and long-term neurobehavioral effects of SSRIs in the newborn infant remain unknown at this time.

Tricyclic Antidepressants

TCAs alter brain catecholamine activity and are used to treat clinical depression and pain syndromes such as migraine and peripheral neuropathy. Tricyclic antidepressants readily cross the placenta, and their safety during pregnancy has not been clearly established. None of the major epidemiologic surveys in the United States, Europe, or Australia found a significant increase in major congenital malformations in infants exposed to TCAs in utero (98–102). Animal studies on teratogenicity are inconclusive (103). Children born to mothers taking these drugs rarely show signs of anticholinergic effects (tachycardia, urinary retention), myoclonus, or withdrawal symptoms (104,105). Although apparently safe, tricyclic antidepressants should be used only when strongly indicated during pregnancy.

Use of TCAs by women who breastfeed is controversial. Because only a small percentage of the maternal serum concentrations is excreted in breast milk and levels of TCAs are usually low or undetectable in the blood of breastfed infants (106,107), TCA use by breastfeeding mothers appears relatively safe. However, because the effects of TCAs on the newborn and infant are unknown, avoidance of breastfeeding has been advocated (16).

Monoamine Oxidase Inhibitors

MAOIs interfere with metabolism of brain catecholamines and are potent drugs used to treat depression. The MAOIs pose greater risks to the pregnant woman and her child than TCAs. Therefore, use of MAOIs during pregnancy should be restricted only to women whose disorder absolutely requires their use. Tyleden (108) and Mortola (18) recommend discontinuing MAOIs in women who become pregnant. The risk of MAOI-induced hypertensive crisis may be especially dangerous to pregnant women because fluid and blood pressure homeostasis are altered during pregnancy. Dietary restrictions must be strictly enforced. The patient, obstetrician, and anesthesiologist must be informed about risks of opiates and general anesthetics during labor and delivery. Also, if a woman is taking an MAOI, beta-adrenergic agonists are contraindicated, thereby eliminating a treatment of choice for tocolysis if premature labor develops. MAOI use may pose cardiovascular problems for the fetus from placental hypoperfusion (20,109).

The teratogenic effects of MAOIs in humans are unknown. In rodents and dogs, high doses reduce the number of viable offspring and cause growth retardation (87). Safety of breastfeeding while taking a MAOI has not been established. Mortola (18) recommends that women should not breastfeed while taking MAOIs.

Atypical Antidepressants

The atypical antidepressants (e.g., bupropion, venlafaxine, nefazodone, and mirtazapine) have varying mechanisms of action and side-effect profiles. These agents provide options for patients who are unresponsive to, or intolerant to, the SSRIs. Bupropion is a norepinephrine and dopamine reuptake inhibitor with no effect on serotonin. It can increase the risk of seizures, especially at doses greater than 450 mg/day. Bupropion is less sedating and causes less sexual dysfunction than the TCAs and SSRIs (91). Altshuler and associates (63) report two cases involving in utero exposure to bupropion. One woman was taking both bupropion and lithium during pregnancy. Following delivery, the infant had coarse tremors and twitching activity that resolved after several hours. Both bupropion-exposed infants were physically normal with no follow-up information available (63).

Nefazodone inhibits presynaptic uptake of both serotonin and norepinephrine and is a potent $5HT_{2A}$ receptor blocker with no effect on dopamine. Adverse effects associated with nefazodone include somnolence, headache, dizziness, and dry mouth. Mirtazapine is a unique presynaptic alpha-2 adrenoreceptor blocker that increases central noradrenergic and serotonergic action. Common side effects include increased appetite, weight gain, and sedation, with minimal effects on sexual function. Mirtazapine may have a faster onset of antidepressant action than SSRIs (110). Venlafaxine potently inhibits serotonin and norepinephrine reuptake. Side effects are similar to those of SSRIs, and at doses higher than 300 mg/day it may elevate blood pressure (81).

Unfortunately, reproductive safety information is lacking for these agents. There are no published controlled clinical trials using these agents during pregnancy or lactation. The Food and Drug Administration has assigned bupropion in a class B risk category. Animal studies with bupropion show no evidence of impaired fertility or fetal harm, and the bupropion pregnancy registry does not show increased fetal anomalies (111). Nefazodone, venlafaxine, and mirtazapine are assigned class C risk category. Because the risk to humans is unknown during pregnancy, labor and delivery, and lactation, caution should be exercised when administering these drugs, and, if possible, they should be avoided until more complete data become available.

Lithium

Lithium carbonate effectively treats mania and stabilizes mood in bipolar disorder. This monovalent cation is distributed throughout the body with excretion similar to sodium.

Lithium use during pregnancy poses potential hazards to the mother and fetus. Lithium should not be used during the first trimester because of its teratogenic potential. Its use during the last two trimesters should be restricted to women who fail treatment with neuroleptics or carbamazepine.

Renal clearance of lithium increases approximately 70% during pregnancy, and dose adjustments may be needed to maintain therapeutic levels (0.7 to 1.2 mmol/L) (112). If diuretics are prescribed or sodium is restricted during pregnancy, lithium toxicity (>1.5 mmol/L) can occur. Lithium toxicity in the mother also can develop during labor and shortly after delivery as clearance returns to baseline. Typical features of toxicity include lethargy, psychomotor slowing, nausea, anorexia, tremor, chorea, and fasciculations.

Lithium effectively crosses the placenta and reaches similar concentrations in the fetal circulation (113). Birth defects, especially cardiac anomalies, are more common among infants whose mothers used lithium during pregnancy (114,115). Ebstein's anomaly of the tricuspid valve is the most common anomaly (115,116), occurring in approximately 3% of exposed babies, with total cardiac anomalies found in up to 8% of exposed infants (117). Shou (118) reported no long-term sequelae in 60 infants exposed to lithium in utero who had no congenital malformations at birth. Neonates exposed to lithium in utero during the last trimester can develop neurologic (impaired reflexes, decreased muscle tone, lethargy), cardiovascular (atrial flutter, tricuspid regurgitation, congestive heart failure, cyanosis), and thyroid (reversible goiter) disorders (119–121).

Lithium should be avoided during pregnancy, if possible. When used during the last two trimesters, we recommend the following (20):

1. Monitor lithium level every 1 to 2 weeks.
2. Obtain ultrasound prior to delivery to exclude fetal goiter.
3. Follow hydration status closely during labor.

4. Decrease lithium dose by 50% during the 2 weeks prior to expected due date.
5. If the mother enters premature labor and is on full-dose lithium, hold one or more doses and reduce subsequent doses pending serum levels and clinical status.
6. Consider early delivery if decreased lithium doses are associated with exacerbation of the psychiatric disorder.

Lithium is excreted in breast milk, with milk-to-serum ratios varying from 1:4 to 3:4 (122). Renal clearance of lithium by the neonate is less than that of adults. Breastfeeding infants have serum lithium levels between 10% to 50% of maternal levels (114–125). Infants breastfed by mothers taking lithium can develop neurologic (decreased tone) and cardiac (T-wave changes, cyanosis) disorders, especially when dehydrated (107,113,114). Therefore, breastfeeding is not recommended for women taking lithium (18,115,116).

Phenothiazines

Phenothiazines were once the most extensively used antipsychotic drugs. Chlorpromazine is one of the most commonly used aliphatic phenothiazines. Phenothiazines cross the placenta and are metabolized by both the fetal and neonatal liver. Use of phenothiazines in pregnancy exemplifies the principle of weighing risk versus benefit.

In women without psychiatric disorders, low doses of phenothiazines have been used during early pregnancy to ameliorate nausea and vomiting and during labor to complement analgesic therapy. Whereas low doses have not been documented to adversely affect the fetus, acute dystonic reactions can occur in the mother. Diphenhydramine (25 to 75 mg intramuscularly) and benztropine (1–2 mg intravenously) are usually effective in aborting this reaction, although diphenhydramine administration occasionally exacerbates dystonia.

Akathisia, parkinsonism, and tardive dyskinesia may first develop during pregnancy for women with longstanding psychiatric disorders taking moderate to high doses of phenothiazines, butyrophenones and other antipsychotic agents. Aliphatic phenothiazines such as chlorpromazine and thioridizine can cause hypotension, which can affect both maternal and fetal circulations. Rodent studies reveal that chlorpromazine exposure in utero can alter both cerebellar Purkinje cell and vascular development and cause behavioral problems (126–128).

In humans, most series and studies have not found increased frequencies of congenital malformations among infants exposed to phenothiazines in utero (129–135). However, several large studies have found a trend towards increased malformations among infants whose mothers received phenothiazines while pregnant (136,137). In one hospital, two babies with major congenital limb deformities were born to mothers treated with prochlorperazine for hyperemesis gravidarum (138).

Infants exposed to phenothiazines in utero may develop extrapyramidal side effects, including coarse tremor, increased tone, motor restlessness and hyperactivity, and impaired suck and other primitive reflexes. This can persist for months (139–144). Hepatic functions also can be altered, causing neonatal enzyme induction, jaundice, and hyperbilirubinemia (132,133).

Breast milk concentrations of chlorpromazine and perphenazine are 30% and 100% of plasma, respectively (122). No adverse effects have been documented in neonates and infants breastfed by mothers taking phenothiazines. These drugs do not represent an absolute contraindication to breastfeeding. Many physicians recommend that women taking these medications should not breastfeed because the safety remains unproven. However, when women breastfeed on these drugs, the infant should be monitored for behavioral or motor effects.

Haloperidol

Haloperidol is a widely used antipsychotic agent that also has been used to treat hyperemesis gravidarum. This high-potency antipsychotic drug has less sedative and hypotensive effects than the lower potency phenothiazines, but it is more likely to cause extrapyramidal side effects.

The frequency of congenital malformations is not increased among women with hyperemesis gravidarum receiving relatively low dosages of haloperidol during the first trimester (145). Although phocomelia developed in one infant of a woman taking haloperidol, ingestion was not during the first trimester (146). In a retrospective survey of infants with phocomelia, no haloperidol exposure in utero was reported (147).

Haloperidol is secreted in breast milk, but the percentage excreted was low in one study (148) and moderate in another (149). Behavioral toxicity has not been demonstrated in breastfed babies (148). The safety of haloperidol to the fetus and breastfed neonate has not been clearly established, although there is no convincing evidence that exposure at either of these stages is dangerous.

Newer (Atypical) Antipsychotics

The new generation of antipsychotic drugs (e.g., clozapine, olanzapine, quetiapine, risperidone, and ziprasidone) is used to treat schizophrenia, bipolar disorder, and other behavioral disorders. The atypical neuroleptics are less likely than traditional neuroleptics to cause extrapyramidal symptoms (EPS) or increases in serum prolactin levels (150). Adverse effects associated with the atypical neuroleptics include weight gain, new-onset diabetes, and hypertriglyceridemia (150–152). However, one small study (*n*=37) by Kingsbury and associates reports short-term use of ziprasidone to lower serum lipid levels (153). Dickson and Hogg (154) present one schizophrenic woman that developed gestational diabetes, possibly exacerbated by treatment with clozapine.

The safety of newer antipsychotics during pregnancy, labor and delivery, and lactation has not been studied extensively. Only case reports and initial pregnancy registries are available. Nagy and colleagues (155) report the birth of a healthy newborn to a young psychotic woman treated with olanzapine after the twenty-fifth week of pregnancy. The Lilly Safety Database, with both prospective and retrospective reports of olanzapine-exposed pregnancies (spontaneous abortion 13%, stillbirth 5%, major malformation 0%, and prematurity 5%), suggests no obvious added risks to the fetus or infant over normal control rates (156). These newer antipsychotic agents should only be used during pregnancy and lactation when the potential benefit justifies the potential risk to the fetus or infant.

Electroconvulsive Shock Therapy

ECT can be administered to pregnant women, but it is usually only considered when serious clinical depression persists despite psychotropic medication use or intolerable or dangerous side effects develop from medication use (157). Only experts should administer ECT during pregnancy.

The first reported use of ECT in pregnancy was in 1941 (140). Several larger series (129, 158) found an increased frequency of fetal death or other complications in ECT-treated subjects compared with control subjects. Among the 318 women treated by Impastato and colleagues (158), there was a 5% complication rate (six cases of developmental defects; three abortions; two cases of prematurity; one neonatal death; one stillbirth; one case of vaginal bleeding; and one term labor shortly after ECT). This complication rate was comparable to untreated pregnant patients with psychosis and the general population. In one severely depressed woman, each ECT was immediately followed by uterine contractions and active uterine bleeding, postulated as recurrent abruptio placentae resulting from maternal hypertension (180–190/90–100 mmHg) (159).

Nurnberg (157), based on a review of the literature (17,158,160,161), recommends the following guidelines for ECT in pregnancy:

1. Complete physical and pelvic examination should be performed.
2. High-risk pregnancies are relative contraindications for ECT. Special precautions are needed.

3. An obstetrician should be present during ECT to monitor fetal status before and after treatment.
4. Adequate muscle relaxation and oxygenation must be maintained throughout ECT.
5. External fetal monitoring for fetal distress must be maintained.
6. Glycopyrrolate is the anticholinergic drug of choice with anesthesia.
7. ECT should be administered in a setting where a premature delivery can be managed safely.

PERIPARTUM PSYCHIATRIC DISORDERS

Although psychiatric disorders do not occur more commonly during pregnancy, the first 2 to 6 postpartum weeks are associated with a marked increase in major psychiatric illness, including depression and psychosis.

Postpartum Depression

Depression is prevalent during the postpartum period. Mild dysphoria during the first 10 days after delivery, referred to as "baby blues," occurs in 50% to 87% of women (162–164). Short and self-limited episodes of sadness, crying, irritability, anxiety, headache, or sleep disorders typically occur 2 to 4 days after delivery (165,166).

Depression occurs in approximately 10% to 15% of new mothers, with usual onset between 2 to 4 months after delivery (166–171). Of these women, approximately one-third manifest depressive symptoms 1 year later, and 30% to 75% are at risk for recurrent postpartum depression (166–172). Eighty-six of 71,378 (0% to 12%) pregnant women in Denmark developed postpartum depression requiring hospitalization (173).

Postpartum depression does not differ clinically from depression in other settings. Feelings of sadness and helplessness, tearfulness, fatigue, poor concentration, and impaired concentration are commonly reported. Vegetative signs such as loss of appetite and insomnia (early morning awakening is common) are often present. Some patients are unaware of "depression" and only report fatigue, anhedonia, and disinterest in the child and other aspects of life. In more severe cases, psychomotor retardation, agitation, confusion, delusions, and auditory (often deprecating) and visual hallucinations occur. If neurobehavioral features such as disorientation, cognitive impairment, hallucinations, or language disorder are present, a systemic or neurologic disorder must be considered, and a careful drug history should be performed.

Pathogenesis

The cause of postpartum depression is multifactorial. Psychosocial factors such as marital conflicts, lack of a close relationship with a significant other, and financial, housing, and other socioeconomic problems may predispose to postpartum depression (168,171). Personal or family history of depression, first pregnancy, cesarean section, and history of premenstrual syndrome are other reported risk factors (16,162,174). Hormonal factors, especially sudden declines in serum estrogen and progesterone levels, may be pathogenetic (174–176) . Several studies implicate autoimmune thyroid disorders (177–179). Harris and colleagues (178) found markedly elevated postpartum depression ratings in women with elevated postpartum thyroid autoantibodies, regardless of thyroid dysfunction. Other potential pathogenetic factors include withdrawal of endogenous opiates (180,181) and altered alpha-2 adrenoreceptor binding (182).

Suicide and Pregnancy

In contrast to epidemiologic studies from the early 20th century (183), the suicide rate of pregnant and postpartum women is not elevated compared to age-matched women in the general population (184). Kleiner and Greston (183) compared 13 studies between 1900 and 1947 and 15 studies between 1943 and 1980. Among completed suicides in women, the percentage of pregnant women declined from 12.8% to 1.8% between these periods. Social changes, including legal abortion, acceptability of single parenthood, marriage during and after pregnancy, as well as social support programs such as Medicaid may have contributed to the dramatic decline in suicides during pregnancy and the puerperium. Although there is a peak in suicides during the first month after delivery, the rate is lower than in control women (184,185). Recent stillbirth and teenage pregnancy remain risk factors for suicide (184).

Therapy

Patients with notable anxiety or depressive symptoms during pregnancy should be observed closely for postpartum depression (186). Early recognition permits prompt intervention. Minor, transient postpartum dysphoria requires support from the family and obstetrician, and, in selected cases counseling or therapy is helpful. Pharmacotherapy is not indicated for such cases. In contrast, major postpartum depression should be treated with psychotherapy as well as psychotropic medications (e.g., tricyclics, MAOIs, SSRIs, or lithium) when indicated. SSRIs often are preferred because they are less likely to cause weight gain and constipation, which are especially troublesome postpartum side effects. However, agitation and insomnia are common in postpartum depressed patients and these serotonergic drugs can exacerbate these symptoms. Therefore, some doctors avoid SSRIs in postpartum depression with agitation or insomnia, especially as the initial treatment. In this setting, sedating tricyclics such as amitriptyline may be helpful. Estrogen replacement shortly after delivery may reduce the rate of recurrent postpartum depression (166). The importance of therapy is highlighted by the observation that postpartum depression can impair interactions between mother and child and is associated with subsequent child behavior problems (187,188).

Postpartum Psychosis

In 1858 Louis Marce (189) reported 44 women with postpartum psychiatric disorders and identified psychosis as a distinct organic entity. Psychosis complicates one to two per 1,000 pregnancies (190–192). During the first postpartum month, women are 22 times more likely to be hospitalized with psychosis than age- and sex-matched controls (193). The vast majority of postpartum psychoses occur within 6 weeks parturition (191)—half within 2 weeks and two-thirds within a month. The recurrence rate of postpartum psychosis is approximately 15% (193).

Postpartum psychosis must be distinguished from psychotic disorders unrelated to pregnancy. Onset of schizophrenia during pregnancy or the postpartum period is rare. Although functional psychoses such as schizophrenia and affective psychosis are uncommon in childbearing women (<2% between ages 18 and 45 years), such psychotic disorders more often worsen than improve during pregnancy (2,194).

Clinical Features

Most postpartum psychoses are affective with manic or depressive features predominating (193,195). Postpartum schizophreniform psychoses are uncommon. Patients who develop postpartum psychosis initially may be euphoric, normal, or emotionally removed during the first days or weeks after delivery. The onset is often abrupt but may be gradual, with psychotic symptoms emerging between 2 and 14 days after delivery. The symptom complex includes delirium with prominent confusion and attention deficit; psychosis; delusions; auditory, visual, and other hallucinations; sleep disorders; and agitation. Delirium often resolves most rapidly after therapy, with affective and psychotic symptoms remaining for variable periods.

Injury to the neonate is a serious concern in postpartum psychosis. Although directed aggression toward the baby is rare (196), accidental injury as a result of neglect, confusion, or delusional acts occurs more often. The mother's delusions often incorporate the baby and vary dramatically in content. For these reasons, psychotic mothers should be supervised carefully.

Pathogenesis

The cause of postpartum psychosis is unknown and probably includes both psychosocial and biologic factors. Risk factors for postpartum psychosis include age, cesarean delivery, fewer children and longer intervals between pregnancies, and family or personal history of psychosis or other psychiatric disorders (191,193). History of bipolar disorder may be the most significant risk factor, with approximately 25% of these women developing postpartum psychosis (193,197).

Tetlow (198) found that psychosocial issues are important. There were significantly ($p<.01$) more women who were single or had pregnancy resulting from extramarital relations with postpartum psychosis than controls. Kendell and colleagues (193) found that lack of a husband at time of the birth and perinatal death are risk factors for postpartum psychosis.

There is little evidence to support hormonal changes in the pathogenesis of postpartum psychosis (88,199). Lindstrom and colleagues (200) found increased cerebrospinal levels of opioid receptor active components in women with postpartum psychosis when compared to healthy lactating women, but the significance of this finding is unclear.

Treatment

Women with postpartum psychosis should be treated with an antipsychotic drug such as a phenothiazine, with butyrophenone, or with one of the newer agents (e.g., risperidone, olanzapine, or quetiapine) with a dose sufficient to reduce acute psychosis and agitation (88). Excessive doses, which impair hydration or nutritional status, should be avoided unless absolutely necessary. Chlorpromazine or thioridizine often were used initially, and the less-sedating haloperidol later was substituted if there has been a good initial response. Currently, newer antipsychotic drugs are used because of the lower risk of extrapyramidal side effects. For patients who do not respond to antipsychotic drugs within 1 week, lithium or ECT should be considered (16,201).

Duration of therapy must be individualized, although most patients should be treated for at least 2 to 3 months with an antipsychotic drug. Unfortunately, many women with postpartum psychosis have disturbed mother–child relationships for more than 4 years after the psychotic episode (202). Therefore, these women and their children may require ongoing follow-up.

REFERENCES

1. Bibring G, Valenstein A: Psychological aspects of pregnancy. *Clin Obstet Gynecol* 1976;19:357–371.
2. McNeil TF, Kaij L, Malmquist-Larsson A. Women with nonorganic psychosis: mental disturbance during pregnancy. *Acta Psychiatr Scand* 1984;70:127–139.
3. McCullough LB. Ethically justified guidelines for family planning interventions to prevent pregnancy in female patients with chronic mental illness. *Am J Obstet Gynecol* 1992;167:19–25.
4. Carmen E, Brady SM. AIDS risk and prevention for the chronic mentally ill. *Hosp Community Psychiatry* 1990;41;652–657.
5. Abernethy V. Sexual knowledge, attitudes, and practices of young female psychiatric patients. *Arch Gen Psychiatry* 1974;30:180–182.
6. Coverdale JH, Aruffo J. Family planning needs of female chronic psychiatric outpatients. *Am J Psychiatry* 1989;146:1489–1491.
7. Wrede G, Mednick SA, Huttunen MO, et al. Pregnancy and delivery complications in the births of an unselected series of Finnish children with schizophrenic mothers. *Acta Psychiatr Scand* 1980;62:369–381.
8. Cohen LS. Psychotropic drug use in pregnancy. *Hosp Community Psychiatry* 1989;40:566–567.
9. Cohen LS, Heller VL, Rosenbaum JF. Treatment guidelines for psychotropic drug use in pregnancy. *Psychosomatics* 1989;30:25–32.
10. McCance-Katz EF. The consequences of maternal substance abuse for the child exposed in utero. *Psychosomatics* 1991;32:268–274.
11. Zax M, Sameroff AH, Babigian HM. Birth outcomes in the offspring of mentally disordered women. *Am J Orthopsychiatry* 1977;47:218–229.
12. Kinney DK. Schizophrenia and major mood disorders (manic-depressive illness). In: Emery AE, Rimoin DL, eds. *Principles and practice of medical genetics.* Edinburgh: Churchill Livingstone, 1990:457–472.

13. Reiss D, Plomin R, Hetherington EM. Genetics and psychiatry: an unheralded window on the environment. *Am J Psychiatry* 1991;148:283–291.

14. American College of Obstetricians and Gynecologists. *Sterilization of women who are mentally handicapped.* ACOG Committee Opinion 63. Washington, DC: ACOG, 1988.

15. Nadelson CC: "Normal" and "special" aspects of pregnancy: a psychological approach. In Nadelson CC, Notman MT, eds. *The woman patient. Medical and psychological interfaces: Vol. 1 Sexual and reproductive aspects of women's health care.* New York: Plenum Publishing, 1978.

16. Downey JI, Whitaker AH. Important psychiatric problems during pregnancy and the postpartum period. In: Reece EA, Hobbins JC, Mahoney MJ, et al, eds. *Medicine of the mother and fetus.* Philadelphia: Lippincott, 1992:1293–1307.

17. Nurnberg HG, Prudic J. Guidelines for treatment of psychosis during pregnancy. *Hosp Community Psychiatry* 1984;35:67–71.

18. Mortola JF. The use of psychotropic agents in pregnancy and lactation. *Psychiatric Clinics North Am* 1989;12:69–87.

19. Gise, LH. Psychiatric implications of pregnancy. In: Cherry SH, Berkowitz RL, Kase NG, et al, eds. *Medical, surgical, and gynecologic complications of pregnancy,* 3rd ed. Baltimore: Williams & Wilkins, 1991: 614–654.

20. O'Grady JP. *Obstetrics: psychological and psychiatric syndromes.* New York, Elsevier Science, 1992.

21. Uvnas-Moberg K. The gastrointestinal tract in growth and reproduction. *Sci Am* 1989;261:78.

22. Fairweather DV. Nausea and vomiting during pregnancy. *Am J Obstet Gynecol* 1968;102:135–175.

23. Robertson GG. Nausea and vomiting during pregnancy. *Lancet* 1946;2:336.

24. Kallen B. Hyperemesis during pregnancy and delivery outcome: A registry study. *Eur J Obstet Gynecol Reprod Biol* 1987;26:291–302.

25. FitzGerald CM: Nausea and vomiting in pregnancy. *Br J Med Psychol* 1984;57:159–165.

26. Fairweather DV. Nausea and vomiting during pregnancy. *Obstet Gynecol Annu* 1978;7:91–105.

27. Harvey WA, Shertey MJ. Vomiting in pregnancy. *Psychosom Med* 1954;16:1.

28. Franko DL, Spurrell EB. Detection and management of eating disorders during pregnancy. *Obstet Gynecol* 2000;95:942–946.

29. Ditto A, Morgante G, la Marca A, et al. Evaluation of treatment of hyperemesis gravidarum using parental fluid with or without diazepam. A randomized study. *Gynecol Obstet Invest* 1999;48:22–236.

30. Weiss E. English OS. *Psychosomatic medicine,* 3rd ed. Philadelphia, WB Saunders, 1957.

31. Freud S. Breuer J: Studies on hysteria. In Freud S, ed. *Complete psychological works, standard edition 2.* London: Hogarth Press, 1955.

32. Katon WJ, Ries RK, Bokan JA, et al. Hyperemesis gravidarum: a biopsychosocial perspective. *Int J Psychiatry Med* 1980–1981;10:151–162.

33. Wolkind S, Zajicek E: Psychosocial correlates of nausea and vomiting in pregnancy. *J Psychosom Res* 1978; 22:1–5.

34. Mednick BR: *Consequences of family structure and maternal state for child and mother's development.* Washington, DC: National Institute for Child Health and Development, 1979.

35. Henker FO: Psychotherapy as an adjunct in treatment of vomiting during pregnancy. *South Med J* 1976;69; 1585–1587.

36. Callahan EJ, Disiderato I. Disorders in pregnancy. In: Blechman EA, Brownell KD, eds. *Handbook of behavioral medicine for women.* New York: Pergamon Press, 1984.

37. Apfel RJ, Kelley SF, Frankel FH. The role of hypnotizability in the pathogenesis and treatment of nausea and vomiting of pregnancy. *J Psychosom Obstet Gynaecol* 1986;5:179–186.

38. Simon EP, Schwartz J. Medical hypnosis for hyperemesis gravidarum. *Birth* 1999;26:248–254.

39. National Research Council Committee on Nutrition of the Mother and Preschool Child. *Alternative dietary practices and nutritional abuses in pregnancy.* Washington, DC: National Academy Press, 1982.

40. Garfinkel PE, Garner DM. *Anorexia nervosa: a multidimensional perspective.* New York: Brunner/Mazel, 1982.

41. Herzog DB, Copeland PM. Eating disorders. *N Engl J Med* 1985;313:295–303.

42. Brinch M, Isager T, Tolstrup K. Anorexia nervosa and motherhood: reproductional pattern and mothering behavior of 50 women. *Acta Psychiatr Scand* 1988; 77:98.

43. Treasure JL, Russell GF. Intrauterine growth and neonatal weight gain of women with anorexia nervosa. *BMJ (Clin Res Ed)* 1988;296:1038.

44. Hediger ML, Scholl TO, Belsky DH, et al. Patterns of weight gain in adolescent pregnancy: effects on birth weight and preterm delivery. *Obset Gynecol* 1989;74: 6–12.

45. Stewart DE Rasking J, Garfinkel PE, et al. Anorexia nervosa, bulimia, and pregnancy. *Am J Obstet Gynecol* 1987;157:1194–1198.

46. Speroff L. Anorexia and bulimia. In O'Grady JP, Rosenthal M, eds. *Psychological and psychiatric syndromes.* New York: Elsevier, 1992.

47. Sichel DA, Cohen LS, Dimmock JA, et al. Postpartum obsessive compulsive disorder: a case series. *J Clin Psychiatry* 1993;54:156–159.

48. Altshuler LL, Hendrick V, Cohen LS. Course of mood and anxiety disorders during pregnancy and the postpartum period. *J Clin Psychiatry* 1998;59:29–33.

49. Maina G, Albert U, Bogetto F, et al. Recent life events and obsessive-compulsive disorder (OCD): the role of pregnancy/delivery. *Psychiatry Res* 1999;13:49–58.

50. Ingram IM. Obsessional illness in mental hospital patients. *J Ment Sci* 1961;107:382–402.

51. Buttolph ML, Holland DA. Obsessive-compulsive disorders in pregnancy and childbirth. In: Jenike MA, Baier L, Minichiello WE, eds. *Obsessive compulsive disorders: theory and management.* Chicago: Year Book Medical Publishers, 1990.

52. Neziroglu F, Anemone R, Yaryura-Tobias JA. Onset of obsessive compulsive disorder in pregnancy. *Am J Psychiatry* 1992;149:947–950.

53. Lo WH. A follow-up study of obsessional neurotics in Hong Kong Chinese. *Br J Psychiatry* 1967;113: 823–832.

54. Davidoff R, O'Grady JP. Disorders of mother-infant

attachment. In: O'Grady JP, Rosenthal M, eds. *Obstetrics: psychological and psychiatric syndromes.* New York: Elsevier Science, 1992.

55. Kumar R, Robson K. A prospective study of emotional disorders in childbearing women. *Br J Psychiatry* 1984;144:35–47.

56. Brockington IF, Winokur G, Dean C. Puerperal psychosis. In: Brockington IF, Kumar R, eds. *Motherhood and mental illness.* London: Academic Press, 1982.

57. Brozovsky M, Falit H: Neonatacide. Clinical and psychodynamic considerations. *J Am Acad Child Psychiatry* 1971;10:673–683.

58. Resnick PJ. Murder of the newborn: a psychiatric review of neonaticide. *Am J Psychiatry* 1970;126:1414–1420.

59. Finnegan P, McKinstry E, Robinson GE. Denial of pregnancy and childbirth. *Can J Psychiatry* 1982;27:672–674.

60. Green CM, Manohar SV. Neonaticide and hysterical denial of pregnancy. *Br J Psychiatry* 1990;156:121–123.

61. Cohen LS, Rosenbaum JF. Psychotropic drug use during pregnancy: weighing the risks. *J Clin Psychiatry* 1998;59:18–28.

62. Wisner KL, Gelenberg AJ, Leonard H, et al. Pharmacologic treatment of depression during pregnancy. *JAMA* 1999;282:1264–1269.

63. Altshuler LL, Cohen L, Szuba MP, et al. Pharmacologic management of psychiatric illness during pregnancy: dilemmas and guidelines. *Am J Psychiatry* 1996;153:592–606.

64. Boobis AR, Lewis FJ. Pharmacokinetics in pregnancy. In: Lewis P, ed. *Clinical pharmacology in obstetrics.* Boston: Wright-PSG, 1983.

65. Davison JM, Hytten FE. Glomerular filtration during and after pregnancy. *J Obstet Gynaecol Br Commonw* 1974;81:558.

66. Maternal adaptations to pregnancy. In: Cunningham FG, Gant NF, Leveno KJ, et al., eds. Williams Obstetrics, 21st ed. New York: McGraw-Hill, 2001:167–200.

67. Gardner DK, Rayburn WF. Drugs in breast milk. In: Rayburn WF, Zuspan FP, eds. *Drug therapy in obstetrics and gynecology.* Norwalk, CT: Appleton-Century-Crofts, 1980:175–196.

68. Giacoia GP, Catz CS. Drugs and pollutants in breast milk. *Clin Perinatol* 1979;6:181–196.

69. Saxen I, Saxen L. Letter. Association between maternal intake of diazepam and oral clefts. *Lancet* 1975;2:496.

70. Aarskog D. Association between maternal intake of diazepam and oral clefts [Letter]. *Lancet* 1975;2:921.

71. Rosenberg L, Mitchell AA, Parsells JL, et al. Lack of relation of oral clefts to diazepam use during pregnancy. *N Engl J Med* 1983;309:1282–1285.

72. Shiono PH, Mills JL. Oral clefts and diazepam use during pregnancy. *N Engl J Med* 1984;311:919–920.

73. Crombie DL, Pinsent RJ, Fleming DM, et al. Fetal effects of tranquilizers in pregnancy. *N Engl J Med* 1975;293:198–199.

74. Hartz SC, Heinonen OP, Shapiro S, et al. Antenatal exposure to meprobamate and chlordiazepoxide in relation to malformations, mental development, and mortality. *N Engl J Med* 1975;292:726–728.

75. Milkovich L, Van den Berg BJ. Effects of the teratogenicity of certain antinauseant drugs. *Am J Obstet Gynecol* 1970;125:244–248.

76. Laegreid L, Olegard R, Wahlstrom J, et al. Abnormalities in children exposed to benzodiazepines in utero. *Lancet* 1987;1:108–109.

77. Barry WS, St Clair SM. Exposure to benzodiazepines in utero. *Lancet* 1987;1:1436–1437.

78. Calabrese JR, Gulledge AD. Carbamazepine, clonazepam use during pregnancy. *Psychosomatics* 1986;27:464.

79. Scher J, Hailey DM, Beard RW. The effects of diazepam on the fetus. *J Obstet Gynaecol Br Commonw* 1972;79:635–638.

80. Shannon RW, Fraser GP, Aitken RG. Diazepam in preeclamptic toxemia with special reference to its effects on the newborn infant. *Br J Clin Pract* 1972;26:271–275.

81. Rowlatt RJ. Effect of maternal diazepam on the newborn. *Br J Anaesthesiol* 1976;1:985.

82. Speight AN. Floppy-infant syndrome and maternal diazepam and/or nitrazepam. *Lancet* 1977;2:878.

83. Rementeria JL, Bhatt K. Withdrawal symptoms in neonates from intrauterine exposure to diazepam. *J Pediatr* 1977;90:123–126.

84. Mazzi E. Possible neonatal diazepam withdrawal: A case report. *Am J Obstet Gynecol* 1977;129:586–587.

85. Athinarayanan P, Pierog SH, Nigam SK, et al. Chlordiazepoxide withdrawal in the neonate. *Am J Obstet Gynecol* 1976;124:212–213.

86. Bitnum S. Possible effects of chlordiazepoxide on the fetus. *Can Med Assoc J* 1969;100:351.

87. Hauser LA. Pregnancy and psychiatric drugs. *Hosp Community Psychiatry* 1985;36:817–818.

88. Robinson GR, Stewart DE. Postpartum psychiatric disorder. *Can Med Assoc J* 1986;134:31–35.

89. Patrick MJ, Tilstone WJ, Reavey P. Diazepam and breast-feeding. *Lancet* 1972;1:542–543.

90. Schiff D, Chan G, Stern L. Fixed drug combinations and the displacement of bilirubin from albumin. *Pediatrics* 1971;8:139–141.

91. Fankhauser MP. Psychiatric disorders in women: psychopharmacologic treatments. *J Am Pharm Assoc (Wash)* 1997;NS37:667–678.

92. Emslie G, Judge R. Tricyclic antidepressants and selective serotonin reuptake inhibitors: use during pregnancy, in children/adolescents and in the elderly. *Acta Psychiatr Scand Suppl* 2000;403:26–34.

93. Nulman I, Rovet J, Stewart DE, et al. Neurodevelopment of children exposed in utero to antidepressant drugs. *N Engl J Med* 1997;336:258–262.

94. Pigott TA. Gender differences in the epidemiology and treatment of anxiety disorders. *J Clin Psychiatry* 1990;60:4–15.

95. Friedman JM, Polifka JE. *The effects of neurologic and psychiatric drugs on the fetus and nursing infant.* Baltimore: The John Hopkins University Press, 1998.

96. Lester BM, Cucca J, Andreozzi L, et al. Possible association between fluoxetine hydrochloride and colic in an infant. *J Am Acad Child Adolesc Psychiatry* 1993;32:1253–1255.

97. American Academy of Pediatrics Committee on Drugs: The transfer of drugs and other chemicals into human milk. *Pediatrics* 1994;93:137–150.

98. Scanlon FJ. Use of antidepressant drugs during the first trimester. *Med J Aust* 1969;2:1077.

99. Crombie DL, Pinsent RJ, Fleming D. Imipramine in pregnancy. *BMJ* 1972;1:745.

100. McBride WG. The teratogenic effects of imipramine. *Teratology* 1972;5:262A.

101. Barson AJ. Malformed infant. *BMJ* 1972;2:45.

102. Idanpaan-Heikkula J, Saxen L. Possible teratogenicity of imipramine-chloropyramine. *Lancet* 1973;2: 282–284.

103. Robson JM, Sullivan FM. The production of foetal abnormalities in rabbits by imipramine. *Lancet* 1963;i: 638–639.

104. Shearer WT, Schreiner RL, Marshall RE. Urinary retention in a neonate secondary to maternal ingestion of nortriptyline. *J Pediatr* 1972;81:570–571.

105. Webster PA. Withdrawal symptoms in neonates associated with maternal antidepressant therapy. *Lancet* 1973;2:318–319.

106. Erickson SH, Smith GH, Heidrich F. Tricyclics and breast feeding. *Am J Psychiatry* 1979;136:1483.

107. Bader TF, Newman K. Amitriptyline in human breast milk and nursing infants' serum. *Am J Psychiat* 1980; 137:855–856.

108. Tyleden E. Pregnancy and monoamine oxidase inhibitors. *BMJ* 1968;2:698.

109. Berkowitz RL, Coustan D, Mochizuki T. *Handbook for prescribing medications during pregnancy*. Boston: Little, Brown and Company, 1981.

110. Quitkin FM, Taylor BP, Kremer C. Does mirtazapine have a more rapid onset than SSRIs? *J Clin Psychiatry* 2001;62:358–361.

111. Marcus SM, Barry KL, Flynn HA, et al. Treatment guidelines for depression in pregnancy. *Int J Gynaecol Obstet* 2001;72:61–70.

112. Schou M, Amdisen A, Steenstrup OR. Lithium and pregnancy. II. Hazards to women given lithium during pregnancy and delivery. *BMJ* 1973;2:137–138.

113. MacKay AV, Loose R, Glen A. Labor on lithium. *BMJ* 1976;1:878.

114. Shou M, Amdisen A. Lithium and pregnancy. III. Lithium ingestion by children breast-fed by women on lithium treatment. *BMJ* 1973;2:138–142.

115. Weinstein MR, Goldfield MD. Cardiovascular malformations with lithium use during pregnancy. *Am J Psychiatry* 1975;132:529–531.

116. Linden S, Rich CL. The use of lithium during pregnancy and lactation. *J Clin Psychiatry* 1983;44: 358–361.

117. Kallen B, Tandberg A. Lithium and pregnancy. A cohort study on manic-depressive women. *Acta Psychiatr Scand* 1983;68:134–139.

118. Shou M. What happened to the lithium babies? *Acta Psychiatr Scan* 1976;54:193–197.

119. Wilbanks GD, Bressler B, Peete HC, et al. Toxic effects of lithium carbonate in a mother and newborn infant. *JAMA* 1970;213:865–867.

120. Woody JN, London WL, Wilbanks GD. Lithium toxicity in a newborn. *Pediatrics* 1971;47:94–96.

121. Strothers JK, Wilson DW, Hoyston N. Lithium toxicity in a newborn. *BMJ* 1973;3:233–234.

122. Wilson JT, Brown RD, Cherek DR, et al. Drug excretion in human breast milk, principles, pharmacokinetics and projected consequences. *Clin Pharmacokinet* 1980;5:1.

123. Kerns LL. Treatment of mental disorders in pregnancy. A review of psychotropic drug risks and benefits. *J Nerv Ment Dis* 1986;174:652–659.

124. Karlsson K, Lindstedt G, Lundberg PA, et al. Transpla-

125. Sykes PA, Quarrie V, Alexander FW. Lithium carbonate and breast-feeding. *BMJ* 1976;2:1299.

126. Hoffeld DR, McNew J, Webster RL. Effect of tranquilizing drugs during pregnancy on activity of offspring. *Nature* 1968;218:357–358.

127. Hannah RS, Roth SH, Spira W. The effects of chlorpromazine and phenobarbital on cerebellar Purkinje cells. *Teratology* 1982;26:21–25.

128. Hannah RS, Roth SH, Spira AW. The effects of chlorpromazine and phenobarbital on vasculogenesis in the cerebellar cortex. *Acta Neuropathol (Berl)* 1982;57: 306–308.

129. Sobel DE. Fetal damage due to ECT, insulin coma, chlorpromazine or reserpine. *Arch Gen Pscyhiatry* 1960;2:606–611.

130. Kris EB, Carmichael DM. Chlorpromazine maintenance therapy during pregnancy and confinement. *Psychiatric Quarterly* 1957;31:690–695.

131. Rawlings WJ, Ferguson R, Maddison TG. Phenmetrazine and trifluoperazine. *Med J Aust* 1963;1:370.

132. Moriarty AJ, Nance NR. Trifluoperazine and pregnancy. *Can Med Assoc J* 1963;88:375–376.

133. Catz CS, Yaffee SJ. *Environmental factors: Pharmacology. I: Prevention of embryonic, fetal and perinatal disease*. Chap. 6. Washington, DC: U.S. Government Printing Office, 1971.

134. Sloane D, Siskind V, Heinonen OP, et al. Antenatal exposure to the phenothiazines in relation to congenital malformation, perinatal mortality rate, birth rate, birth weight, and intelligence quotient score. *Am J Obstet Gynecol* 1977;128:486–488.

135. Milkovich L, van den Berg BJ. Effects of prenatal meprobamate and chlordiazepoxide hydrochloride on human embryonic and fetal development. *N Engl J Med* 1974;291:1266–1271.

136. Rumeau-Rouquette C, Goujard J, Huel G. Possible teratogenic effects of phenothiazines in human beings. *Teratology* 1977;15:57–64.

137. Edlund MJ, Craig TJ. Antipsychotic drug use and birth defects: an epidemiologic reassessment. *Compr Psychiatry* 1984;25:32–37.

138. Rafla N. Limb deformities associated with prochlorperazine. *Am J Obstet Gynecol* 1987;156:1557.

139. Desmond MM, Rudolph AJ, Hill RM, et al. Behavior alterations in infants born to mothers on psychotropic medication during pregnancy. In: Farrel G, ed. *Congenital mental retardation*. Austin: University of Texas Press, 1967.

140. Falterman LG, Richardson DJ. Small left colon syndrome associated with maternal ingestion of psychotropic drugs. *J Pediatr* 1980;97:300–310.

141. Levy W, Wisniewski K. Chlorpromazine causing extrapyramidal dysfunction. *N Y State J Med* 1974;74: 684–685.

142. Hill RM, Desmond MM, Kay JL. Extrapyramidal dysfunction in an infant of a schizophrenic mother. *J Pediatr* 1966;69:589.

143. O'Connor M, Johnson GM, Jamis DI. Intrauterine effects of phenothiazines. *Med J Aust* 1981;1:416.

144. Tammer A, McKay R, Arias D, et al. Phenothiazine induced extrapyramidal dysfunction in the neonate. *J Pediatr* 1969;75:479.

145. Van Waes A, Van de Velde EJ. Safety evaluation of

haloperidol in the treatment of hyperemesis gravidarum. *J Clin Pharmacol* 1969;9:224–227.

146. McCullar FW, Heggeness L. Limb malformations following maternal use of haloperidol. *JAMA* 1975; 231:62–64.

147. Hanson JW, Oakley GP. Haloperidol and limb deformity. *JAMA* 1975;231:26.

148. Stewart RB, Karas B, Springer PK. Haloperidol excretion in breast milk. *Am J Psychiatry* 1980;137: 849–850.

149. Whalley L. Blain PG, Prime JK. Haloperidol secreted in breast milk. *BMJ* 1981;282:1746.

150. Goldstein JM. The new generation of antipsychotic drugs: how atypical are they? *Int J Neuropsychopharmacol* 2000;3:339–349.

151. McIntyre RS, McCann SM, Kennedy SH. Antipsychotic metabolic effects: weight gain, diabetes mellitus, and lipid abnormalities. *Can J Psychiatry* 2001; 46:273–281.

152. Meyer JM. Novel antipsychotics and severe hyperlipidemia. *J Clin Psychopharmacol* 2001;21:369–374.

153. Kingsbury SJ, Fayek M, Trufasiu D, et al. The apparent effects of ziprasidone on plasma lipids and glucose. *J Clin Psychiatry* 2001;62:347–349.

154. Dickson RA, Hogg L. Pregnancy of a patient treated with clozapine. *Psychiatr Serv* 1998;49:1081–1083.

155. Nagy A, Tenyi T, Lenard K, et al. [Olanzapine and pregnancy.] *Orv Hetil* 2001;142:137–138.

156. Goldstein DJ, Corbin LA, Fung MC. Olanzapine-exposed pregnancies and lactation: early experience. *J Clin Psychopharmacol* 2000;20:399–403.

157. Nurnberg HG. An overview of somatic treatment of psychosis during pregnancy and postpartum. *Gen Hosp Psychiatry* 1989;11:328–338.

158. Impastato DJ, Gabriel AR, Lardara HH. Electric and insulin shock therapy during pregnancy. *Dis Nerv Syst* 1964;25:542–546.

159. Sherer DM, D'Amico ML, Warshal DP, et al. Recurrent mild abruptio placentae occurring immediately after repeated electroconvulsive therapy in pregnancy. *Am J Obstet Gynecol* 1991;165:652–653.

160. Resnick RA, Maurice WL. ECT in pregnancy. *Am J Psychiatry* 1978;135:761–762.

161. Fink M. Convulsive therapy today. *Psychiatry Lett* 1986;4:7–12.

162. Yalom ID, Lunde DT, Rudolf H, et al. "Postpartum blues" syndrome. *Arch Gen Psychiatry* 1968;18:16–27.

163. Pitt B. Maternity blues. *Br J Psychiatry* 1973;122: 541–545.

164. Brandon S. Depression after childbirth. *BMJ* 1982; 284:613–614.

165. Maloney JC. Postpartum depression or third-day depression following childbirth. *New Orleans Child and Parent Digest* 1952;6:20–32.

166. Ziporyn T. Postpartum depression: True blue? *Harvard Health Lett* 1992;17:1–3.

167. Braverman J, Roux JF. Screening for the patient at risk for postpartum depression. *Obstet Gynecol* 1978;52: 731–736.

168. Paykel ES, Emms EM, Fletcher J, et al. Life events and social support in puerperal depression. *Br J Psychiatry* 1980;136:339–346.

169. Cox JL, Connor Y, Kendell RE. Prospective study of the psychiatric disorders of childbirth. *Br J Psychiatry* 1982;140:111–117.

170. Kumar R, Robson KM. A prospective study of emotional disorders in childbearing women. *Br J Psychiatry* 1984;144:35–47.

171. Watson JP, Elliott SA, Rugg AJ, et al. Psychiatric disorder in pregnancy and the first postnatal year. *Br J Psychiatry* 1984;144:453–462.

172. Garvey MJ, Tuason VB, Lumry AE, et al. Occurrence of depression in the postpartum state. *J Affect Disord* 1983;5:97–101.

173. David HP, Rasmussen NK, Holst E. Postpartum and postabolition psychotic reactions. *Fam Plann Perspect* 1981;13:88–92.

174. Nott PM, Frankin M, Armitage C, et al. Hormonal changes and mood in the puerperium. *Br J Psychiatry* 1967;128:379–383.

175. Tulchinsky D, Ryan KJ. *Maternal-fetal endocrinology.* Philadelphia: WB Saunders Co, 1980:144–166.

176. Brockington IF, Kumar R, eds. *Motherhood and mental illness.* London: Academic Press, 1982:1–65.

177. Hayslip CC, Fein HG, O'Donnell VM, et al. The value of serum antimicrosomal antibody testing in screening for symptomatic post-partum thyroid dysfunction. *Am J Obstet Gynecol* 1988;159:203–209.

178. Harris B, Othman S, Davies JA, et al. Association between postpartum thyroid dysfunction and thyroid antibodies and depression. *BMJ* 1992;305:152–156.

179. Harris B, Fung H, Johns S, et al. Transient post-partum thyroid dysfunction and postnatal depression. *J Affect Disord* 1989;17:243–249.

180. Newnham JP, Tomlin S, Ratter SJ, et al. Endogenous opioid peptides in pregnancy. *Br J Obstet Gynaecol* 1983;90:535–538.

181. Newnham JP, Dennett PH, Ferron SA, et al. A study of the relationship between circulating beta-endorphin-like immunoreactivity and post partum "blues." *Clin Endocrinol* 1984;20:169–177.

182. Metz A, Stump K, Cowen PJ, et al. Changes in platelet alpha 2-adrenoceptor binding post partum: possible relation to maternity blues. *Lancet* 1983;1:495–498.

183. Kleiner GJ, Greston WM. *Suicide in pregnancy.* Boston: John Wright, 1984.

184. Appleby L. Physiology of pregnancy, labor and puerperium: suicide during pregnancy and in the first postnatal year. *BMJ* 1991;302:137–140.

185. Kendall RE. Suicide in pregnancy and the puerperium. *BMJ* 1991;302:126–127.

186. Dean C, Kendell RE. The symptomatology of puerperal illness. *Br J Psychiatry* 1981;139:128–133.

187. Ghodsian M, Zajicek E, Wolkind S. A longitudinal study of maternal depression and child behavior problems. *J Child Psychol Psychiatry* 1984;25:91–109.

188. Billings AF, Moos RH. Children of parents with unipolar depression: a controlled 1-year followup. *J Abnormal Child Psychol* 1985;14:149.

189. Marce LV. Traite de la folie des femmes enceintes, des nouvelles accouchees et des nourrices. Paris: Bailliere, 1858.

190. Paffenbarger RS. Epidemiological aspects of parapartum mental illness. *Br J Preventive Soc Med* 1964; 18:189–195.

191. Paffenbarger RS, McCabe LJ. The effect of obstetric and perinatal events on risk of mental illness in women of childbearing age. *Am J Public Health* 1966;56: 400–407.

192. Paffenbarger RS. Epidemiological aspects of mental

illness associated with childbearing. In: Brockington JF, Kumar R, eds. *Motherhood and mental illness.* New York: Grune & Stratton, 1982.

193. Kendell RE, Chalmers JC, Platz C. Epidemiology of puerperal psychoses. *Br J Psychiatry* 1987;150:662.

194. Robins LN, Helzer JE, Weissman MM, et al. Lifetime prevalence of specific psychiatric disorders in three sites. *Arch Gen Psychiatry* 1984;41:949.

195. Brockington IF, Cernik KF, Schofield EM, et al. Puerperal psychosis. Phenomena and diagnosis. *Arch Gen Psychiatry* 1981;38:829.

196. Margison F. Pathology of the mother-child relationship. In: Brockington IF, Kumar R (eds). *Motherhood and mental illness.* London: Academic Press, 1982:1–65.

197. Reich T, Winokur G. Postpartum psychosis in patients with manic depressive disease. *J Nerv Ment Dis* 1970; 151:60.

198. Tetlow C. Psychoses of childbearing. *J Ment Sci* 1955;101:629–639.

199. Brockington IF, Winokur G, Dean C. Puerperal psychosis. In: Brockington IF, Kumar R (eds). *Motherhood and mental illness.* London: Academic Press, 1982:1–65.

200. Lindstrom LH, Nyberg N, Terenius L, et al. CSF and plasma beta-casomorphin-like opioid peptides in postpartum psychosis. *Am J Psychiatry* 1984;141: 1059–1066.

201. Oates MR. The treatment of psychiatric disorders in pregnancy and the puerperium. *Clin Obstet Gynecol* 1986;13:385–389.

202. Uddenberg N, Engelsson I. Prognosis of postpartum mental disturbance. A prospective study of primiparous women and their 4-1/2 year old children. *Acta Psychiatr Scand* 1978;58:201–209.

Neurological Complications of Pregnancy, Second
Edition, edited by Brian Hainline and Orrin Devinsky.
Lippincott Williams & Wilkins, Philadelphia, © 2002.

21

Cocaine and Alcohol Use

Joan T. Moroney and *Machelle H. Allen

*Department of Neurosciences, Royal College of Surgeons, Ireland, and Department of Neurology,
Beaumont Hospital, Dublin, Ireland; *Department of Obstetrics and Gynecology,
New York University School of Medicine, Bellevue Hospital, New York, New York, U.S.A.*

Although drug and alcohol use during pregnancy adversely affects both mother and fetus, medical literature is weighted heavily toward fetal and neonatal complications of maternal drug use. A clear understanding of the complications of cocaine and alcohol use during pregnancy is hampered by several factors: (a) polysubstance abuse is common among cocaine and alcohol abusers; (b) prospective, reliable screening for drug and alcohol use among pregnant women is scant and unreliable; and (c) society's punitive approach to maternal drug and alcohol users leads many women to avoid counseling or treatment.

Drug abuse is the second most common psychiatric disorder among young women aged 18 to 24 (1). Traditionally, alcoholism and other forms of drug abuse have been studied as discrete, isolated disorders. However, polysubstance abuse has become recognized as an increasingly common pattern. Alcoholics and cocaine abusers often abuse tobacco, tranquilizers, depressants, and marijuana. The concept of polysubstance abuse implies that there may be similarities between addictive disorders that transcend specific pharmacologic properties of abused drugs. An improved synthesis of existing information about alcohol and drug abuse should reveal the extent to which there are common processes in the development and maintenance of polysubstance abuse (2).

This chapter reviews maternal, fetal, and neonatal complications of cocaine and alcohol use during pregnancy. Suggestions for future management of women who use these substances are offered.

COCAINE

Epidemiology

In 2000, an estimated 1.2 million Americans were cocaine users, 20% of whom smoked crack cocaine (3). The highest number of initiates of cocaine occurred in the late 1970s and early 1980s, with approximately 1.0 to 1.5 million new users each year. The number of new users of cocaine fell to a low in the early 1990s, but there has been an upward trend during the past few years, especially for youths aged 12 to 17. Since 1965, the highest annual rate of first use among youths occurred in 1998, with 14.5 per 1,000 potential new users (3).

The last detailed epidemiologic study of drug use in pregnancy was in 1992 (4), although there are some pertinent statistics from the 2000 National Household Survey on Drug Abuse (3). In 1999 and 2000, among pregnant women aged 15 to 44 years, 3.3% used illicit drugs in the previous month. The rate of illicit drug use was higher among African-American pregnant women (7.1%) than among white (2.9%) or Hispanic (2.1%)

pregnant women. In 1992, more than 5% of the 4 million women who gave birth in the United States used illegal drugs during pregnancy; 1.1% used cocaine. African-American pregnant women had a higher rate of cocaine use (4.5%) compared to white (0.4%) and Hispanic (0.7%) pregnant women (4). Up to 30% of pregnant women who live in the inner city and seek medical care through the hospital emergency room use cocaine (5).

Among women who smoked cigarettes or drank alcohol during pregnancy, 9.5% used cocaine. Conversely, among women who neither smoked nor drank during pregnancy, only 0.1% used cocaine (4). Such data confirm that polysubstance abuse during pregnancy is a major problem that needs to be addressed.

Methodologic Considerations

Determining the effects of intrauterine cocaine exposure in isolation from other variables is problematic because there is no single sensitive and specific test to detect exposure to cocaine in utero. Detection of intrauterine exposure to cocaine depends on a combination of testing maternal urine for cocaine and its metabolites and interviewing the mother. Frank and colleagues (6) elegantly illustrated the limitations of using only one of these approaches. They prospectively studied 1,226 mothers for cocaine use by interview and urinalysis. Interview alone would not have detected 24% of exposed infants, whereas urinalysis alone would have failed to detect 47% of exposed infants. Furthermore, urine testing in neonates provides evidence only of recent exposure to cocaine. The duration of intrauterine exposure cannot be determined from laboratory analysis.

Another methodologic difficulty is the presence of confounding influences in the life of the cocaine-exposed fetus and infant. Pregnant women who abuse cocaine often abuse other drugs, are undernourished, and fail to seek prenatal care (1). During a 3-month period in 1990, an anonymous universal screening assessment of all pregnant women presenting for evaluation at New York University Medical Center revealed that 15% of these women had evidence of recent drug use; 80% of drug users tried cocaine. Although urine was not screened for drug use, these results confirm the prevalence of drug use, specifically cocaine, among pregnant urban women.

Pharmacology

Cocaine (benzoylecgonine) is an alkaloid derived from the leaves of coca plants. The first extraction yields coca paste, a raw and generally impure product consumed mostly in South America. Further extraction with hydrochloric acid yields cocaine hydrochloride, which is usually diluted and either snorted or used intravenously. If the hydrochloride salt is treated with a base such as sodium bicarbonate and then re-extracted with a solvent such as ether, the "free-base" form is obtained. Cocaine's systemic and brain effects are mediated by alterations in synaptic transmission. Cocaine blocks the presynaptic reuptake of norepinephrine and dopamine, producing an excess of transmitter at postsynaptic receptor sites.

Cocaine plasma levels peak in about 15 to 60 minutes after snorting and in about 45 to 90 minutes after oral ingestion. Peak levels of cocaine are reached within seconds after smoking or intravenous use. Cocaine crosses lipid membranes easily and can accumulate in the brain (7). Cocaine is metabolized by serum and hepatic cholinesterases to water-soluble metabolites (benzoylecgonine and ecgonine methylester) that are excreted in the urine (7). Plasma cholinesterase activity is much lower in fetuses, infants, elderly men, patients with liver disease, and pregnant women (8). Cocaine has a plasma half-life of about 1 hour, and its metabolites may be present in the urine of adults from 12 to 24 hours after use to as long as 3 weeks, depending on the route of administration, cholinesterase activity, and frequency of use (7,9,10).

Following cocaine ingestion, individuals typically become less fatigued and more talkative and develop a general sense of euphoria and well-being. Cocaine's behavioral effects are mediated through the reward and reinforcing circuitry of the mesocortical and mesolimbic dopaminergic system (11). The potent reinforcing effects of cocaine may be related to specific cocaine brain receptor sites (12). Cocaine-induced dysphoria occurs minutes to hours following acute intoxication and is attributed to presynaptic dopamine depletion. Cocaine craving in relatively naive users results from attempts to alleviate dysphoric symptoms; in chronic users, cocaine craving is related to the development of receptor site supersensitivity. Acute cocaine intoxication may cause hypertension, cardiac arrhythmias, and seizures from systemic and central sympathetic overdrive (11).

Obstetric Complications

The pharmacologic characteristics of cocaine enhance its potential for adverse effects on the fetus. It readily crosses the placenta and the fetal blood–brain barrier because of its low molecular weight and high water and lipid solubility (2). Obstetric complications attributed to cocaine use are numerous and extend throughout pregnancy. Spontaneous abortions and premature separation of the placenta (abruptio placentae) are the most frequently described (13–15). Chasnoff and colleagues (16) state that the spontaneous abortion rate in pregnant women using cocaine is 38%, whereas the rate for pregnant heroin users is 16%. The incidence of abruptio placentae in pregnant women using cocaine alone or with opiates is 17% and 18%, respectively. Cocaine use in pregnancy increases the rate of stillbirths by a factor of 10 over women who use no drugs during pregnancy (16).

These obstetric complications result from increased sympathetic tone following uptake of cocaine into monoaminergic nerve terminals. A sudden rise in maternal blood pressure, enhancement of uterine activity, or both occurs from increased blood catecholamines. Uterine artery spasm and placental vasoconstriction interfere with transport of oxygen and other nutrients to the fetus. Such changes have been confirmed by catheterization of maternal and fetal arteries and veins in pregnant ewes and their fetuses (17). Although inferences to human responses should be made with caution, research in pregnant ewes clearly documents the risks of cocaine use for both mother and fetus. Furthermore, these observed changes occur following one-time doses, whereas pregnant women using cocaine are subject to such hemodynamic effects repeatedly.

Intrauterine Growth Restriction

Cocaine exposure has been independently linked to intrauterine growth restriction (IUGR), even after statistical consideration of other confounding variables (18). A prospective study of 17,466 pregnancies in the University of Illinois perinatal network assessed the risk of prematurity and IUGR at 87% when cocaine was used during pregnancy (19). Bingol and colleagues (20) reported that infants with a history of intrauterine cocaine exposure had an average birthweight of 2,275 g compared to 3,121 g in control infants.

An important factor in the pathogenesis of impaired fetal growth is the disturbance in the transfer of oxygen and other nutrients to the fetus because of impaired placental blood flow (17). In addition, a rise in fetal catecholamines can accelerate metabolism and deplete fetal nutrient stores. IUGR correlates with poorer developmental outcome; the emerging evidence of the independent impact of cocaine on intrauterine growth, especially head circumference, indicates a need for continued investigation of these interactions on subsequent adverse neurobehavioral outcomes.

Teratogenicity of Cocaine

Although the relationship between maternal cocaine use and obstetric–gestational complications is clear, the possible teratogenic effects of cocaine remain controversial. The incidence of congenital malformations in infants born to cocaine-abusing mothers is 10%, compared to 2% among control infants (8). Major and minor malformations have been described, including bilateral cryptorchidism, hydronephrosis, bone defects, ossification delay, eye defects, and exencephaly (8).

Cocaine and the Developing Human Brain

Microcephaly (head circumference of 2 standard deviations below the mean for gestational age) is the most common brain abnormality described in infants of cocaine-abusing mothers. Both intrauterine brain growth and somatic growth are impaired (21). Disturbances of midline prosencephalic development and neuronal migration occur. A series (22) of seven infants exposed to cocaine in utero found varying combinations of agenesis of the corpus callosum, absence of the septum pellucidum, schizencephaly, and septo-optic dysplasia in three of the infants. Neuronal heterotopias (collections of neurons in cerebral white matter due to impairment of neuronal migration) also were described.

Cocaine-induced disturbances of neuronal differentiation in cerebral, diencephalic, and brainstem structures are supported by animal research (23). Prenatal cocaine exposure in rats results in persistent defects in the hippocampus, the nigrostriatal pathway, and the mesolimbic dopaminergic system. Thus, exposure to cocaine during the earliest phases of neuronal differentiation in laboratory animals causes profound and permanent effects on the function of many neuronal systems.

The pathophysiology of cocaine's effects on neuronal differentiation remains unclear. Because all of these pathways use monaminergic neurotransmitters or are themselves the targets of neurons using monoamines as neurotransmitters, derangements of neurotransmitters is a plausible hypothesis (24). These neurotransmitters appear early in brain development and have important regulatory roles in the development of neuronal circuitry. The specific nature of these derangements in the cocaine-exposed fetus requires further definition.

Cerebral Infarction and Intracranial Hemorrhage in the Cocaine-Exposed Fetus

In utero exposure of the fetus to cocaine may lead to serious destructive brain lesions. The first clear example (25) was the demonstration of middle cerebral artery infarction in a newborn whose mother had snorted large doses of cocaine for 3 days prior to delivery. Subsequent reports (26) have linked cerebral infarction in the distribution of major cerebral vessels with exposure to cocaine in utero. All such lesions appear to have been prenatal, but the timing of infarctions has varied from hours to months before delivery according to radiographic and clinical criteria (26). Dixon and Bejar (27) found ultrasonographic evidence of subarachnoid, subependymal, or intraventricular hemorrhage in 12% of infants exposed to cocaine.

The mechanisms of ischemic and hemorrhagic brain lesions associated with intrauterine cocaine exposure are probably multifactorial. Abrupt increases in blood pressure due to placentally transferred catecholamines and increased fetal catecholamine secretion may lead to brain hemorrhages (17). Vasospasm may be causative in brain ischemia. Cocaine-induced vasoconstriction may be a direct effect mediated through sodium channels. Support for this hypothesis is derived from animal studies whereby cocaine-induced arteriolar constriction, with resultant decrease in cerebral blood flow, was blocked by tetrodotoxin, a local anesthetic antagonist, but not by phentolamine, an adrenergic antagonist (28).

Neuronal excitotoxicity is another possible mechanism of neuronal injury in the cocaine-exposed fetus. Catecholamine excess can cause neuronal death in cell cultures by acting as glutamate agonists (28). Glutamate receptor antagonists markedly reduced the occurrence of cocaine-induced seizures and death in mice exposed to cocaine in utero.

Neonatal Neurologic Manifestations

Several studies (8,29–32) address the clinical features of neonates exposed to cocaine in utero. Neonatal differences in neurobehavioral functioning are important because they may be early signals of possible long-term neuropsychiatric effects of cocaine. Alternatively, they may impair caretaker–infant interactions and adversely affect developmental outcome indirectly (30).

A minority of infants exposed to cocaine in utero have a neonatal neurologic syndrome characterized by abnormal sleep patterns, tremors, poor feeding, irritability, and seizures. This syndrome is usually not severe, is most apparent on the second day, and is relatively short lasting (29). Abnormal electroencephalograms and brainstem-evoked potentials have been described that disappear 1 to 6 months after birth (33); neurologic and cognitive outcomes are unclear. Current conventional testing of neurologic and cognitive development is not suitable to detect the potential abnormalities in cocaine-exposed infants. The experimental data that emphasize the role of the monoaminergic system suggest that the function of the limbic, hypothalamic, and extrapyramidal systems should be assessed carefully. Thus, studies of infant development must effectively quantify arousal, attention, emotional control, and related behaviors.

Cocaine is excreted in the breast milk. Breastfeeding infants of cocaine-using mothers can develop symptoms and signs of acute intoxication (34).

Maternal Complications

Henderson (35) reported a case of a ruptured intracranial aneurysm in a 24-year-old pregnant woman who smoked crack cocaine. Alvaro (36) reported a 25-year-old woman who suffered a postpartum intracerebral hemorrhage following cocaine use. The pregnancy was complicated by repeated crack cocaine use, poor fetal growth, and diminished amniotic fluid volume. She underwent an uneventful cesarean section. Four days later, she suddenly became euphoric, irritable, and hypertensive and suffered a generalized tonic-clonic seizure. The working diagnosis was postpartum eclampsia; urine toxicology 15

hours later was negative. The patient admitted to smoking crack cocaine, and a brain computed tomography scan revealed intracerebral hemorrhage in the left frontal lobe. Selective carotid angiography showed no evidence of aneurysm or vascular malformation.

Levine (10) reported 28 patients from four medical centers that had cerebral vascular accidents temporally related to crack cocaine use. Two patients were pregnant women. The 28 patients suffered the following: 18 cerebral infarctions, five subarachnoid hemorrhages, four intraparenchymal hemorrhages, and one primary intraventricular hemorrhage. One pregnant woman developed intracerebral hemorrhage after using intranasal cocaine, and the other suffered a middle cerebral artery infarct. Pathogenesis of cerebral infarcts from cocaine use is likely cerebral vasospasm. Most patients with brain hemorrhage have preexisting cerebral aneurysms or arteriovenous malformations, although acute hypertension may be causative. Pregnant women also are susceptible to other acute and chronic effects of cocaine use, although the literature offers little assessment of this phenomenon.

Management

Pregnant women who use cocaine are high-risk pregnancy patients and deserve careful monitoring, including testing maternal urine for cocaine and its metabolites. Strict monitoring of positive cases along with preventive education and drug treatment may contribute toward a much-needed reduction in maternal and perinatal morbidity and mortality associated with cocaine use during pregnancy. Unfortunately, the deleterious impact of maternal drug use on the infant and child has shifted management of high-risk patients from education and drug treatment to criminal prosecution. Furthermore, social and medical services are often unavailable for those patients most in need. As an example, 87% of drug treatment programs in New York City in 1989 refused to provide services to pregnant women who were addicted to crack cocaine and on Medicaid (37).

Hopefully, this punitive attitude will shift because comprehensive treatment for pregnant users of crack cocaine yields beneficial results. The Parent and Child Enrichment (PACE) program in New York City is an inpatient, multidisciplinary program for drug treatment during pregnancy. For long-stay patients, fetal exposure to cocaine decreased dramatically, and infants had greater mean birthweights, less low birthweight, and less IUGR than infants of nontreated mothers (38). Chemical addiction is a medical illness, and criminal prosecution is counterproductive (see Chapter 23). Untreated chemical dependency during pregnancy inflicts emotional and physical harm on the mother, child, and other family members and should be the driving force toward public health policy reform.

ALCOHOL

Epidemiology

Alcohol occupies a unique position in Western civilization as the only potent pharmacologic agent legally available and socially acceptable for the purpose of self-intoxication (10). In 2000, almost half of Americans aged 12 and older reported being current users of alcohol; 5.6% of this population are heavy drinkers (five or more drinks on the same occasion at least five different days in the prior 30 days). Among these 12.6 million heavy drinkers, 30% are current illicit drug users. In 1998, approximately 5.1 million people initiated the use of alcohol—the highest rate of new users since the early 1970s. Among pregnant women aged 15 to 44 years in 1999 and 2000 combined, 12.4% used alcohol and 3.9% were binge drinkers. These rates are substantially lower than in nonpregnant women of the same age (48.7% and 29.9%, respectively) (3).

The 1992 National Institute on Drug Abuse study demonstrated that 18.8% of pregnant women drank alcohol. Alcohol use during pregnancy was higher among white women (23%) than among African-American (15.8%) and Hispanic (8.7%) women (4). An ethnic comparison of cocaine use versus alcohol use during pregnancy points to the importance of attending to social–cultural–ethnic issues in assessing for and managing drug and alcohol use in women of childbearing ages.

Pharmacology

Alcohol (ethanol) is a simple 2–C structure (see Fig. 21.1) (11). Ethanol is rapidly absorbed from the gastrointestinal system to the circulation, is widely distributed to all organs and fluid compartments, and diffuses freely across the placental barrier. Peak blood levels can be achieved within 45 minutes on an empty stomach. More than 90% of ethanol is oxidized to acetaldehyde, the major metabolite (39). The rate of metabolism is constant with time and is little affected by the absolute blood level. Blood alcohol levels decline on average at a rate of 10 to 20 mg/dL per hour. Women have higher blood alcohol concentrations than men after consuming comparable amounts of alcohol. Furthermore, epidemiologic evidence indicates that women are more susceptible than men to the adverse effects of alcohol. Research studies have documented a significant "first pass" metabolism of gastric alcohol dehydrogenase activity as measured in endoscopic gastric biopsy (40). An explanation for the sex-related difference in blood alcohol concentration after ingestion is the decreased gastric oxidation of alcohol in women. This contributes to the enhanced vulnerability of women to both acute and chronic effects of alcohol (41).

Alcohol has been described as a drug without a receptor. Meyer (42) proposed that

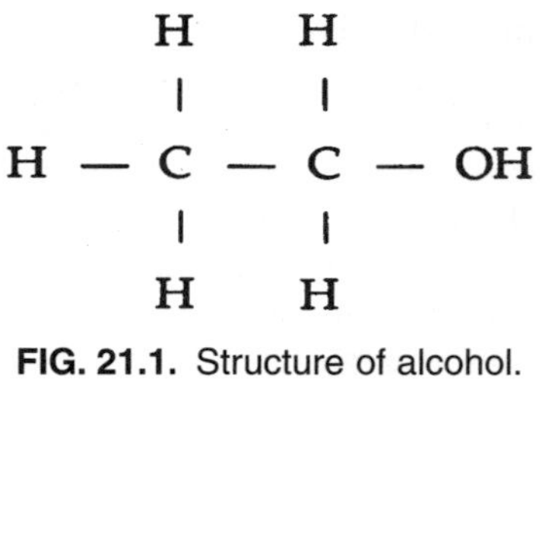

$$H - C - C - OH$$

(with H atoms above and below each C)

FIG. 21.1. Structure of alcohol.

ethanol produces intoxication through alteration of membrane lipids. Physiologically attainable concentrations of alcohol (25 to 100 mmol) significantly increase the "fluidity" of all membrane lipids (43). Ethanol-induced sedation correlates with these changes in membrane fluidity. However, although alcohol does not interact with a brain receptor in the classical sense, specific molecular sites of action have been identified. These sites include particular areas of lipid "microdomains" within neuronal membranes and hydrophobic "receptive" regions of membrane-bound proteins (44) (Table 21.1).

The central nervous system is the primary target for the physiologic effects of alcohol. Effects are in general proportional to the blood concentration of alcohol (11). Impairment of sensory perceptions, cognitive function, and motor coordination occur with alcohol concentrations between 31 and 65 mg/dL. Clinical intoxication occurs with blood levels of 50 to 150 mg/dL, whereas lethargy and/or coma supervene with concentrations greater than 200 mg/dL. Legal intoxication is defined as blood alcohol levels of greater than 100 mg/dL. On average, one drink (1 oz 50% hard liquor, 12 oz 4% beer, 3 oz wine) results in maximum blood concentration of 20 mg/dL (10) (see Tables 21.2 and 21.3.

The Fetal Alcohol Syndrome

The initial recognition of alcohol as a teratogen hinged on the specificity of a clinically recognizable phenotype. Fetal alcohol syndrome (FAS) was first described in France by Lemoine (45) and subsequently by Jones and Smith (46). The incidence of FAS worldwide is about 119 per 1,000 live births. Using these estimates, the number of FAS children born annually in the United States is about 7,000. The incidence of FAS varies and is dependent on socioeconomic and geographic considerations. In areas with mostly white, middle-class mothers the rate of FAS is 0.6 per 1,000 live births. The rate increases to 2.6 per 1,000 live births in areas with predominantly African-American women of low socioeconomic status, and peaks at 3.1 per 1,000 live births in American Indian women in the southwestern United States (47).

FAS is characterized by a triad of signs (48,49):

IUGR
Central nervous system involvement
Characteristic facial dysmorphology

Key facial features are short palpebral fissures, hypoplastic upper lips with thinned vermilion, diminished or absent philtrum, and midfacial and mandibular growth deficiencies

TABLE 21.1. *Evidence for specificity of central nervous system effects of ethanol*

System receptors and receptor-effector coupling	Membrane-bound enzymes
A. Gamma-aminobutyric acid–benzodiazepine–barbiturate receptor–chloride ionophore Ethanol affects binding only to chloride ionophore B. Catecholamine receptor–adenylate cyclase Ethanol primarily affects G8 function C. Receptor mediated polyphosphoinositide (PI) breakdown Ethanol affects muscarinic-cholinergic-receptor-stimulated PI breakdown D. Opiate receptor binding Ethanol preferentially inhibits ligand binding to delta in comparison to mu receptors. Kappa receptors are resistant to ethanol.	A. Monoamino oxidase (MAO) Ethanol selectively inhibits MAO-B activity B. NA$^+$/K$^+$ ATPase Activity of neuronally located form of the enzyme is sensitive to ethanol

From Woods JR, Plessinger MA, Kenneth EC. Effects of ethanol on uterine blood flow and fetal oxygenation. *JAMA* 1987;257. Reprinted with permission.

TABLE 21.2. *Clinical effects and blood levels in acute alcoholism*

Symptoms	Blood level (mg/dL)
Euphoria, giddiness, verbosity	25–100
Impaired mental status	
Prolonged reaction time	
Nystagmus	
Hypalgesia to noxious stimulation	
Boisterousness, ataxia	100–200
Nystagmus, dysarthria	
Pronounced hypalgesia	
Nausea, vomiting, drowsiness	200–300
Diplopia, wide sluggish pupils	
Marked ataxia and clumsiness	
Hypothermia, amnesic stupor	>200
Severe dysarthria	
Anesthesia to noxious stimulation	
Hypoventilation, coma, death	

(46). Other anomalies include cardiac septal, skeletal, and urogenital defects. Structural and developmental anomalies of the brain and spinal cord have been found.

Ethanol adversely affects neuronal proliferation and migration in offspring of ethanol-fed rats (50). These defects, along with errors in cortical differentiation, probably account for the structural abnormalities underlying mental retardation and motor dysfunction in children with FAS. Additional clinical studies have emphasized that prenatal alcohol exposure accounts for hearing, language, and visual disorders and results in hyperactivity and attention deficit disorders (51).

Fetal Alcohol Effects

Prenatal alcohol exposure results in a spectrum of fetal effects. The more severe outcomes generally are associated with higher

TABLE 21.3. *Approximate blood alcohol content per drink*

Drink	mg/dL
12-oz beer	20
3-oz wine	20
1-oz hard liquor (whiskey, vodka)	20
3.5-oz martini/manhattan	40
4-oz daiquiri	30
8-oz highball	30

maternal alcohol intake. Children with FAS represent the extreme end of a continuum of effects. Lesser alcohol-related teratogenic effects are termed "fetal alcohol effects," of which the major manifestation is IUGR (46). Alcohol abuse alone results in a 2.4-fold increase in IUGR. Children born to alcoholic women who drink during pregnancy weigh 490 g below normal, whereas children of alcoholic women who abstained during pregnancy weigh about 260 g less than control infants (52). Other factors associated with alcohol use during pregnancy may contribute to IUGR. For example, combined tobacco smoking and alcohol use during pregnancy results in a 3.9-fold increase in IUGR (46).

Pathophysiology of FAS

The maternal–placental–fetal unit is a complex pharmacologic model. Each compartment is an independent and dependent contributor to the overall picture of drug disposition and toxicity. Rapid bidirectional transfer of ethanol takes place through the placenta, producing near-identical maternal and fetal blood concentrations within minutes (53). Amniotic fluid accumulation is slower, reaching equilibrium with blood level in approximately 3 hours. The human placenta oxidizes ethanol to acetaldehyde and releases it into the fetal perfusate. The amniotic fluid sac serves as an ethanol reservoir; a 1 g/kg dose is cleared in approximately 12 hours (54). The implication is clear: the fetus shares the same concentration of ethanol present in the maternal blood.

The weight of current evidence suggests that alcohol is a teratogen in several species. Controversy over the teratogenic effects of alcohol exists because the mother of a child with FAS often uses other drugs, is malnourished, and has inadequate medical care during pregnancy. Specific attribution of birth defects to alcohol requires strict control of malnutrition and polysubstance abuse.

Animal models address these issues. Macaque monkeys were administered alcohol in doses of 2.5 to 4.1 g/kg once weekly from 40 days postconception to delivery (55).

These doses produced average blood alcohol levels between 240 and 415 mg/dL within 2 hours after alcohol ingestion. This regimen resulted in one spontaneous abortion and three live births. Infants were followed for a period of 6 months and compared with age- and sex-matched controls. Prenatal exposure to the highest alcohol dose (4.1 g/kg) resulted in neurologic developmental and facial anomalies similar to those described in human FAS infants. Behavioral exam showed profound mental retardation. Neuropathology revealed cerebral asymmetry, minimal cortical organization, and hydrocephalus *ex vacuo*. One of two surviving infants exposed to a lower dose (2.5 g/kg) of alcohol prenatally had no developmental or neuropathologic abnormalities. The other surviving infant was hyperkinetic and showed evidence of developmental retardation and brain abnormalities.

The alcohol-exposed Macaque monkeys differs from human FAS infants in two respects: (a) all were abnormally large at birth, whereas low birthweight is common in human FAS infants (nutritional status was undoubtedly better in the Macaque mothers than in most alcoholic women); and (b) none showed malformations of heart, kidney, and other organs. The absence of organ malformations is probably because alcohol was not administered to the mother until the end of the organogenic period.

Fetal circulating ratio of betahydroxy-butyrate to acetoacetate, plasma proteins, and liver triacylglyceride content are similar in ethanol-fed rats, pair-fed rats, and normal controls fed *ad libitum* (56). These results and those of the Macaque monkeys suggest that certain teratogenic effects specifically result from ethanol rather than undernutrition.

The most devastating effects of alcohol are on the developing brain. Animal research has been used to identify the mechanisms underlying such damage. Prenatal exposure to alcohol in rats reveals that ethanol alters the plasma membrane structure of astrocytes, especially during periods of proliferation and differentiation in primary cultures (57). Biochemical brain modifications in pups born to alcohol-consuming rats were investigated (58). Superoxide dismutase, enolase isoenzymes, glutamine synthetase, and acetaldehyde dehydrogenase were analyzed. Activities of all these enzymes were decreased in the brain even when alcohol was later withdrawn from the mother's diet during either pregnancy or lactation. The authors conclude that the alterations observed in experimental FAS are from toxicity of alcohol and its metabolites, with resultant free radical formation following decreased superoxide dismutase activity. Alcohol-induced damage to the developing brain encompasses a longer developmental timeframe, affects more cell populations, occurs at lower levels of exposure, produces greater numbers of permanent effects, and is modulated by more factors than initially appreciated.

Alcoholics are frequently malnourished. Regardless of maternal nutritional status, however, ethanol can be placentotoxic, impairing the normal transfer of essential fetal nutrients. Ethanol and acetaldehyde inhibit placental uptake and transfer of amino acids, zinc, and glucose (59). Therefore, maternal ethanol ingestion may cause fetal injury by at least two mechanisms: (a) directly by fetotoxicity from alcohol or acetaldehyde, and (b) indirectly by ethanol-induced placental injury and selective fetal malnutrition (59).

Although it seems likely that alcohol is a specific teratogen, the extent to which the human FAS is specific to alcohol remains unresolved. Other drugs are also fetotoxic, and polysubstance abuse during pregnancy can result in a profile of low birthweight, delayed development, and brain malformation similar to that reported for alcohol abuse.

Maternal Complications

The medical literature is virtually silent regarding maternal complications of alcohol use. Given the number of women with drinking problems, acute and chronic adverse effects must not be uncommon. The most serious acute side effect of alcohol intoxication is poor judgment. Intoxicated pregnant women are at high risk of fatal motor-vehicle accidents and related problems because of impaired judgment and motor coordination (11). Chronic alcohol-abusing pregnant women are at risk of alcohol withdrawal if drinking is stopped suddenly; this presents a risk for both mother and fetus, especially if delirium tremens develops. Alcoholics often are undernourished, which may be particularly problematic during pregnancy. Chronic alcohol ingestion by women may cause numerous long-term medical and neurologic adverse health effects, which are beyond the scope of this chapter.

Management

No screening tests identify FAS early in pregnancy, and treatment of alcoholism often is limited and unsuccessful. Mental retardation, a major component of FAS, usually is identified only several years after birth. The actual impairment of alcohol on a child's development is immense, accounting for 10% of children in our society with mental retardation. Thus, FAS is as prevalent as Down's syndrome (60). Public and professional education are the only available preventive measures. Despite great clinical and research interest, comparatively little attention has been paid to preventive strategies and appropriate policy development. Such strategies should include general publicity and counseling for pregnant women.

Pregnant women should be questioned about alcohol intake during routine antenatal visits, and they should be advised accordingly. Previous use of alcohol or cigarettes, including during the month prior to pregnancy, most differentiates pregnant alcohol users from nonusers (61). Pregnant women will reduce alcohol intake through learning health information and corresponding behavior strategies (62).

Routine urine toxicology and measurement of liver function enzymes during prenatal visits are other approaches to identity pregnant women at risk for carrying a child with FAS. Attention must be paid to characteristics of patients for whom intervention is targeted, and the underlying social and psychologic factors that maintain drinking in these pa-

tients need to be examined (63). Individuals with comorbid alcohol and drug use disorders are at particularly high risk for psychiatric disorders and poor treatment outcomes. Miles and colleagues (64) found that drug-dependent pregnant women with comorbid alcohol dependence have greater psychopathology than drug-dependent women without comorbid alcohol dependence.

Because there are no clear relationships between quantity of alcohol consumed during pregnancy and the severity of FAS, it is reasonable to assume that factors such as maximum blood alcohol concentration, stage of gestational development, nutritional adequacy, and smoking and other drug use contribute to the severity of FAS. Attempts have been made to establish a "safe level" of alcohol, but with so many uncertainties, such information is speculative. The safest recommendation is to abstain from drinking during pregnancy (65). As with cocaine, providing a protective environment in which the mother can receive sound education and treatment should be the driving force toward public health policy reform (66).

REFERENCES

1. Streissguth AP, Grant TM, Barr HM, et al. Cocaine and the use of alcohol and other drugs during pregnancy. *Am J Obstet Gynecol* 1991;64:1239–1243.
2. Jaffe JH. Drug addiction and drug abuse. In: Goodman LS, Gilman A, Rall TW, et al, eds. In: *The pharmacological basis of therapeutics.* 8th ed. New York: Macmillan, 1990:522–573.
3. Substance Abuse and Mental Health Services Administration. *Summary of findings from the 2000 National Household Survey on Drug Abuse.* Rockville, MD: Office of Applied Studies, 2001; NHSDA Series H-13, DHHS Publication No. (SMA) 01-3549.
4. *National Pregnancy and Health Survey—Drug use among women delivering live births: 1992.* Rockville, MD: National Clearinghouse for Drug and Alcohol Information, 1992; NCADI publication No. BKD192.
5. Ness RB, Grisso JA, Hirschinger N, et al. Cocaine and tobacco use and the risk of spontaneous abortion. *N Engl J Med* 1999;340:333–339.
6. Frank DA, Zuckerman BS, Amaro H, et al. Cocaine use during pregnancy: prevalence and correlates. *Pediatrics* 1988;82:888–895.
7. Farrar HC, Kearns GL. Cocaine: clinical pharmacology and toxicology. *J Pediatr* 1989;115:665–675.
8. Volpe J. Review article: mechanisms of disease—effect of cocaine use on the fetus. *N Engl J Med* 1992;327:399–407.
9. Cregler LL, Mark H. Medical complications of cocaine abuse. *N Engl J Med* 1986;315:1495–1500.

10. Levine SR, Brust JC, Futrell N, et al. Cerebrovascular complications of the use of the "crack" form of alkaloidal cocaine. *N Engl J Med* 1990;323:699–704.
11. Wadler GI, Hainline B. *Drugs and the athlete.* Philadelphia: FA Davis Co, 1989.
12. Ritz ML. Cocaine receptors on dopamine transporters are related to self-administration of cocaine. *Science* 1987;237:1219–1221.
13. Miller JM, Boudreaux MC, Regan FA. A case-control study of cocaine use in pregnancy. *Am J Obstet Gynecol* 1995;172:180–185.
14. Little BB, Snell LM, Trimmer KJ, et al. Peripartum cocaine use and adverse pregnancy outcome. *Am J Human Biol* 1999;11:598–602.
15. Addis A, Moretti ME, Ahmed Syed F, et al. Fetal effects of cocaine: an updated meta-analysis. *Reprod Toxicol* 2001;115:341–369.
16. Chasnoff IJ, Burns WJ, Schnoll SH, et al. Cocaine use in pregnancy. *N Engl J Med* 1985;313: 666–672.
17. Woods JR, Plessinger MA, Kenneth EC. Effects of cocaine on uterine blood flow and fetal oxygenation. *JAMA* 1987;257:957–962.
18. Zuckerman BS, Frank DA, Hingson R, et al. Effects of maternal cocaine use on fetal growth. *N Engl J Med* 1989;320:762–768.
19. Handler A, Kistin N, Davis F, et al. Cocaine use during pregnancy: prevalence and perinatal outcomes. *Am J Epidemiol* 1991;133:818–825.
20. Bingol N, Fuchs M, Diaz V, et al. Teratogenicity of cocaine in humans. *J Pediatr* 1987;110:93–96.
21. Little BB, Snell IM. Brain growth among fetuses exposed to cocaine in utero: asymmetrical growth retardation. *Obstet Gynecol* 1991;77:361–364.
22. Dominguez R, Vila-Coro AA, Slopis JM, et al. Brain and ocular abnormalities in infants with in utero exposure to cocaine and other street drugs. *Am J Dis Child* 1991;145:688–695.
23. Dow-Edwards DL. Cocaine effects on fetal development: a comparison of clinical and animal research findings. *Neurotoxicol Teratol* 1991;13:347–352.
24. Wyatt RJ, Karoum F, Suddath R, et al. Persistently decreased brain dopamine levels and cocaine. *JAMA* 1988;259:2996.
25. Chasnoff IJ, Bussey ME, Savich R, et al. Perinatal cerebral infarction and maternal cocaine use. *J Pediatr* 1986;108:456–459.
26. Chasnoff IJ, Griffith DR, MacGregor S, et al. Temporal patterns of cocaine use in pregnancy: perinatal outcomes. *JAMA* 1989;261:1741–1745.
27. Dixon SP, Bejar R. Echoencephalographic findings in neonates with maternal cocaine and methamphetamine use. *J Pediatr* 1989;115:770–778.
28. Lien R, Goplerud JM, Kurth CD, et al. Interaction of cocaine with sympathetic modulation of regional cerebral blood flow in newborn piglets. *Ped Res* 1991;29:222x.
29. Neerhof MG, MacGregor SN, Retzky SS, et al. Cocaine abuse during pregnancy: perinatal outcome. *Am J Obstet Gynecol* 1989;161:633–638.
30. Doberczak TM, Shanzer S, Senie RT, et al. Neonatal neurologic and electroencephalographic effects of intrauterine cocaine exposure. *J Pediatr* 1988;113:354–358.
31. Singer LT, Hawkins S, Huang J, et al. Developmental outcomes and environmental correlates of very low birthweight, cocaine-exposed infants. *Early Hum Dev* 2001;64:91–103.
32. Schuler ME, Nair P. Brief report: frequency of maternal cocaine use during pregnancy and infant neurobehavioral outcome. *J Pediatr Psychol* 1999;24:511–514.
33. Rosenak D, Diamant YZ, Yaffe H, et al. Cocaine: maternal use during pregnancy and its effect on the mother, the fetus and the infant. Review. *Obstet Gynecol Surv* 1990;45:348–359.
34. Cocaine found in breast milk of nursing mother who used drugs. *Am Med News* 1988:42.
35. Henderson CE, Torbey M. Rupture of intracranial aneurysm associated with cocaine use during pregnancy. *Am J Perinatol* 1988;5:142–143.
36. Mercado A, Johnson G Jr, Calver D, et al. Cocaine, pregnancy, and postpartum intracerebral hemorrhage. *Obstet Gynecol* 1989;73:467–468.
37. Chavkin W. Drug addiction and pregnancy: policy crossroads. *Am J Public Health* 1990;80:483–487.
38. McMurtrie C, Rosenberg KD, Kerker BD, et al. A unique drug treatment program for pregnant and postpartum substance-using women in New York City: results of a pilot project, 1990–1995. *Am J Drug Alcohol Abuse* 1999;25:701–713.
39. Mello NK. Alcohol abuse and alcoholism. In: Meltzer H, ed. *Psychopharmacology: the third generation of progress.* New York: Raven Press, 1987:15–20.
40. Frezza M, di Padova C, Pozzato G, et al. High blood alcohol levels in women. The role of decreased gastric alcohol dehydrogenase activity and first-pass metabolism. *N Engl J Med* 1990;322:95–99.
41. Schenker S, Speig VK. The risk of alcohol intake in men and women. *N Engl J Med* 1990; 322:127–129.
42. Meyer HH. *Arch Exp Pathol Pharmacol* 1901;46: 388–386.
43. Harris RA, Schroeder F. Membrane effects of alcohol. *Mol Pharmacol* 1981;20:128–137.
44. Tabakoff B, Hoffman PL. Biochemical pharmacology of alcohol. In: Meltzer H, ed. *Psychopharmacology: the third generation of progress.* New York: Raven Press, 1987;1521–1526.
45. Lemoine P, Harousseau H, Borteyru JP, et al. Les enfants de parents alcooliques: anomalies observes a prefes de 27 cas. *Oest Med* 1968;25:477.
46. Jones KL, Smith DW. Recognition of the fetal alcohol syndromes in early infancy. *Lancet* 1973;2:999.
47. Abel EL, Sokol RJ. Incidence of the fetal alcohol syndrome (FAS) and economic impact of FAS related anomalies. *Drug Alcohol Depend* 1987;51:51–70.
48. Clarren SK, Smith DW. The fetal alcohol syndrome. *N Engl J Med* 1978;298:1063.
49. Prenatal exposure to alcohol. *Alcohol Res Health* 2000; 24:32–41.
50. Lewis G. Effects of alcohol on the generation and migration of cerebral cortical neurons. *Science* 1986;233: 1308–1311.
51. Church MV, Gerkin KP. Hearing disorders in children with the fetal alcohol syndrome: findings from case reports. *Pediatrics* 1988;82:147–154.
52. Little RE, Graham JM, Samson HH. Fetal alcohol effects in humans and animals. *Adv Alcohol Subst Abuse* 1982;1:103–125.
53. Brien JF, Clarke DW, Richardson B, et al. Disposition of ethanol in maternal blood, fetal blood, and amniotic fluid of third trimester pregnant ewes. *Am J Obstet Gynecol* 1985;152:583–590.
54. Karl PL, Gordon BH, Lieber CS, et al. Acetaldehyde production and transfer by the perfused human placental cotyledon. *Science* 1988;242:273–275.

55. Clarren SK, Bowden DM. A primate model of the fetal alcohol syndrome. *J Pediatr* 1982;101:819–824.

56. Testar X, Llobera M, Herrera E. Comparative metabolic effects of chronic ethanol intake and undernutrition in pregnant rats and their fetuses. *Alcohol Clin Exp Res* 1988;12:197–200.

57. Renau-Piqueras J, Guerri C, Burgal M, et al. Prenatal exposure to ethanol alters plasma membrane glycoproteins of astrocytes during development in primary culture, as evidenced by concanavalin A binding and 5'-nucleotidase activity. *Glia* 1992;5:65–74.

58. Ledig M, Tholey G, Kopp P, et al. An experimental study of fetal alcohol syndrome in the rat: biochemical modifications in brain and liver. *Alcohol Alcohol* 1989; 24:231–240.

59. Fisher SE, Karl PL. Maternal ethanol use and selective fetal malnutrition. *Recent Dev Alcohol* 1988;6:277–289.

60. Crepin G, Dehalne P, Samaille C. Clinical aspects and epidemiology of fetal alcoholism: a current daily problem. *Bull Acad Natl Med* 1989;173:572–582.

61. Chasnoff IJ, Neuman K, Thornton C, et al. Screening for substance use in pregnancy: a practical approach for the primary care physician. *Am J Obstet Gynecol* 2001: 184:752–758.

62. Strychar IM, Griffith WS, Conry RF. The relationship among learning, health beliefs, alcohol consumption and tobacco use of primigravidas. *Can J Public Health* 1990;81:462–467.

63. Waterson EJ, Murray-Lyon IM. Preventing alcohol related birth damage: a review. *Soc Sci Med* 1990;30:349–364.

64. Miles DR, Svikis DS, Kulstad JL, et al. Psychopathology in pregnant drug-dependent women with and without comorbid alcohol dependence. *Alcohol Clin Exp Res* 2001;25:1012–1017.

65. Mills JL, Grauband BI. Is moderate drinking during pregnancy associated with an increased risk for malformations? *Pediatrics* 1987;80:309–314.

66. Hankin J, McCaul ME, Heussner J. Pregnant, alcohol-abusing women. *Alcohol Clin Exp Res* 2000;24: 1276–1286.

Neurological Complications of Pregnancy, Second Edition, edited by Brian Hainline and Orrin Devinsky. Lippincott Williams & Wilkins, Philadelphia, © 2002.

22

Complementary and Alternative Medicine

Steven M. Rosman and *Brian Hainline

*Complementary Medicine, ProHEALTH Care Associates; and *Neurology and Integrative Pain Medicine, ProHEALTH Care Associates, Lake Success, New York, U.S.A.*

Complementary and alternative medicine (CAM) increasingly is becoming integrated with mainstream medicine. CAM is characterized as "treatment that is generally not used or recommended within the context of the mainstream biomedical community" (1). As such, CAM is dependent on the prevailing acceptance of the culture. CAM also is defined as a "broad domain of healing resources that encompass all health systems, modalities, practices, and their accompanying theories and beliefs, other than those intrinsic to the politically dominant health system of a particular society or culture in a given historical period" (2). The American Holistic Health Association characterizes the unifying principles of CAM: "Rather than focusing on illness or specific parts of the body, holistic health considers the whole person and how it interacts with its environment.... An individual is a whole made up of interdependent parts, which are the physical, mental, emotional and spiritual. When one part is not working at its best, it will impact all the other parts of that person" (3).

CAM encompasses a wide variety of modalities and techniques, including but not limited to acupuncture, acupressure, massage therapy, relaxation therapy and biofeedback, spiritual healing, nutritional and herbal therapy, homeopathy, folk remedies, chiropractic, chelation therapy, kinesiology, energy medicine, and magnetic field therapy. In a follow-up to his landmark study, Eisenberg followed trends in CAM used in the United States from 1970 through 1990 (4). The use of at least one type of CAM therapy during the previous year increased from 33.8% in 1990 to 42.1% in 1997. The therapies increasing the most included herbal medicine, massage, megavitamins, self-help groups, folk remedies, energy healing, and homeopathy. The probability of users visiting a CAM practitioner increased from 36.3% to 46.3%. CAM therapies were used most frequently for chronic conditions. Only 38.5% of patients using CAM therapies disclosed such use to their physicians. Ranzini and colleagues (5) assessed the use of CAM therapies among obstetric patients. In 463 postpartum patients surveyed, 31.3% used one or more forms of CAM therapy. The most frequent reasons for pregnant women using CAM therapy included gastrointestinal dysfunction, anxiety, nausea and vomiting, and urinary tract problems. Similarly, Gibson studied the use of herbal and other CAM therapies during pregnancy (6). Of patients, 9% reported using herbal supplements during pregnancy, and 13.3% used other forms of CAM.

Whereas in 1993 the National Institutes of Health (NIH) declared that CAM therapies were not taught widely in American medical schools, currently more than 50% of medical schools, including Harvard, Stamford, and Johns Hopkins, teach some courses in CAM (1). Criticism of CAM often alleges that many complementary therapies are not scientific and have no grounding in good research. Proponents of CAM counter that a number of treatments have been subjected to stiff scientific scrutiny. The truth, as with many accepted allopathic techniques, may lie somewhere in between. However, with a more widely accepted CAM therapy, such as acupuncture, NIH panels have examined its efficacy and have developed a consensus statement about its applications, safety, and efficacy (7). The German government's Commission E, an expert committee of physicians, pharmacologists, toxicologists, and others, have evaluated commonly used herbal medicines and published 330 monographs presenting their research findings. These monographs have been translated into English by the American Botanical Council (8). Similarly, monographs have been prepared by the British Herbal Pharmacopeia, British Herbal Compendium, the European Scientific Cooperative on Phytotherapy, and the World Health Organization (8). Thus, as CAM becomes more widely available, it also is becoming more widely subjected to the scientific scrutiny of other medical treatments.

CAM research does present some methodologic difficulties with regard to the scientific method. Conventional biomedicine tends to understand disease treatment in terms of a single intervention that is expected to have a direct and observable disease-specific outcome. In contrast, many CAM therapies consist of multiple interventions directed at correcting multiple imbalances or stimulating the body's own defenses (8). In addition, placebo controls are difficult for some complementary treatments such as acupuncture; even "sham" acupuncture may have a therapeutic effect, and it is a challenge to achieve blinding for treatments such as acupuncture and massage therapy (9).

This chapter will examine the role of CAM in a pregnant patient. In particular, we will explore possible roles for acupuncture, acupressure, chiropractic, massage and relaxation therapies, and nutritional and herbal therapies. Such treatments will be discussed within the context of pregnant patients suffering with nausea and vomiting, low back pain, and migraine. In addition, the possible role of CAM in breech presentation and labor induction will be discussed. When available, prospective, double-blinded, placebo-controlled trial studies will be presented. Many of the treatments discussed lack such strict control, but the reader is cautioned not to use this as a reason for rejecting outright any proposed treatments. Otherwise, many such treatments that are discussed in conventional medical textbooks would be considered invalid. Medicine is art and science, and the physician, at any point in time, must choose the most appropriate treatment for his or her patient based on the best available evidence and the prevailing medical wisdom.

ACUPUNCTURE

Acupuncture has been used as a mainstream therapy for at least 4,000 years in China. Acupuncture involves the insertion of sterile needles into key points of the body and often manipulating these needles to achieve a desired effect. Most practitioners use disposable needles, and the authors view this as the acceptable manner in which to practice acupuncture. The U.S. Food and Drug Administration (FDA) recently acknowledged that acupuncture needles are not experimental (7). The NIH declared that acupuncture may effectively relieve pain following dental surgery and may relieve nausea and vomiting in association with surgery, cancer chemotherapy, and pregnancy (8). The NIH further notes that the data in support of acupuncture are as strong as those for many accepted Western medical therapies. Acupuncture may be used in conjunction with heat produced by burning specific herbs, such as moxibustion, and also may be used with a form of surface stimulation called acupressure.

The seminal principle of acupuncture is Qi. Traditional Chinese medicine (TCM) holds that Qi compromises all of the essential life forces, including the spiritual, emotional, mental, and physical, that course through the human body. Although Qi is difficult to conceptualize for most Western-trained practitioners, at a simplistic level the notion of Qi may be considered the defining principle in a corpse versus a living human body. Traditional Chinese medicine holds that health is maintained by a normal flow of Qi, and disease results when Qi flow is either excessive, deficient, obstructed, or otherwise imbalanced. Traditionally, Qi is described as flowing through meridians or pathways that are analogous to nerve and vascular pathways. There are 14 primary meridians, and countless others have been described. Acupuncture points are locations in which Qi can be assessed and influenced. Research has described these sites of electrical conductions. Insertion of the fine acupuncture needles at these points, along with proper manipulation, helps regulate and restore a normal flow of Qi.

Because Qi is a difficult notion for most Western-trained physicians and scientists, more traditional research has focused on neuroendocrine and immune function alterations with acupuncture. Research studies demonstrate that acupuncture may work by any of the following mechanisms, alone or in combination (10–15):

1. Endorphin modulation
2. Enhancement of immune function
3. Alteration in antiinflammatory and cyclo-oxegenase pathways
4. Reduction in myofascial tension

In clinical practice, acupuncture needle insertions may follow standard "point prescriptions," or they may be based on what TCM calls the "pattern of illness" (16). In addition, there are other schemes that guide the acupuncturist in the formulation of point prescription, including the five element theory, French energetics, Japanese meridian theory, and others (17).

There are few well-designed prospective research studies demonstrating the clinical utility of acupuncture. Ezzo (18) conducted a retrospective study of randomized trials of acupuncture in the treatment of pain. Using MEDLINE, two complementary medicine databases, 69 conferences proceedings, and the bibliographies of other articles and reviews, 51 studies met inclusion criteria. Three-fourths of the studies received a low-quality score for scientific design. High-quality studies clustered in designs using sham acupuncture as the control group. Sham acupuncture itself has been documented to benefit patients in ways similar to a strong placebo response. Whether there are additional factors influencing sham treatment is not clear.

Nausea and Vomiting

Nausea and vomiting is a common complication of pregnancy, especially during the first trimester. This is usually a self-limiting condition, but when protracted, severe electrolyte imbalance and dehydration may adversely affect the patient, the developing fetus, or both. In addition, persistent nausea and vomiting can considerably impair the pregnant woman's quality of life. Medications to control nausea and vomiting generally are avoided during pregnancy because most are category C drugs. Both acupuncture and acupressure (which is stimulation of an acupuncture point without use of a needle) use the P6 or Neiguan acupuncture point for treatment of nausea and vomiting during pregnancy. P6 is located on the volar surface of the forearm approximately three finger breaths rostral to the wrist.

Dundee (19) compared three treatment groups in pregnant patients with nausea and vomiting. P6 acupressure was compared to acupressure at a point near the right elbow and to no treatment. Only the P6 groups showed a significant reduction in morning sickness, although there was also a reduction in symptomatology in the sham acupressure group when compared to the control. Knight (20) studied 55 patients during the first trimester, comparing traditional versus sham acupuncture for treatment of nausea. With a 95% power to detect significant differences in nausea scores, both acupuncture and sham treatment significantly reduced nausea symptomatology, but there was no difference in treatment outcome between these two groups. In a prospective, randomized, blinded study, Belluomini (21) demonstrated that P6 acupressure treatment significantly reduces nausea when compared to sham acupressure.

In patients receiving spinal anesthesia for cesarean section, acupressure is as effective as intravenous metoclopramide in preventing intraoperative nausea in the awake patient (22). Bilateral stimulation of P6 by way of acupressure also can significantly reduce the incidence of nausea and vomiting following epidural morphine administration for postcesarean section pain relief (23).

Pain

The medical literature is rather silent on the use of acupuncture for common pain syndromes during pregnancy, including low back pain and headache. Ternov and colleagues (23a) retrospectively assessed the efficacy and side-effect profile of acupuncture for low back pain and pelvic pain during the second and third trimesters of pregnancy. The cause of pain was not specified. Of 167 consecutive patients, 72% obtained good or excellent pain relief. One patient developed transient premature labor, and 21% of patients noticed transient dizziness or tiredness—a common accompaniment of acupuncture. Although the results of this study are encouraging and suggest that acupuncture is safe and effective as a treatment for low back and pelvic pain during pregnancy, controlled prospective studies are needed to confirm these findings and to better define appropriate acupuncture candidates.

In the authors' experience, acupuncture is a viable and safe alternative for treatment of noncomplicated low back pain during pregnancy, including muscle fatigue and sacroiliac dysfunction. When low back pain, neck pain, or headache are strongly correlated with muscle spasm, specific acupuncture techniques, which involve spinning the needle, lead to a clinical outcome known as myofascial release. Muscle groups initially contract and then move into a more relaxed state.

There are a few studies on the analgesic effects of acupuncture during childbirth. Ternov (24) studied 180 women, half of whom received acupuncture and the other half of whom received no treatment during labor. Acupuncture-treated patients obtained 58% pain relief without need of other treatments such as epidural analgesia or narcotics, compared to 14% in the control group. There were no side effects in the acupuncture-treated group. Methodologically, this study has limitations, and at this point, such treatment cannot be recommended for widespread use during labor.

Uterine Effects

Acupuncture can have a direct effect on the uterus. In TCM, the LI 4 acupuncture point controls uterine motility. When the LI 4 point is stimulated in pregnant rats, uterus motility is reduced 75%, and this is believed to be from an inhibition of COX-2 enzymes (25). Acupuncture also can be used to enhance uterine contractility, and, with this in mind, acupuncture is not to be taken lightly in the pregnant patient and must be performed only by an experienced acupuncturist. Dunn (26) studied the effectiveness of transcutaneous electrical stimulation at acupuncture points in 20 postdate pregnant women. Treatment patients were compared to sham patients, in which equipment was attached but not activated. The "spleen 6" (lower leg) and "liver 3" (foot) acupuncture points were used. A significant increase in frequency and strength of the uterine contractions occurred in the electrostimulated patients when compared to the placebo group. Other studies have demonstrated that electrical acupuncture significantly increases uterine contractions without maternal or fetal side effects (27,28).

In an intriguing study of pregnant patients with breech presentation between 33 and 35 weeks gestation, Cardini and Weixin (29) performed a randomized, controlled, open clinical trial. Of the 260 pregnant patients with breech presentation studied, 130 were treated with moxibustion of the BL 67 acupuncture point. At 35 weeks, 75% of the treatment group and 48% of the controls were vertex. At 35 weeks, all women who remained breech were offered external cephalic version. Risks of rupture of membranes and premature labor were more likely in the control group. Fetal movement counts were significantly higher in the treatment group, suggesting that version occurs because of increased fetal movement in this group.

CHIROPRACTIC

Chiropractic, although based on several health care traditions such as bonesetting and magnetic healing, is about 100 years old in the form it is currently known and practiced. Theoretically, chiropractic is based on the notion that mechanical impediments such as vertebral misalignment, joint immobility, and poor posture can obstruct the pathway of the body's "innate intelligence" through the human nervous system (30). Chiropractic may be summarized by a commonly-held chiropractic belief that function follows form.

That chiropractic is used widely is almost self-evident. Its acceptance, however, is much more controversial, especially among established medical practitioners. Despite its controversy, medical practitioners need to be mindful of the usefulness of chiropractic in treating low back pain, as well as the satisfaction among patients who receive such treatment. When outcome measures are assessed for patients treated with acute low back pain, there is no difference whether treatment is provided by a primary care practitioner, chiropractor, or orthopedic surgeon. However, satisfaction is greatest among patients treated by chiropractors (31). Chiropractic therapy and physical therapy provide similar effects and costs in patients with low back pain (32,33).

With regard to pregnancy and chiropractic, data are sparse. At least 5% of pregnant patients use a chiropractor (5). In a survey of certified nurse–midwives, 57% of nurse–midwives recommended chiropractic as a treatment strategy to their pregnant patients (34).

No prospective, randomized study of chiropractic care for low back pain or other symptomatic treatment during pregnancy has been performed. In a retrospective analysis of pregnant patients who sought chiropractic care and who were compared to standard obstetric care, there were no noted differences in the rates of obstetric interventions used during labor or delivery (35). In the authors' view, chiropractic is a safe and effective treatment for uncomplicated low back pain during pregnancy. Well-designed, prospective studies are needed, but the reader should be advised that although there is paucity of data for chiropractic care during pregnancy, there are also few well-designed studies for physical therapy as a treatment modality during pregnancy.

MASSAGE AND RELAXATION THERAPIES

Massage Therapy

Massage therapy is a very general description of a soothing technique in which the practitioner uses his or her hands to loosen, stimulate, or invigorate muscles and myofascial connections. There are numerous different massage therapy styles, and none has been prospectively studied in relation to one another. Field and colleagues (36) examined the comparative effects of massage and relaxation therapy on 26 pregnant women over the course of 5 weeks. Although both groups reported reduction in anxiety and leg pain, the massage therapy group alone reported a reduction in anxiety, improved mood, better sleep, and less back pain by the last day of the study. In the massage therapy group, urine norepinephrine levels decreased, and the women suffered fewer complications, including preeclampsia and premature birth. The type of massage therapy is not specified.

Perineal Massage

Perineal massage is a more specific technique in which the pregnant patient massages the perineum in an attempt to lessen the frequency, the complications, or both from epi-siotomies. When massage and stretching of the perineum with a water-soluble lubricant is limited to the second stage of labor, there is no outcome difference regarding episiotomy, pain, dyspareunia, or urinary and fecal problems (37). However, for primiparous versus multiparous patients, perineal massage beginning at 34 weeks leads to a significant reduction in perineal trauma. A dose-response relationship exists in that patients with better compliance have better results (38).

Biofeedback

Biofeedback is a technique that involves self-regulation. The patient is hooked up to a computerized device and, by way of constant feedback signals, the patient learns to regulate his or her physiology. Generally, mental imagery and relaxation techniques are used, and endpoints include measures such as an increase in limb skin temperature or a decrease in surface electromyographic (EMG) activity. Although biofeedback is more commonly accepted than other CAM therapies among neurologists, there are few prospective well-designed studies regarding biofeedback and neurologic conditions. There are even fewer in the pregnant patient. For hypertensive pregnant patients, biofeedback, without or with relaxation therapy, leads to a significant decrease in hospital admissions during pregnancy. Biofeedback-treated patients alone, or in combination with relaxation therapy, had significantly lower systolic and diastolic pressures than a control group (39). For childbirth pain, pregnant patients trained in biofeedback using surface EMG electrodes report significantly less pain than controls from the time of admission to labor and delivery and 24 hours postpartum. Biofeedback-treated patients also labored an average of 2 hours less and used 30% fewer medications (40).

Hypnotherapy

Although hypnosis is not commonly used by traditional physicians, many are comfort-able with the concept that their patients may use hypnosis as an aid to discontinue cigarette smoking. Hypnosis is provided by skilled practitioners who bring the susceptible patient into a trancelike state and then provide the patient with mental imagery or suggestions. The idea is that these suggestions then will become manifest at a targeted time during the patient's awake state. Schauble and colleagues (41) describe their experience with more than 3,000 deliveries using hypnosis. Although they provide an excellent overview of hypnosis in general for use during labor and delivery, they provide no prospective, well-designed studies of this matter. In their experience, patients experience much less need for anesthesia, have fewer premature deliveries, and have less perinatal morbidity and mortality. Studying patients who are invited to undergo hypnosis (42) and who are compared to age-match controls, significant differences are noted in both primigravid and parous women. The mean lengths of the first stage of labor and second stage of labor are both significantly diminished in the hypnotized group. In addition, the use of analgesics is reduced significantly among hypnotized patients when compared to controls.

NUTRITIONAL SUPPLEMENTATION

In the Western world, it is commonplace for obstetricians to recommend a multivitamin supplementation with folic acid and iron to their pregnant patient. Iron supplementation helps to prevent pregnancy-induced anemia (43,44). Folic acid significantly reduces the incidence of neural tube defects, especially in patients taking anticonvulsants (45). Whereas these supplements are commonplace, few practitioners raise their eyebrows regarding the lack of FDA control over vitamin, iron, and folic acid supplementation. Most align themselves with a reliable brandname product.

Other, less traditional dietary supplements may be more widespread than is commonly recognized by the unsuspecting obstetrician. Tsui and colleagues (46) documented a 13%

use of dietary supplements during pregnancy, with the most common products being echinacea, pregnancy tea, and ginger. Most patients use these supplements to help relieve nausea and vomiting. Similarly, Gibson and colleagues (47) documented a 9% use of herbal supplements during pregnancy, with the most commonly used herbs being garlic, aloe, chamomile, peppermint, ginger, echinacea, pumpkin seeds, and ginseng. Although nutritional supplementation is used more commonly for relieving nausea and vomiting, side-effect profiles are unknown from these two studies. (45,47).

The greatest difficulty the practitioner faces with regard to CAM nutritional supplementation is that available medical databases are virtually silent with regard to the safety of herbal and other nutritional supplementation during pregnancy. Although herbal remedies often are labeled as drug-free and therefore safe, the dearth of original research related to safety indicates that these compounds should be used with caution (48). Despite these shortcomings, some products deserve special mention.

Ginger

Ginger (zingiber officinale) is beneficial as a treatment for nausea during pregnancy. Ginger has become more commonly used among obstetricians. In a survey of 488 physicians, 52% recommended ginger to their patients who suffered with nausea and vomiting. Women physicians were more likely to recommend ginger and less likely to prescribe an antiemetic medication (49). Fischer-Rasmussen and colleagues demonstrated significant subjective and objective improvement in symptoms over 4 days for participants taking ginger when compared to placebo (50). Ginger may be even more effective when used in conjunction with vitamin B6 supplementation, 100 to 400 mg daily (49–51). In rat studies, ginger tea supplementation results in increased early embryo loss with increased growth in surviving fetuses (52). However, Weidner and Sigwart found no maternal or fetal toxicity when ginger was administered at daily doses of up to 1,000 mg/kg body weight during organogenesis (53). Overall, ginger supplementation appears to reduce nausea and vomiting during pregnancy without significant side effects.

Magnesium

Intravenous magnesium supplementation has an accepted, albeit somewhat controversial, role in the emergency treatment of preeclampsia. Oral magnesium supplementation during pregnancy has been used for other conditions. For pregnant patients with leg cramps, magnesium supplementation has a demonstrable benefit in decreasing leg cramp distress (54). Makrides and Crowther (55) note that many women, especially those from disadvantaged backgrounds, have intakes of magnesium below recommended levels; magnesium supplementation during pregnancy may reduce fetal growth restriction and preeclampsia in such patients. In their review of six trials involving 2,637 women, only one was judged to be of high quality. When compared with placebo, oral magnesium treatment from before the 25th week of gestation was associated with a lower incidence of preterm birth, fewer maternal hospitalizations, fewer cases of antepartum hemorrhage, and a lower incidence of low birthweight and small-for-gestational-age infants. The poor quality of these trials likely resulted in a bias favoring magnesium supplementation. Sibai and colleagues (56) found no significant difference in treatment versus control groups when prospectively assessing magnesium treatment for incidences of preeclampsia, fetal growth restriction, preterm labor, birthweight, gestational age at delivery, or number of infants admitted to the special care unit. Thus, the efficacy of magnesium supplementation during pregnancy for prevention of fetal outcome measures is, at best, equivocal.

Other

The role of antioxidants in pregnancy is unclear. In one randomized, prospective-con-

TABLE 22.1. *Nutritional supplement
contraindications during pregnancy*

Alder buckthorn
Aloes
Angelica
Arnica
Autumn crocus
Barberry
Bethroot
Black cohosh
Broom
Butternut
Calamus
Calendula
Cascara sagrada
Coltsfoot
Cowslip
Damiana
Dong quai
Ephedra (ma huang)
Feverfew
Ginseng (Panax quinquefolia)
Goat's rue
Goldenseal
Gotu kola
Ipecac
Juniper berries
Licorice
Lily of the valley
Lobelia
Male fern
Mandrake
Mistletoe
Mugwort
Nutmeg
Pennyroyal
Periwinkle
Peruvian bark
Pleurisy root
Poke root
Rue
Rhubarb
Sage
Sarsaparilla
Senna
Shepherd's purse
Stillingia
Tansy
Thuja
Wormwood
Yarrow

trolled trial, vitamin C and vitamin E supplementation were used in patients with increased risk of preeclampsia. Markers of vascular endothelial activation and placental insufficiency were significantly reduced in the treated group. Preeclampsia developed in 18% of treated patients compared to 78% of controls. There were no reported side effects

of supplementation. This study, although showing some promise, does not have large statistical power (57).

Calcium supplementation has been studied as a treatment for pregnancy-induced hypertension. When compared with controls, supplementation with calcium (2 gm daily) showed significant results in lowering the incidence of pregnancy-induced hypertension. Larger studies are needed to confirm these results (58).

A Note of Caution

Because of the lack of research in the area of botanical medicine in pregnancy, a good rule is that nutritional and herbal supplementation, especially during the first trimester, should be used in pregnancy only when necessary (59). Although negative effects or contraindications of nutritional supplements during pregnancy receive little attention in the literature, Table 22.1 lists those products that should not be used during pregnancy (59). It is important for the obstetrician to discuss nutritional supplements with her or her patient to be certain that any supplements are being used in accordance with good medical care.

CONCLUSION

It is undeniable that there are few rigorously designed, double-blinded, placebo-controlled studies regarding the use of CAM during pregnancy. Despite this lack of conventional evidence, there is ample, credible documentation of some CAM treatments that offer efficacy and safety for the pregnant patient. Especially in light of the risk that many conventional medical treatments pose to the developing fetus and mother, some CAM modalities represent viable and safe options. Future research is faced with the task of adapting current experimental guidelines to account for the unique considerations of CAM studies. Because well-established trends among patients and within medical schools make it clear that an interest in CAM will continue to grow during this new century, it is up to us to provide evidenced-based guidance for its safe and effective use.

REFERENCES

1. Ko G. Practical overview of "complementary & alternative" medicine. *Natural Medicine Journal* April 1999: 16–20.
2. Aikins Murphy P. Alternative therapies for nausea and vomiting of pregnancy. *Obstet Gynecol* 1998;91: 149–155.
3. Pizzorno JE, Murray MT, eds. *Textbook of natural medicine.* New York: Churchill Livingstone, 1999.
4. Eisenberg DM, Davis RB, Ettner SL, et al. Trends in alternative medicine used in the United States. *JAMA* 2000;283:884–886.
5. Ranzini A, Allen A, Lai Y. Use of complementary medicines and therapies among obstetric patients. *Obstet Gynecol* 2001;97:S46.
6. Gibson PS, Powrie R, Star J. Herbal and alternative medicine use during pregnancy: a cross sectional survey. *Obstet Gynecol* 2001;97:44–45.
7. Hsu DT. Acupuncture. A review. *Reg Anesth* 1996;21: 361–370.
8. Murphy PA, Kronenberg F, Wade C. Complementary and alternative medicine in women's health. Developing a research agenda. *J Nurse Midwifery* 1999;44: 193–194.
9. Murphy PA. Alternative therapies for nausea and vomiting of pregnancy. *Obstet Gynecol* 1998;91:151–153.
10. Syrop S. Acupuncture: a scientific review and clinical applications. *Ann Dent* 1998;2:4–5,9.
11. Pomeranz B. Scientific research into acupuncture for relief of pain. *J Altern Complement Med* 1996;2:53–60.
12. Sommers B. Chinese medicine and acupuncture in the treatment of AIDS. *Sidahora* 1995;Oct–Nov:37–38.
13. Wu B, Zhou RX, Zhou MS. Effect of acupuncture on immunomodulation in patients with malignant tumors. *Zhongguo Zhong Xi Yi Jie He Za Zhi* 1996;16:139–141.
14. Wu B. Effect of acupuncture on the regulation of cell-mediated immunity in the patients with malignant tumors. *Zhen Ci Yan Jiu* 1995;20:67–71.
15. Petti F, Bangrazi A, Liguori A, et al. Effects of acupuncture on immune response related to opioid-like peptides. *J Tradit Chin Med* 1998;18:55–63.
16. Dahlgren C. Acupuncture. *STEP Perspect* 1998;98: 19–20.
17. Diehl D. Acupuncture for gastrointestinal and hepatobiliary disorders. *J Altern Complement Med* 1999;5: 28–30.
18. Ezzo J, Berman B. Is acupuncture effective for the treatment of chronic pain? A systemic review. *Pain* 2000; 86:217–225.
19. Dundee JW, Sourial FB, Ghaly RG, et al. P6 acupressure reduces morning sickness. *J R Soc Med* 1998;81: 456–457.
20. Knight B, Mudge C, Openshaw S, et al. Effect of acupuncture on nausea of pregnancy: a randomized, controlled trial. *Obstet Gynecol* 2001;97:184–188.
21. Belluomini J, Litt RC, Lee KA, et al. Acupressure for nausea and vomiting of pregnancy: a randomized, blinded study. *Obstet Gynecol* 1994;84:245–248.
22. Stein DJ, Birnbach DJ, Danzer BI, et al. Acupressure versus intravenous metoclopramide to prevent nausea and vomiting during spinal anesthesia for cesarean section. *Anesth Analg* 1997;84:342–345.
23. Ho CM, Hseu SS, Tsai SK, et al. Effect of P-6 acupressure on prevention of nausea and vomiting after epidural morphine for post-cesarean section pain relief. *Acta Anaesthesiol Scand* 1996;40:372–375.
23a. Ternov NK, Grennert L, Aberg A, et al. Acupuncture for lower back and pelvic pain in late pregnancy: a retrospective report on 167 consecutive cases. *Pain Medicine* 2001;2:204–207.
24. Ternov K, Nilsson M, Lofberg L, et al. Acupuncture for pain relief during childbirth. *Acupunct Electrother Res* 1998;23:19–26.
25. Kim J, Shin KH, Na CS. Effect of acupuncture treatment on uterine motility and cyclooxygenase-2 expression in pregnant rats. *Gynecol Obstet Invest* 2000; 50:225–230.
26. Dunn PA, Rogers D, Halford K. Transcutaneous electrical nerve stimulation at acupuncture points in the induction of uterine contractions. *Obstet Gynecol* 1989; 73:286–290.
27. Yip SK, Pang JC, Sung ML. Induction of labor by acupuncture electro-stimulation. *Am J Chin Med* 1976; 4:257–265.
28. Kubista E, Kucera H, Muller-Tyl E. Initiating contractions of the gravid uterus through electro-acupuncture. *Am J Chin Med* 1975;3:343–346.
29. Cardini F, Weixin H. Moxibustion for correction of breech presentation: a randomized controlled trial. *JAMA* 1998;280:1580–1584.
30. Kaptchuk TJ, Eisenberg DM. Chiropractic: origins, controversies, and contributions. *Arch Intern Med* 1998; 158:2215–2224.
31. Carey TS, Garrett J, Jackman A, et al. The outcomes and costs of care for acute low back pain among patients seen by primary care practitioners, chiropractors, and orthopedic surgeons. *N Engl J Med* 1995;333:913–917.
32. Cherkin DC, Deyo RA, Battie M, et al. A comparison of physical therapy, chiropractic manipulation and provision of an educational booklet for the treatment of patients with low back pain. *N Engl J Med* 1998;339: 1021–1029.
33. Skargren EI, Carlsson PG, Oberg BE. One-year follow-up comparison of the cost and effectiveness of chiropractic and physiotherapy as primary management for back pain. Subgroup analysis, recurrence, and additional health care utilization. *Spine* 1998;23: 1875–1883.
34. Krantz CK. Chiropractic care in pregnancy. *Midwifery Today Int Midwife* 1999;52:16–17.
35. Phillips CJ, Meyer JJ. Chiropractic care, including craniosacral therapy, during pregnancy: a static-group comparison of obstetric interventions during labor and delivery. *J Manipulative Physiol Ther* 1995;18:525–529.
36. Field T, Hernandez-Reif M, Hart S, et al. Pregnant woman benefit from massage therapy. *J Psychosom Obstet Gynaecol* 1999;20:31–38.
37. Stamp G, Kruzins G, Crowther C. Perineal massage in labour and prevention of perineal trauma: randomized controlled trial. *BMJ* 2001;332:1277–1280.
38. Labrecque M, Eason E, Marcoux S, et al. Randomized controlled trial of prevention of perineal trauma by perineal massage during pregnancy. *Am J Obstet Gynecol* 1999;180:593–600.
39. Little BC, Hayworth J, Benson, P, et al. Treatment of hy-

pertension in pregnancy by relaxation and biofeedback. *Lancet* 1984;1:865–867.

40. Duchene P. Effects of biofeedback on childbirth pain. *J Pain Symptom Manage* 1989;4:117–123.

41. Schauble PG, Werner WE, Rai SH, et al. Childbirth preparation through hypnosis: the hypnoreflexogenous protocol. *Am J Clin Hypn* 1998;40:273–283.

42. Jenkins MW, Pritchard MH. Hypnosis: practical applications and theoretical considerations in normal labour. *Br J Obstet Gynaecol* 1993;100:221–226.

43. de Onis M, Villar J, Gulmezoglu M. Nutritional interventions to prevent intrauterine growth retardation: evidence from randomized controlled trials. *Eur J Clin Nutr* 1998;52:S83–S93.

44. Villar J, Gulmezoglu AM, de Onis M. Nutritional and antimicrobial interventions to prevent preterm birth: an overview of randomized controlled trial. *Obstet Gynecol Surv* 1998;53:575–585.

45. Nulman I, Laslo D, Koren G. Treatment of epilepsy in pregnancy. *Drugs* 1999;57:535–544.

46. Tsui B, Dennehy CE, Tsourounis C. A survey of dietary supplement use during pregnancy at an academia medical center. *Am J Obstet Gynecol* 2001;185:433–437.

47. Gibson PS, Powrie R, Star J. Herbal and alternative medicine use during pregnancy: a cross-sectional survey. *Obstet Gynecol* 2001;97:44–45.

48. Wilkinson JM. What do we know about herbal morning sickness treatments? A literature survey. *Midwifery* 2000;16:224–228.

49. Jewell D, Young G. Interventions for nausea and vomiting in early pregnancy. *Cochrane Database Syst Rev* 2000;2:CD000145.

50. Fischer-Rasmussen W, Kjaer SK, Dahl C, et al. Ginger treatment of hyperemesis gravidarum. *Eur J Obstet Gynecol Reprod Biol* 1991;38:19–24.

51. Power ML, Holzman BG, Schulkin J. A survey on the management of nausea and vomiting in pregnancy by obstetrician/gynecologists. *Prim Care Update Ob Gyns* 2001;8:69–72.

52. Wilkinson JM. Effect of ginger tea on the fetal development of Sprague-Dawley rats. *Reprod Toxicol* 2000; 14:507–512.

53. Weidner MS, Sigwart K. Investigation of the teratogenic potential of a zingiber officinale extract in the rat. *Reprod Toxicol* 2001;15:75–80.

54. Dahle LO, Berg G, Hammar M, et al. The effect of oral magnesium substitution on pregnancy-induced leg cramps. *Am J Obstet Gynecol* 1995;175:223–224.

55. Makrides M, Crowther CA. Magnesium supplementation in pregnancy. *Cochrane Database Syst Rev* 2000; 2:CD000937.

56. Sibai BM, Villar MA, Bray E. Magnesium supplementation: a double-blind randomized controlled clinical trial. *Am J Obstet Gynecol* 1989;161:115–119.

57. Chappell LC, Seed PT, Briley AL. Effect of antioxidants on the occurrence of pre-eclampsia in women at increased risk: a randomized trial. *Lancet* 1999;354: 810–816.

58. Cong K, Chi S, Liu G. Calcium supplementation during pregnancy for reducing pregnancy induced hypertension. *Chin Med J (Engl)* 1995;108:57–59.

59. Yarnell E. Botanical medicine in pregnancy and lactation. *Alternative and Complementary Therapies* 1997;3: 93–99.

Neurological Complications of Pregnancy, Second
Edition, edited by Brian Hainline and Orrin Devinsky.
Lippincott Williams & Wilkins, Philadelphia, © 2002.

23

Legal Issues: Roles of Physicians in Preventing Fetal Harm

H. Richard Beresford

Department of Neurology, University of Rochester School of Medicine, Rochester, New York, U.S.A.

The public interest in protecting the human fetus is strong and enduring. *Roe v. Wade* (1) affords constitutional protection to the liberty of a woman to choose to abort her fetus. Nonetheless, Supreme Court decisions also empower states to limit the exercise of this fundamental right once a fetus is deemed viable (1–3). The boundaries of state power in this regard remain somewhat ill defined. There is little doubt, however, that states have the constitutional power to enact and enforce laws designed to prevent fetal harm. These include laws requiring that licensed medical professionals be involved in the process of abortion, laws regulating the prescription of fetotoxic drugs, and laws enabling civil and criminal actions against persons charged with wrongfully harming a fetus. This chapter will focus on the role physicians play in the operation of such laws, whether they be laws of general application or laws explicitly aimed at fetal protection. Two dimensions of this role will be considered: (i) the physician as a target of social control and (ii) the physician as an agent of social control. The illustrative legal paradigms are a medical malpractice case that invokes the doctrine of informed consent as a device for achieving fetal protection and state regulatory statutes that enlist physicians in coercive programs with respect to pregnant women who are substance abusers or are infected with human immunodeficiency virus (HIV).

PHYSICIANS AS TARGETS OF SOCIAL CONTROL

Malpractice Claims

Physicians who care for women who are or may become pregnant hardly need reminding of legal overtones. A pregnancy that results in unwanted fetal loss or a deformed or diseased child can produce emotional devastation, financial hardship, and anger at treating physicians. Such consequences can be potent stimuli for malpractice claims (4). Although defendants in medical malpractice cases more often than not prevail, the loss rate and median jury awards tend to be higher in cases where harm to the fetus or neonate is asserted than in other medical injury cases (5). The high malpractice insurance premiums obstetricians pay accordingly reflect the large damage awards and out-of-court settlements with respect to claims for prenatal or neonatal injuries (6). Indeed, concerns about the undesirable fiscal and social impact of huge awards and settlements deriving from these claims have provoked calls for caps on damages and other reforms (7). Also, some states legislatures have enacted special laws for adjudicating fetal injury claims and spreading the costs of compensating for fetal and neonatal injuries among other medical providers and the public (8).

The crux of any malpractice claim is an assertion that a physician failed to meet reasonable or accepted standards of medical practice. Put another way, the defendant allegedly has committed an error that a prudent physician would have avoided. The error can be one of three general types: (i) a *technical* error (e.g., slip of the scalpel, illegible prescription), (ii) a *judgmental* error (e.g., misdiagnosis, inappropriate treatment), (iii) or a *normative* error (e.g., ethical lapse). Obviously, not all errors constitute medical malpractice. Some are difficult for even careful and competent professionals to avoid. Some do not result in demonstrable harm to patients and are therefore not compensable. Some are of the sort that no qualified medical expert is willing to call them malpractice. Errors most likely to sustain malpractice litigation are those that produce demonstrable physical or psychologic injury, generate large medical expenses or loss of income, or are committed by physicians who are perceived as inept or uncaring (7). Among such errors is a failure to obtain informed consent with respect to a choice that turns out badly. An error of this genre will serve to illustrate how law can be applied to target physicians in a way that promotes fetal protection.

The Harbeson Case: Informed Consent As Fetal Protection

Harbeson v. Parke Davis, Inc. (9) displays a sharp judicial response to an alleged failure of physicians to disclose information crucial to a reproductive choice. At issue was an alleged adverse effect of phenytoin on fetal development. However, the case has broad implications for a range of clinical situations involving care of women of childbearing age.

The suit was brought by parents in their own capacity and as representatives of their afflicted children. Mrs. Harbeson had developed generalized epilepsy in 1970 while pregnant with Michael, her first child. Phenytoin (Dilantin) was prescribed, seizures did not recur, and a healthy Michael was born in 1971. In 1972 and 1973, Mrs. Harbeson told two different physicians at an Army hospital where she was receiving care that she was considering having more children but was concerned about the fetal risks of taking phenytoin during pregnancy. Each physician told her that hirsutism and cleft palate were potential complications, but neither mentioned "fetal hydantoin syndrome" as a potential risk nor conducted further inquiry into the potential toxicity of phenytoin. She then elected to continue taking phenytoin and had two more children, Elizabeth in 1974 and Christine in 1975. Each subsequently was diagnosed as having fetal hydantoin syndrome, manifested as growth and developmental retardation, hypoplastic digits, and craniofacial dysmorphism.

Mrs. Harbeson and her husband then filed suit in federal court in the state of Washington, naming as defendants the federal government (as employer of the physicians) and the manufacturer of phenytoin. The core of their claim was that the Army physicians carelessly assessed the fetal risks of phenytoin and thereby infringed their rights as parents to make an informed choice about further childbearing. As remedies for these alleged wrongs, the Harbesons sought damages for themselves for the "wrongful birth" of Elizabeth and Christine and, on their daughters' behalf, for "wrongful life." After hearing expert medical testimony that fetal hydantoin syndrome is a known risk of ingesting phenytoin during pregnancy, the federal court concluded that the physicians had been negligent and that the government should pay damages to the Harbesons. For guidance in calculating damages, the federal court asked the Washington Supreme Court to provide an opinion as to whether state law permitted assessing damages for "wrongful birth" or "wrongful life."

The Washington court determined that damages were payable for such claims. It underscored the failure of the Army physicians to learn more about the fetal risks of phenytoin and the pivotal effect incomplete disclosure had on the parental decision to have more children. In other words, the physicians were held blameworthy because they did not bother to seek more information about phenytoin when they knew—or should have known—that the parents were relying on them for help in making a childbearing decision. As to the calculation of damages, the Washington court decided that the parents were entitled to recover medical and special educational expenses in excess of those projected for raising two normal daughters. They also were found entitled to an award for the pain and suffering linked to the bearing and raising of their impaired daughters. For the daughters "wrongful life" claim, the court restricted assessable damages to the costs of treatment and training beyond those required for normal children once they have reached adulthood. The court declined to approve damages for the daughters' pain and suffering. It reasoned that such damages were incalculable because of the impossibility of quantifying the difference between the value of impaired life and no life at all.

The Constitutional Aspect of Reproductive Choice

In a narrow sense, *Harbeson* is merely one more medical malpractice case in which physicians were found to have violated accepted standards of practice, thereby causing harm to persons whom they owed a duty of care. Yet *Harbeson* is more than an ordinary malpractice case. The wrong to the parents was characterized as a violation of their right to make an informed choice about childbearing, a matter of fundamental personal significance. Were it not for *Roe v. Wade*—even as diluted by later decisions of the Supreme Court (2,3)—the claim of the parents for compensation keyed to infringement of reproductive choice might have seemed less compelling. Given the constitutional protection afforded reproductive choice, however, the Washington court's willingness to allow the parents damages for their own pain and suffering is more readily comprehended. In this respect, *Harbeson* is a potentially valuable precedent for any malpractice claimant who is asserting that a physician's misconduct impaired her right to make informed decisions about pregnancy or childbearing.

Harbeson did not, of course, explicitly implicate abortion rights. At issue was a parental decision whether to have more children, not whether to terminate a pregnancy. Yet the Washington court recognized the import of *Roe v. Wade* in conferring special status on the right of parents to make the "difficult moral choice" to avoid the birth of a defective child. In this respect, the reasoning of *Harbeson* parallels that of judicial decisions in several states other than Washington that permit "wrongful birth" actions for negligent failure to diagnose or predict disorders amenable to prenatal diagnosis, such as chromosomal trisomies, neural tube defects, and Tay-Sachs disease (10). Parents in some of these cases asserted that had timely prenatal diagnosis been made, they would have opted for abortion to avoid bearing defective children.

Partly because cases of this sort raise the divisive issue of abortion rights, some legislatures have sought to constrain or bar claims for "wrongful birth" or "wrongful life" (11). For example, a Minnesota statute bars claims based on an allegation that, but for a medical provider's wrongful act or omission, an impaired child would have been aborted (12). The state Supreme Court upheld the constitutionality of this statute as applied to a suit by parents of a child born with Down syndrome (13). The parents had alleged that physicians were negligent in failing to perform amniocentesis despite the mother's relatively advanced age, and that, if amniocentesis had confirmed the chromosomal trisomy, the mother would have opted for abortion. The court reasoned that the statute did not, on its face, impair her constitutional liberty to obtain an abortion, but merely limited the grounds on which civil suits could be brought in state courts. Critics of the Minnesota law, and other similar statutes, understandably view them as a barely concealed effort to undermine reproductive freedom by selectively barring a legal remedy that could deter attempts to undermine that freedom by knowingly withholding information that could influence parental choice.

Standard of Care

Constitutional questions aside, *Harbeson* confronts the issue of what constitutes acceptable standards of care for woman contemplating reproductive decisions. Both federal and state courts perceived normative error on the part of Mrs. Harbeson's attending physicians. Their failure to better inform themselves about the risks of phenytoin was found professionally wanting. That they communicated what they did know about its adverse effects was not enough. In the courts' view, they should have gone to the books or asked more knowledgeable colleagues for help. The implication was that they would have learned about fetal hydantoin syndrome and that disclosing what they learned to the potential parents was part of the professional standard of care. It is interesting to speculate what weight the courts would have attached to a disclosure that phenytoin had a no greater than 5% risk of causing specific physical or cognitive impairments (including the ones that actually materialized) but that omitted mention of fetal hydantoin syndrome. Such a disclosure should be legally sufficient, despite the apparent special significance the courts seemed to attach to the notion that the parents were not told of a specific "syndrome."

To be entitled to damages on a claim alleging failure to obtain informed consent, claimants ordinarily must prove they would have made a different choice had adequate disclosure been provided (14,15). The mere assertion by the Harbesons that they would have deferred further childbearing if properly informed does not seem proof enough. Indeed other parents have chosen to have children after adequate disclosures about fetal risks of phenytoin. However, parents will predictably differ in risk tolerance, and courts will take this into account in weighing post-hoc assertions about the decisional impact of inadequate disclosure of risk. In *Harbeson,* both the state and federal courts accepted the parents' version of what they would have done in response to being told of the risk of fetal hydantoin syndrome. The judges apparently believed that knowledge of a small risk of this disorder would be a reasonable basis for a parental decision to have no more children. One message of *Harbeson*, therefore, is that, even if the experience of physicians has been that most adequately informed prospective parents choose to accept a particular genetic or other risk, that risk should nevertheless be disclosed if neither remote nor trivial.

A common justification for wrongful birth actions is that they deter physicians from negligence in prenatal diagnosis and counseling. This is a facet of the familiar—but empirically unsubstantiated—contention that the threat of a malpractice suit has social utility beyond compensating victims of iatrogenic harm. In the realm of prenatal care, the threat of suit arguably induces physicians to inquire more carefully into genetic and other risks and to use available diagnostic technologies more appropriately. The inference is, of course, that without such a threat physicians will be less scrupulous in observing prevailing professional standards of care. Although this argument may have an intuitive appeal, it is difficult to validate. It also does not take into account how imprecise, costly, and inefficient malpractice litigation is as a way of exercising social control over the conduct of physicians.

Calculating Damages for Fetal Harm

The approach of the state court in *Harbeson* was to compensate the parents for the incremental costs of caring for their afflicted children and for their own pain and suffering as parents of such children. As for the affected children, they were held entitled to the projected costs of their specialized care as adults. They were denied recovery for their own pain and suffering. The court conceded they had been wronged by the physicians to the extent of being born with a condition that necessitated compensable special care. It found it impossible, however, to calculate in monetary terms the pain and suffering resulting from their births, reasoning that such a calculation would necessitate comparing impaired life with nonexistence.

Other courts have taken a different tack in calculating damages for wrongful birth or wrongful life. For example, one approach is to award damages to parents only for *their* pain and suffering (16). The rationale here is that the essential harm is the infringement of parental liberty that inheres in nondisclosure of fetal risks. Calculating damages attributable to being born in an impaired state is seen as too speculative or as reflecting a socially unacceptable view that life with a disability is of less value than a "normal" life. A contrasting approach is to award parents only economic damages, such as incremental medical and custodial costs, because of the problem of measuring the suffering of parents who have borne a child they claim they would have aborted or not conceived had they been properly informed (17). Courts that permit impaired children to recover damages for wrongful life generally follow *Harbeson* in limiting recovery to economic damages and denying payment for pain and suffering. However, a dissenting judge in a recent New Jersey case involving a child with congenital rubella advocated paying damages to the child for suffering attributable to his "impaired childhood" (18). These differing judicial responses reflect the lingering controversy over whether wrongful birth and wrongful life claims should serve purely compensatory goals or should include elements of deterrence or retribution as well.

PHYSICIANS AS AGENTS OF SOCIAL CONTROL

Context

Pregnant women who abuse drugs or decline treatment for infection with HIV risk substantial harm to their fetuses (19–23). This understandably has evoked calls for interventions that would reduce the risk, including aggressive outreach, timely treatment, and coercive laws. All such interventions require participation of physicians if they are to be effective. The most problematic from a legal viewpoint are coercive laws that pit the rights of pregnant women to be free from unwanted or unsought personal intrusions against the public interest in fetal protection (24). At the center of any such conflict are physicians and other health care providers. They will identify and quantify risks, make required disclosures to law enforcement officials, and deliver mandated treatments. In this sense, they are asked to conflate their clinical roles with their public duties and become agents of social control. Some clinicians will be uncomfortable in this role but may accept it because of the overriding importance of trying to protect a fetus from potentially avoidable harms.

A public choice to use coercion against pregnant women implies a consensus that coercion is a productive strategy for controlling drug abuse or other forms of self-preferring behaviors. On a more basic level, opting for coercion may satisfy a civic desire to punish those who selfishly disregard the interests of their unborn children, regardless of whether the threat of detention or punishment actually influences the targeted behavior. From either perspective, it may be of little significance that there is no consensus on the proposition that a threat of punishment deters drug use or other antisocial behavior. Pregnant women are arguably a special case because they can be presumed to have a strong interest in protecting their unborn children and, therefore, may be more responsive to measures that have little impact on other drug users or HIV-infected persons.

The centerpiece of the ensuing discussion is the decision of the U.S. Supreme Court in *Ferguson v. City of Charleston* (25). The decision promises to have a considerable impact on future lawmaking aimed at achieving fetal protection and on the role of physicians in this effort.

The *Ferguson* case was decided on a backdrop of two contrasting formulations of the relationship between mother and fetus. In one, the mother and fetus are seen as separate legal persons, one a wrongdoer and one an innocent victim. In this formulation, the public interest—and that of law and medicine—is to protect the innocent victim. The mother thus becomes a target for social control through the legal system, and her physician assumes a role different from that of a conventional caregiver. The mother's liberty to ingest or inject whatever she wishes or cannot resist, or her liberty to decline unwanted treatment, is no longer a purely private matter. Also, her physician is no longer bound to respect her autonomy or confidentiality with respect to actions designed to protect the fetus.

An alternative formulation envisions mother and fetus as an integrated entity to whom society owes special solicitude. In this construct, mother and fetus are seen as too closely joined to allow for a conflict between maternal and fetal rights. Practitioners of law and medicine thus should collaborate in efforts to assure that mother and fetus together receive the best care society has to offer. These efforts might include specialized education and counseling by physicians and other qualified people, legislative appropriation of funds adequate to support programs of treatment and rehabilitation, and removal of legal or other obstacles that discourage women from seeking prenatal care or treatment for substance abuse or HIV infection.

Choice of formulation could influence the shape of public policies affecting substance abuse or HIV infection in pregnant women, and the nature of these policies would do much to define the physician's role. If a predominantly coercive approach that emphasizes maternal–fetal conflict were chosen, the state would expect physicians to collaborate in identifying women who are endangering their fetuses and in implementing measures to protect the unborn. If a more therapeutically oriented approach were selected, the challenge for physicians would be the more familiar one of trying to secure compliance with treatments for women whose capacity to control their own conduct may be severely compromised.

Control Through Coercion:
Ferguson v. City of Charleston

The Regulatory Program

The focus of judicial attention in this case was a joint effort of clinicians at the Charleston medical center of the Medical University of South Carolina (MUSC) and local law enforcement officials. The goal of the collaboration was to identify pregnant users of cocaine and to induce them, through threat of arrest and criminal prosecution, to accept referral for treatment. Under South Carolina law, the transplacental delivery of cocaine or other illicit drugs from mother to a viable fetus (24 weeks or older) is punishable as criminal child neglect (26). The collaboration originated from concerns of some clinicians about an apparent increase in cocaine use among pregnant women being cared for at MUSC.

Under the policy first implemented in the fall of 1989, urine samples of all pregnant women seeking maternity care at MUSC were screened for cocaine if any of the following indicia of cocaine use was present: (a) placental separation from uterine wall, (b) intrauterine fetal death, (c) no prenatal care, (d) prenatal care beginning after 24 weeks, (e) fewer than five prenatal visits, (f) preterm labor without obvious cause, (g) history of cocaine use, (h) unexplained birth defects, or (i) intrauterine growth retardation without obvious cause.

If a urine test was positive for cocaine, the result was reported to the South Carolina Police Department or the Solicitor's Office for the judicial circuit encompassing Charleston. Before early 1990, a woman who tested positive was arrested and charged with the crime of distributing cocaine to a minor child. Thereafter, she was offered a choice between arrest and drug treatment. If she opted for treatment, the test result was not forwarded to law enforcement officials and no arrest was made unless she tested positive for cocaine during treatment or failed to comply with treatment obligations. An arrested woman could avoid actual prosecution by successfully completing a drug treatment program, whereupon the criminal charges would be dropped.

The Legal Challenge

Ten women who had been arrested pursuant to this policy brought suit in federal district court against the City of Charleston as owner of the medical center, several individual physicians involved in implementing the policy, and various law enforcement officials. For none of the claimants had a warrant been obtained before urine testing or before results were turned over to law enforcement officials. Moreover, the consent forms the women signed for urine testing did not disclose that drug test results would be shared with law enforcement officials. The plaintiffs alleged several theories of liability. For purposes of discussion here, the most pertinent allegations were (a) infringement by the state upon constitutionally protected privacy (liberty) and (b) violation by the state of the prohibition against unreasonable searches and seizures embodied in the Fourth Amendment to the Constitution.

The Judicial Response

The federal trial court ruled, as a matter of law, that plaintiffs were not entitled to damages for violation of privacy. Jury trial was held with respect to the Fourth Amendment claim, and the jury returned a verdict for the defendants. These rulings were upheld by the 8th Circuit Court of Appeals (186 F. 3d 469). On the Fourth Amendment claim, the circuit court conceded that urine testing amounted to a "search" in the constitutional sense, but ruled that no warrant was required prior to urine testing because the MUSC officials had "special needs" for the information the searches yielded. The court emphasized the "documented health hazards of maternal cocaine use and the resulting drain on social resources" as factors underlying the "substantial" state interest in testing. It also underscored the effectiveness of urine testing for documenting maternal cocaine use and the minimal intrusiveness of this mode of testing. On the privacy issue, the court ruled that interests of the claimants in preserving confidentiality of their personal medical information was outweighed by the "compelling" governmental interest in identifying maternal cocaine use. In reaching this conclusion, it also stressed the nonpublic nature of the disclosure of results of drug testing.

The Supreme Court Decision

In pressing the Supreme Court to hear an appeal, the Center for Reproductive Law and Policy, representing the ten original plaintiffs, argued that the circuit court decision would, if left standing, allow law enforcement agencies to engage in searches without a warrant to gain evidence for prosecution merely by citing a health or safety justification. In this vein, Center lawyers emphasized that most applications of criminal law serve some health or safety purpose (27).

The Supreme Court, by a vote of 7–2, reversed the decision of the circuit court (25). In an opinion written by Justice Stevens, the Court held that urine tests were "searches" under the Fourth Amendment and that reporting of positive test results to the police made the searches unreasonable unless the women had consented to the reporting of test results. The case was thereupon remanded to the federal trial court for a determination of whether the women had consented to what would otherwise have been unlawful searches. The Court rejected the argument that the searches were justified by "special needs" and emphasized their law enforcement purpose. The dissenting justice viewed the searches as consensual because the women had consented to providing urine samples and argued that the state's program had legitimate health benefits independent of its law enforcement goal.

As a result of the Supreme Court's ruling, lawmakers in other states may conclude that a coercive approach of the type attempted by South Carolina with respect to pregnant drug users is no longer feasible. The impact is less clear, however, with respect to state laws that mandate testing of pregnant women for HIV infection or that mandate treatment with antiretroviral agents to prevent intrauterine or perinatal transmission of HIV. In the first place, equating maternal substance abuse with maternal HIV infection poses factual and conceptual difficulties. Women presumably do not choose to become infected with HIV, however reckless they may be in exposing themselves to the risk of infection, and they clearly do not gain any psychic or other rewards from being infected. However, both cocaine abusers and HIV-infected women can substantially reduce the risk of harm to their fetuses if they accept timely treatment, either by participating in a drug treatment program or accepting enough zidovudine or other antiretroviral drug to prevent intrauterine or perinatal transmission (22).

Two recent state appellate court decisions that address the rights of pregnant women to reject medical treatments are of interest here. In one, an Illinois court upheld the right of a pregnant woman with a placental defect to decline a cesarean section that her attending physician and a consultant believed was necessary to prevent her child from dying or incurring severe hypoxic brain injury (28). The woman had cited strongly held religious beliefs as the basis for refusing surgery. In explaining its ruling, the court asserted that "a woman is under no duty to guarantee the mental and physical health of her child at birth, and thus cannot be compelled to do or not do anything merely for the benefit of her unborn child." Similarly, a District of Columbia court ruled that a pregnant woman with end-stage cancer could not be compelled to undergo cesarean section to give her unborn child a better chance of survival (29). She had declined the surgery out of fear it would hasten her own death. The court declared that the determinative factor was the woman's competent choice and that it would be legally inappropriate to try to balance the interests of the fetus against those of the mother.

These cases suggest that a competent pregnant woman cannot be forced to accept risky treatments that could protect her unborn child from neurologic or other harms. It can be argued, of course, that ingesting antiretroviral drugs is sufficiently distinguishable from undergoing major surgery as to make the rulings in these cases irrelevant to the question of whether coerced treatment with antiretroviral agents is lawful. Thus, being forced to take

antiretroviral agents could be analogized to a coercive blood transfusion, which one appellate court has held can be administered over the objections of a pregnant Jehovah's Witness so as to protect her unborn child (30). Although most courts have ruled otherwise with respect to nonconsensual transfusions, some lawmakers may view forced pill-taking to prevent transmission of HIV as a public health measure akin to nonconsensual vaccination against communicable diseases, an intrusion that the Supreme Court long ago held to be a constitutionally permissible exercise of a state's police power (31).

Control Through Coercion: Civil Detention

Rather than subjecting pregnant substance abusers or HIV-infected women to the burden and stigma of criminal prosecution, lawmakers might opt for some sort of civil detention. Existing state laws already permit the involuntary commitment of certain mentally ill persons to public hospitals or treatment programs. These laws are constitutional so long as procedural due process is observed (32) and an appropriate level of treatment is provided (33). However, substance abuse may not qualify as a mental illness of the sort that would justify involuntary detention, and the constitutional adequacy of institutional compulsory drug treatment programs may be contestable. Moreover, infection with HIV would not in itself qualify as a mental illness for purposes of involuntary commitment. Thus, existing involuntary commitment laws probably would have to be amended, or new targeted statutes would have to be enacted, before civil detention can be used as a way of forcing pregnant substance abusers or HIV-infected women to undergo treatment. State legislators may find this approach more palatable than trying to use deterrence-oriented criminal statutes against pregnant women. For example, a bill proposed to the New York legislature in 1999 to create a crime of reckless endangerment of public health by knowingly engaging in conduct that risks transmission of HIV specifically excludes birthing women who transmit HIV to their children (34). Even if civil detention is seen as a preferred approach, however, the enabling statutes must contain adequate procedural protections for targeted women and provide for treatment that will serve the goal of fetal protection.

Control Through Coercion: Removal of Custody

Once a child has been born to a woman who abused drugs during pregnancy or is HIV-infected, existing child abuse and neglect laws may enable public officials to assume custody of the newborn (35). Some form of judicial proceeding ordinarily will be necessary before custody can be transferred. In such a proceeding, the question may arise as to whether maternal drug use or HIV infection in and of itself warrants removal of the child from the mother. The answer may depend on the court's view of the purpose of removal. If punishment of the mother is seen as the primary purpose, the court may place less emphasis on the actual fitness of the mother for childrearing and instead weigh whether punishment for putting her child at risk is a lawful justification for removal of custody under a civil statute. However, if the focus of the custody proceeding is the traditional one of trying to determine whether a mother is fit to care for her child, a court might take into account factors other than proof that the mother put her unborn child at risk by taking illicit drugs or by avoiding treatment for HIV infection. In this context, past maternal "misconduct" is less relevant to the custody decision than predicted fitness to care for her child. Thus, the outcome of the custody proceeding should not turn on whether the drug a mother took during pregnancy was licit or illicit or on the social connotations of the particular infection the mother carries. A mother who abuses a lawful drug (e.g., alcohol) or has a nonstigmatizing infection (e.g., tuberculosis) may endanger her child more than one who has used cocaine or is HIV-infected.

Constitutional and Social Policy Perspectives

Adopting coercive measures to constrain maternal drug use or to override a refusal to accept treatment for HIV raises important constitutional and social policy issues (24). A full discussion of these issues is beyond the scope of this chapter, but a few comments will be offered concerning implications these issues may have for physicians engaged in the care of pregnant women.

If one views constitutional law as establishing a balance between the rights of individual citizens and the interests of the public ("the state"), a first step is to identify and weigh these rights and interests. The more fundamental or compelling they are, the more decisive their impact in situations of conflict. *Roe v. Wade* and the later "abortion rights" decisions have affirmed both the liberty of women to make reproductive choices and the interest of the state in protecting the unborn. That the balance remains an uneasy one is less important here than is the consensus that the state has a valid interest in the outcome of pregnancy, which it can express through properly drawn laws. In this context, laws that are rational in the sense of articulating a valid public interest in fetal protection and laying out a plausible methodology for achieving that goal will satisfy constitutional norms—unless they place an undue burden on maternal rights (3). Surely there is no constitutional right to use illicit drugs or to disseminate an infectious disease, and the right to unconstrained abortion in early pregnancy does not logically include the freedom to willfully or recklessly endanger the fetus a woman has elected to carry. Thus, a carefully drawn law that aims to force a pregnant woman to refrain from conduct that intentionally or recklessly endangers her unborn child could well survive an attack on its constitutionality.

Whether such a law is good public policy is another question entirely. Fetal harm from maternal drug use probably will have already occurred by the time a coercive law is invoked against a particular woman. Hence, a coercive law directed at maternal drug use might only serve to punish the offending woman. Conceivably, it might have social value as a signal to other women that they risk criminal prosecution or other sanctions if they use unlawful drugs during pregnancy. However, it also might dissuade them from seeking prenatal care so as to avoid detection, conduct that in itself will put the fetus at risk. Similarly, a law that threatens criminal prosecution of HIV-infected pregnant women who refuse antiretroviral therapy may discourage them from seeking prenatal care or agreeing to HIV testing.

Coercive strategies for confronting drug abuse or HIV infection in pregnant women obviously implicate physicians. Thus, if existing child abuse laws are amended to include fetal abuse, physicians likely would incur a statutory duty to report instances of maternal drug usage to public agencies. If controlled substance laws are amended or interpreted to permit prosecution of women for transplacental delivery of illicit drugs to a fetus, physicians likely would be required to report the fact of a positive drug screen in the same manner as they are now required to report gunshot or knife wounds. If criminal laws are expanded to allow prosecution of HIV-infected pregnant women for recklessly endangering their fetuses through refusal to accept treatment, physicians presumably would be called on to report positive HIV tests of their pregnant patients to public agencies (34).

Even if new laws are not enacted, the public debate about how to handle maternal substance abuse of HIV infection may lead physicians to believe they have some sort of legal or ethical duty to identify and report affected women to law enforcement or public health officials. Many physicians, particularly those in the mental health field, are aware of the so-called *Tarasoff doctrine* (36), the crux of which is that physicians have a lawful duty to breach confidentiality once they have determined that a patient poses a danger to an identifiable third person. In a paradigm that casts women and their unborn children as separate legal persons, a fetus may be viewed as that third person for the purpose of applying the Tarasoff doctrine.

One aspect of the controversy engendered by the Tarasoff ruling seems particularly germane here. Critics of the ruling have contended that a legal rule encouraging physicians to breach confidentiality to serve public ends, even one as important as protecting third persons from harm, might in the long run prove counterproductive (37). The gist of the argument is that the very patients who most need help in coping with their violent impulses would be deterred from seeking psychiatric help for fear of being involuntarily committed to a mental hospital or being reported to law enforcement officials. Thus, if pregnant women who use drugs or are HIV-infected come to believe that their physicians will conspire with law enforcement to coerce or punish them, they will either not seek prenatal care or will seek to conceal their drug use or infection. The net effect arguably would be to actually increase the risk of fetal injury, as well as miss an opportunity to channel affected women into appropriate treatment.

The argument that coercive laws are antitherapeutic lacks empiric support. It seems at least plausible, however, that a coercive approach to maternal substance abuse or HIV infection actually may achieve less fetal protection than the current disorderly, inadequately funded, and minimally coercive approach (24). If this is true, rather than supporting more intrusive laws, physicians can best serve their patients and the public interest by educating their own patients about the fetal risks of maternal substance abuse and untreated HIV infection and by advocating for stronger education, wider outreach, and more effective treatment programs.

REFERENCES

1. *Roe v. Wade,* 410 US 113 (Sup Ct 1973).
2. *Webster v. Reproductive Health Services,* 492 US 490 (Sup Ct 1990).
3. *Planned Parenthood v. Casey,* 505 US 833 (Sup Ct 1992).

4. Rostow VP, Osterweis M, Bulger RJ. Medical professional liability and the delivery of obstetrical care. *New Engl J Med* 1989;321:1057–1060.

5. Marcotte P. Medical verdicts tightrope. *J Amer Bar Assn* 1989:29–30.

6. Jacobson PD. Medical malpractice and the tort system. *JAMA* 1989;262:3320–3327.

7. Hickson GB, Clayton EW, Githens PB, et al. Factors that prompted families to file medical malpractice claims following perinatal injuries. *JAMA* 1992;267: 1359–1363.

8. Note: Innovative tort reform for an endangered specialty. *Virginia Law Rev* 1988;74:1487–1500.

9. *Harbeson v. Parke Davis,* 656 P 2d 483 (WN Sup Ct 1983).

10. Furrow BR. Impaired children and tort remedies: the emergence of a consensus. *Law Med Health Care* 1983;11:148–154.

11. Note: Wrongful birth actions: the case against legislative curtailment. *Harvard Law Rev* 1987;100: 2017–2034.

12. MINN STAT sec 145.424 (1987 Supp).

13. *Hickman v. Group Health Plan,* 396 NW 2d 10 (MN Sup Ct 1986).

14. *Canterbury v. Spence,* 464 F 2d 772 (DC Cir 1972), *cert den* 409 US 464.

15. *Arato v. Avedon,* 858 P 2d 598 (CA Sup Ct 1993).

16. *Berman v. Allan,* 404 A 2d 8 (NJ Sup Ct 1979).

17. *Becker v. Schwartz,* 386 NE 2d 807 (NY Ct App 1978).

18. *Procanik v. Cillo,* 478 A 2d 755 (NJ Sup Ct 1984), dissenting opinion.

19. Volpe JJ. Effect of cocaine use on the fetus. *New Engl J Med* 1992;327:399–407.

20. Zuckerman B, Frank DA, Hingson R, et al. Effects of maternal marijuana and cocaine use on fetal growth. *New Engl J Med* 1989;320:762–768.

21. Phibbs CS, Bateman DA, Schwartz RM. The neonatal costs of maternal cocaine use. *JAMA* 1991;266: 1521–1526.

22. Lindegren JL, Byers RH Jr, Thomas P, et al. Trends in perinatal transmission of HIV/AIDS in the United States. *JAMA* 1999;282:531–538.

23. DeCock KM, Fowler MG, Mercier E, et al. Prevention of mother-to-child HIV transmission in resource-poor countries. *JAMA* 2000;283:1175–1182.

24. Legal interventions during pregnancy. Court-ordered medical treatments and legal penalties for potentially harmful behavior by pregnant women. *JAMA* 1990;264: 2663–2670.

25. *Ferguson v. City of Charleston,* 121 S. Ct. 1281 (2001).

26. *Whitner v. State,* 492 SE 2d 777 (SC Sup Ct 1997), *cert den* 118 S Ct 1857 (1998).

27. *http//www.washingtonpost. comwp-dynarticlesA44040–2000Fed28.html.*

28. *In re Baby Boy Doe,* 632 NE 2d 326 (IL App 1994), *cert den* 114 S Ct 1198 (1994).

29. *In re AC,* 573 A 2d 1235 (DC App 1990).

30. *Raleigh-Fitkin Hospital v. Anderson,* 201 A 2d 537 (NJ Sup Ct 1964), *cert den* 84 S Ct 1894 (1964).

31. *Jacobson v. Massachusetts,* 197 US 11 (Sup Ct 1904).

32. *Addington v. Texas,* 441 US 418 (Sup Ct 1979).

33. *O'Connor v. Donaldson,* 422 US 563 (Sup Ct 1975).

34. Kromm D. HIV-specific knowing transmission statutes: a proposal to help fight an epidemic. *St John's J Legal Commentary* 1999;14:253–277.

35. O'Flynn M. The Adoption and Safe Families Act of 1997: changing child welfare policy without addressing parental substance abuse. *J Contemp Health Law Policy* 1999;16:243–271.

36. *Tarasoff v. Regents of University of California,* 551 P 2d 334 (CA Sup Ct 1976).

37. Stone A. The *Tarasoff* decisions: suing psychotherapists to safeguard society. *Harvard Law Rev* 1976;90: 358–385.

Subject Index

Note: Numbers in italics are figures; page numbers followed by t indicate tables.